THE EXCEPTIONAL BRAIN

The Exceptional Brain
Neuropsychology of Talent
and Special Abilities

Edited by

Loraine K. Obler, Ph.D.
*Graduate School and University Center
  of the City University of New York, and
Boston University School of Medicine*

Deborah Fein, Ph.D.
*Boston University School of Medicine, and
University of Connecticut*

Foreword by Howard Gardner, Ph.D.

The Guilford Press
New York   London

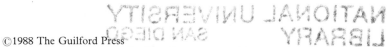

©1988 The Guilford Press
A Division of Guilford Publications, Inc.
72 Spring Street, New York, N.Y. 10012

Printed in the United States of America

Library of Congress Cataloging-in-Publication Data

The Exceptional Brain.

  Includes bibliographies and index.
1. Intellect. 2. Ability—Physiological aspects.
3. Genius—Physiological aspects. 4. Neuropsychology.
I. Obler, Loraine K. II. Fein, Deborah.
[DNLM: 1. Aptitude. 2. Intelligence.
3. Neuropsychology. BF 431 E96]
QP398.E93   1988   153.9   86–27136
ISBN 0–89862–701-X

Contributors

Martin L. Albert, MD, PhD. Department of Neurology, Section of Behavioral Neuroscience, Boston University School of Medicine, Boston, Massachusetts; and Boston Veterans Administration Medical Center, Boston, Massachusetts.

Ann L. Aldershof, ScB. Boston University School of Medicine, Boston, Massachusetts.

Dorothy M. Aram, PhD. Department of Pediatrics, Case Western Reserve University, Rainbow Babies and Childrens Hospital, Cleveland, Ohio.

Camilla P. Benbow, PhD. Study of Mathematically Precocious Youth, Iowa State University, Ames, Iowa.

Lola Bogyo, PhD. North Shore Children's Hospital, Salem, Massachusetts.

Evan Brown, PhD. Department of Psychology, University of Nebraska, Omaha, Nebraska.

Neil Charness, PhD. Department of Psychology, University of Waterloo, Waterloo, Ontario, Canada.

Jane Clifton, PhD. Department of Psychology, University of Waterloo, Waterloo, Ontario, Canada.

Lee D. Cranberg, MD. Department of Neurology, Section of Behavioral Neuroscience, Boston University School of Medicine,

Boston, Massachusetts; and Boston Veterans Administration Medical Center, Boston, Massachusetts.

Susan Curtiss, PhD. Department of Linguistics, University of California at Los Angeles, Los Angeles, California.

Kenneth Deffenbacher, PhD. Department of Psychology, University of Nebraska, Omaha, Nebraska.

G. Robert DeLong, MD. Massachusetts General Hospital and Harvard Medical School, Boston, Massachusetts.

Chantal Desmarais, MA. School of Human Communication Disorders, McGill University, Montreal, Quebec, Canada.

Ronald Ellis, PhD. Boston University School of Medicine, Boston, Massachusetts.

K. Anders Ericsson, PhD. Department of Psychology, University of Colorado, Boulder, Colorado.

Irene A. Faivre, PhD. Department of Psychology, University of Colorado, Boulder, Colorado.

Deborah Fein, PhD. Laboratory of Neuropsychology, Boston University School of Medicine, Boston, Massachusetts; and Department of Psychology, University of Connecticut, Storrs, Connecticut.

Howard Gardner, PhD. Harvard University, Boston University School of Medicine, and Boston Veterans Administration Medical Center, Boston, Massachusetts.

Steven Greenberg, PhD. Harvard Medical School, Cambridge, Massachusetts.

Lyn R. Haber, PhD. Department of Psychology, University of Illinois at Chicago, Chicago, Illinois.

Ralph Norman Haber, PhD. Department of Psychology, University of Illinois at Chicago, Chicago, Illinois.

Jane M. Healy, PhD. Hathaway Brown School, Cleveland State University, Cleveland, Ohio.

Adele Holevas, PhD. League School of Boston, Newton, Massachusetts.

Tedd Judd, PhD. Department of Psychiatry and Behavioral Medicine, Pacific Medical Center, Seattle, Washington.

Edith Kaplan, PhD. Department of Neurology, and Division of Psychiatry, Boston University School of Medicine, Boston, Massachusetts.

Yvan Lebrun, PhD. Neurolinguistics Department, Free University of Brussels, School of Medicine, Brussels, Belgium.

Dorothy Lucci, PhD. Laboratory of Neuropsychology, Boston University School of Medicine, Boston, Massachusetts.

Lyle MacDonald, MA. Algoma District Mental Retardation Service, Sault Ste. Marie, Ontario, Canada.

Steven Matthysse, MD. Mailman Research Center, McLean Hospital, Belmont, Massachusetts.

Loriana Novoa, MA. Department of Curriculum and Instruction, College of Education, Florida International University, Miami, Florida.

Loraine K. Obler, PhD. Program in Speech and Hearing Sciences, Graduate School and University Center of the City University of New York, New York, New York; and Aphasia Research Center of the Boston University School of Medicine, Boston, Massachusetts.

Marlene Oscar-Berman, PhD. Psychology Service, Boston Veterans Administration Medical Center, Boston, Massachusetts; and Department of Neurology and Division of Psychiatry, Boston University School of Medicine, Boston, Massachusetts.

Bernard Rimland, PhD. Institute for Child Behavior Research, San Diego, California.

Elizabeth Rosenblatt, EdM. Harvard Project Zero, Harvard University, Cambridge, Massachusetts.

Eta I. Schneiderman, PhD. Department of Linguistics, University of Ottawa, Ottawa, Ontario, Canada.

Avraham Schweiger, PhD. Psychology Department, University of California at Los Angeles, Los Angeles, California.

Steven Smith, PhD. Private practice, Wenatchee, Washington.

Henri Szliwowski, MD. Neurology Unit, University Hospital, Brussels, Belgium.

Claudie Van Endert, MD. Free University of Brussels, School of Medicine, Brussels, Belgium.

Lynn Waterhouse, PhD. Child Behavior Study, Trenton State College, Trenton, New Jersey.

Ellen Winner, PhD. Psychology Department, Boston College, Chestnut Hill, Massachusetts; and Harvard Project Zero, Harvard University, Cambridge, Massachusetts.

Jeremy M. Wolfe, PhD. Department of Psychology, Massachusetts Institute of Technology, Cambridge, Massachusetts.

Foreword

The topic of this fascinating collection of papers would have raised few eyebrows during the 19th century. During its initial stirrings in the days of phrenology, and during its early history at the time of Paul Broca's epoch-making discoveries, the field of brain–behavior relations comfortably embraced the major issues being examined here. That is, the range of human abilities, talents, and proclivities was considered a suitable subject for study, and the belief that these capacities had specific neural representations was quite widely held.

Why, then, would this topic have seemed so suspect just a few decades ago? Why have we had to wait until this moment for a comprehensive collection of papers on the neuropsychology of talent? In the history of science, events (or, for that matter, nonevents) rarely have a single cause. Any review of the past century of neurological and psychological studies would disclose at least the following factors that contributed to the delay in focusing on the neuropsychological approach: the widespread (and sometimes ideologically based) lack of interest in neural representation entailed in the behaviorist revolution; the precipitous decline of interest in localization following the First World War and the concomitant ascendance of holistic and gestalt positions; the psychometric tyranny that placed "general intelligence" on a pedestal and dictated one way of measuring it; the restriction of psychological studies to populations of normal subjects (unreflectively particularized as Norwegian rats or college sophomores), with individual differences and developmental progressions essentially ignored; and the well-intentioned but naive belief that all minds were (or could be trained to be) essentially alike.

An introductory essay is scarcely the appropriate place for a critique of these items of faith to which so many of our predecessors adhered, often with surprising and ill-supported tenacity. What must be stressed, however, is that each of these perspectives has been gradually undermined by the cognitive and neurobiological revolutions. Cognitive science has sanctioned the study of the full range, and the highest reaches, of human cognitive capacities; there has been a willingness to examine covert thoughts and internal representations as well as observable behaviors; a multifaceted view of the human intellect has increasingly been endorsed, and it is considered appropriate to examine a variety of factors using a range of research methods. Analogously, within the neurobiological disciplines there is universal recognition that the nervous system is highly differentiated, with specific capacities exhibiting their own characteristic structural and functional organizations; that there are regular and perhaps systematic differences in the morphology of brain organization in different populations and subpopulations; and that the nervous system undergoes a characteristic development that is influenced by extrinsic as well as intrinsic factors.

Suffice it to say, then, that the zeitgeist is extremely friendly to the appearance now of a volume that surveys a wide sweep of talents—from eidetic imagery to chess—in a broad range of populations—from autistic children to skilled scientists—and does so from a variety of disciplinary perspectives and theoretical allegiances. Thanks to the work described in this book, and to other research being carried on in the same tradition, we will soon have excellent descriptions of a variety of human talents, preliminary accounts of the computational processes that underlie these talents, and promising taxonomies of the neural substrates and systems that undergird these individually striking behaviors. Moreover, by fully proposing a research agenda, this book should prove invaluable to researchers and clinicians, who will henceforth be on the lookout for evidence supporting—or refuting—the accounts offered here. Happily, this volume is comprehensive and compelling; it touches on the principal lines of study undertaken in this new area, and it leaves the reader with an excellent sense of what has been accomplished and what remains to be done.

Because the remainder of this volume will allow readers to survey what has been done, I would like to comment on the task that lies ahead. I believe that the focus on talents and special abilities marks but the beginning of a larger scientific agenda—a story of complexity and importance which ultimately needs to be told. Human capacities do not, in most cases, exist and unfold in a vacuum. Rather, they evolve within a particular cultural setting to serve certain individual and collective needs, and whether and how they come to be expressed is as much a social and cultural phenomenon as it is an issue of individual neuroanatomy and expression. To be sure, there are people in whom special talents exist in splendid or terrifying isolation. Much can be learned from studying these exceptional individuals. But for the most part, talents exist in people who have definite goals and purposes, who have been molded to exercise their abilities in one way or another, and whose ultimate performances are accepted or rejected, channeled or thwarted, by the social groups in whose company they live.

Because unusual talents and abilities unfold in such a context, we need to view them from at least five different perspectives. First, there is the *neurobiological substrate* of unusual abilities, and second, there are the *cognitive or informational processes* by which these abilities are expressed. These perspectives, deriving from the cognitive and neurobiological sciences, are well reflected in these pages.

The third perspective focuses on the *personality characteristics and personal dynamics* that enable certain individuals to persevere in developing their talents, while others are diverted from, or self-consciously choose to abandon, their endeavors. These aspects of purpose, will, and mission, which determine whether the potential talent can even be detected by others, are the concern of psychologists of personality and motivation.

Fourth, we must take into account the content of the *domain of knowledge* (Feldman, 1980). Not even the most gifted individuals can excel in chess if the game does not exist; individuals cannot create polyphonic music if they live in a monophonic society; nor can talented persons practice physics if they are reared in a preliterate or prescientific culture. Such epistemological issues must be addressed not only by philosophers or experts in a particular domain (linguists or musicologists) but by anyone who studies the expression of talent within a given cultural setting.

Finally, there is the *social context or field* in which abilities are fostered, tolerated, or thwarted (Robinson & Csikszentmihalyi, 1986). Individuals may be extremely talented and highly motivated, and they may have access to an appropriate domain of knowledge or performance; but unless they effect the proper affiliations within their culture, advance through appropriate networks, and become identified as members of their guild or profession, their only options are to create their own fields of expertise or to remain obscure. These are the concerns of sociologists or historians, but neuroscientists ignore them at their peril.

In touching upon such concerns as the domain of knowledge and the field of expression, I am going beyond the stated scope of this book. Indeed, I am addressing the differences between gifted *potential* and the *expression of a talent* in ways valued by the culture. In my view, however, this is an important step. Talented individuals may be of theoretical interest in the abstract, but unless they become of some consequence within the society, they are likely to be ignored. No doubt countless special abilities are possessed across the population—perhaps each of us has dozens of unique talents—and yet they would not be noticed, let alone singled out for study, unless on some account they matter. Just why certain talents have mattered in the past, and how they may matter even more in the future, is part of the story that any examination of this subject must encompass. And why some individual talents are expressed chiefly for one's personal amusement, whereas others become mobilized by society for constructive or destructive ends, is a question that none of us can afford to ignore—in our stances as scientists as well as in our roles as citizens. We need to understand the relationships—and the differences—among the isolated idiot savant, the gifted technician, and the radically creative genius.

Obviously, no one scientist can address all of these concerns, but it is important not to lose sight of the ensemble. My own bias, like that of many of the authors collected here, is to begin with the biological bases of talent. Toward that end, in the spring of 1984, I and several of my colleagues at the Social Science Research Council organized what may have been the first conference on the biological bases of giftedness. During the conference, we discussed issues even more purely biological than those treated here: the roles of the most basic levels of anlaysis, including individual neurons and the connections among nerve cells; aspects of neural development; various genetic and epigenetic models of the expression of a talent; and animal models of talent (see Gardner & Dudai, 1985, for a summary of the results of this conference). Following the conference, its organizers agreed that the most relevant contributions to a neurobiological account of human talents had been made by the noted neurologist Norman Geschwind, who was to die suddenly just a few months after the meeting.

I am sure I will not be alone among readers of this book in missing the words of Norman Geschwind. More so than any other single researcher, he called attention to the issues discussed here and devised some of the most fruitful ways of thinking about the neuropsychological and the neuroanatomical aspects of unusual human capacities. Perhaps not coincidentally, he himself epitomized the individual of unusual talents who was able to direct them toward the advancement of knowledge and that sharpening of issues that may lead to improvements in the human condition. Ideally, he should have written this introduction; indeed, he should have written this book. We should keep in mind his example as we ponder the ideas in this volume and try to build upon them in our future work.

Howard Gardner, Ph.D.
Harvard University
Boston University School of Medicine
Boston Veterans Administration Medical Center

References

Csikszentmihaly, M., & Robinson, R. (1986). Culture, time, and the development of talent. In R. Sternberg (Ed.), *Conceptions of giftedness*. New York: Cambridge University Press.

Feldman, D. H. (1980). *Beyond universals in cognitive development*. Norwood, NJ: Ablex.

Gardner, H., & Dudai, Y. (1985). Biology and giftedness. *ITEMS* (Social Science Research Council) *39*, 1–6.

Preface

The idea for this book began when LKO attended the 1982 NATO Conference on Dyslexia in Maratea, Italy. She was struck by the case of a hyperlexic autistic young man with musical abilities reported by Dorothy Aram; the case appeared to provide an opportunity to invert the standard neuropsychological paradigm and focus on special talents rather than specific disabilities. R. Malatesha Joshi and Harry Whitaker are to be thanked for organizing that conference under a warm October sun by an exquisite coast, and at the relaxed pace of a ten-day conference which permitted the idea behind the book to capture the imagination.

Deborah Fein then agreed to co-work on the project; her commitment to understanding the neuropsychological underpinnings of autism had generated in her a prior interest in *idiots savants*. We decided to attempt to collect in one volume current thinking and research on the neuropsychology of talent, sharing both the intellectual burden and the excitement with our authors. We are most grateful to them for the high caliber of work and enthusiasm they put into their contributions.

The ground for our seed of an idea had already been prepared for us at the Boston Veterans Administration Medical Center, a truly remarkable center for study of neuropsychology. In his regular case presentations at the Aphasia Research Center Aphasia and Neurobehavior Grand Rounds, Norman Geschwind shared the important neuroimmunoendocrinological theory he was developing. On the 14th floor in Psychology Research, as well as at Harvard, Howard Gardner was elaborating his theory of multiple intelligences which was to influence our thinking for this book. And on 7-D, Edith Kaplan trained DF, and served as a model for both of us in the keen observation of ability and disability. All three of them gave this project support in its developmental stages.

We are deeply grateful to LKO's research partner, Martin Albert and to DF's research partner Lynn Waterhouse for their general encouragement and for fruitful discussions in the course of the project, as well as their agreeing to set their minds to address the difficult questions we posed for them in their chapters.

Boston more generally has served as a stimulating environment for us. Phyllis Fisher's help was invaluable in preparing our prospectus for the book. LKO received much valuable inspiration from the Feminist Research Methodology Group and DF much from her lab chief, Marlene Oscar-Berman.

Grants that have funded our research projects on language and autism in the course of work on this book (VA Project 001 to Albert and Obler; NIMH 28605 to Waterhouse and Fein; NIMH 40162 to Fein and Waterhouse; NINCDS 20489 to Fein as part of the CNS-INS Task Force on Nosology of Higher Cerebral Function Disorders in Children, R. David, P.I.) have enabled us to undertake it, as have our affiliations with Boston University School of Medicine and the Boston Veterans Administration Medical Center, and now the City University of New York Graduate School (LKO) and the University of Connecticut (DF).

We are appreciative of the contributions made by Suzanne Ruscitti on the index, and by Margaret Humes-Bartlo and Ann Aldershof in helping proofread the manuscript.

And as always, we are grateful to our life partners Margaret Fearey and Joseph Berger for the intellectual stimulation and support they bring to our lives.

Loraine K. Obler
Deborah Fein

Contents

24. *What's Exceptional About Exceptional Abilities?*   *436*
K. Anders Ericsson and Irene A. Faivre

25. *Special Talents of Autistic Savants*   *474*
Bernard Rimland and Deborah Fein

26. *Speculations on the Neuroanatomical Substrate*   *493*
of Special Talents
Lynn Waterhouse

I

INTRODUCTION

1

Neuropsychological Study of Talent: A Developing Field

DEBORAH FEIN
LORAINE K. OBLER

A Definition of Terms

Talent, it sometimes appears, lies in the eyes of the beholding culture. In the West the abilities to draw or paint, to create music, and to write in vivid and compelling language have long been considered talents. Only recently, however, have we considered the ability to write a brilliant computer program a talent, though it is accorded somewhat less status than being talented in the arts. The ability, after puberty, to learn a second language like a native speaker may be considered a talent in American society where so few have the opportunity to learn languages in childhood, but it is less valued in countries such as Denmark or India, where everyone speaks several languages from a young age.

Moreover, in our culture the ability to find four-leaf clovers, to speak backwards or read upside down, or to calculate quickly what day of the week July 12, 1948, was, is considered a mere curiosity, not worthy of the label "talent." Broader calculating ability, whereby an exceptional person can multiply two 10-digit numbers by each other in a minute or two, is an example of a talent that is no longer so highly respected since computers can perform the same operations; at one time people with this skill could make a living by performing their calculating feats.

For our purposes in this book, we intend to include a full range of outstanding abilities under the concept "talent." Though in fact we will cover only those abilities for which some neuropsychological research exists, we would certainly include in this range talents in the performing arts, athletics, handicrafts, and games such as bridge, as well as abilities in such areas as simultaneous translation, abacus operation, and telegraphy. For each of these fields, it is the case that some people are unable to learn the skill at all well, many can learn it with a fair amount of training and practice, and a few excel at the skill, learning it with surprising ease. Among the talented individuals will be both prodigies and specialized geniuses—

Deborah Fein. Laboratory of Neuropsychology, Boston University School of Medicine, Boston, Massachusetts; and Department of Psychology, University of Connecticut, Storrs, Connecticut.
Loraine K. Obler. Program in Speech and Hearing Sciences, Graduate School and University Center of the City University of New York, New York, New York; and Aphasia Research Center of the Boston University School of Medicine, Boston, Massachusetts.

the early and speedy acquisition of the ability by the prodigy may or may not continue into adulthood; the exceptionally high quality of the genius's contribution to society may or may not derive from early or speedy acquisition of the talent.

The performance of a talented individual is deemed to be outstanding in one of two ways. Either it is outstanding by comparison to the performances of others in society, as the term "talent" is generally applied, or, of equal interest to neuropsychologists, it is outstanding for the individual in question. Individuals with a single outstanding talent may be of otherwise normal ability, or they may be autistic or retarded, a group traditionally termed "idiot savants." (This is a somewhat problematic term, as a number of our contributors have pointed out, because of the connotations, in English, of the word "idiot.") For the purposes of this volume, our definition of talent is deliberately broad. Curtiss (Chapter 20) offers the most extreme example of our nonstandard use of the term "talent" in her report of children for whom the mere learning of language must be considered a special ability since their retardation in all other areas is so severe.

Our contributors have dealt with definitional, methodological, and conceptual issues in different ways. Charness and his colleagues (Chapter 14) have chosen the term "mono-savants" to describe individuals in whom one skill stands out above all others; Judd (Chapter 6) has chosen the term "savantism." We have imposed no editorial fiats, no arbitrary limit such that an individual must be in the top 1% of a field to be considered talented, or, in the case of an idiot savant, that a special ability has to be two standard deviations above performance in one's other abilities. We feel that such quantification at this early stage would be misleading since the parameters to be measured, and the ways of measuring them, have yet to be determined. We assume that there is fair consensus among our readers as to who counts as talented, and we have certainly ensured that our contributors clarify on what basis talents or special abilities have been assumed to exist.

Historical Context of the Discussion of Talent

In the history of Western thinking, the discourse on talent has occurred primarily within the fields of philosophy and education. At the end of the last century, with the emergence of the fields of anthropology, psychology, and neuropsychology, the discussion of talent was embedded in a discussion of intelligence that was relatively more prominent than it subsequently was during the first half of this century. One crucial issue in this discussion was whether intelligence was unitary or whether it might be divided into a set of talents (see Waterhouse, Chapter 26, this volume). Last century's phrenologists, for example, were clearly among those analysts who identified subcomponents of human cognition and intelligence.

Out of their work, the field of anthropology developed initially for the purpose of studying the range of human shapes and sizes. Paul Broca, the famous neurologist credited with discovering that the left hemisphere of the brain was responsible for language, was a member of the Anthropological Society of Paris. One aspect of this society's discussion of intelligence, Gardner (1983) and Gould (1981) report, was its encouragement of members to donate their brains after death.

These were then studied in fairly gross ways—such as by weighing them—according to the technology of the time. As Gould reports, enthusiasm for the comparison of brain weights diminished when it was discovered that some geniuses had extremely light brains at death, whereas some morons had brains as heavy as any of the geniuses studied, or when it was discovered that women's brains *relative to their body weights* were no smaller than those of men.

Late 19th century neuropsychologists undertook just slightly more sophisticated measurements, by counting the number of convolutions in the brains of polyglots, but their work eventually fell into disrepute. Only recently, with Geschwind's proposal of a neuroanatomical theory of talent and Galaburda's cytoarchitectonic studies (Geschwind & Galaburda, 1985a, 1985b, 1985c), have we been encouraged to perform the sort of neuroanatomical and neurophysiological work that our current technology permits. Leaders in the field are M. Diamond and A. Scheibel, whose work on the sections of Einstein's brain has even been described in the popular press (e.g., the science section of *The New York Times*, July 28, 1985). They have studied such phenomena as neuronal branching and the percentage of glial cells in Einstein's brain, in the brain of a nongenius control, and in the brains of numerous rats whose life conditions have been either enriched or kept dull. They have concluded that there is a greater degree of neuronal branching in the brain of a genius (i.e., Einstein's) and in the brains of rats living in enriched environments, which presumably reflects greater speed in thinking and, for the human at least, the ability to make connections not made by the rest of us.

Galaburda's work on the brains of dyslexics, some of whom have relatively exceptional visuo-spatial abilities (one, for example, was an engineer), takes the architectonic approach. He notes that there are different sorts of cells and cell clusters in the brains of these individuals, which can actually be demonstrated at a relatively gross level. For the six dyslexic males he examined (but not for the one female seen), the planum temporale in the left hemisphere (strongly implicated as a site for normal persons' language), is the same size as that in the right hemisphere, whereas for normal, right-handed persons this site is almost invariably smaller in the right hemisphere. This finding, we note, is the first to apparently contradict the notion within neurolinguistics that larger is better. For example, it has regularly been assumed that because the planum temporale on the left is larger, that is why it is a crucial seat for language. Galaburda proposes rather that it is the smallness of the right hemisphere in normal persons that somehow permits the learning of language by the left.

Between the neuroanatomical theorizing and gross counting of the last century and that of the past 5 years, mainstream neuropsychology developed by way of case studies of brain-damaged patients. Most of these studies were of aphasic patients, in whom language was disturbed in one or more ways in the context of relatively spared abilities for other cognitive tasks such as memory and visuo-spatial performance. In addition to the case studies, which present the specifics of the language impairment against a background of spared abilities, there have been numerous studies of series of cases, and group studies, which in similar fashion articulate dissociations between spared and impaired abilities. The underlying assumption in interpreting these case studies is that, through study of the abilities impaired by selective brain damage, we can develop a theory of the operation of the normal brain. Virtually no one has pretended to use such a methodology to develop a theory of the exceptionally talented brain except Luria, whose book, *The Mind of a Mnemonist* (1968), is discussed in this volume by Brown and Deffenbacher (Chapter 8).

In her psychological discourse on intelligence, Bronner (1921) anticipated some of the ways of thinking that Gardner proposes in his book *Frames of Mind: The Theory of Multiple Intelligences* (1983). Bronner reported several cases where the ability to use language reasonably well stood out in the context of retardation; the case of a male for whom reading was the special ability, one for whom memory abilities stood out, and one for whom number work was far beyond his other scholastic abilities; and, finally, three males for whom the ability to work with concrete materials was outstanding, a category Gardner calls "kinesthetic intelligence." Gardner's volume culminates that discussion in psychology with his identification of seven intelligences: musical, logical–mathematical, linguistic, bodily-kinesthetic, spatial, knowledge of self, and knowledge of others. Most crucially, he puts forward the argument, which we develop here, that the study of talents and special abilities provides a methodological lever to understanding not only an exceptionally talented person but also, potentially, the performance of the given ability by a normal person.

The Current Questions

As we see it, the current questions are as follows:

1. *Is there a neurological substrate for talent?* Of course, as neuropsychologists we hypothesize that there must be such a substrate and would hardly think to relegate talent somehow to "mind." What evidence currently exists would be the results of the work on Einstein's brain discussed previously. Some indirect evidence may be derived from the phenomenon of critical ages for the acquisition of specific abilities (Lenneberg, 1967). There appears, for example, to be a critical age for first-language acquisition, which may be neurologically determined. Studies such as Curtiss's study of Genie (1977; see also Chapter 20, this volume) indicate that, in the rare instance when a person of normal intelligence is not exposed to language until past puberty, the ability may never be fully developed. Broader evidence for a critical period for first-language acquisition comes from those children who are brain damaged in their left hemispheres in childhood and who lose language but then recover it quite quickly, indeed, quicker than true learning could account for, thus suggesting that the right hemisphere's abilities for language production are available to them. After puberty, however, such apparent plasticity diminishes, and there is often little recovery of language in the older adult aphasic.

A similar notion of critical age appears to be acting in the development of a number of the talents discussed in this book. For example, Smith's comprehensive collection of the great mental calculators (1983; see also Chapter 2, this volume) indicates that those who have auditory calculating abilities learn them by around the age of 8, while those who have visual calculating abilities may learn them later. Likewise among chess masters, those who learned the game at the age of 14 or 15 are considered to be great exceptions because they learned the game so late, and no chess master has been reported to learn it later. Precisely what makes the second-language acquirers exceptional (Novoa, Obler, & Fein, Chapter 15) is that they escape the apparent critical period for second-language acquisition, after which (again, around puberty) the ability to learn a second language like a native speaker, particularly with regard to accent, falls off in the normal population. The argument concerning critical age, then, would be that puberty appears to be a crucial point with respect to the development of talent, and that the hormonal influences, presumably on the brain, can facilitate development of the talent for a few but inhibit it for all others.

2. *Assuming that there is a neurological substrate for talent, where is it?* Some of the history of neuroanatomical theories of talent, including the current work by Scheibel and Diamond on brain weight and branching patterns, is reviewed by Waterhouse (Chapter 26, this volume). The recent revolutionary theory of Geschwind and Behan (1982) and Geschwind and Galaburda (1985a, 1985b, 1985c), linking familial immune disorders, handedness, neuropsychological deficits and special talents, and brain development, is evaluated in some detail in the chapters on second-language acquisition (Novoa, Fein, & Obler, Chapter 15; Schneiderman & Desmarais, Chapter 5) and in an article on mathematical talent (Benbow, Chapter 3). This theory should predict that most special talents are attributable to the superior functioning of the right hemisphere; indeed, several authors in this book explicitly suggest that the talents they focus on are related to right-hemisphere functioning, including such talents as chess (Cranberg & Albert, Chapter 7), music (Lucci, Fein, Holevas, & Kaplan, Chapter 17; Charness, Clifton, & MacDonald, Chapter 14), the special abilities of autistics (Rimland & Fein, Chapter 25), pattern recognition (Waterhouse, Chapter 18), and artistic design (Schweiger, Chapter 16). In fact, the question of why most special talents seem to be in skill areas usually attributed to right-hemisphere functioning is discussed explicitly by Rimland and Fein and by Charness, Clifton, and MacDonald. It may be, as Charness and his colleagues suggest, that individuals with left-hemisphere deficits and right-hemisphere preservation come to professional attention much more regularly. Or it may rest on a more concrete neurological base, as Geschwind's theory of slowed left hemisphere development would suggest.

Several new neuropsychological theories are presented in this volume. Notions about changes in cortical architecture lending themselves to particular talents are suggested by Waterhouse (Chapter 26), Matthysse and Greenberg (Chapter 23), and Rimland and Fein (Chapter 25). Theories about chemical and electrical predisposition to hyperfunction leading to special abilities are developed with reference to memory (Oscar-Berman, Chapter 9), music (Lucci, Fein, Holevas, & Kaplan, Chapter 17), and special skills in autism (Rimland & Fein, Chapter 25). Of course, not all ideas and observations about neurological abnormality and giftedness could be covered in a single volume, and creativity per se and its suggested connection with epilepsy are not dealt with in detail in any chapter.

It should be noted that all of the theories about hyperfunction developed in this volume relate to structures in the temporal lobe. We recently came across one particularly suggestive anecdote in Oliver Sacks's fascinating book *The Man Who Mistook His Wife for a Hat* (1985):

> The "secret" of Shostakovich('s talent for composition), it was suggested—by a Chinese neurologist, Dr. Dajue Wang—was the presence of a metallic splinter, a mobile shell-fragment, in his brain, in the temporal horn of the left ventricle. Shostakovich was very reluctant, apparently, to have this removed: Since the fragment had been there, he said, each time he leaned his head to one side he could hear music. His head was filled with melodies—different each time—which he then made use of when composing. X-rays allegedly showed the fragment moving around when Shostakovich moved his head, pressing against his "musical" temporal lobe, when he tilted, producing an infinity of melodies which his genius could use. (p.135)

3. Assuming that there is a neurological substrate for talent that is distinct from that of the normal person, what caused the difference? A key question that underlies many of the fundamental issues discussed in this book is whether (or which forms of) special ability rests on some form of neurological difference, or whether anyone (within certain neurological limits) could perform at an outstanding level given the requisite environmental stimulation, drive state, opportunity for practice, or personality traits. This is not, strictly speaking, a distinction between biology and environment, since experience may shape the brain, and personality traits or drive states may rest on neurological factors. Nevertheless, there is a fundamental difference in point of view between (1) those authors who suggest that no innate differences exist between accomplished and unaccomplished individuals, but that their accomplishments are primarily attributable to motivation and practice (a position taken most unequivocally by Ericsson and Faivre, but also considered in some detail by Charness *et al.*, Smith, and Brown & Deffenbacher), and (2) those authors who present a neurological theory of talent. It would appear from cognitive psychological studies of a number of the talents, especially memory and chess, that practice is necessary in any case. In the limiting case, even persons with a predisposition to acquire a talent would not acquire it if they were never exposed. As Mead puts it, "The gifted child cannot go beyond the limits of his culture" (Metraux, p. 129). It would appear that what practice does at least in part is to permit chunking of greater amounts of information as well as to promote automatization of ability, which permits performance of the ability either at greater speeds or at higher levels, or both.

But is practice enough? Is it the case that any one of us who practiced as much as the chess master could achieve chess mastery? With respect to certain memory tasks, it appears that it is possible to achieve great proficiency, but with respect to other tasks such as music or chess, we suspect that practice alone is not enough. There may need to be some genetic predisposition to learn and perhaps to excel in a given talent, on top of which practice is overlaid. This predisposition is probably related in some way to the structure of the knowledge area; it is not an "across the board" predisposition to be talented. Someone who has become a chess player might have become a mathematician, but it is probably less likely that he or she would have become an exceptional musician, dancer, or inventor.

Clearly, genetic factors need not be explicitly inherited from the family of the talented individual. Chess players, Cranberg and Albert (Chapter 7, this volume) report, show no family history of exceptional chess playing. Geschwind and Galaburda's theory provides one explanation, in their discussion of "the pathology of excellence." They argue that certain phenomena—including talents and a set of characteristics relating more obviously to brain lateralization such as handedness and dyslexia—cluster in certain families. They theorize that the fetal hormonal environment accounted for the unusual development of cortical connections in individuals in these families. In particular, Galaburda suggests that testosterone levels interact with the "normal" development of the two hemispheres (i.e., the right hemisphere in advance of the left), resulting in a different developmental pattern of the hemispheres. Cells "destined" for one area of the brain, by this analysis, either end up elsewhere or die off in patterns different from those that usually follow birth (Galaburda, 1983). These cellular diversions, then, would account for combinations of talent and disability in certain individuals, such as the dyslexics who have particularly good mathematical or visuo-spatial abilities.

This theory would permit the unusual assignment of cells that Waterhouse's schema accounting for talent in the brain suggests, and it would also permit Judd's explanation (personal communication, 1986) that talents at least in idiot savants are explainable by something like a watershed lesion. Traditionally in neuropsychology, these lesions occur around the language area of the brain, so that they spare basic language abilities such as articulation and repetition, but any language abilities requiring information from elsewhere in the brain (such as the ability to describe what is seen or to initiate a conversation) are impaired.

Geschwind and Galaburda's theory would also account for some of the gender disparity seen in certain talents. One sees more boys with prodigious mathematical skills (Benbow, Chapter 3 this volume), but more girls with exceptional language abilities. Geschwind and Galaburda (1985) explain these sex differences by the level of testosterone excreted by the male fetus in addition to that contributed by the mother. They take great pains to emphasize that their theory is not simply a deterministic one. Stating that a talent or disability is biologically or genetically based does *not* mean that it will necessarily develop or fail to develop regardless of the conditions under which a child grows up. Certain environmental factors are crucial for the manifestation of talent, as they are for the manifestation of disability (Geschwind, 1983). It is clear that among the case studies in this book there are a number, if not all, in which the families evidence some of the phenomena that Geschwind indicates (e.g., Novoa, Fein, & Obler, Chapter 15).

What we suspect is that a certain biological predisposition for a talent or a cluster of talents develops in some cases for hormonal reasons and in other cases for familial non-hormonal reasons. Along with it, a biological predisposition for concentrating permits development of special abilities in the case where the subject is (1) exposed to the necessary knowledge-base materials, (2) encouraged to learn—or at least not discouraged from learning—the materials, and (3) encouraged to practice—or at least not discouraged from practicing—the ability.

What exactly these predispositions look like, what exactly the practice does to brain structures and chemicals, and what automaticity looks like in the brain (and how it develops) remain to be studied.

4. What are the cognitive psychological components of the abilities or talents that permit them to appear as outstanding—either speedily performed and quickly automatic, or performed in a qualitatively superior way? Among the answers that have been proposed in this book are "chunking," as discussed in the literature on memory and chess playing, and "pattern recognition." "Pattern recognition," we note, is probably too broad a term since the ability to recognize qualitatively different parts of patterns can be distinguished. A calculator's ability to recognize mathematical patterns is not the same as the ability of a mathematical genius to recognize such patterns, and the ability to recognize chess patterns is certainly not necessarily related to the ability of good therapists to recognize patterns in their clients' behavior. The chapters in Smith's book (1983) on the mathematical shortcuts employed by a number of calculators indicate that special mathematical processes are developed and discovered and then employed in calculators' abilities. In Obler's unpublished 1985 interview with the calculator Wim Klein, however, the latter clarified that the development of an algorithm is not enough to produce prodigious performance, but rather, the calculator must engage in a fair amount of practice in order to decrease the performance time. At the age of 62, Klein had decided to learn to take the 13th root of a 100-digit number when he read that a German in Mexico could do it in 40 minutes. Klein subsequently developed one algorithm that permitted him to do it in 25 minutes and then developed another, which, after substantial practice, permitted him to do it in 3 minutes.

5. How should one go about studying these behaviors from a neuropsychological perspective? The goal of neuropsychological study is to understand the relation between human behavior and the brain substrate underlying it. The neuropsychologist wants to know what is going on in the brain of an adult performing an activity and how the brain developed to permit that individual to perform the cognitive activity. The major methodology for studying these relations has been to observe and analyze the deficient behaviors of the brain-damaged patient and then to draw conclusions about normal activity. For example, if the aphasic patient has difficulty with production of speech but not with comprehension as a result of the brain-damage, then we conclude that production and comprehension are dissociable components in the healthy performance of speech and language abilities. If the child, but not the adult, recovers language fully after a severe left-hemisphere lesion, we conclude that in the normal, non-brain-damaged child the right hemisphere is able to take over language processing, but that this ability is then lost sometime in young adulthood.

This paradigm has been applied to some case studies of individuals with exceptional talents who became brain damaged. Schweiger (Chapter 16, this volume), for example, mentions several visual artists who lost the ability to draw three-dimensional figures, or who changed from a linear style to a more abstract style, after a stroke. Judd (Chapter 6) reviews the case of a composer who lost the ability to synthesize musical elements into a unified piece and who was no longer able to experience music affectively after a right-hemisphere stroke.

In most instances such studies have not yet questioned whether the components of the ability discovered through brain damage would be those found in any normal person who spent some time composing or painting, say, or whether they are components of the ability in the famous and highly skilled artist, which have developed as a result of either biological proclivities or years of exercising the ability.

A second, newer approach to the study of talents reverses the standard neuropsychological methodology. Instead of looking at the components of deficient abilities against the background of spared abilities, we analyze the exceptional ability against the background of merely normal abilities in the prodigy, or against the less-than-normal abilities in the case of the idiot savant.

Gardner exemplifies this methodology in *Frames of Mind: The Theory of Multiple Intelligences* (1983). Gardner's point in this book was to demonstrate that the seven types of "intelligence" he isolated do exist as independent categories. One of the arguments he used to support his thesis was the example of prodigies and idiot savants. If we have reports, such as those in Gardner (1983), of an autistic boy who can build sophisticated electric devices or recall music, or of a young girl such as Nadia who draws like a talented adolescent, and these individuals have few or no other exceptional or even normal abilities, we have a good argument for the fact that these abilities are isolatable ones. This should be true even for other individuals in whom the abilities do not stand out so starkly, but rather are seen in the context of other normal abilities.

Smith's book *The Great Mental Calculators: The Psychology, Methods, and Lives of Calculating Prodigies, Past and Present* (1983) demonstrates, as his chapter in this book indicates, that calculating abilities can occur in idiot savants as well as in apparently normal individuals, and even in mathematical geniuses such as Gauss and von Neumann. Had we studied only the mathematical geniuses with the skill, we might have spent a long time looking for the connection between mathematical genius and calculating ability. Once we recognize that some mathematical geniuses have exceptional calculating ability and that others do not, we can appreciate that it is probably an independent skill.

In addition to demonstrating the independence of the skills and talents, however, it will be useful to conduct more detailed neuropsychological testing of prodigies and idiot savants in order to discover the components of their talent and the other neuropsychological skills that may be dissociated from, or associated with the talent. Two sorts of case studies can be useful. In one sort, cognitive neuropsychological tasks are devised to determine the components of a skill. Chapter 14 (this volume), by Charness and colleagues, exemplifies such a study. Chapter 15, by Novoa, Fein, and Obler, exemplifies the other sort of case study, in which a battery of neuropsychological tests given to C. J., an exceptional second-language learner, is analyzed.

Such case studies, it must be noted, are particularly good at showing *dissociations*. We can tentatively conclude, on the basis of the single case study of C. J., that IQ, as it is normally measured, and the ability to abstract grammatical rules are not crucial for exceptional second language learning. But the evidence for *associations* between certain abilities and the ability under examination is more circumstantial. While it makes sense that a specific ability to remember words apart from their meaning categories is important in C. J.'s language-learning ability, it is conceivable that the next talented second-language learner we study will not have this skill. Thus to demonstrate associations, unlike dissociations, we need large group studies.

Certain hints that there may be linked phenomena are reported in this volume. For example, the Benbow study indicates a clear link between prodigious mathematical abilities, left-handedness and disorders of the autoimmune system, as Geschwind's theory would predict. With respect to the calculators, there is clearly no association with mathematical abilities across the board, but Smith (Chapter 2, this volume) reports a high incidence of hyperactivity in the auditory calculators and of homosexuals among the calculators, both of which are phenomena included in the Geschwind cluster. Benjamin Rush (1812) reported on a calculator, Thomas Fuller, whose face recognition was so poor that he did not recognize on the next day the people who had been testing him for several hours the day before. Another calculator, Wim Klein, mentioned in an interview with Loraine Obler that his face-recognition abilities were also poor. In addition, he evidenced a surprising lack of familiarity with the visual aspects of Amsterdam, a city he had lived in at least half of his life.

If talents and deficits are found empirically to be linked, there are several classes of explanations. Neurological explanations could be put forth, such as the Geschwind theory that language deficits based in the left hemisphere and talents based in the right hemisphere are linked by a common neurological mechanism. However, one must also consider purely psychological explanations, such as the idea advanced by Waterhouse (Chapter 26, this volume) and by Selfe (1977) that language deficits may lead to nonlinguistically based perception and memory, leading to more faithful and powerful visual pattern recognition and reproduction, or the idea that individuals with deficits in one area devote themselves, in compensation, to areas in which they have the potential to excel.

In addition to the question of deficits being linked to talents, there is the question of which talents tend to co-occur. Co-occurrence of particular talents can suggest either (1) common or contiguous brain substrates or (2) common underlying psychological processes, such as when Gardner (1983) suggests that music requires a kind of spatial thinking. In this volume the linkage or isolation of particular abilities is considered for hyperlexic children (Aram & Healy, Chapter 4), eidetikers (Haber & Haber, Chapter 10), mathematically gifted children (Benbow, Chapter 3), and chess masters (Cranberg & Albert, Chapter 7). Several authors explore whether a certain minimum general intellectual ability is necessary for the full development of certain talents; this question is treated for persons with linguistic abilities (Curtiss, Chapter 20; Novoa, Fein, & Obler, Chapter 15), mnemonists (Brown & Deffenbacher, Chapter 8), calculators (Smith, Chapter 2), and those who excel in chess, music, and physics (Charness, Chapter 22; Cranberg & Albert, Chapter 7).

The association of talent in a given domain with exceptional memory for that domain arises again and again, and the importance of this association probably cannot be overestimated. Exceptional domain-specific memory is mentioned in almost all of the case histories and is dealt with in detail in the cases by Novoa, Fein, and Obler (Chapter 15); Lucci, Fein, Holevas, and Kaplan, (Chapter 17); Waterhouse, (Chapter 18); and Bogyo and Ellis (Chapter 13). The role and importance of memory in particular kinds of talent are explored in detail for music (Judd, Chapter 6), hyperlexia (Aram & Healy, Chapter 4), linguistic skills (Curtiss, Chapter 20), and art (Rosenblatt & Winner, Chapter 19), and across skills (Charness, Chapter 22). Mechanisms for particular kinds of memory are explored by Haber and Haber (Chapter 10), Wolfe (Chapter 11), Brown and Deffenbacher (Chapter 8), and Oscar-Berman (Chapter 9).

Overview of the Book

Because we offer this book as an opportunity to further develop a young field of study, we solicited review chapters, in Part II, on those abilities for which there was enough literature to survey and an expert or team of experts prepared to speculate on the basis of that literature. Parts III and IV consist of a set of case studies and a set of small group studies, respectively, presented as examples of the different ways in which such studies can contribute to this field. In Part V we offer discussion on topics that cut across the different abilities.

We invited our authors to consider definitions of the talent or talents they describe, theories about how a given skill is performed by talented individuals or how it develops, and what the components of the skill seem to be. Questions regarding the cognitive processes underlying such mysterious talents and abilities as calendar calculating, eidetic imagery, and musical composition, and the roles that memory and experience play, are explored in depth by Charness (music, chess, and physics; Chapter 22), Matthysse and Greenberg (calculating; Chapter 23), Smith (calculating; Chapter 2), Brown and Deffenbacher (memory; Chapter 8), and Haber and Haber (eidetic imagery; Chapter 10). Other contributors, such as Judd (music; Chapter 6) and Schweiger (artistic design; Chapter 16), consider in detail the component skills making up the talent.

We asked what was known about the standard neuropsychological parameters accompanying the skill, such as gender, handedness, birth history, and hemispheric dominance. Variables such as handedness, sex, and age of onset are dealt with in some detail by many of the authors. An increased incidence of left-handedness is reported for many types of skills, and the implications of this for the Geschwind and other neurological theories are drawn by Benbow (Chapter 3) and by Cranberg and Albert (Chapter 7). The differential incidence of various abilities for males and females is also reported by several authors (Benbow, Chapter 3; Rosenblatt & Winner, Chapter 19; Brown & Deffenbacher, Chapter 8; Cranberg & Albert, Chapter 7), and the implications for neurological versus cultural theories are considered. The frequent early appearance of talents is considered in many of the case histories (Waterhouse, Chapter 18; Lucci, Fein, Holevas, & Kaplan, Chapter 17; Bogyo & Ellis, Chapter 13) and is discussed in reviews by Rimland and Fein (autism; Chapter 25), Smith (calculation; Chapter 2), Cranberg and Albert (chess; Chapter 7), and Charness (music; Chapter 14).

We also asked our authors to speculate about the brain structures or processes that may underlie the ability to perform the talent, and to record those research questions that currently can be, but have not yet been, addressed, as well as research questions that could be asked if we had additional knowledge or technology.

Future Research

Research strategies for the future are suggested by many of the authors in this volume, some explicitly, and some by the studies, serving as excellent illustrations of a particular mehod. The neuropsychological case method, where full cognitive evaluations reveal associations with, and dissociations from the talent in question, is illustrated by Lebrun, Van Endert, and Szliwowski (Chapter 12); Waterhouse (Chapter 18); Lucci, Fein, Holevas, and Kaplan (Chapter 17); Novoa, Fein, and Obler (Chapter 15); and Bogyo and Ellis (Chapter 13). Case studies of brain-damaged individuals who premorbidly showed a high degree of certain talent are illustrated by Schweiger (Chapter 16) and reviewed by Cranberg and Albert (Chapter 7). Studies of family histories of traits associated with particular talents (such as those of DeLong & Aldershof, Chapter 21, and Smith, Chapter 2) will certainly be fruitful in understanding genetic linkages between talents and other traits. Studies of the subcomponents of talents—such as the fine-grained analysis of musical talent by Judd (Chapter 6) and the discussion of linguistic dissociations by Curtiss (Chapter 20) and by Aram and Healy (Chapter 4)—will pave the way for more refined catalogs of skills to be studied. Detailed cognitive investigations of how skills are performed by different individuals are presented by Haber and Haber (Chapter 10), Brown and Deffenbacher (Chapter 8), and Matthysse and Greenberg (Chapter 23). Chapter 23, in particular, takes a delimited problem, lays out several ways in which the skill could theoretically be performed, and proposes specific tests by which the issue could be resolved. The observation by Smith (Chapter 2) about concomitant motor and vocal activity in calculators suggests the possibility of adapting, for the study of talented performance, the current neuropsychological method of studying what kinds of motor activity interfere with the performance of a skill. Chapter 11, by Wolfe, on the visual system in eidetic imagery and Chapter 9 by Oscar-Berman, on brain systems underlying memory serve as an illustration of how detailed phenomenological description (as given by Haber & Haber, Chapter 10 and Brown and Deffenbacher, Chapter 8) can be used as a basis for speculating about what brain systems could be involved.

Finally, some specific physiological methods are proposed. Electroencephalographic and radiological methods are suggested by Matthysse and Greenberg (Chapter 23), and a beginning has been made of adapting these to the study of talent, as described by Cranberg and Albert (Chapter 7), who observed EEG activation in chess players. The architectonic speculations raised in a number of chapters naturally suggest cytoarchitectonic brain studies of talented individuals, along the lines of those that Galaburda and Kemper (1979) used for the study of dyslexic individuals.

We agree with Waterhouse (Chapter 26) that attempts to find the neurological structures and mechanisms underlying talent should not be considered reductionistic. No one can deny the important influences of environment and attitudes, both individual and societal, on the development or underdevelopment of a given person's talents. With all our contributors, however, we share a belief that we can learn more about the range of possibilities of the human brain, and how it operates, through consideration of the neuropsychology of talent.

References

Benbow, C., & Stanley J. (1983). Sex differences in mathematical reasoning ability: More facts. *Science, 222,* 1029–1031.

Bronner, A. F. (1921). *The psychology of special abilities and disabilities.* Boston: Little, Brown.

Curtiss, S. (1977). *Genie: A psycholinguistic study of a modern-day wild child.* New York: Academic Press.

Diamond, M. C., & Scheibel, A. B. (1985, July 28). Research on the structure of Einstein's brain. In W. Reich, The stuff of genius. *The New York Times Magazine,* pp. 24–25.

Galaburda, A. (1983). Definition of the anatomical phenotype. In C. Ludlow & J. Cooper (Eds.), *Genetic aspects of speech and language disorder.* New York: Academic Press.

Galaburda, A. M., & Kemper, T. (1979). Cytoarchitectonic abnormalities in developmental dyslexia—A case study. *Annals of Neurology, 6,* 94–100.

Gardner, H. (1983). *Frames of mind: The theory of multiple intelligences.* New York: Basic Books.

Geschwind, N. (1983). Genetics: Fate, chance, and environmental control. In C. Ludlow & J. Cooper (Eds.), *Genetic aspects of speech and language disorder.* New York: Academic Press. 21–36.

Geschwind, N., & Behan, P. (1982). Left-handedness: Association with immune disease, migraine, and developmental learning disorder. *Proceedings of the National Academy of Sciences, USA, 79,* 5097–5100.

Geschwind, N., & Galaburda, A. M. (1985a). Cerebral lateralization: Biological mechanisms, associations and pathology: 1. A hypothesis and a program for research. *Archives of Neurology, 42,* 428–459.

Geschwind, N., & Galaburda, A. M. (1985b). Cerebral lateralization: Biological mechanisms, associations and pathology: 2. A hypothesis and a program for research. *Archives of Neurology, 42,* 521–552.

Geschwind, N., & Galaburda, A. M. (1985c). Cerebral lateralization: Biological mechanisms, associations and pathology: 3. A hypothesis and a program for research. *Archives of Neurology, 42,* 634–654.

Gould, S. J. (1981). *The mismeasure of man.* New York: W. W. Norton.

Lenneberg, E. (1967). *Biological foundations of language,* New York: Wiley.

Metraux R. (Ed.). (1979). *Margaret Mead: Some personal views.* New York: Walker.

Rush, B. (1812). *Medical inquiries and observations upon the diseases of the mind.* Philadelphia: Kimber & Richardson.

Sacks, O. (1985). *The man who mistook his wife for a hat and other clinical tales.* New York: Simon & Schuster.

Selfe, L. (1977). *Nadia.* New York: Harcourt Brace Jovanovich.

Smith, S. (1983). *The great mental calculators: The psychology, methods, and lives of calculating prodigies, past and present.* New York: Columbia University Press.

II

SURVEYING SPECIFIC AREAS OF TALENT

2

Calculating Prodigies

STEVEN B. SMITH

Calculating prodigies (also sometimes called "lightning calculators") are those rare individuals with astonishing abilities for mental calculation. Exactly what qualifies as "astonishing" I leave open. Anyone who can multiply two arbitrary three-digit numbers together mentally in 30 seconds or so certainly qualifies. But though this is a sufficient condition for being a calculating prodigy, it is not a necessary one. Some calculators are distinguished not by the speed but by the size of the calculations they can carry out. Furthermore, there are cases of retarded prodigies who are incapable of solving any arithmetic problems, but who can supply the day of the week for remote dates in the future or past.

In *The Great Mental Calculators* (Smith, 1983; henceforth TGMC) I argue that the calculating ability of prodigies is based on the same faculty as that for speech. A consequence is that any child capable of speech is a potential calculating prodigy.

The fundamental neurological question to be answered about calculating prodigies is whether they are in any way neurologically distinct (and if so, how and why). In the case of one type of calculating prodigy at least (auditory calculators, described subsequently), there is reason to believe that they do tend to be different. The question then is, can a talent that is largely restricted to a neurologically peculiar subset of the population be potentially within the province of any ordinary child? The answer is yes, but the how and why will require some background.

Types of Calculators

Calculators may be classified by the way in which they imagine numbers. There are two primary types: those who "see" numbers in the mind's eye, and those who "hear" them (sometimes literally, since they are often given to muttering while calculating). The former are traditionally termed "visual" and the latter "auditory."

Steven B. Smith. Wenatchee, Washington.

Auditory calculators have certain typical traits, namely:

1. Some sort of verbalizing while calculating—muttering numbers and the like. This is frequently accompanied by exaggerated motor activities—pacing, head shaking, hand wagging, and nervous tics. For this reason auditory prodigies have sometimes been referred to as "auditory–motor" or even "acoustic–rhythmic–motorial." Visual prodigies are usually, by comparison, placid.

2. Self taught, left-to-right methods of calculation. Visual calculators typically use cross multiplication.

3. Precocity. Most learned to calculate before learning written numbers. Visual prodigies must of course know written numbers in order to calculate, but there are visual prodigies who did not begin serious mental calculation until they were in their 20s.

Visual calculators fall into groups, depending upon the way in which they imagine numbers. The members of one group always see numbers in their own handwriting, regardless of the mode of presentation. One of the most interesting cases is that of Salo Finkelstein, of whom Bousfield and Barry (1933) noted:

(a) The numbers appear as if written with chalk on a freshly washed blackboard. (b) The numbers are in Mr. Finkelstein's own handwriting regardless of the form of presentation. (c) Ordinarily the numbers appear to be from 5 to 7 cm. in height. (d) The images normally appear to be at a distance of 35 to 40 cm. from the eyes. (e) The span of imagery includes about six figures with a definite preference for their horizontal arrangement. If, for example, a list of 200 numbers has been memorized, at any one moment any group of about six figures may be made to stand out clearly. (f) When the figures are visualized on a ground at a distance of about 1 1/2 m., they are about 30% smaller and less distinct (p. 355).

Although Finkelstein could obtain images with his eyes closed, he preferred to have them open. "Finkelstein says that he opens his eyes wide as an aid to concentration. He has the impression that it helps him. He thinks that with his eyes he sees the book or blackboard, and above his eyes he sees the numbers. This may be only a subjective illusion. But so he feels" (Weinland, 1948, p. 255).

There are other visual calculators who apparently "see" numbers exactly as presented to them, though in the process of calculating they must generate their own images. In the latter case, Gottfried Rückle, a 19th-century German mathematician, said that he saw numbers in his handwriting.

When the contemporary Indian calculator Shyam Marathe gave a demonstration at the Rand Corporation he ran into difficulty because he had run out of room on the blackboard and had therefore written the numbers at the bottom very small. When trying to visualize them, he found that those numbers were so small that he had a hard time making them out.

There are also calculators who are neither auditory nor visual. Louis Fleury, who was blind, moved his fingers over imaginary "cubarithms" (Tocquet, 1957, p. 24), counting symbols used by the blind.

The brilliant 20th-century mathematician Alexander Craig Aitken (1954) seems to have had no number imagery when calculating: "I myself can visualize if I wish, and at intervals in a calculation, and also at the end when all is done, the numbers come into focus; but mostly it is as if they were hidden under some medium, though being moved about with decisive exactness with regard to order and ranging" (p. 302).

Nature of the Ability

Mental calculation involves several components: (1) basic operations of arithmetic; (2) more complex algorithms, often iterative, using the operations of arithmetic; (3) special memorized data (such as logarithms or the number of seconds in a year), which are used in the algorithms; and (4) retaining results, which serve as input to further stages of the algorithm. The operations involved tend to become increasingly unconscious with practice, particularly those of basic arithmetic.

The algorithms often bear a striking resemblance to computer programs, although many were devised before the days of calculating machines. The major problem is the limitations of short-term memory, in which results, interim or final, must be stored. (It is possible to calculate in long-term memory, as did Jedediah Buxton, who sometimes took months to complete a calculation, but for the most part entering and retrieving data is too slow and unreliable to be of much use in rapid mental calculation.)

The fundamental operation for calculating prodigies is multiplication. George Parker Bidder (1856), a child calculating prodigy and later a prominent 19th-century British engineer, said, "I propose therefore . . . first to take you through the process of multiplication; and I begin with that rule because it is the basis of all calculations" (p. 257). Frank D. Mitchell (1907), psychologist and mental calculator, pointed out the reason for this:

> It has been suggested above that in the earlier stages the "natural" calculator who begins with counting—as distinguished from the "artificial" calculator who begins relatively late in life, using book-methods from the start—is interested mainly in *properties* of numbers and of simple series. Now these properties are revealed not by addition, but by multiplication (p. 103).

Auditory prodigies typically multiply from left to right. This seems natural from the point of view of speech, since spoken numbers are directional in a way in which written numbers are not. This method was discovered independently by almost all auditory calculators. Figure 2-1 illustrates how it works.

Bidder (1856) remarked of this method: "Now . . . it must be apparent, and must be received as an established fact, that reduced to paper, mental processes do not recommend themselves as expeditious; but that, on the contrary, they are very often prolix; they are, in reality, solely designed to facilitate the registration in the mind" (p. 261).

Visual prodigies, on the other hand, generally use cross multiplication. This method is particularly effective if the calculator is given the problem in written form and can write the answer from right to left as it is obtained. This is quite another matter, however, from doing a problem entirely mentally, when even the

```
Steps in multiplying 373 by 279:

200 × 300 =  60,000
200 ×  70 =  14,000
       sum   74,000
200 ×   3 =     600
       sum   74,600
 70 × 300 =  21,000
       sum   95,600
 70 ×  70 =   4,900
       sum  100,500
 70 ×   3 =     210
       sum  100,710
  9 × 300 =   2,700
       sum  103,410
  9 ×  70 =     630
       sum  104,040
  9 ×   3 =      27
       sum  104,067    Final product
```

FIGURE 2-1. Left-to-right multiplication.

problem must be memorized and the answer given in left-to-right order. Around five digits by five digits is probably the upper limit for such a problem, unless the intermediate steps are laboriously memorized, and three digits by three digits is, according to Bidder, the point past which one should give up on mental multiplication and get out pencil and paper. Using cross multiplication with the problem in view and writing down the answer as it is obtained, 10 digits by 10 digits is certainly possible, or even 12 digits by 12 digits. (Bear in mind we are here talking about multiplying two different numbers—squaring numbers requires less memory and allows the use of special short-cuts.)

Wim Klein, who worked for many years as a "human computer" at the Center for Nuclear Research (CERN) in Geneva, was an auditory calculator, but he used cross multiplication in performances because it allowed him to do large calculations rapidly.[1] He also multiplied two digits at a time, the only calculator known with certainty to have done so. Figure 2-2 illustrates Klein's method for multiplying two nine-digit numbers.

Mental calculators, no less than other mortals, are subject to short-term memory limitations. Where they differ is in their ability to treat groups of digits as single items in memory. For Bidder (1856) three digits constituted one item in memory, just as a word, regardless of length, constitutes one memory item:

> I believe that much of the facility of mental calculation, and also of mastery over numbers, depends on having the idea of numbers impressed upon the mind, without any reference to symbols. The number 763 is represented symbolically by three figures

1. The order in which numbers are spoken in Dutch may have something to do with this. In Dutch one does not say the equivalent of 'twenty-four," but "four-and-twenty." Thus left-to-right multiplication of two-digit numbers in spoken Dutch corresponds to cross multiplication in written arithmetic. The situation is different when larger numbers are involved, but if the method of cross multiplication is firmly ingrained in the child on the basis of two-digit numbers, it may be naturally extended to more complex calculations.

7–6–3; but 763 is only one quantity,—one number,—one idea, and it presents itself to my mind just as the word "hippopotamus" presents the idea of one animal. . . . Each set, or series of 3 figures, constitutes a step in numbers, 787 is one series,—the second series is 787 thousand, the next series 787 millions, the next 787 thousand millions, and the next 787 billions. Therefore, at the change beyond each third figure, another idea must be seized by the mind; and though it is but one idea, yet with all the training I have had, when I pass three figures, and jump from 787 to 1,787, I cannot realize to myself that it is but one idea;—in fact there are two, and this increases the strain on the registering powers of the mind (p. 263).

Calculating prodigies have discovered remarkable algorithmic methods closely resembling steps in a computer program. One such example is an iterative

		Current partial product		
1. 78 × 26 = 2,028	28	6. carry 109		
2. carry 20		13 × 2 = 26		
78 × 95 = 7,410		sum 135		
sum 7,430		39 × 14 = 546		
13 × 26 = 338		sum 681		
sum 7,768	6828	75 × 84 = 6,300		
3. carry 77		sum 6,981		
78 × 84 = 6,552		5 × 95 = 475		
sum 6,629		sum 7,456	564827786828	
13 × 95 = 1,235		7. carry 74		
sum 7,864		39 × 2 = 78		
39 × 26 = 1,014		sum 152		
sum 8.878	786828	75 × 1 = 1,050		
4. carry 88		sum 1,202		
78 × 14 = 1,092		5 × 84 = 420		
sum 1,180		sum 1,622	22564827786828	
13 × 84 = 1,092		8. carry 16		
sum 2,272		75 × 2 = 150		
39 × 95 = 3,705		sum 166		
sum 5,977		5 × 14 = 70		
75 × 26 = 1,950		sum 236	3622564827786828	
sum 7,927	27786828	9. carry 2		
5. carry 79		5 × 2 = 10		
78 × 2 = 156		sum 12	123,622,564,827,786,828	
sum 235			Final product	
13 × 14 = 182				
sum 417				
39 × 84 = 3,276				
sum 3,693				
75 × 95 = 7,125				
sum 10,818				
5 × 26 = 130				
sum 10,948	4827786828			

FIGURE 2-2. Cross Multiplication. Method used by Wim Klein to multiply 214,849,526 times 575,391,378 in 48 seconds in a test conducted in 1953 by Fred Barlow.

method worked out by Bidder as a child for computing compound interest. (I don't mean to imply that Bidder was the first to discover this method—only that he did so independently.) It is based on the binomial theorem, though Bidder had no awareness of this when he worked it out.

Although the general calculative scheme of prodigies is often cast in a form similar to a computer program, the actual implementation is another matter. Calculating prodigies have vast stores of information, acquired largely unintentionally, simply from doing so many calculations. This information is brought to bear in particular cases. As Wim Klein says, "The computer doesn't know when to skip things. The human being just sees it and knows it. You have to tell the computer every damn thing."

That mental calculation tends to become unconscious is borne out by the testimony of various calculators, as in this statement by Aitken (1954):

> I have noticed at times that the mind has anticipated the will; I have had an answer before I even wished to do the calculation; I have checked it, and am always surprised that it is correct. This, I suppose (but the terminology may not be right), is the subconscious in action; I think it can be in action at several levels; and I believe that each of these levels has its own velocity, different from that of our ordinary waking time, in which our processes of thought are rather tardy (p. 302).

And Hunter (1962) remarked on the inadequacy of Aitken's descriptions of his procedures: "An absolutely complete description was never possible: in part because much calculative activity was unavailable to self-observation, in part because much that was available could not be put readily into words" (p. 245).

Genesis

In the case of many prodigies, interest in calculation was stimulated by counting. In fact, in some cases mental calculators taught themselves to multiply armed with only a knowledge of counting.

Jedediah Buxton, a retarded 18th-century Derbyshire farm laborer, experimentally determined that a cubic inch contained the following (Holliday, 1751): 200 grains of barley, 300 grains of wheat, 512 grains of rye, 180 grains of oats, 40 peas, 25 beans, 30 vetches, 100 lentils, and 2,304 hairs one inch long. When Buxton was taken to see *Richard III* at the Drury Lane playhouse, he spent his time counting the number of steps taken by the actors and the number of words spoken by Garrick (The Life of Jedediah Buxton. 1754).

Thomas Fuller, a Virginia slave, explained the role of counting in the development of his calculating ability to Thomas Wistar (Rush, 1789):

> He informed the first-mentioned gentleman that he began his application to figures by counting ten, and that when he was able to count an hundred, he thought himself (to use his own words) "a very clever fellow." His first attempt after this was to count the number of hairs in a cow's tail, which he found to be 2872. He next amused himself with counting, grain by grain, a bushel of wheat and a bushel of flax-seed (p. 62).

Bidder (1856) also started his calculating career through counting:

My Father was a working mason, and my elder Brother pursued the same calling. My first and only instructor in figures was that elder Brother, who was some years since removed from among us by death; the instruction he gave me was commenced by teaching me to count up to 10. Having accomplished this he induced me to go on to 100, and there he stopped. Having acquired a certain knowledge of numbers, by counting up to 100, I amused myself by repeating the process, and found that by stopping at 10, and repeating that every time, I counted up to 100 much quicker than by going straight through the series. I counted up to 10, then to 10 again = 20, 3 times 10 = 30, 4 times 10 = 40, and so on. This may appear to you a simple process, but I attach the utmost importance to it, because it made me perfectly familiar with numbers up to 100; they became as it were my friends, and I knew all their relations and acquaintances (pp. 257–258).

Bidder subsequently taught himself the multiplication table up to 10 by 10, by arranging shot in rectangles.

Emile Jacoby (n.d.) gives a remarkable description of the relationship of counting to calculation in the case of Henri Mondeux (translation by the author):

If he went into the fields, he walked with his eyes closed and counted until an accident or fear of an accident forced him to open his eyes. Then he would take a step with his eyes open for the first five steps taken with his eyes closed, two for the second five, three for the third five, and so on. He had thus to divide by five the number of steps taken with his eyes closed, then to take the sum of the series of natural numbers from one up to the number of times he had taken five steps with his eyes closed. In this way, he says, he tried to take the largest number of steps possible with his eyes closed so as to be able to take a greater number with his eyes open. And if by chance he sat in a chair, he would lean back, balancing the chair as long as possible and counting until it fell down again on its front legs. Then from the numbers so obtained, he would make summations of series or raise them to the second or third power, or sum a series of squares or cubes, without being conscious of what he was doing, nor the processes he used to arrive at the goal he proposed to reach. (p. 117)

The great mathematician Karl Friedrich Gauss remarked upon his habit of unconscious counting (Gauss & Schumacher, 1861):

From time to time as I am walking I begin to count my steps mentally (incidentally always when I am walking rhythmically). So I count up to 100 and then I begin from one again. I do all this, once it has started, unconsciously. I think of other things, observe whatever happens to catch my eye; the only thing I am not able to do is speak during that time. And then only after a certain amount of time do I become aware that I am continuing to count rhythmically . . . and always accurately, naturally however without knowing whether or how often I have reached 100 (p. 298).

The vaudeville performer Arthur Griffith also first became interested in numbers through counting (Bryan & Lindley, 1941): "Before his fifth year he was able to keep a mental record of the number of grains of corn fed the chickens. The total for three years, according to his childish count, was 42,173. He says he could remember weeks afterward how many grains he fed the chickens on a given day" (p. 24).

At least two auditory calculators had a talent for rapid counting. For example, Henry P. Curtis, who knew Truman Henry Safford (later a prominent astronomer) as a child, said that Safford's friends

> used to ply him with all sorts of questions *in numbers*. Out in the country they would ... ask him how many sticks there were in a long fence, over there, and he would sweep his eye over it, and say right off 147, and they would go and count the palings and would find sure enough 147. Then they would turn around to another fence, and ask for the number of palings in that new one, and passing his eyes along it would say without delay 274, and they would find that the correct number (Lewis & Plotkin, 1982, p. 54).

Zacharias Dase was a performer and later a compiler of mathematical tables. Schumacher (Gauss & Schumacher, 1861) noted of him: "If you take a handful of peas and throw them on a table it's enough for him to take just a quick glance at them to give their number. He did something similar here with the dots on dominoes, at which he took merely a glance and was able to give their sum (117)" (p. 277).

Counting leads naturally to the discovery of multiplication, and then to raising to powers. For example, if one arranges pebbles in rectangles, one discovers that the total number of pebbles is the product of the number of pebbles in one row and the number in one column, and that if the number of pebbles is such that they cannot be arranged in a rectangle (except that rectangle represented by a simple string), then that number is prime.

And one soon learns that it is more rapid to count, not by ones, but in higher multiples. If one counts in 3's, counting becomes three times as fast. One further learns that, if one counts by 3 six times, the result is 18. So 6 *times* 3 is 18. In fact, Bidder (1856) stressed the importance of the common English terminology in his learning to multply:

> When I commenced seriously to calculate, my vocabulary was so restricted, that I did not even know the meaning of the word "multiply." The first time I was asked to "multiply" some small affair, say 23 by 27, I did not know what was meant:—and it was not until I was told that it meant 23 times 27 that I could comprehend the term. I believe, however, that it is not unimportant, that I should have begun without knowing the meaning of the conventional term "multiply," because the words "23 times 27" had to my comprehension a distinct meaning; which was—that 23 times 27 meant 20 times 20 plus 20 times 7, and 3 times 7 plus 20 times 3. It must be evident then, that the powers I possess are derived from careful training; which resulted very much from accident at first, and I think this want of knowledge of terms was one of the accidents, that particularly favoured my progess in arithmetic (p. 261).

Mitchell (1907) gives a good account of how counting can progress to calculation:

> To understand this precocity we must note, first of all, that arithmetic is the most independent and self-sufficient of all the sciences. Given a knowledge of how to *count*

and later a few definitions, as in Bidder's case, and any child of average ability can go on, once his interest is accidentally aroused, and construct, unaided, practically the whole science of arithmetic, no matter how much or how little he knows of other things (pp. 97–98).

Exaggerated Motor Activity

There exist a number of reports of auditory calculators who display exaggerated motor activity, particularly when children and particularly when calculating. This may relate to a general tendency toward hyperactivity on the part of auditory calculators, but at least one such calculator (Jacques Inaudi) was described as having a mild temperament.

I summarize what is known in this connection about various auditory calculators.

As a child, Zerah Colburn was internationally known for his calculating ability. He remarks in his *Memoir* (Colburn, 1833):

Since the author commenced writing this book, he has met with some gentlemen who saw him when quite a child, who have mentioned a circumstance, of which, if it ever existed, he has no recollection. It was in relation to his personal appearance, when engaged in studying out the answer to a question:—that his body immediately assumed certain contortions, as if he were affected with what is called St. Vitus's dance, which continued until he obtained the result (p. 173).

Professor MacNeven (1811), who saw Colburn perform at the age of 6, noted, "His movements are precipitate, and he is incessantly active" (p. 22).

Truman Henry Safford was interviewed at age 10 by a mathematician, Chester Dewey (*Chambers's Edinburgh Journal*, 1847), who described his antics while calculating: "He flew around the room like a top, pulled his pantaloons over the top of his boots, bit his hand, rolled his eyes in their sockets, sometimes smiling and talking, and then seeming to be in agony" (p. 266).

The 19-century French calculator Henri Mondeux was certainly mentally disturbed and possibly mentally retarded. As a child, he was usually described as a veritable savage. Today he would no doubt be diagnosed as hyperactive and learning disabled. His teacher and promoter, Emile Jacoby (n.d.), described Mondeux while calculating:

Then his features, calm in solitude, take on a thousand diverse expressions. First his brow darkens, his eyes have a frightening fixity, his lips move ceaselessly and his movements are abrupt and hurried; his fingers seem to clench; he imparts to his body a balance like that of a clapper of a church bell. He doesn't see anything, nor hear anything; he is completely withdrawn into himself; this is when he is grappling with a problem. Then his eyes rise slowly, he looks over the audience, his mouth is smiling, his complexion takes on color, there is in all his being an expression that is not without charm—the difficulty is overcome and he seems to look for inspiration in the heavens (p. 146).

Jacques Inaudi, a performer studied by Alfred Binet, (1894) also displayed sundry nervous mannerisms while calculating: "During the calculations, he makes various gestures, tics without importance and, moreover, very variable . . . ." (p. 37). But Binet (1894) describes him as calm and tranquil, with a mild and modest character. Binet does mention, however, that as a child Inaudi was very mischievous.

Jakobsson (1944) reported on a 21-year-old mentally retarded woman, Gullan B., who had an unusual ability for mental multiplication. He noted, "As a child she manifested 'a nervous twitch' of the arms and face" (p. 180).

Charles and George (no last name given), identical twin idiot savants, were described in *Life* magazine by Dora Jane Hamblin (1966; see also Horwitz, Kestenbaum, Person, & Jarvik, 1965). The twins were born 2 months premature and had a twin sister who died within 12 hours of birth. Hamblin (1966) remarks: "They did not walk until they were $2\frac{1}{2}$ years old, and the moment they got up on their feet they seemed bent upon destruction. They banged their heads, they bit their hands, they threw things" (p. 108). When the twins were 9, they were sent to a state mental institution because they had become intolerable at home.

At the time of the *Life* article, the twins, then 26, were still given to occasional violent, self-destructive outbursts: "But then, one day, Charles or George turns up with a scarred forehead or a bandaged forearm and it turns out that he has, in the twins' own words, 'gone on a toot' and engaged in violence. The last time Charles went on a toot was when a nurse absent-mindedly picked up the morning papers and delivered them herself" (Hamblin, 1966, p.110).

And like other hyperactives, sitting still was difficult: "Too nervous to sit still very long, they are not interested in television, reading or playing games. They like to keep moving" (Hamblin, 1966, p. 111).

Wim Klein and his brother Leo are particularly interesting because both were exceptional calculators. A variety of tests dealing with both words and numbers conducted in Amsterdam during the war by Berthold Stokvis (1949) revealed that Wim's memory was essentially auditory, while Leo's was visual. Of particular interest was the difference in their demeanors while memorizing: "It was noticed that WILLIAM [Wim] made pantomimic expression movements: while memorizing, his torso, arms and legs move rhythmically; he shakes his head and moves his lips. LEO, on the contrary, would remain sitting or standing completely rigid as he listened to the task set him or stare at the paper before his eyes" (Stokvis, 1949, pp. 81–82).

Wim Klein was an anthill of agitation. His friend, Hans Eberstark, a visual calculator, exudes monolithic placidity. As Wim described Hans: "He's great, He's absolutely daft, also. He does not smoke. He does not drink. He's big and fat. He's so quiet. He never gets nervous. Just the opposite from me."

Joel Kupperman was the youngest (he first appeared when he was 5) and most popular of the children on the "Quiz Kids" radio show in the early 1940s. He was specially adept at mathematical problems. Beatty (1943) gave the following description of him: "His main trouble [on radio shows] is in keeping still. When he is doing a mathematical problem he writhes in his chair, kicks his feet, rubs his head with his hands, and sways so much it is necessary to have a man on hand to shove the microphone back and forth" (p. 142).

The contemporary American calculator Arthur Benjamin was diagnosed as hyperactive and took medication for this through the eighth grade. He was also asthmatic and was found at age 3 to have an abnormal EEG. Doctors advised his father not to enroll him in public school because his attention span was too short to function effectively. But he proved too much of a discipline problem at preschool and wound up in public school by default.

He says of his childhood: "In elementary school I was not an easy child to deal with. I couldn't sit still—I still have trouble sitting still."

However, at least one visual prodigy displayed the sort of nervous mannerisms typical of auditory prodigies:

> Concomitant with the more extensive processes of memorization and calculation, one notes in Mr. Finkelstein a large amount of motor activity such as pacing to and fro, gesticulation, and facial contortion. Before writing the sum of a column of figures or the product of two large numbers written on the blackboard, he invariably draws a line through them. A definite kinesthetic component is here involved. There is a feeling of inhibition when these movements are suppressed (Bousfield & Barry, 1933, p. 355).

What of other visual prodigies? We have already seen that Leo Klein and Hans Eberstark display no unusual motor activity when calculating. Shyam Marathe also appears calm (personal observation). Binet (1894) makes no mention of any nervous activity in the case of Pericles Diamandi (visual) as he does in the case of Jacques Inaudi (auditory).

Hunter (1962) wrote of Aitken, who had no imagery while calculating, but who could visualize the answers if he so chose, ". . . . the thinker uses no gestures but sits, relaxed and still, while calculating" (p. 244).

Childhood Illness and Injury

There are a number of reports of severe childhood illness, or injury to calculating prodigies. In the cases of several idiot savants, their retardation has been attributed to such incidents.

At 4 years, Henri Mondeux contracted scarlet fever and was severely ill. Because of complications, his entire body swelled and remained swollen for 3 weeks, with his life in doubt. It was toward the end of this period that he first suffered one of the nervous attacks that were to afflict him throughout his life. Jacoby (n.d.) wrote:

> Henri Mondeux, who is solidly constituted, who seems built more for handling a plough than holding a pen, is tormented by nerves. He is subject to violent and frequent nervous attacks, which in an instant cause him to lose his strength and his reason. This is the true reason, the true cause of the atrophy of his reason (p. 156).

This loss of strength and reason from nervous attacks suggests epilepsy.

Luigi Pierini, born in 1878, was a shepherd boy who became a professional calculator. Mitchell (1907) noted that Pierini "learned late to speak and to walk, suffered from many children's diseases, and was an epileptic" (p. 87).

Sabine W., a 22-year-old retarded calculator described by Wizel (1904), contracted a severe case of typhus at the age of 4. Her retardation reportedly stemmed from this incident; prior to this she was a normal child attending school. She subsequently suffered from epilepsy and hypochondria. She alternated between periods of apathy, in which she would sit in the sun in summer or by the stove in winter, and extreme manic states.

Bryan and Lindley (1941) remark of Arthur Griffith, "When seven years old, after a severe illness, he became epileptic" (p. 24). Griffith died of a stroke at the age of 31.

Mohammed Ismail Turki El Attar died in 1934 at age 19 in a mental hospital in Cairo. As a child, he made money by performing mental calculations in cafes. Dudgeon and Hurst (1934) wrote: "The autopsy disclosed that he had a softened patch, probably an old haemorrhage, in the right occipital region of the brain, about the size of a small hen's egg. A recent haemorrhage at the same place was the cause of his death" (p. 579).

When Gullan B., a moderately retarded calculator described by Stig Jakobsson (1944) "was about 2 or 3 years old she contracted a trauma of the skull associated with a loss of consciousness. . . . As long as she could remember she had felt a weakness in her right arm and leg. . . . The neurological examination revealed a mild right-sided spastic hemiparesis. She was left-handed" (p. 180).

If the neurological peculiarities typical of some calculators can be the result of illness or injury, then genetic predilection becomes a much less viable explanation.

It is possible that some people are calculating prodigies because of genetics and that others arrive at the same point as a result of explicit brain injury.

I do not believe that brain damage could create a talent, but rather that the talent must always have been latent. It seems to me more likely that brain damage eliminates some of the competition. If this is so, we have a couple of possibilities. The first is that this talent, for biological reasons, could never have been accessed (or only very imperfectly accessed) were it not for the trauma. This is conceivable, but a view I would adopt only in the face of a lot of evidence. The second possibility, to which I subscribe, is that environment can channel interest in the same manner as biological damage.

Suppose there are talents that cannot, in the general case (i.e., the nongenetic case), be realized in the absence of brain damage. This would seem to say something rather strange about evolution: that we have talents that we can only get to in the case of a major foul-up. (It's true that female canaries have a latent talent for song that can be realized only by pumping them full of male hormones, but I think this situation is different. You can't get them to sing by infecting them with a variety of different illnesses or by banging their brains in a number of different ways—at least I don't think you can.)

It seems to me much more likely that talent for mental calculation is not normally stimulated except in the case of individuals who cannot (for various reasons—psychological, physiological, and sociological) participate in more commonplace distractions.

Spatial Inabilities

In the case of two calculators, Thomas Fuller and Henri Mondeux, there is evidence of prosopagnosia, or the inability to recognize faces.

Rush (1812) wrote of Fuller: "The famous African calculator Thomas Fuller, of Virginia, whose memory was exercised exclusively upon numbers, had so little recollection of faces, that he was unable to recognise [sic] the persons who had spent hours in conversing with him, and listening to his calculations, the next day after he saw them" (p. 282).

It appears, however, that Fuller had a good memory for other spatial matters: "With a little instruction he would have been able to cast up [reckon] plats (sic) of land. He took great notice of the lines of land which he had seen surveyed" (*Columbian Centinel*, 1790). And Rush (1789) noted:

> From this he was led to calculate with the most perfect accuracy, how many shingles a house of certain demensions [sic] would require to cover it, and how many polls [sic] and rails necessary to inclose, and how many grains of corn were necessary to sow a certain quantity of ground. From this application of his talents, his mistress has often derived considerable benefit (pp. 62–63).

Whether Fuller's inability to recognize faces was of long standing is unknown. At the time he was interviewed by Rush's acquaintances, Fuller was about 80 and "he said his memory began to fail him" (Rush, 1789, p. 63). It would also be interesting to know whether he "forgot" the faces of those he had encountered the previous day or whether he forgot the encounter altogether.

Jacoby (n.d.) alludes to serious difficulties in recognizing faces and geometric figures on the part of Mondeux: "Mondeux could never draw a line, [or] retain the form of a geometric figure; he is incapable of orienting himself alone in a city and he never recognizes people whom he has seen a thousand times. I caught him in the same day mistaking one of my friends, whom he had encountered very often, for three different people" (p. 150). And, "It was the same with people who came every day to the house; he could never remember their names, or recognize them" (p. 126).

When Jacoby tried to teach Mondeux written arithmetic, he encountered some peculiar difficulties:

> I would give him an addition to do. He sat down at the table and here is how he proceeded: he mentally added up each column, put each successive result in a corner of the blackboard one after the other, but not in its respective place: the units were in the place of the hundreds of thousands, the tens in the place of tens of thousands and reciprocally, such that the order of digits entirely reversed, and what was more curious, was that he had also reversed the form of the characters, so that a six resembled a nine (Jacoby, n.d., p. 125).

This suggests dyslexia, but there are other considerations. Mondeux was already 12 years old when he began to learn to write numbers and letters. That he mentally added from left to right and that Jacoby expected him to add from right to left may have further confused him.

Mondeux did eventually learn to cope with written words, though probably not numbers, since mental arithmetic was far easier and more interesting for him: "He reads badly, he writes legibly, but his writing is neither regular nor rapid; he is beginning to understand a little the proper spelling of words and to apply some grammatical rules" (Jacoby, n.d., p. 132).

Mondeux was even induced to keep a journal at Jacoby's (n.d.) request:

> What does he say in these curious narrations? He will say for example that a person presented him a problem and that he could not stop laughing because this person, according to him, did not know how to calculate. He will say that the streets are long and badly paved; or that he was well or badly greeted by such and such a person to whom he was presented (pp. 137–138).

Jacoby often complains of Mondeux's inability to remember things in general (apart from numbers), not merely spatial matters:

> Henri has not retained the name or the aspect of the countries he has visited. . . . The impressions that with other people are never erased: such as a service received of a friend, a stormy night in the mountains, a blizzard, the view of Mount Blanc, a beautiful sunset on Lake Geneva, a squall weathered at sea; all this slips through his memory and does not leave a trace (p. 137).

It is certain, however, that Mondeux's memory was not as devoid of content as Jacoby is inclined to suggest. The early portions of Jacoby's *Biographie de Henri Mondeux* are based largely on information supplied by Mondeux. And Mondeux did retain certain recent events: "The *queen* of the ball had the ambition to do a contra-dance with the shepherd of the Touraine; and Henri was so proud of it, that he later sometimes recalled it, with a certain pride" (Jacoby, n.d., pp. 94–95).

Furthermore, Mondeux's interest seems to have been attracted to matters of no interest to Jacoby (n.d.) and conversely:

> When he is asked what he saw of beauty in traveling, when he is asked what he remarked of beauty in some important city that he visited, he saw nothing, or at least he remembers nothing, absolutely nothing. In a city, he perceives only the length of the streets and the quality of the paving. As to monuments, he sees in the Madeleine, for example, only a very long building flanked by large columns, in the bell tower of Strasbourg only a very high pile of stones, in the Champs-Elysees only a vast lost piece of earth—and he calculates how many people one could feed with the wheat that could be cultivated if this promenade were converted into a vast field which was sown every year (p. 132).

There is evidence that Mondeux's ability to orient himself in space, at least under certain circumstances, could not have been too bad. He was a cowherd, an occupation that requires taking animals out to the fields and bringing them back.

Mondeux was once caught stealing fruit by a farmer. Jacoby (n.d.) quotes Mondeux:

> The farmer took me by one ear which he pulled a little too hard, but I knew that his cows had not come back from the wood and that they had been sought for nearly an hour, and the idea came to me to profit from this circumstance to get out of my difficulty. "Beat me as much as you like, but I promise you that you will not find your cows again." "All right, if you tell me where they are," replied the farmer, "no harm will come to you." "Then let me go and I will take you." He gave me my liberty; I walked to the side of the wood that I knew hadn't been searched. Luck was with me and I found the cows right away. I was saved; the event caused an uproar, and I was definitely looked upon as having relations with the devil (p. 35).

Notice that Mondeux was familiar with all the places that had previously been searched and knew that this was not among them.

Two other auditory calculators seem to have had difficulties in orienting themselves in cities. Wim Klein had a moderate amount of difficulty in finding his way about. In any case his brother Leo, who was a visual calculator, was vastly superior in this regard. Leo would come into a town, buy a map, scan it briefly, and know his way about. Klein remarked of his brother: "He would say to a waiter in a pub, 'I have to go there.' The chap would say, 'Well, you go like this.' My brother says, 'And if you go like this, is it not shorter?' The waiter says, 'Yes, sir.' There were hundreds of examples like this. Funny, eh? This visualizing. I cannot do it at all."

Jacques Inaudi also seems to have been generally forgetful and recognized towns with difficulty: "His impresario often remarked that he did not recognize a city to which he had already come to give performances. More than another person, he forgets his gloves and his cane when visiting, and appointment times. Perhaps there is a little malice in this, to give himself the opportunity for easy jokes" (Binet, 1894, p. 32).

It is possible that right-hemisphere debilities such as prosopagnosia can lead to an interest in calculation. If the ability to recognize things as a whole, the forte of the right hemisphere, is compromised, then the left hemisphere may have to take over a task for which it is ill prepared. It may undertake to identify things by a point-by-point comparison against certain stored information. Such a comparison could easily involve counting specific features, such as the number of spots on the left side of a cow, the number of moles on a person's forearm, and so forth. Counting could thus become central to maintaining a coherent world.

Environment

Calculating prodigies are typically physically or psychologically isolated from their peers. As Mitchell (1907) observed:

> Several of the calculators—Mondeux, Mangiamele, Pierini, Inaudi—were shepherd-boys, an occupation which, since it requires an ability to count and affords ample

leisure, is peculiarly favorable for practicing calculation, several, again,—Grandmange (born without arms or legs), Safford, Pierini, the present writer,—were sick or otherwise incapacitated for active play to a greater or less extent, and thus enjoyed an equally good opportunity to practice calculation. Fuller and Buxton, on the other hand, whether precocious or not, were men of such limited intelligence that they could comprehend scarcely anything, either theoretical or practical, more complex than counting; and their purely manual occupations left their minds free to carry on almost without limit their slow and laborious calculations (pp. 98–99).

Heredity

There is no evidence that an ability for mental calculation is inherited. It does not run in families as did, say, Colburn's supernumerary digits (see Supernumerary Digits section).

There are a few cases in which there was more than one mental calculator in the same family, but in every case they were members of the same household, and one was the instigator, while the other was an inferior emulator.

George Parker Bidder and his son of the same name were both mental calculators, but the father was much the superior calculator. Furthermore, he was an auditory calculator and multiplied from left to right; his son was a visual calculator and used cross multiplication, a more artificial technique.

Wim Klein and his brother Leo were also both outstanding mental calculators, but, again, Wim was auditory while Leo was visual.

There is also the case of the identical twins, George and Charles, who do calendar calculations. Horwitz *et al.* (1965) stated: "Although Charles is completely accurate only for this century, George can project his calendar identifications to centuries before and centuries beyond our present perpetual calendars" (p. 1075). And it was George who first showed an interest in calendar calculations. This case is particularly telling, since one would expect identical twins to have comparable calculating talents.

Several members of Aitken's family were good at arithmetic, and he was of the opinion (which, of course, I do not share) that "there was heredity in it" (Aitken, 1954, p. 307). Of his daughter he said (paraphrase of remarks following a lecture):

> She could work out square numbers as quickly as he could without trouble. If she thought it worth while, she could do some of the things he did, but she did not think it worth while. He thought it could be developed by small degrees, but he thought it developed exponentially and that each step was more rewarding, after a while. In the end one got clean away from the ordinary distribution which one would imagine to be among the populace (Aitken, 1954, p. 307–308).

If anyone can perform extraordinary feats of mental calculation, why should emulators be inferior to their models? Emulators are likely to be much more poorly motivated than the models (they may also begin at an older, and less flexible, age), as the comments by calculating prodigies about their relatives suggest. If you set out to teach yourself ancient Greek simply because your older sister taught herself ancient Greek (such people are probably nearly as rare as calculating prodigies), you are likely to fail. Nonetheless, both you and your sister would have learned ancient Greek had you been ancient Greeks.

Take the case of Wim Klein and his brother Leo, where it is plain that Leo was not nearly so well motivated as Wim. Wim said, "As soon as I started multiplying four digits [by four digits] my brother said, 'Oh, forget it, man.' He was a little bit infected by me. Because I did it he had to do it."

Gender

Though there are few reported cases of female calculating prodigies, they are not unknown. They include the contemporary calculator Shakuntala Devi, Lady Frederica Murray, the French performer Mlle. Osaka (possibly retarded), and two retarded calculators, Sabine W. and Gullan B., described previously; in the category of retarded calculators, there are no doubt many more of whom I am unaware. In Smith (1983) I suggested that "the apparent discrepancy in the frequency of male and female calculating prodigies can probably be ascribed to underreporting, lack of opportunity to develop the talent, and lack of encouragement for continued development (perhaps outright discouragement)" (p. 44).

One of the editors of this volume, Loraine K. Obler, took issue with me on this matter, arguing in a review of TGMC the following:

> S[mith] maintains that calculating is like juggling: any child can acquire calculating skills, as virtually everyone acquires language. But with exceptional calculating abilities (or juggling), not everyone bothers to. I suspect that S. is wrong. The overrepresentation of males among calculators (38 males vs. 3 females in this comprehensive book), suggests unusual brain development in calculators (Obler, 1985, p. 511).

It is true that not everyone bothers to learn to perform amazing feats of mental calculation any more than everyone bothers to learn Lithuanian—unless one happens to be surrounded by people speaking Lithuanian, the bother is going to be considerable, and only a very oddly motivated person is likely to undertake it. If such a person turned out to be neurologically peculiar, I don't think it would come as a great shock. Peculiar activities are likely to be the province of peculiar people. But this does not affect the fact that any child placed in the appropriate circumstances will learn Lithuanian.

Juggling turned out to be a more apt analogy than I initially supposed. Obler is prepared to grant that anyone can learn to juggle. This also seems to be the view of professional jugglers, who agree that anyone can learn the basics, and that from there it is just a matter of practice until it becomes "second nature," like walking or talking. But women with top-notch skills are exceedingly rare in the juggling fraternity—there are perhaps a dozen, as opposed to hundreds of males. When I questioned a professional juggler about the reason for this, he said that it was because women "prefer to do something real."

There are many hypotheses we could entertain regarding the rarity of female jugglers, just as in the case of calculating prodigies. I think the fact that baton twirling, which has much in common with juggling, is practiced almost exclusively by girls suggests an environmental explanation, even if that explanation is not immediately evident. (One wonders about the incidence of hyperactivity among jugglers. It wouldn't seem to be an amusement for phlegmatic individuals.)

In this connection the views of the brilliant contemporary mathematician Paul Erdös seem to me relevant. Erdös (1970), who certainly cannot be accused of being nonsexist because he refers to women as "bosses" and to men as "slaves," wrote:

> Lovasz and Posa [child prodigy mathematicians—see Mathematical Ability section] when they still went to high school once asked me why are there so few girl mathematicians. I told them: Suppose the slave children (boys) would be brought up with the idea that if they are very clever the bosses (girls) will not like them—would there be then many boys who do mathematics? Both said: well perhaps not so many (p. 15).

Erdös's mother, incidentally, was a mathematician.

Intelligence

The ability to do complex, if not necessarily sophisticated, mental calculations is often confused with genius, say, of the sort manifested by Mozart in writing symphonies as a child.

It is not at all clear that an ability for menal calculation can, in and of itself, be taken as evidence of intelligence. To begin with, we are loathe to acknowledge any sort of intelligence on the part of computers. But if sheer calculating ability is taken as evidence of intelligence, then, in that respect at least, computers are far smarter than any human beings. There are those who would agree to that, possibly even revel in it, but who is ready to grant intelligence to a pocket calculator or even an old-fashioned mechanical desk-top machine? However, as Aitken (1954) remarked:

> The machine, whether desk, hand or electric, or electronic, is bound to have a deleterious effect on mental calculation. When I came from New Zealand thirty years ago and first used an arithmometer, even of the antiquated types then available, I saw at once how useless it was, how gratuitously useless, to carry out for myself any mental multiplication of large numbers. Almost automatically I cut down my faculty in that direction, though I still kept up squaring and reciprocating and square-rooting, which have a more algebraic basis and a statistical use. But I am convinced that my ability deteriorated after that first encounter (pp. 302–303).

There is something that I believe might reasonably be identified as "calculating intelligence": the ability to discover novel methods of calculation suitable to the limitations of the human mind, or to adapt mathematical discoveries for similar purposes. This can take particularly creative forms when one has a variety of methods at one's command and adopts the most apt method, or combination of methods, for a given situation. In this sense calculating intelligence is similar to that exercised by an expert programmer.

Calculating prodigies exist at all intelligence levels, and, contrary to popular belief, most are not idiot savants but intelligent people with varied interests. But the brilliant and retarded do appear overrepresented in the ranks of calculating prodigies. In part, this reflects the nature of our sample. For the most part calculating prodigies fall into three groups: brilliant mathematicians, professional performers, and the mentally retarded.

Brilliant mathematicians leave behind a lot of writings and are often the subjects of biographies. Professional performers are written up in the popular press. The mentally retarded often end up in institutions, where they come to the attention of psychologists, who then describe them in journals.

Still, many people come to public attention, and apart from a few mathematicians, hardly any of them are calculating prodigies. (Richard Whately, Archbishop of Dublin from 1831 to 1863, was one, but he lost his ability for calculation when he entered grammar school.) And it also seems likely that calculating prodigies occur more frequently among the retarded than they do in the general population.

In TGMC I suggest the following:

> There is a property, shared by those at either end of the mental spectrum, which would account for such an unequal distribution—a tolerance for what ordinary folk find intolerably dull. This is a common characteristic of the retarded, who often specialize in memorizing great quantities of data on some subject or other. . . People on either end of the intelligence scale seem to be less limited in what they may find interesting. Perhaps this is because they are already regarded as so peculiar that peer support for their interests is not required, or perhaps it is because the brilliant and retarded are not required to shoulder the responsibility of nurturing and transmitting popular culture (Smith, 1983, pp. 81–82).

Cerebral Dominance

As is well known, in right-handed people and in most left-handers the left hemisphere of the brain is dominant for language, and the right hemisphere, for spatial functions. In about a third of left-handers, this situation is reversed. According to the thesis developed in TGMC, the calculating ability of prodigies, at least in the case of auditory ones, should be a left-hemisphere function.

That the calculations have a verbal component—virtually all auditory prodigies do some kind of talking while calculating—provides presumptive evidence for this view, but it is not conclusive. The language of calculation is limited and odd, and the right hemisphere has some language capability, particularly involuntary oaths (when Wim Klein, who was Dutch, ran into difficulty while calculating, his muttering was liberally sprinkled with *Gott ver dammer*), so that it is conceivable that such calculation is a right-hemisphere process. In any case, there is a pressing need for studies of both auditory and other calculating prodigies to determine in which hemisphere they compute.

As far as I know, only two attempts have been made to determine the hemisphere in which prodigies calculate. At my instigation, Shyam Marathe, a visual calculator, agreed to EEG testing. On October 30, 1978, in the Department of Neurosciences of the School of Medicine at the University of California, San Diego, an EEG was taken under the general direction of Dr. R. G. Bickford; Dr. D. F. Scott conducted the actual testing. Unfortunately, apart from showing that Marathe did not suffer from a brain tumor, the tests were inconclusive, for a variety of reasons.

First, although Marathe is seemingly right-handed, he uses his left hand for some things, such as cutting with scissors or combing his hair. Furthermore, there is a cultural prohibition in India against the use of the left hand for eating, and writing with the left hand would probably have been discouraged in Marathe's generation. This leads to the possibility that he may actually be left-handed and, like some one-third of all left-handers, dominant for speech in the right hemisphere.

The EEG does, in fact, suggest just this. Dr. Scott, in a letter to me, pointed out:

> The alpha activity, the brain waves characteristic of the alert adult with eyes closed, appears a bit more prominently over the posterior part of the left hemisphere than the right. This is the reverse of what is seen in the right-handed individual and suggests that the subject is left-handed, and his right hemisphere dominant for speech. During all tasks including the calculations, etc., the alpha activity virtually disappears. Of great interest is the observation that when the subject is giving the answers to number problems, the alpha activity reappears over the left hemisphere. When the answer is complete, and the subject is told it is correct, the alpha activity returns to its resting state over the right hemisphere. This would again imply that the subject's right hemisphere is dominant for speech (personal communication, D. F. Scott, November 9, 1978).

The uncertainty over which hemisphere is dominant for speech might have presented a serious problem in interpretation had it been possible to determine in which hemisphere Marathe calculates, but this could not be done.

Marathe was given two tasks typical of left- and right-hemisphere mental activities, respectively, to serve as a baseline for evaluating calculations. The first was the repetition of certain rhymes tapped out with a pencil, and the second involved repeating some sentences in English. But as Dr. Scott remarked: "The sentences would generally be a left-hemisphere task in most individuals, and the tapping task, a right-hemisphere one. In the present subject one could not conclude which hemisphere was in action during these tasks as there was no differential blocking of alpha activity." The same difficulty existed in the case of the calculations.

Marathe finds it necessary to calculate with his eyes open in order to "see" the numbers. Keeping the eyes open during an EEG also tends to eradicate the differential blocking of alpha activity.

Burling, Sappington, and Mead (1983) report on "a 24-year-old, moderately retarded and clearly right-handed male" who "was capable of identifying the correct day of the week for any given date into the remote past or future" (p. 326). The investigators attempted to determine, through observations of lateral eye movement, the degree of hemispheric specialization for the calendar and other tasks. They found that "the results indicate strongest left hemisphere specialization for the perpetual calendar task, moderate left hemisphere specialization for the mathematical questions, and no specialization for the musical and spatial questions. Such findings extend previous research documenting a relationship between ability and the degree of lateralization (p. 327).

Compulsive Practice

Calculating prodigies certainly practice a lot, particularly when they are acquiring the skill. Whether this practice qualifies as "compulsive" (a term with some pejorative connotations) depends partly on one's point of view. Does a child who is learning to speak practice speech "compulsively?" I suspect that a child who does not is in serious difficulty.

The following comment by Aitken, however, suggests some compulsiveness in the matter of factoring numbers:

> If I go for a walk and if a motor car passes and it has the registration number 731, I cannot but observe that is 17 times 43. But as far as possible, I shut that off because it interferes with thought about other matters. And after one or two numbers like that have been factorized, I am conditioned against it for the rest of my walk (Hunter, 1962, p. 247).

He further remarked that he sometimes squared numbers he happened to see: "This isn't deliberate, I just can't help it" (p. 247).

Birth Order

The birth order of calculating prodigies is often hard to come by. Sometimes it can be determined in part through comments about other matters. For example, we know that Bidder was taught to count by his oldest brother, meaning, presumably, that he had at least two older brothers. We also know that he sent two younger brothers through college, but this is all we know. He may have had five other brothers and seven sisters. (No doubt this information is available somewhere, but I will leave it to others to compile.) Here, briefly, is what I know. Of the nine calculators for whom I have data, four were the oldest children: Aitken (oldest of seven), Griffith (oldest of six), Arthur Benjamin (older of two), and von Neumann (eldest of three boys). Then we have Colburn (fifth of seven), Bidder (at least two older and two younger brothers), Mondeux (two older brothers and two yet older half brothers), Inaudi (a number of brothers, at least one of whom was older), and Gauss (second of three sons). Diamandi had 14 brothers and sisters, but where he ranked among them I don't know.

Supernumerary Digits

It is a bizarre fact that two calculating prodigies had six fingers on each hand: Zerah Colburn (who also had six toes on each foot) and Arumogam. Colburn was a 19th-century Vermont farm boy who traveled about the British Isles as a natural phenomenon. Arumogam performed as a lad in Ceylon in the early part of this century.

There are various possible explanations for this strange fact: that Colburn and Arumogam were related, that people with six fingers are genetically predisposed toward mental calculations (though this did not befall any of Colburn's six-fingered relations), or that having six fingers provokes one to ponder counting and the nature of the decimal number system (Colburn did calculate in decimal). Sheer coincidence is perhaps the most likely answer.[2]

Handedness

Nothing is known regarding the handedness of calculators in the past, but two contemporary calculators, Wim Klein and Shyam Marathe, seem to have been left-handed originally and then were switched to the right hand. Marathe's case is not so clear (see Cerebral Dominance section), but Klein remarked when he saw me writing with my left hand, "That was my idea also, but they wouldn't let me do it."

When I tried to determine what other things Klein did with his left hand, I had a difficult time. I asked him with which hand he would throw a ball, or with which foot he would kick one. He was completely nonplussed.

I did establish, however, that Klein fillips peanuts in restaurants with his left hand.

Second-Language Ability

There are many reasons for acquiring a second language, such as living in a foreign country, societal and familial expectations, or the need for certain information that is otherwise unavailable. Though these are relevant considerations in the case of calculating prdigies, it is nevertheless striking how often they display extraordinary second-language abilities.

Leonhard Euler, the great Swiss mathematician and calculating prodigy, studied Greek and Hebrew with an eye to entering the church. He later published in Latin, German, French, and Russian.

---

2. Loraine Obler has pointed out to me in correspondence that Norman Geshwind and Albert Galaburda proposed in lectures "that the same fetal hormonal levels which result in unusual hemispheric organization for reading as in dyslexia and for mathematical abilities, also interact differentially with developing bodily organs, and results in skeletal abnormalities ranging from scoliosis to an extra digit." I remain skeptical.

Karl Friedrich Gauss, possibly the greatest mathematician in history, was also a calculating prodigy. When he first went to the university, he considered a career in philogy. Eric Temple Bell (1956) wrote of him:

> The facility with which he mastered languages in his youth stayed with Gauss all his life. Languages were rather more to him than a hobby. To test the plasticity of his mind as he grew older he would deliberately acquire a new language. The exercise, he believed, helped to keep his mind young. At the age of sixty two he began an intensive study of Russian without assistance from anyone. Within two years he was reading Russian prose and poetical works fluently, and carrying on his correspondence with scientific friends in St. Petersburg wholly in Russian. In the opinion of Russians who visited him in Göttingen he also spoke the language perfectly (p. 329).

That Gauss's spoken Russian was perfect is no doubt untrue, but what Russian mathematician visiting Gauss in Göttingen was likely to say otherwise?

Zerah Colburn's obituary notes that he was "Professor of the Latin, Greek, French, and Spanish Languages, and English Classical Literature." He also penned an eloquent autobiography (Colburn, 1833).

Pericles Diamandi spoke five languages: Greek, Rumanian, French, German, and English.

Alexander Craig Aitken took first-class honors in Latin and French and taught languages at Otago Boys' High School in New Zealand before becoming a mathematician. He maintained an intense interest in literature and could recite long passages from Milton and Virgil.

Wim Klein spoke fluent Dutch, English, French, and German (but that's not so uncommon for a Dutchman).

Hans Eberstark is a simultaneous translator and speaks some 15 languages with varying degrees of fluency.

John von Neumann, one of the outstanding mathematicians of the 20th century, was described in the following terms by S. Ulan (1958): "Among other accomplishments, Johnny was an excellent linguist. He remembered his school Latin and Greek remarkably well. In addition to English, he spoke German and French fluently. His lectures in this country were well known for their literary quality" (p. 6).

Shakuntala Devi and Shyam Marathe, native speakers of Hindi, both speak English extremely well.

Mathematical Ability

The term "mathematics" means different things to different people. To a grammar school child, mathematics is solving problems using arithmetic; to a high school student or college undergraduate, mathematics is solving problems using geometry, algebra, logarithms, calculus, and other forms of "higher math." (Proofs are typically regarded as a particularly onerous form of problem solving.) To a mathematician, mathematics is proving theorems (general mathematical truths) from axioms and previously discovered theorems. (It has been said that a mathematician is a machine for turning coffee into theorems.) Whether or not a given prodigy can be said to be good at mathematics depends on how that term is construed.

Calculating prodigies, with a few exceptions (such as some retarded calculators who do only calendar calculations), are good at arithmetic. Even quite unsophisticated calculators can solve, by trial and error, problems that appear to require elaborate application of algebra when the answer can be assumed to be an integer.

The interest of a great many calculators, however, was pretty much limited to integer arithmetic, and some, like Buxton, never advanced even to the level of using decimal fractions (they simply announced a remainder, if any), much less to a comprehension of any "higher" mathematics.

There does appear to be an antipathy on the part of most auditory calculators (except those who became mathematicians) for geometry.

Then there are those who are able to use at least some aspects of "higher" mathematics in their calculations. In fact, Zacharias Dase computed pi to 205 places (of which the first 200 were correct) and computed tables of logarithms and factors. In spite of this, Schumacher (Gauss & Schumacher, 1861) wrote to Gauss on April 7, 1847, that Dase "cannot comprehend the first elements of mathematics . . . but his ability for numerical reckoning now astounds everyone" (p. 295).

There have been cases of child prodigies in mathematics, just as in music. Paul Erdös (1970) wrote a paper on child mathematicians he had known (who in no way should be confused with calculating prodigies). Of one he wrote:

> I will start to talk about Posa who is now 22 years old and the author of about eight papers. I met him before he was twelve years old. When I returned from the United States [to Hungary] in the summer of 1959 I was told that there is a little boy whose mother is a mathematician and who knows all that there is to be known in high school. I was very interested and next day I had lunch with him. . . . While we had lunch and Posa was eating his soup I told him the following problem. Prove that if you have $n + 1$ integers less than or equal to $2n$ then there are always two of them which are relatively prime. It is quite easy to see that the theorem is not true for n integers because if you take the multiples of 2 there are n of them not exceeding $2n$ and no two of them are relatively prime. Actually I discovered this simple result some years ago but it took me about ten minutes until I found the very simple proof. Posa ate his soup, and then said, "If you have $n + 1$ integers less than or equal to $2n$ two of them are consecutive and therefore they are relatively prime." It was needless to see [sic] that I was very much impressed. . . . Our first joint paper was written when he was fourteen and one half years old. . . . Posa wrote many significant papers also by himself. Some of which still have a great deal of effect. His best known and most quoted paper is on Hamiltonian lines and he wrote it when he was fifteen. Unfortunately since about 4 or 5 years he has not proved and conjectured much and I often comment sadly that he is dead, but I very much hope that he will come back to Life soon. I got first worried about him when he told me when he was 16 that he rather would be Dostojewsky [Dostoevski] than Einstein (Erdös 1970, pp. 3–6).

I think it is evident that this sort of thing has nothing to do with computing, say, the number of vetches required to fill a cubical bin a mile on each side (as did Buxton). But there is one area of mental calculation that bears some relationship to true mathematics—the discovery of general relationships between numbers, which relates to the theory of numbers. Henri Mondeux, for example, discovered that every odd natural number is the difference between the squares of two successive natural numbers. This may be trivial, but it does involve mathematical insight. True mathematics begins when one finds proofs for mathematical facts, a step Mondeux could never have taken.

Further Research

Very little research has been done on calculating prodigies. There are various reasons for this, but the most obvious is that subjects are so hard to come by. One has to find calculating prodigies (no easy task), pay transportation costs, and possibly pay them substantial sums of money to make up for lost earnings. Furthermore, they may have a lot of ego invested in mental calculation and not wish to be compared with their peers. There is also a tendency to regard calculating prodigies in the category of charlatans, suitable only for the *National Enquirer*.

But the very rarity of calculating prodigies makes research on them all the more critical. We cannot today go back and do studies on Buxton, Colburn, Bidder, Mondeux, Dase, Klein and so forth. I hope in the future it will not be said that we missed our opportunity to study contemporary prodigies.

Unanswered questions about calculating prodigies are legion. A high-priority item would be the experimental determination of lateralization of calculation (and other tasks) for both auditory and visual calculators. All sorts of tests can and should be done on calculating and memory load for various operations. We should reconstruct mental processes for various computations and try to determine which parts of the processes are unconscious (or perhaps semiconscious). Even in the case of entirely unconscious processes there may be ways of figuring out what is going on. We should also try to determine to what extent mental calculation is learnable by ordinary children and adults who are motivated by such mundane considerations as money.

Conclusions

In TGMC I argue that the rarity of calculating prodigies can be accounted for by opportunity and inclination. By "inclination" I had in mind some personality traits, innate and/or acquired, that would lead a child to pursue mental calculation, an activity for which there is little peer interest or support. I suggested that "if mental calculation were even as popular as, say, surfing, we would have calculating prodigies in abundance" (Smith, 1983, p. 5).

My claim is thus that every child has the capacity to become a calculating prodigy, but that few children have the motivation. We are not surrounded by people doing mental calculation as we are by people speaking; therefore only a peculiar and highly motivated child is likely to practice such calculation.

Although genetic factors certainly contribute to an individual's interests, it is clearly no simple matter. What impels one child to astronomy, another to tightwire walking, and a third to the study of Bulgarian? What accounts for the fact that one of America's top rodeo cowboys is Bobby Del Vecchio from the Bronx? Some combination of environment and genetics, no doubt, but the way in which these ingredients are mixed to produce a butcher, a surfer, or a calculating prodigy surpasses my understanding.

Some critics of the book took issue with me on this point. For instance, John Cohen (1983) wrote:

> Smith's original contribution lies in his theory . . . that the superiority of his prodigies is to be sought in their being able to tap "some of the same unconscious capacity that underlies speech." . . . This thesis carries the corollary that any speaking child is a latent calculating prodigy. But surely, if so, one might just as well say that any child that can chant *Sing a Song of Sixpence* is a potential Mozart (p. 819).

Though Cohen's comment almost caused me to fall off my chair laughing, it belies a serious misconception. The ability of some children to do complex mental calculation is not remotely comparable to Mozart's juvenile musical genius.

That a talent can be acquired by any child does not mean that it is trivial or that there are not differing levels of skill involved. Any child can learn English, an astonishingly complex matter—but few of us learn English in such a way as to become masters of English prose or poetry. In fact, few even learn to be outstanding tellers of jokes or stories. When I say that anyone can become a calculating prodigy, I do not mean that we might all become Aitkens or Kleins any more than I mean that, because we are all capable of learning English, we might all become Brontës. Any child is capable of learning to play "The Moonlight Sonata," but not all are capable of learning to play it in such a way as to attract a willing audience.

I have remarked on certain neurological peculiarities of auditory calculators. But neurology has environmental consequences. First, it affects the way people treat us. This is immediately evident to (almost) everyone in the case of race, sex, age, and certain physical handicaps, but it is also true of hyperactivity, myopia, epilepsy, height, amount of body fat, shape of nose, and so forth. So we must consider the possibility that people with neurological peculiarities characteristic of auditory prodigies may be treated differently, in a way that sometimes promotes an interest in numbers.

Second, our neurobiological make-up not only affects the way people treat us, it is an unavoidable part of our environment. If a person's legs are deformed for genetic reasons, and if that person develops exceptional upper-body strength, we are not inclined to regard this as an example of genetic predilection. For one thing, we can see some plausible causal connection, for another, we know that people whose legs are deformed for reasons that are not genetic are also inclined to develop unusual upper-body strength. So we must also consider whether the traits common to auditory calculators might be such as to encourage them to find solace in numbers.

I think both internal and external neuro–environmental factors play a role in determining who will become a calculating prodigy.

Consider the personality of a typical auditory calculator: nervous; verbal; likes to be the center of attention; has nervous "twitches" (sometimes even epilepsy) which may put people off; may be inclined toward violence directed at himself or herself or at others.

What do we do with such children? Give them something to do that isn't likely to be dangerous or annoying to the neighbors. Tell them to go count how much wood is in the woodpile and get back to you. For example, Bryan and Lindley (1941) wrote that Griffith's mother "would give him sticks, pebbles, potatoes, and the like to count, in order to keep him still" (p. 28).

And if their tempers are about to blow and they are ready to smash something? Tell them to count to 10, and if that doesn't work to 100, and if that doesn't work to 1,000.

But calculation itself is likely to prove much more interesting. It is no accident that calculating prodigies regard multiplication as the central operation. It is only through multiplication and allied operations that the properties of numbers that make them so endlessly fascinating are uncovered. A highly nervous, isolated child who likes to be the center of attention is badly in need of friends, and calculating prodigies are clear on this point—numbers are their friends.

We may be inclined to treat this as merely a metaphor for familiarity with figures, but I think wrongly. For calculating prodigies, numbers really are their friends.

Why numbers? They are always there, day or night. And they have characteristics, even characters, of their own, which can be discovered. Bidder (1856) said of learning to count to 100: "It made me familiar with the numbers up to 100; they became as it were my friends, and I knew all their relations and acquaintances" (p. 258). Wim Klein said: "Numbers are friends for me, more or less. It doesn't mean the same for you, does it, 3,844? For you it's just a three and an eight and a four and a four. But I say, 'Hi, 62 squared.'"

And, like people, some numbers are fascinating, some dull, and others perhaps downright unpleasant. For instance, Salo Finkelstein thought that 214 was a "beautiful" number and that 8,337 was "very nice," but zero was his "pet aversion" (Weinland, 1948, pp. 253–254).

Hans Eberstark remarked:

> I wouldn't go as far as some of my fellow calculators and indiscriminately welcome all numbers with open arms: not the horny-handed, rough-and-tough bully 8 or the sinister 64 or the arrogant, smug, self-satisfied 36. But I do admit to a very personal affection for the ingenious, adventurous 26, the magic, versatile 7, the helpful 37, the fatherly, reliable (if somewhat stodgy) 76 (Smith, 1983, pp. xii–xiii).

Aitken made the amazing (to me) observation: "Sometimes a number has almost no properties at all, like 811, and sometimes a number, like 41, is deeply involved in many theorems that you know." It is a most unusual mathematician who would know a number of theorems in which the 41 is deeply involved.

And numbers are reliable, absolutely consistent. You can depend on them. As Hans Eberstark says: "Life in this irrational world is chaotic, confusing, unfair.

The response to love is contempt; backbreaking efforts go unrewarded; results seem to bear little relation to input. In the world of numbers all comes out right in the end. Figures never fail you" (Smith, 1983, p. xiii). What more could one ask of a friend?

References

Aitken, A. C. (1954). The art of mental calculation: With demonstrations. *Transactions of the Society of Engineers, 44,* 295–309.

Beatty, J. (1943, August). Baby miracle. *American Magazine,* pp. 140–142.

Bell, E. T. (1956). *The prince of mathematicians. The world of mathematics.* New York: Simon & Schuster.

Bidder, G. P. (1856). On mental calculation. *Minutes of Proceedings, Institution of Civil Engineers (1855–56), 15,* 251–280.

Binet, A. (1894). *Psychologie des grands calculateurs et joueurs d'échécs.* Paris: Hachette.

Bousfield, W. A., & Barry, H. (1933). The visual imagery of a lightning calculator. *American Journal of Psychology, 45,* 353–358.

Bryan, W. L. & Lindley, E. H. (1941). *On the psychology of learning a life occupation* (Science Series. No. 11). Bloomington: Indiana University Press.

Burling, T. A., Sappington, J. T., & Mead, A. M. (1983). Lateral specialization of a perpetual calendar task by a moderately mentally retarded adult. *American Journal of Mental Deficiency, 88,* 326–328.

Chambers's Edinburgh Journal. (1847, July–December). Truman Henry Safford, *8,* 265–267.

Cohen, J. (1983, December 15). What makes a calculating prodigy? *New Scientist,* 819.

Colburn, Z. (1833). *A memoir of Zerah Colburn: Written by himself.* Springfield, MA: G. & C. Merriam.

Columbian Centinel (1790, December). Obituary of Thomas Fuller (no title). Vol *14.*

Dudgeon, H. W., & Hurst, H. E. (1934). An arithmetical prodigy in Egypt. *Nature, 133,* 578–579.

Erdös, P. (1970, November). *Child prodigies.* Paper presented at the Third CSMP International Conference of the Teaching of Algebra at the Pre-college Level, Co-sponsored by Southern Illinois University at Carbondale & Central Midwestern Regional Educational Laboratory.

Gauss, K. F., & Schumacher, H. C. (1861). *Briefwechsel zwischen Gauss und Schumacher.* Altona, Germany.

Hamblin, D. J. (1966, March 18). They are "idiot savants"—Wizards of the calendar. *Life,* pp. 106–108.

Holliday, T. (1751). Account of Jedediah Buxton. *Gentlemen's Magazine, 21,* 347–349.

Horwitz, W. A., Kestenbaum, C., Person, E., & Jarvik, L. (1965). Identical twins—"Idiot savants"—Calendar calculators. *American Journal of Psychiatry, 121,* 1075–1079.

Hunter, I. M. L. (1962). An exceptional talent for calculative thinking. *British Journal of Psychology, 53,* 243–258.

Hunter, I. M. L. (1968). Mental calculation. In P. C. Wason & P. N. Johnson-Laird (Eds.), *Thinking and reasoning* (pp. 341–351). Middlesex, England: Penguin Books.

Jacoby, E. (n.d.) *Biographie de Henri Mondeux.* Paris: Charpentier.

Jakobsson. S. (1944). Report on two prodigy mental arithmeticians. *Acta Medica Scandinavica, 119,* 180–191.

Lewis, K. R., & Plotkin, H. (1982, September–October). Truman Henry Safford, the remarkable "lightning calculator". *Harvard Magazine,* pp. 54–56.

The life of Jedediah Buxton. (1754). *Gentlemen's Magazine, 24,* 251–252.

MacNeven. (1811). An account of Zerah Colburn, the wonderful calculator. *The New York Medical and Philosophical Journal.* New York: T. & J. Swords, *3,* pp. 19–23.

Mitchell, F. D. (1907). Mathematical prodigies. *American Journal of Psychology, 18,* 61–143.

Obler, L. (1985). [Review of *The great mental calculators*]. *Language, 61,* 510–511.

Prime, S. I. (1875). *Life of S. B. Morse.* New York: Appleton.

Rush, B. (1789). Account of a wonderful talent for arithmetical calculation in an African slave, living in Virginia. *American Museum, 5,* 62–63.

Rush, B. (1812) *Medical inquiries and observations upon the diseases of the mind.* Philadelphia: Kimber & Richardson.

Smith, S. B. (1983). *The great mental calculators: The psychology, methods, and lives of calculating prodigies, past and present.* New York: Columbia University Press.

Stokvis, B. (1949). A medico-psychological account, followed by a demonstration of a case of supernormal aptitude. In I. C. van Houte & B. Stokvis (Eds.), *Proceedings of the Second International Congress on Orthopedagogics.* (pp 79–89). Amsterdam: Systemen Keesing.

Tocquet, R. (1957.) *The magic of numbers* (D. Weaver, Trans.). New York: A. S. Barnes.

Ulam, S. (1958). John von Neumann 1903-1957. *Bulletin of the American Mathematical Society. 64*(3), 1–49.

Weinland, J. D. (1948). Memory of Salo Finkelstein. *Journal of General Psychology, 39,* 243–257.

Wizel, A. (1904). Ein Fall von phänomenalen Rechentalent bei einem Imbecillen. *Archiv fur Psychiatrie und Nervenkrankheiten, 38:*122–155.

3

Neuropsychological Perspectives on Mathematical Talent

CAMILLA PERSSON BENBOW

An overwhelming majority of events that have been described by Kuhn (1962) as "scientific revolutions" can be ascribed to the work of mathematicians or mathematically brilliant men (Cohn, 1980). Moreover, Krutetskii (1976) stated that

> The increased development of mathematics is necessary for the progress and effectiveness of a whole series of major fields of knowledge.... [T]he development of the sciences has been characterized recently by a tendency for them to become more mathematical, and this applies not only to physics, astronomy, and chemistry but also to such sciences as modern biology, archaeology, medicine, meteorology, economics, planning, linguistics, and others. Mathematical methods and the mathematical style of thinking are penetrating everywhere. It is hard to find a field of knowledge to which mathematics would not be related. With each year mathematics will find broader applications in various fields of endeavor. In principle, the realm of applications of mathematics is unlimited (p. 6).

Because mathematics is of such import, gaining a clearer understanding of the concept of mathematical talent is of real significance. Yet very little work has been done in this area. The intent of this chapter is to provide a review of the nature and associated characteristics of mathematical talent. The main thrust of the chapter will be to explore those studies relating to the neuropsychology of mathematical talent.

Definitions of Mathematical Talent

Werderlin (1958) characterized mathematical talent as the "ability to understand the nature of mathematical (and similar) problems, symbols, methods, and proofs; to learn them, to retain them in memory and to reproduce them; to combine them with other problems, symbols, methods, and proofs; and to use them when solving mathematical (and similar) tasks" (p. 13).

Camilla Persson Benbow. SMPY, Iowa State University, Ames, Iowa.

According to Davis (1983), complex mathematical cognition involves thoughtfulness, the rethinking of old assumptions, intelligent guessing, insight, and shrewd planning. A crucial aspect is intuition.

Gardner (1983) postulates the existence of seven kinds of intelligences, one of which is logical–mathematical intelligence. He views mathematical talent as "the ability to handle skillfully long chains of reasoning" (p. 139). Moreover, mathematical talent "requires the ability to discover a promising idea and then to draw out its implications" or "the ability to recognize significant problems and then solve them" (p. 143). Other components of mathematical talent are the ability to discover relationships among analogies and the making of patterns using ideas.

One of the major works defining mathematical talent is *The Psychology of Mathematical Abilities in School Children* (Krutetskii, 1976). Through a qualitative analysis of the processes that students used to solve various experimental problems that were new to them, Krutetskii formulated the following components of mathematical talent: formulized perception of mathematical material; logical thinking in mathematical spheres, including thinking in symbols; rapid and broad generalization ability, curtailment of reasoning and thinking; reversibility of mathematical thinking; striving for economy; flexibility of thinking; and generalized mathematical memory. In addition, Krutetskii also identified a mathematical cast of mind, which was a tendency to see the world through mathematical eyes. Speed of mental processing, computational ability, spatial ability, the ability to visualize abstract mathematical relationships, and memory for symbols, numbers, and formulae were not viewed as being important. Thus, Krutetskii believed that mathematical talent is defined by qualitatively different psychological processes, as shown in Table 3-1.

The Study of Mathematically Precocious Youth (SMPY), now located at Johns Hopkins University, and Iowa State University, was founded by Dr. Julian C. Stanley in 1971 with the express purpose of identifying mathematically talented seventh graders in order to provide some much needed educational intervention (Stanley, 1977). Its methods and procedures have become widely replicated nationally and internationally. Even though it is one of the largest studies dealing with mathematically talented students, it has not concerned itself much with conceptualizing mathematical talent. Because there are many children who are clearly talented mathematically and who need educational assistance, SMPY has concentrated its efforts instead on devising novel educational alternatives for them. The chief aim of SMPY is not to help youths learn to think like mathematicians but to help them acquire early and well the mathematical tools that scientists need.

The indicator of mathematical talent used by SMPY is simply a high score at an early age on the mathematics section of the College Board's Scholastic Aptitude Test (SAT-M). Although narrow, this indicator is simple and objective. Moreover, few would argue that such an ability does not indicate a high level of cognitive functioning.

What does such a high score on SAT-M mean? The SAT-M was designed for above-average high school students to measure their mathematical reasoning ability (Donlon & Angoff, 1971). It has been used by SMPY, however, to test seventh graders (who are approximately 4 to 5 years younger) who have already scored in

TABLE 3-1.   Comparison of Selected Cognitive Characteristics of Mathematically
Gifted and Nongifted Students

Gifted students	Nongifted students
Perceive mathematical material in a problem analytically and synthetically	Perceive mathematical material in a problem only as disconnected data and have difficulty synthesizing data
Generalize quickly and broadly both the content of a problem and the method of solution	Acquire generalizations slowly
Curtail processes for solving similar problems with relatively little exposure to them	Curtail processes for solving similar problems only after repeated exposure
Switch easily from one cognitive process to another	Have inflexible thinking
Do not depend on conventional solution techniques	Are hindered by previous solution techniques
Strive for elegant solutions	Are satisfied with any solution
Reverse reasoning processes easily	Experience great difficulty in working backwards or backtracking
Thoroughly investigate aspects of difficult problems before directly attempting to solve them	Are goal-directed
Remember generalized and curtailed structures associated with problems and their solutions	Remember contextual details of problems instead of structural features
Tire both mentally and physically less readily during mathematical activity than during other kinds of lessons	Have a tendency to tire easily if a problem is difficult or involves a large number of steps to solve
View the world mathematically	Have no apparent tendency to mathematize everyday experiences

Note. This summary is based on Lester and Schroeder (1983).

the top 3% on standardized mathematics achievement tests. Few of the SMPY students had received formal opportunities to develop their abilities in algebra and beyond (Benbow & Stanley, 1982a, 1982b, 1983). For example, it was found that, among the top 10% of the SMPY students (i.e., those eligible for fast-paced summer programs in mathematics), a majority did not know even first-year algebra well. Thus they began their mathematics studies with Algebra I.

Yet, although demonstrably unfamiliar with mathematics from algebra onward, many of them were able to score highly on a difficult test of mathematical reasoning ability. Presumably, this could occur only by the use of extraordinary ability at the "analysis" level of Bloom's (1956) taxonomy. Thus it was concluded that the SAT-M functions far more at an analytical reasoning level for talented seventh graders than it does for high school juniors and seniors (Benbow & Stanley, 1981, 1983). We (Minor & Benbow, 1986) have found support for this contention in a study contrasting the factorial structure of the SAT-M of high school students with that of gifted seventh graders. Pollins (1984), using a different methodological paradigm, also came to the conclusion that the SAT-M was a test of mathematical reasoning ability for young, talented students. Based on this evidence, SMPY has defined mathematical talent as a high level of mathematical reasoning ability manifested at an early age. Such a definition does not imply that most young high scorers on the SAT-M become mathematicians. Instead, many such students will be ideally suited for careers in the physical or biological sciences, computer science, medicine, law, economics, and so forth.

Lester and Schroeder (1983) feel that the position taken by such programs as SMPY falls short of the mark regarding the ways used to identify talented students. They claim that standardized tests include conventional, routine problems that require convergent thinking. Such an approach also does not provide any information about how the student thinks, the authors claim. Clearly, the use of the SAT-M at an age much earlier than the conventional age with students who have not been taught the content of the test cannot be subject to the first criticism. Moreover, the SMPY approach has shown that mathematically talented students think like older, less talented students. They are precocious. For example, it is not unusual for a mathematically talented student to have entered Piaget's stage of formal operations by grade five (Keating, 1975; Keating & Schaefer, 1975). This is much earlier than is typical. Nonetheless, investigations in this area are in progress.

In conclusion, the definitions of mathematical talent surveyed here are quite diverse, and few similarities can be found among them. Yet all of them seem to deal with higher level cognitive processes that require reasoning ability. Computational ability is not of much direct concern. Thus Gardner's (1983) position that mathematical talent involves the ability to handle long chains of reasoning may best represent the consensus.

Development of Mathematical Talent

Not much research has been done on how mathematical talent develops. Even Krutetskii, whose explicit aim was to study the development of mathematical talent, did not provide such information. He tended to focus on conceptualizing the learning strategies utilized by mathematically talented students. The focus of SMPY is to study what the consequences are of being mathematically talented, using a longitudinal design similar to that of Terman's classic study of children with IQ's of at least 135 (Burkes, Jensen, & Terman, 1947; Oden, 1968; Sears, 1977; Sears & Barbee, 1977; Terman, 1925; Terman & Oden, 1947, 1959). Thus SMPY does not know how its students became mathematically talented, although several retrospective studies have provided some suggestions (e.g., Benhow, 1986b; Fox, Brody, & Tobin 1982; Raymond & Benbow, 1986).

Gardner (1983) stated, however, that logical–mathematical intelligence develops through a confrontation with the world of objects, as postulated by Piaget.

The roots of the highest regions of logical, mathematical, and scientific thought, he believes, can be found in the simple actions of young children upon the physical objects in their worlds. In handling objects, ordering them, and assessing their quantity, the initial and most fundamental knowledge is gained. Logical–mathematical intelligence, however, soon becomes remote from the world of objects. The child becomes more capable of appreciating the actions that one can perform upon objects, the relations among those actions, statements about possible actions, and their interrelationships. Children proceed from objects to statements, from actions to relations among actions, from the stage of sensorimotor to pure abstraction.

In contrast to Piaget's notion of the self-directed equilibration of logical thought in the course of development, there is Vygotsky's (1962, 1978) historical–cultural determinism. Saxe and Posner (1983), when contrasting these points of view, stated that Piaget and Vygotsky were both partially correct in describing the development of mathematical thinking. They concluded that, although economic and cultural forces shape some aspects of mathematical cognition, individuals, regardless of cultural background, engage in self-directed activities that develop their own concept of number and produce cognitive universals.

Riley, Greeno, and Heller (1983) studied the development of children's problem-solving ability in arithmetic word problems. They suggested that a child's conceptual knowledge of the relations between quantities in a word problem is related to the acquisition of more efficient counting procedures. Necessity and efficiency are two motivators for acquiring more advanced schemata. Moreover, procedural knowledge leads to the acquisition of schemata, and these schemata in turn are involved as intermediate steps in acquiring more advanced procedures. Of relevance to the development of mathematical talent, Riley, Greeno, and Heller (1983) state that children who are more skilled have acquired schemata that act as principles for organizing the information in a problem and that override distracting, irrelevant factors.

Moreover, Krutetskii (1976) stated:

> In all cases we studied, the development of abilities in mathematics began with the formation of the initial component: the ability to generalize mathematical objects, relationships, and operations. The ability to curtail reasoning, the generalizing memory, and the striving for economy and rationality in solutions were formed at later stages. There is reason to believe that these components of mathematical abilities are formed on the basis of the initial ability to generalize mathematical material. But, of course, this question still requires special study (pp. 340–341).

In terms of mathematically talented students, the components seem to emerge at an earlier age. This is similar to the SMPY conception of mathematical precocity. As for the the nature–nuture question, Krutetskii's (1976) view is: "And to the sacramental question, 'Can anyone become a mathematician or must one be born one?' we would hypothetically give the following answer: 'Anyone can become an ordinary mathematician; one must be born an outstanding, talented mathematician'" (p. 361).

Bloom (1982) postulated that the family, selected teachers, and sometimes the peer group are important influences on the development of talent. Mathematics learning arises from the talented student's interaction with books and observation of others rather than from interaction with, or direct instruction by, teachers.

Brody (1984) studied the effects of course work on the development of precocious mathematical reasoning ability. She found that intensive course work in a short period of time in algebra and geometry had no effect on the mathematical reasoning ability of seventh graders, as measured by the SAT-M. Thus the development of precocious mathematical reasoning ability does not appear to depend upon the amount of formal instruction in mathematics received, which is consistent with the earlier hypothesis made by Benbow and Stanley (1980, 1981, 1982a, 1983). Brody & Benbow (1986) however, found that coursework and achievement over a long period of time do relate to score gains on the SAT-M.

In conclusion, there is not much information on how mathematical talent develops in a child. Some of the studies on the development of mathematical thinking in average children (e.g., Ginsburg, 1983) may be relevant, especially since it seems that a major difference between the mathematically talented and other students appears to be that the talented acquire skills and competencies at an earlier age (Robinson, 1983; Stanley, 1977; Stanley & Benbow, 1986). There are, of course, some cognitive characteristics that differentiate the talented and other students (see Table 3-1), but just the amount of mathematics instruction does not appear to be a relevant variable.

Abilities Correlating with Mathematical Talent

Almost all investigators of the nature of mathematical talent have concluded that computational ability is not related to mathematical talent (Krutetskii, 1976; Stanley, 1977; Stanley & Benbow, 1986). Of course, one must know how to compute, but rapid calculators are not necessarily considered mathematically talented.

Some investigators have proposed that spatial ability is related to mathematical aptitude (Harris, 1978; Maccoby & Jacklin, 1974; McGee, 1979; Sherman, 1967, 1977; Smith, 1964.) Sherman (1967), for example, postulated that sex differences in spatial ability can account for the sex differences found in mathematical reasoning ability (to be discussed later). Support for this hypothesis is somewhat mixed. Armstrong (1981) did not find that sex differences in mathematics achievement were related to sex differences in spatial ability. Moreover, Becker (1978) found that the three-way interaction of spatial ability, sex, and item performance on the SAT-M was not significant for the seventh graders in a SMPY mathematics talent search. Spatial ability was found, however, to be related to superior performance on the SAT-M as a whole. Sherman (1977), cited evidence that sex differences in mathematical ability could be attributed in part to sex differences in spatial ability. Burnett, Lane, and Dratt (1979) found that sex difference on SAT-M was no longer significant after controlling for spatial ability among a college sample. Finally, McGee (1979) concluded that "sex differences in various aspects of perceptual-cognitive functioning (e.g., mathematics and field independence) are secondary consequences of differences with respect to visualization and spatial orientation abilities" (p. 909).

In view of these results, the possibility that mathematical reasoning ability and spatial ability are related deserves serious consideration. This may be especially true for the mathematically talented. When the most mathematically precocious students identified by SMPY from 1972 to 1979 were retested (in 1979) with a battery of cognitive tests, a verbal and a spatial factor accounted for their performance (Benbow, Stanley, Zonderman & Kirk, 1983). Through such testing sessions, we have also found that mathematically talented students tend to score highly in nonverbal reasoning, verbal reasoning, mechanical comprehension, abstract reasoning, and spatial ability (Benbow, 1978; Benbow, Stanley, Zonderman & Kirk, 1983, Cohn, 1977, 1980, Pollins, 1984). Moreover, in contrast to high performance on the verbal section of the SAT (SAT-V) at an early age, precocious ability measured by the SAT-M does not necessarily predict overall high ability. That is, the SAT-M does not appear to be an especially strong measure of g (general intelligence). Moreover, Pollins (1984) found evidence to indicate that the distinction between those who score highly on SAT-V and those who score high on SAT-M at an early age is one between students with a wealth of knowledge (SAT-V), perhaps the product of excellent learning skills, and students who reason extremely well (SAT-M).

Certain cognitive styles may also relate to mathematical talent. Field independence versus field dependence may be such a dimension. A field-independent cognitive style is characterized by an analytical approach to a situation that consists of the ability to overcome the influence of an embedding context while inferring the salient features. A field-dependent (or field-sensitive) cognitive style is a general approach that is highly influenced by the situational context (Witkin, Moore, Goodenough, & Cox, 1975). A field-independent person is more adept at situations requiring high analytical ability, such as mathematics (Vaidya & Chansky, 1980). These researchers found a positive relationship between a field-independent cognitive style and mathematics achievement among second- through fourth-grade children. Bien (1974) found, among fourth-grade students, similar findings with word problems but not with computation.

Krutetskii (1976) suggested a further dimension, according to which individuals can be divided on the basis of their style in processing information in mathematics. The first type of individual is the analytical type, who prefers the verbal-logical to the visual-pictorial modes. The second is the geometric type, who prefers the visual-pictorial to the verbal-logical mode. The third, the harmonic type, uses both modes freely. Webb (1979) and Moses (1977, 1980) found that visualizers obtained higher scores on a problem-solving inventory, whereas Lean and Clements (1981) found superior performance for those who utilize a verbal-logical mode.

The resolution of this apparent inconsistency may lie in the nature of the problem. Kosslyn and Jolicoeur (1980) postulated that speed and ease of retrieval from memory of an object's properties and associations determines whether an image is consulted when answering a question. For the case of mathematics, if the problem is routine and involves well-learned concepts, then a verbal-logical mode would be utilized. If the problem is unfamiliar, however, an image would be consulted. Interestingly, in the conflicting studies just cited concerning imagery and mathematics performance, the studies that employed unfamiliar mathematics problems revealed that the use of imagery was an important component in predicting performance. In contrast, when routine and familiar problems were used, a verbal-logical approach was superior.

Because the seventh-grade SMPY students who take the SAT have little formal training in algebra and beyond (Benbow & Stanley, 1982a, 1982b; 1983), and because course work was found not to relate to SAT performance at that age (Brody, 1984), the problems on the SAT-M are novel and appear to be measuring reasoning. We therefore hypothesized that students who score highly on the SAT-M at an early age and are thus mathematically talented use imagery.

Blum-Zorman (1984) investigated the cognitive style of mathematically precocious adolescents. She found two cognitive styles to be characteristic: (1) literal, systematic, microscopic orientation or (2) literal, systematic, telescopic orientation. These styles were found to be consistent with findings from research mathematicians. In contrast, students who were not mathematically precocious were found to be unsystematic and sometimes also projective in orientation. Blum-Zorman (1984) concluded that logicism and intuitionism may apply not only to adult mathematicians but also to mathematically precocious children.

Osborne (1981) listed the following factors as being associated with successful problem solving: an appreciation of uniqueness, existence, and universality; a tendency to see mathematics in the ordinary and commonplace; flexibility in considering alternative strategies; and the ability to recognize unproductive strategies quickly. Greenes (1981) extends this list by adding that mathematically talented children have excellent memory and high verbal and reasoning skills, and are very capable in spontaneously formulating problems, organizing data, interpreting problem information in original ways, transferring ideas to new contexts, and generalizing quickly.

Neuropsychological Parameters of Mathematical Talent

Sex Differences

One striking characteristic of the mathematically highly talented is that they are much more frequently male than female (Benbow & Stanley, 1980, 1981, 1982a, 1983, 1984). This find was based on the SMPY mathematics talent searches conducted in 1972, 1973, 1974, 1976, 1978, and 1979, which involved 9,927 mathematically able junior high school students between 12 and 14 years of age. Students attending schools in the Middle Atlantic States had been eligible to participate in a SMPY talent search if they had scored in the upper 5% (1972), 2% (1973 and 1974), or 3% (1976, 1978, and 1979) in mathematical ability based on national norms of a standardized achievement test administered in the regular testing program of the students' schools. Thus both male and female talent-search participants had been selected by equal criteria for high mathematical ability before entering the program. Girls constituted 43% of the participants in those searches.

As part of the talent search, these participants took the SAT-M and the SAT-V under standard conditions. Although there were no sex differences in verbal test scores, a large sex difference in mathematical reasoning ability was observed in every talent search (Benbow & Stanley, 1980). On the average, the boys scored about one-half of a standard deviation better than did the girls. There were also some indications that the sex difference was especially great at the upper ranges of mathematical reasoning ability.

These results were limited by the fact that only selected, mathematically able, highly motivated students were tested. Also, too few cases of extremely high scoring students were obtained to conclude whether greater differences existed at the high end of the scoring scale of the SAT-M.

These issues were addressed later, in a second series of studies. Benbow and Stanley (1983) presented findings from a broader sample of 40,000 intellectually talented students (i.e., the top 3% in mathematical, verbal, or overall ability on standardized, grade-appropriate, achievement tests) who had been tested in the seventh grade with the SAT through a Johns Hopkins talent search conducted by the Center for the Advancement of Academically Talented Youth. A national sample of individuals who scored extremely high on the SAT-M (i.e., ≥ 700 before age 13) was also studied. Although this time the sample contained students talented in verbal, mathematical, and overall ability, the mean sex difference on the SAT-M remained the same. This mean difference in SAT-M scores, however, was not considered the most important finding. Rather, the ratios of high-scoring boys to high-scoring girls were of major significance.

For example, the ratio of boys to girls scoring ≥ 500 on the SAT-M (495 was the SAT-M mean of 1983-84 college-bound 12th grade males) was 2.1. to 1, based on 5,325 cases; at ≥ 600 on the SAT-M (78th percentile of such 12th-grade males) the ratio was 4.1 to 1 for the 806 students scoring that high; and, finally, at ≥ 700 on the SAT-M (the 95th percentile of college-bound 12th-grade males) the ratio was 12.9 to 1 for the 278 reported cases (Benbow & Stanley, 1983). These high ratios of boys to girls were found even though equal numbers of boys and girls took the test, and even though the boys and girls had been matched on previous ability, age, grade, and talent-search entry. Moreover, in a subsequent set of studies, these sex differences in mathematical reasoning ability were found to persist over a number of years and to relate to later differences in mathematics and science achievement in high school and college (Benbow & Stanley, 1982a, 1984).

We can conclude, then, that there are many more mathematically talented boys than girls, especially at the higher levels. Similar differences have been found in an international study of achievement or aptitude (Kelly, 1978; Stanley, Huang & Zu, 1986). A series of studies on the SMPY population indicates that almost certainly these differences are not entirely the result of socialization or environmental factors (Benbow, 1986b, Benbow & Benbow, 1984; Benbow & Stanley, 1980, 1981, 1982a, b, 1984; Fox, Benbow, & Perkins, 1983; Fox, Brody, & Tobin, 1982; Raymond & Benbow, 1986). Some of the studies cited in the sections that follow support a hypothesis emphasizing biological as well as environmental factors.

Left-Handedness

An increased frequency of left-handedness has recently been noted among college mathematics students and teachers (Annett & Kilshaw, 1982). Moreover, Burnett, Lane, and Dratt (1982) found that in a college population the highest scores on a spatial ability measure were obtained by individuals who had left-handed relatives and whose handedness scores were in the range considered mixed or slightly right-handed. As a result of an article by Geschwind and Behan (1982), we independently began to investigate, along with some other physiological characteristics, the frequency of left-handedness among SMPY's most intellectually talented students. Preliminary findings were reported in Benbow and Benbow (1984), and final results in Benbow (1986).

We studied students who had scored at least 700 on the SAT-M or at least 630 on the SAT-V before the age of 13. These students represented the top 1 in 10,000 in their age group in the respective abilities. At the time of the investigation, the students were mostly between the ages of 12 and 15. The Edinburgh Handedness Inventory of Oldfield (1971) was mailed to the students and their parents. In addition to the parents' completing the inventory for themselves, they were requested to report on the handedness of their other children. Scores on the Oldfield inventory are designated as laterality quotients (LQ) and range from -100 (complete left-handedness) to $+100$ (complete right-handedness). In that study an individual with LQ < 0 was considered left-handed; ambidextrous individuals were not included in this range. Geschwind and Behan (1982) found that, in the general adult population they studied in Glasgow, 7.2% were left-handed by this criterion, a finding that is similar to the Oldfield (1971) results.

The frequency of left-handedness in SMPY's extremely precocious students was more than twice that of the general population figure of 7.2% (Benbow, 1986a). Both mathematically and verbally precocious students were more likely to be left-handed than less able students. Moreover, the frequency of left-handedness among our mathematically or verbally precocious students was higher than it was among their mothers, fathers, or siblings (Benbow, 1986a). The rate of left-handedness among family members was similar to that found among a comparison group of low-scoring gifted students—those whose combined SAT-M and SAT-V score as seventh graders was ≤ 540 (Benbow, 1986a). The students in this comparison group scored least well on the SAT, whereas the extremely precocious students we were studying were at the other end of the SAT scale as seventh graders. Clearly, left-handedness is a characteristic of the extremely precocious mathematical and/or verbal reasoners.

In addition, the extremely precocious students tended to be either (1) familial left-handers or (2) right-handers with a family history of left-handedness. Many of the students were ambidextrous. As a matter of fact, about 50% of the extremely precocious students were left-handed, mixed-handed, or right-handed with left-handed family members. The significance of this is that such individuals have been shown to be more likely to have different brain organization from complete right-handers; specifically, they tend to have more bilateral representation of cognitive functions (see reviews by Bradshaw & Nettleton, 1983; Bryden, 1982; Herron,

1980; Springer & Deutsch, 1981). Because approximately half of the extremely precocious students exhibited signs of such bilateral representation, I (Benbow, 1986a) proposed that bilateralization itself is associated with extreme mathematical and/or verbal reasoning ability. This hypothesis is in contrast to previous beliefs that greater specialization of the hemispheres leads to superior spatial or mathematical reasoning ability (Bradshaw & Nettleton, 1983; Bryden, 1982; Springer & Deutsch, 1981). Moreover, it was previously hypothesized that boys do better on spatial or mathematical reasoning tasks because males exhibit greater specialization of their hemispheres (Levy, 1972). It is difficult to reconcile our data, and the findings of the Burnett, Lane, and Dratt (1982) study, with this hypothesis.

We have completed a pilot study in which the extremely precocious students were tested on a spatial and a letter-matching task by a computer simulation of a tachistoscope (Benbow & Benbow, 1986). Results indicate that these students have right hemisphere or bilateral representation of language and spatial abilities. A control group, however, has not yet been tested with these same tasks.

Immune Disorders and Hormones

Because Geschwind and Behan (1982) had found high rates of immune disorders among left-handers, we investigated the frequency of such disorders among the extremely precocious students we studied. Using a survey designed by Dr. Franklin Adkinson, a specialist in allergies, it was found that over 50% of the extremely precocious students had allergies (Benbow, 1986a). This was more than twice the frequency found in the general population with the use of this instrument. Furthermore, the extremely precocious students had allergies more frequently than their parents, their siblings, or the comparison group of less gifted students.

Geschwind and Behan (1982) suggested that left-handedness and immune disorders may be related to exposure in fetal life to high levels of testosterone or to high fetal sensitivity to it. They hypothesized that testosterone slows the development of the left hemisphere and simultaneously affects immune development. Diminution of the size of one area in the cortex may lead to enlargement in the homologous region of the opposite side and in areas adjacent to the one whose development is impaired (Goldman-Rakic & Rakic, 1984). This has been shown in the fetal monkey. Spatial abilities, which may be important in mathematics, depend on parts of the right hemisphere and on the left-sided region just behind the posterior language area (Benton, 1979; Lezak, 1983). Nonetheless, prenatal testosterone exposure may lead to enhanced right-hemisphere functioning.

It is interesting, therefore, that both of the postulated consequences of being exposed prenatally to high levels of testosterone were found for the extremely intellectually talented students. Thus precocious mathematical and verbal *reasoning* ability may be related to prenatal exposure to testosterone, and this may have subsequently affected the organization or structure of the brains of individuals with those talents. Much further research is needed, however, before this conclusion can be accepted.

Consistent with this hypothesis of fetal exposure to sex hormones is our extension of the findings of Maccoby, Doering, Jacklin, and Kraemer (1979). Reinisch (1974) and Reinisch, Gandelman, and Spiegel (1979) had shown that prenatal exposure to sex hormones may affect cognitive functioning. Then Maccoby *et al.* (1979) found that concentrations of testosterone in the umbilical cord were significantly greater in males than in females, whereas no differences in concentrations were found for the other four sex hormones. Moreover, in both sexes, firstborns had significantly more progesterone and estrogen, with progesterone showing the largest birth-order effect. Among male infants, however, firstborns also had higher concentrations of testosterone. These results were not a consequence of maternal age, length of labor, or birth weight, but were related to the temporal spacing of childbirths. Later borns who were closely spaced in relation to their next older siblings had lower concentrations of hormones. Maccoby *et al.* (1979) related these findings to possible hormone depletion and suggested that this may be a factor in explaining why firstborns tend to have higher intellectual aptitude than later borns. Interestingly, most (over 60%) of our extremely intellectually precocious students were firstborns (Benbow & Benbow, 1986). The remaining tended to be well spaced. This is consistent with the Maccoby *et al.* (1979) contention and with the hypothesis that extreme intellectual precocity relates to prenatal exposure to high levels of testosterone.

Myopia

In the course of studying the extremely precocious SMPY students, we noted that many wore glasses. This observation and the results of some previous studies (Karlsson, 1975; Sofaer & Emery, 1981) led us to investigate the possibility that extremely precocious students would be myopic in elevated frequency. I (Benbow, 1986a) found that the extremely precocious mathematical and verbal reasoners were approximately four times more likely to be myopic than high school students in general. They were also more frequently myopic than their parents, their siblings, and the comparison group of gifted students who had scored lowest on the SAT. Interestingly, there was a sex difference in myopia. Girls were more frequently myopic than boys, and verbally talented students were more frequently myopic than mathematically talented students. Finally, the average age at which myopia was diagnosed was extremely early. Thus onset of myopia at an early age seems to be another characteristic of the extremely gifted. Cohn, Cohn and Jensen (in press) have confirmed my results and extended them. Their paper provides some insights as to possible explanations.

Physiological Correlates and Mathematical Talent

At first it may appear rather confusing to find that those physiological traits characterizing mathematically talented individuals also characterized those who were verbally talented. Our results may be due to the fact that we studied verbal *reasoning* ability. Verbal reasoning ability may be more directly affected by right-hemisphere processes than language production or syntactical aspects of verbal

ability, because verbal reasoning ability involves comprehension and the understanding of difficult words and their relationships (Caramazza, Gordon, Zurif, &
DeLuca, 1976; Eisenson, 1962; Gardner, Brownell, Wapner, & Michelow, 1983).

Seemingly even more confusing was that verbally talented males were more
frequently left-handed than the mathematically talented males. Benbow (1986a)
offered this explanation:

> This may have something to do with the frequency of mathematical and verbal talent
> in the population when the effects of testosterone are eliminated. In that case, one
> might expect to find sex differences favoring males in mathematical reasoning ability
> but none or perhaps a slight female advantage in verbal reasoning ability. It appears,
> however, that there are nonetheless slightly more males than females with extremely
> high verbal reasoning ability and many more with extremely high mathematical rea-
> soning. The proportion of testosterone-exposed (and, thus, left-handed) males among
> the extremely high verbal reasoners, we speculate, may therefore be higher than
> among the extremely high mathematical reasoners (p. 723).

In sum, Benbow (1986a), and Benbow and Benbow (1984) identified three
physiological correlates of mathematical talent: left-handedness, immune disorders, and myopia. The first two of these traits *may* be related to prenatal exposure
to high levels of testosterone and their possible effect on the development of the two
hemispheres of the brain which may be two additional physiological correlates.
Nevertheless, it seems that mathematically talented individuals are also likely
to have bilateral representation of cognitive functions and are more likely to be
male than female. Finally, Witelson's (1985) finding that the corpus callosum
is larger in left- and mixed-handers than in right-handers is intriguing in this
connection.

Brain Structures or Processes and Mathematical Talent

Much of the work described in the previous sections is applicable to this topic. To
recapitulate, it seems widely accepted that spatial ability is a right-hemisphere
function (see reviews by Bradshaw & Nettleton, 1983; Bryden, 1982; Springer &
Deutsch, 1981). Not such a clear consensus exists for mathematics. Actually, computation and the ability to read and produce signs in mathematics are usually
considered left-hemisphere functions (e.g., Zolog, 1983). The understanding of
numerical relations and concepts, however, appears to be largely mediated by the
right hemisphere (Dahmen, Hartje, Bussing, & Sturm, 1982; Gardner, 1983;
Troup, Bradshaw, & Nettleton, 1983; Warrington, 1982). The posterior areas of
the left hemisphere have been implicated in the recognition of ordered arrays and
patterns (Benton, 1979; Gardner, 1974; Lezak, 1983). Such spatial ability has been
clearly related to mathematical ability, as discussed previously in this chapter.
Moreover, Grafman, Passafuime, Faglioni, and Boller (1982) illustrated the
importance to mathematics and logic of the left parietal lobes and the occipital
association areas contiguous to them. There is no strong consensus on this last
point, however.

These above conclusions were derived from studies on individuals with dyscalculia, or learning disabilities in mathematics. My studies on physiological correlates of mathematical talent, however, provide support for the possible importance of these same brain structures in high-level mathematical thinking as well. A strong indication from my data is that bilateral representation of cognitive functions is associated with mathematical talent. This is consistent with Gervais (cited in Gardner, 1983) and with Kraft, Mitchell, Languis, & Wheatley (1980), who have documented that activation of both hemispheres occurs during the solution of mathematics problems.

Biological Bases to Mathematical Talent

There are many indications that mathematical talent is at least in part under biological influences, which supports Krutetskii's belief that anybody can become an ordinary mathematician but that one has to be "born" a great one. In this section I summarize the evidence for this point.

That spatial ability, which has been related to mathematical ability, is under some genetic influence has been clearly demonstrated by several studies (DeFries *et al.*, 1978; DeFries *et al.*, 1979; McGee, 1979). Moreover, among the SMPY population of mathematically talented individuals, we have found evidence supporting the familiality of specific cognitive abilities (Benbow, Zonderman, & Stanley, 1983). Extreme giftedness, however, cannot be predicted reliably as solely a result of the mating of bright parents. High spatial ability showed the greatest influence of genetic factors and may therefore be suggestive of the role of genetics in mathematics. Unfortunately, mathematical reasoning ability could not be tested in that study. Cohn, Cohn and Jensen (in press) tested speed of information processing among mathematically talented youths and their siblings. The mathematically talented students had faster reaction times than their siblings. Thus, Cohn, Cohn and Jensen concluded that this was evidence in support of a genetic model of intelligence.

Attacking this issue from a different perspective, the role of training in causing mathematical talent has not been substantiated. Brody (1984) studied students participating in a Johns Hopkins talent search who had taken the SAT as seventh graders and then attended a special mathematics, science, or verbal class the following summer. Most of these students had not mastered even Algebra I before the summer program. In the mathematics class the students studied, in a fast-paced manner, as much precalculus mathematics as they could in 3 weeks of intensive, all-day instruction. Only precalculus mathematics not already known was studied. Even though these students focused directly on subject matter considered prerequisite for the SAT-M, their SAT-M scores did not improve more than did the scores of students in the other classes or in a control group. Supporting these findings, the majority of talent-search participants themselves reported learning most of their mathematics in the regular classroom (Benbow & Stanley, 1982b). There were no indications that the mathematically talented students identified by SMPY had undergone intensive training programs.

Moreover, Raymond and Benbow (1986) studied the involvement of parents in various aspects of the education of their mathematically or verbally talented children. It was found that fathers were more involved in quantitative areas, whereas mothers were more involved in verbal areas. There was, however, no greater involvement overall of fathers with mathematically talented students than with verbally talented students. Thus this aspect of socialization did not appear to be influencing the emergence of mathematical talent. Finally, a lack of effect of certain toys (e.g., construction toys, blocks) on mathematical talent was also found (Benbow, 1986b).

In contrast, the possible role of biology in mathematical talent became evident when its physiological correlates (i.e., left-handedness, immune disorders, myopia, etc.) were discovered. It would be difficult to conclude logically that all of these physiological traits exhibited by the mathematically talented are solely the result of environmental factors.

Finally, a series of studies has shown that the main environmental hypotheses proposed to account for sex differences in mathematical reasoning ability do not entirely explain the results obtained for SMPY's mathematically talented individuals (Benbow, 1986; Benbow & Benbow, 1984; Benbow & Stanley, 1980, 1981, 1982a, 1982b, 1983, 1984; Raymond & Benbow, 1986). It was proposed in these studies that these sex differences are the result of both endogenous and exogenous factors. The finding of physiological correlates of mathematical talent lends credence to this claim.

Summary

In the many and diverse definitions of mathematical talent I reviewed, few commonalities could be found. Yet all of them dealt with higher level cognitive processing requiring mathematical reasoning ability. Computational ability was not viewed as an essential aspect of mathematical talent. If one were to seek a consensus, it seems that mathematical talent can best be defined as the ability to handle long chains of reasoning.

The development of mathematical talent in children has, unfortunately, received little study. Because a major difference between the mathematically talented and other students appears to be that the talented acquire skills and competencies at an earlier age, studies of the development of mathematical thinking in average children may be relevant, especially since SMPY has found that mathematically talented children remain talented as adults. Mathematics instruction or training does not relate much to the development of mathematical reasoning ability.

In contrast, many researchers have investigated which cognitive abilities or characteristics correlate with mathematical talent. The following factors were identified: spatial ability, field independence, use of images, logicism, intuition, flexibility, the ability to recognize unproductive strategies, excellent memory, and high verbal and reasoning skills.

A striking neuropsychological parameter of mathematical talent is sex. We have shown that many more males than females are mathematically talented, especially at the upper end of the scale. These sex differences are important and are predictive of later sex differences in achievement in mathematics and the sciences. In addition, we have tried to determine why these sex differences in mathematical reasoning ability occur. Our results are inconsistent with an explanation that is entirely environmental.

In a separate series of studies, we found that mathematically talented individuals tend to be left-handed, ambidextrous, or right-handed with their immediate family members tending to be left-handed. The significance of this finding is that such individuals have been shown to be more likely to have different brain organization from that of complete right-handers; they tend to have more bilateral cognitive representation. I therefore proposed that bilateralization is associated with extreme mathematical reasoning ability.

Moreover, extremely mathematically talented students suffer much more frequently from immune disorders (e.g., allergies). Because these students tend much more frequently to be left-handed and to have allergies, it is possible that they were exposed prenatally to high levels of testosterone. Geschwind and Behan (1982) cited evidence supporting the hypothesis that left-handedness and immune disorders are related to prenatal exposure to high levels of testosterone.

Another physiological correlate of mathematical talent is myopia, although its basis is obscure. Finally, further evidence was presented that supported a genetic component to mathematical talent.

In conclusion, I view this chapter as a beginning towards better understanding the neuropsychology of mathematical talent. Although not much is known, the studies cited should serve as useful indicators of the most fruitful directions for future research. Furthermore, there are many different types of mathematics and mathematicians. Each uses or requires a unique set of abilities. How this relates to brain functioning may be an especially interesting topic to explore in the future.

Another interesting area of study is how training or experience in mathematics affects brain functioning. As problem-solving strategies become incorporated, do the relative contributions of the two hemispheres change? It has been found, for example, that there are differences between 7th and 12th graders in the factorial structure accounting for the performance on the SAT-M (Minor & Benbow, 1986). Could this possibly relate to a shift in the relative activation of the two hemispheres? For example, in very simplistic terms, when listening to music, untrained listeners tend to rely more on their right hemispheres, whereas the reverse is true for trained musicians (Bever & Chiarello, 1974; Kellar & Bever, 1980; Shannon, 1980; see Bradshaw & Nettleton, 1983, for a review). Moreover, we postulated earlier that the novelty of the task may relate to a greater contribution of the right hemisphere in cognitive processing. Does this imply that trained and experienced mathematicians would rely more on left- rather than on right-hemisphere processes and that the opposite would be true for less-experienced mathematicians? If such differences in brain functioning were found, would they relate to the finding that the most important contributions in mathematics tend to be made at an early age (Lehman, 1953)? Are such contributions made at a time when the individual is relying more on the right hemisphere for solving problems rather than on the left? All of these comments are highly speculative, of course, but perhaps they can serve as suggestions for future work.

References

Annett, M., & Kilshaw, D. (1982). Mathematical ability and lateral asymmetry. *Cortex*, *18*(4), 547–568.

Armstrong, J. M. (1981). Achievement and participation of women in mathematics: Results of two national surveys. *Journal for Research in Mathematics Education, 12,* 356–372.

Becker, B. J. (1978). *The relationship of spatial ability to sex differences in the performance of mathematically precocious youths on the mathematical section of the Scholastic Aptitude Test.* Unpublished master's thesis, Johns Hopkins University, Baltimore.

Benbow, C. P. (1978). Further testing of the high scorers from SMPY's 1978 talent search. *ITYB* (Intellectually Talented Youth Bulletin), *5*(4), 1–2.

Benbow, C. P. (1986a). Physiological correlates of extreme intellectual precocity. *Neuropsychologia, 24,* 719–725.

Benbow, C. P. (1986b, April). *Toys and home environments: Their relationship to aptitude and gender.* Paper presented at the Annual Meeting of the American Educational Research Association. San Francisco, CA.

Benbow, C. P., & Benbow, R. M. (1984). Biological correlates of high mathematical reasoning ability. In G. J. DeVries, J. P. C. DeBruin, H. B. M. Vylings, & M. A. Corner (Eds.), *Sex differences in the brain: The relation between structure and function. Progress in Brain Research, 61,* (pp. 469–490). Amsterdam: Elsevier Science Publishers.

Benbow, C. P. & Benbow, R. M. (1986). Extreme mathematical talent: A hormonally induced ability? *Proceedings from the Wenner-Gren Center International Symposium on the Dual Brain.* Houndsmill, England: The MacMillan Press, Ltd.

Benbow, C. P., & Stanley, J. C. (1980). Sex differences in mathematical ability: Fact or artifact. *Science, 210,* 1261–1264.

Benbow, C. P., & Stanley, J. C. (1981). Mathematical ability: Is sex a factor? *Science, 212,* 118–119.

Benbow, C. P., & Stanley, J. C. (1982a). Consequences in high school and college of sex differences in mathematical reasoning ability: A longitudinal perspective. *American Educational Research Journal, 19,* 598–622.

Benbow, C. P., & Stanley, J. C. (1982b). Intellectually talented boys and girls: Educational profiles. *Gifted Child Quarterly, 26*(2), 82–88.

Benbow, C. P., & Stanley, J. C. (1983). Sex differences in mathematical reasoning ability: More facts. *Science, 222,* 1029–1031.

Benbow, C. P., & Stanley, J. C. (1984). Gender and the science major. In M. W. Steinkamp & M. L. Maehr (Eds.), *Advances in motivation and achievement* (Vol. 2, 139–164). Greenwich, CT: JAI Press.

Benbow, C. P., Stanley, J. C., Kirk, M. K., & Zonderman, A. B. (1983). Structure of intelligence in intellectually precocious children and in their parents. *Intelligence, 7,* 129–152.

Benbow, C. P., Zonderman, A. B., & Stanley, J. C. (1983). Assortative marriage and the familiality of cognitive abilities in families of extremely gifted students. *Intelligence, 7,* 153–161.

Benton, A. (1979). In K. Heilman & E. Valenstein (Eds.), *Clinical neuropsychology*. New York: Oxford University Press.

Bever, T. G., & Chiarello, R. J. (1974). Cerebral dominance in musicians and nonmusicians. *Science, 185,* 137–139.

Bien, E. C. (1974). *The relationship of cognitive style and structure of arithmetic materials to performance in fourth-grade arithmetic.* Unpublished doctoral dissertation, University of Pennsylvania, Philadelphia.

Bloom, B. S. (Ed.) (1956). *Taxonomy of educational objectives. Handbook I: The cognitive domain.* New York: David McKay.

Bloom, B. S. (1982). The role of gifts and markers in the development of talent. *Exceptional Children, 48*(6), 510–522.

Blum-Zorman, R. (1984). Cognitive controls, cognitive styles and mathematical potential among gifted preadolescents. Doctoral dissertation, *Dissertation Abstracts International, 44,* 3656A.

Bradshaw, J. C., & Nettleton, N. C. (1983). *Human cerebral asymmetry.* Englewood Cliffs, NJ: Prentice-Hall.

Brody, L. E., & Benbow, C. P. (1986). *The effects of high school coursework on SAT scores.* Paper presented at the annual meeting of the American Psychological Association, Washington, D.C.

Brody, L. E. (1984). *The effects of an intensive summer program on the SAT scores of gifted seventh graders.* Unpublished doctoral dissertation, Johns Hopkins University, Baltimore.

Bryden, M. P. (1982). *Laterality: Functional asymmetry in the intact brain.* New York: Academic Press.

Burkes, B. S., Jensen, D. W., & Terman, L. M. (1947). The promise of youth: Follow-up studies of a thousand gifted children. *Genetic studies of genius* (Vol. 3). Stanford, CA: Stanford University Press.

Burnett, S. A., Lane, D. M., & Dratt, L. M. (1979). Spatial visualization and sex differences in quantitative ability. *Intelligence, 3,* 345–354.

Burnett, S. A., Lane, D. M., & Dratt, L. M. (1982). Spatial ability and handedness. *Intelligence, 6,* 57–68.

Caramazza, A., Gordon, J., Zurif, E. B., & Deluca, D. (1976). Right-hemispheric damage and verbal problem-solving behavior. *Brain and Language, 3,* 41–46.

Cohn, S. J. (1977). Cognitive characteristics of the top-scoring participants in SMPY's 1976 talent search. *Gifted Child Quarterly, 22*(3), 416–421.

Cohn, S. J. (1980). Two components of the Study of Mathematically Precocious Youth's intervention studies of educational facilitation and longitudinal follow-up. Unpublished doctoral dissertation, Johns Hopkins University, Baltimore.

Cohn, S. J., Cohn, C. M. G., & Jensen, A. R., (in press). Speed of information processing and myopia in academically gifted youths and their siblings. *Intelligence.*

Dahmen, N., Hartje, W., Bussing, A., & Sturm, W. (1982). Disorders of calculation in aphasic patients—spatial and verbal components. *Neuropsychologia, 20*(2), 145–153.

Davis, R. B. (1983). Complex mathematical cognition. In H. P. Ginsburg (Ed.), *The development of mathematical thinking* (pp. 254–291). New York: Academic Press.

DeFries, J. C., Ashton, G. C., Johnson, R. C., Kuse, A. R., McClearn, G. E., Mi, M. P., Rashed, M. N., Vandenberg, S. G., & Wilson, J. R. (1978). The Hawaii Family Study of Cognition: A reply. *Behavior Genetics, 8,* 281–288.

DeFries, J. C., Johnson, R. C., Kuse, A. R., McClearn, G. E., Polovina, J., Vandenberg, S. G., & Wilson, J. R. (1979). Familial resemblance for specific cognitive abilities. *Behavior Genetics, 9*(1), 23–43.

Donlon, T. F., & Angoff, W. H. (1971). The Scholastic Aptitude Test. In W. Angoff (Ed.), *The College Board Admissions Testing Program.* Princeton, NJ: College Entrance Examination Board.

Eisenson, J. (1962). Language and intellectual modifications associated with right cerebral damage. *Language and Speech*, *5*, 49–53.

Fox, L. H., Brody, L. E., & Tobin, D. (1982, January). *The study of social processes that inhibit or enhance the development of competence and interest in mathematics among highly able young women*. Report to the National Institute of Education. Baltimore: Department of Education, Johns Hopkins University.

Gardner, H. (1974). *The shattered mind: The person after brain damage*. New York: Vintage.

Gardner, H. (1983). *Frames of mind*. New York: Basic Books.

Gardner, H., Brownell, H. H., Wapner, W. & Michelow, D. (1983). Missing the point. The role of the right hemisphere in the processing of complex linguistic materials. In E. Perecman (Ed.), *Cognitive processing in the right hemisphere* (pp. 169–191). New York: Academic Press.

Geschwind, N., & Behan, P. (1982). Left-handedness: Association with immune disease, migraine, and developmental learning disorder. *Proceedings of the National Academy of Sciences, USA 79*, 5097–5100.

Ginsburg, H. P. (Ed.). (1983). *The development of mathematical thinking*. New York: Academic Press.

Goldman-Rakic, P. S., & Rakic, P. (1984). Experimental modification of gyral patterns. In N. Geschwind & A. M. Galaburda (Eds.), *Cerebral dominance: The biological foundations* (pp. 179–192). Cambridge, MA: Harvard University Press.

Grafman, J., Passafuime, D., Faglioni, P., & Boller, F. (1982). Calculation disturbances in adults with focal hemisphere damage. *Cortex*, *18*, 37–50.

Greenes, C. (1981). Identifying the gifted child in mathematics. *The Arithmetic Teacher*, *28*(6), 14–17.

Harris, L. J. (1978). Sex differences in spatial ability: Possible environmental, genetic, and neurologic factors. In M. Kinsbourne (Ed.), *Asymmetrical function of the brain* (pp. 405–522). Cambridge: Cambridge University Press.

Herron, J. (Ed.). (1980). *Neuropsychology of left-handedness*. New York: Academic Press.

Karlsson, J. L. (1975). Influence of the myopia gene on brain development. *Clinical Genetics*, *8*, 314–318.

Keating, D. P. (1975). Precocious cognitive development at the level of formal operations. *Child Development*, *46*, 276–280.

Keating, D. P., & Schaefer, R. A. (1975). Ability and sex differences in the acquisition of formal operations. *Developmental Psychology*, *11*(4), 531–532.

Kellar, L. A., & Bever, T. G. (1980). Hemispheric asymmetries in the perception of musical intervals as a function of musical experience and family handedness background. *Brain and Language*, *10*, 24–38.

Kelly, A. (1979). *Girls and Science: An international study of sex differences in school science achievement*. Stockholm, Sweden: Almqvist & Wiksell International.

Kosslyn, S. M., & Jolicoeur, P. (1980). A theory-based approach to the study of individual differences in mental imagery. In R. E. Snow, P. A. Federico, & W. E. Montague (Eds.), *Aptitude, learning, and instruction* (Vol. 2). Hillsdale, NJ: Erlbaum.

Kraft, R. H., Mitchell, D. R., Languis, M. L., & Wheatley, G. H. (1980). Hemispheric asymmetries during six-to-eight-year-olds' performance of Piagetian conservation and reading tasks. *Neuropsychologia*, *18*, 637–643.

Krutetskii, V. A. (1976). *The psychology of mathematical abilities in school children*. Chicago: University of Chicago Press.

Kuhn, T. S. (1962). *The structure of scientific revolutions*. In *International encyclopedia of unified science* (Vol. 2, No. 2). Chicago: University of Chicago Press.

Lean, G., & Clements, M. S. (1981). Spatial ability, visual imagery and mathematical performance. *Educational Studies in Mathematics*, *12*, 267–299.

Lehman, H. C. (1953). *Age and achievement*. Princeton, NJ: Princeton University Press.

Lester, F. K., & Schroeder, T. L. (1983, May). Cognitive characteristics of mathematically gifted children. *Roeper Review* pp. 26–28.

Levy, J. (1972). Lateral specialization of the human brain: Behavioral manifestations and possible evolutionary basis. In J. A. Kiger (Ed.), *The biology of behavior* (pp. 159–180). Corvallis, OR: Oregon State University Press.

Lezak, M. D. (1983). *Neuropsychological assessment* (2nd ed.). New York: Oxford University Press.

Maccoby, E. E., Doering, C. H., Jacklin, C. N., & Kraemer, H. (1979). Concentrations of sex hormones in umbilical-cord blood: Their relation to sex and birth order of infants. *Child Development, 50,* 632–642.

Maccoby, E. E., & Jacklin, C. N. (1974). *The psychology of sex differences*. Stanford, CA: Stanford University Press.

McGee, M. G. (1979). Human spatial abilities: Psychometric studies and environmental, genetic, hormonal, and neurological influences. *Psychological Bulletin, 86,* 889–918.

Minor, L., & Benbow, C. P. (1986, April). *Construct validity of the SAT-M: A comparative study of high school students and gifted seventh graders*. Manuscript submitted for publication. Paper presented at the annual meeting of the American Educational Research Association, San Francisco.

Moses, B. E. (1977). *The nature of spatial ability and its relationship to mathematical problem solving*. Unpublished doctoral dissertation, Indiana University, Bloomington.

Moses, B. E. (1980, April). *The relationship between visual thinking tasks and problem-solving peformance*. Paper presented at the annual meeting of the American Educational Research Association, Boston.

Oden, M. H. (1968). The fulfilment of promise: 40-year follow-up of the Terman gifted group. *Genetic Psychology Monographs, 77,* 3–93.

Oldfield, R. C. (1971). The assessment and analysis of handedness: The Edinburgh Inventory. *Neuropsychologia, 9,* 97–113.

Osborne, A. (1981). Needed research: Mathematics for the talented. *The Arithmetic Teacher, 28*(6), 24–25.

Pollins, L. D. (1984). *The construct validity of the Scholastic Aptitude Test for young gifted students*. Unpublished doctoral dissertation, Duke University, Durham, NC.

Raymond, C. L., & Benbow, C. P. (1986). *Gender differences in mathematics: A function of student sex-typing and parental support*. Developmental Psychology, 22, 808–819.

Reinisch, J. M. (1974). Fetal hormones, the brain, and human sex differences: A heuristic, integrative review of the recent literature. *Archives of Sexual Behavior, 3*(1), 51–96.

Reinisch, J. M., Gandelman, R., & Spiegel, F. S. (1979). Prenatal influences on cognitive abilities: Data from experimental animals and human and endocrine syndromes. In M. Wittig & A. C. Petersen (Eds.), *Sex-related differences in cognitive functioning: Developmental issues* (pp. 215–240). New York: Academic Press.

Riley, M. S., Greeno, J. G., & Heller, J. I. (1983). Development of children's problem-solving ability in arithmetic. In H. P. Ginsburg (Ed.), *The development of mathematical thinking* (pp. 153–164). New York: Academic Press.

Robinson, H. B. (1983). A case for radical acceleration: Programs of The Johns Hopkins University and The University of Washington. In C. P. Benbow & J. C. Stanley (Eds.), *Academic precocity: Aspects of its development* (pp. 139–159). Baltimore: The Johns Hopkins University Press.

Saxe, G. B., & Posner, J. K. (1983). The development of numerical cognition: Cross-cultural perspectives. In H. P. Ginsburg (Ed.), *The development of mathematical thinking* (pp. 292–318). New York: Academic Press.

Sears, P. S., & Barbee, A. H. (1977). Career and life satisfaction among Terman's gifted women. In J. C. Stanley, W. C. George, & C. H. Solano (Eds.), *The gifted and creative: A fifty-year perspective* (pp. 28–65). Baltimore: The Johns Hopkins University Press.

Sears, R. R. (1977). Sources of life satisfaction of the Terman gifted men. *American Psychologist, 32,* 119–128.

Shannon, B. (1980). Lateralization effects in musical decision tasks. *Neuropsychologia, 18,* 21–31.

Sherman, J. A. (1967). The problem of sex differences in space perception and aspects of individual functioning. *Psychological Review, 75,* 290–299.

Sherman, J. A. (1977). Effects of biological factors on sex-related differences in mathematics achievement. In *Women and mathematics: Research perspectives for change* (NIE Papers in Education and Work, No. 8). Washington, DC: National Institute of Education.

Smith, I. M. (1964). *Spatial ability.* London: University of London Press.

Sofaer, J., & Emery, A. (1981). Genes for super-intelligence. *Journal of Medical Genetics, 18,* 410–413.

Springer, S. P., & Deutsch, G. (1981). *Left brain, right brain.* San Francisco: W. H. Freeman.

Stanley, J. C. (1977). Rationale of the Study of Mathematically Precocious Youth (SMPY) during its first five years of promoting educational acceleration. In J. C. Stanley, W. C. George, & C. H. Solano (Eds.), *The gifted and the creative: A fifty-year perspective* (pp. 75–112). Baltimore: The Johns Hopkins University Press.

Stanley, J. C., & Benbow, C. P. (1986). Youths who reason exceptionally well mathematically. In R. J. Sternberg & J. Davidson (Eds.), *Conceptions of Giftedness* (pp. 361–387). Cambridge University Press.

Stanley, J. C., Huang, J. & Zu., X. (1986). SAT-M scores of highly selected students in Shanghai tested when less than 13 years old. *College Board Review, 140,* 10–13, 28–29.

Terman, L. M. (1925). Mental and physical traits of a thousand gifted children. In *Genetic studies of genius* (Vol. 1), Stanford, CA: Stanford University Press.

Terman, L. M., & Oden, M. H. (1947). The gifted child grows up: Twenty-five years' follow-up of a superior group. In *Genetic studies of genius* (Vol. 4). Stanford University Press.

Terman, L. M., & Oden, M. H. (1959). The gifted group at mid-life: Thirty-five years' follow-up of the superior child. In *Genetic studies of genius* (Vol. 5). Stanford, CA: Stanford University Press.

Troup, G. A., Bradshaw, J. L., & Nettleton, N. C. (1983). The lateralization of arithmetic and number processing. A review. *International Journal of Neuroscience, 19*(1–4), 213–242.

Vaidya, S., & Chansky, N. (1980). Cognitive development and cognitive style as factors in mathematics achievement. *Journal of Educational Psychology, 72,* 326–330.

Vygotsky, L. S. (1962). *Thought and language.* Cambridge, MA: The MIT Press.

Vygotsky, L. S. (1978). *Mind in society: The development of higher psychological processes.* Tran. M. Cole, V. John-Steiner, S. Scribner, & E. Souberman (Eds.), Cambridge, MA: Harvard University Press.

Warrington, E. K. (1982). The fractionation of arithmetic skills: A single case study. *Quarterly Journal of Experimental Psychology, 34A,* 31–51.

Webb, N. L. (1979). Processes, conceptual knowledge and mathematical problem-solving ability. *Journal for Research in Mathematics Education, 10,* 83–93.

Werderlin, I. (1958). *The mathematical ability*. Lund, Sweden: Gleerups.

Witelson, S. F. (1985). The brain connection: The corpus callosum is larger in left-handers. *Science, 229,* 665–668.

Witkin, H. A., Moore, C. A., Goodenough, D. R., & Cox, P. W. (1975). *Field-dependent and field-independent cognitive styles and their educational implications* (Research Bulletin 75-24). Princeton, NJ: Educational Testing Service.

Zolog, A. (1983). Speech disturbances in parietal lobe lesions. *Neurologie et Psychiatrie, 21*(3), 165–167.

4

Hyperlexia: A Review
of Extraordinary Word Recognition

DOROTHY M. ARAM
JANE M. HEALY

Children with extraordinary reading skills despite serious linguistic, cognitive, and behavioral disorders have been described for many years. It was not until 1967 that the term "hyperlexia" was coined by Silberberg and Silberberg to refer to children's ability "to recognize words . . . on a higher level than their ability to comprehend and integrate them" (p. 41). Subsequently, case studies, descriptions of small numbers of children, and a few experimental studies have confirmed the existence of this unusual developmental syndrome. While the neurophysiological basis for this remarkable developmental discrepancy in skill attainment is far from clear, several attempts have been made to offer explanatory theory and data. In this chapter we will review a number of behavioral and neurological findings associated with hyperlexia, discuss several explanatory theories, and propose directions for research to illuminate our understanding of this unique condition.

The Data: Studies Reviewed

Studies of hyperlexic children are chiefly individual cases or descriptive studies of small groups. A few recent studies have also tested diverse explanatory hypotheses, providing evidence from various experimental tasks. For this review, we have somewhat arbitrarily grouped studies into three broad types: individual case studies, which may or may not involve experimental measures; descriptive studies, which rely predominantly on reports of group characteristics and standardized psychometric findings; and experimental studies of various hypotheses tested with standardized and experimental measures. Table 4-1 summarizes the principal studies reviewed in this chapter.

Dorothy M. Aram. Department of Pediatrics, Case Western Reserve University, Rainbow Babies and Childrens Hospital, Cleveland, Ohio.
Jane M. Healy. Hathaway Brown School, Cleveland State University, Cleveland, Ohio.

Case Studies of Individual Children

Probably the earliest reports of children with amazing word recognition were of idiot savants who exhibited islands of extraordinary skills despite severe intellectual limitations. Phillips (1930) is frequently cited for one of the earliest descriptions of a hyperlexic among three "talented imbeciles," one with a talent for numerical calculation, a second with marked mechanical ability, and a third, Gordon, who at 10 years of age was near "the zero point in the scale of social 'efficiency' " and a low-grade imbecile on the mental scale, yet was endowed with a conspicuous gift for words and tunes. He was able to repeat short stories almost verbatim, was talented in audiomotor memory, and had a "love of literature," which was not further clarified.

The case of L., an idiot–savant child described in exquisite detail by Scheerer, Rothman, and Goldstein (1945), is also an early report of hyperlexia, although L.'s well-developed reading skills were overshadowed by his extraordinary talents in spelling, calculations, memory for music and rhythms, and calendar knowledge. Although many of the characteristics described are similar to those reported in other cases of hyperlexia, L.'s reading was but one of an array of "talents" and, unfortunately, not fully documented.

Child psychiatrists have also observed advanced reading skills in severely disturbed children. Cain (1969) described special "isolated" abilities in several severely psychotic children, one of whom was said to read and spell, presumably without understanding, at a fifth-grade level despite the fact that most other aspects of ego development were arrested at an 18-month level. Goodman (1972) described Sam, an "autistic–savant," providing vivid details of this child's obsessional preoccupation with reading.

Since Silberberg and Silberberg's 1967 description, several case studies of individuals labeled as hyperlexic have appeared, including those of Silberberg and Silberberg (1968), Elliott and Needleman (1976), and Aram, Rose, and Horwitz (1984). The earlier case descriptions detailed general cognitive and behavioral characteristics, whereas more recent studies focused upon various aspects of reading.

Descriptive Studies of Small Groups

Descriptive studies of groups of hyperlexic children within the past 15 years have ranged from exemplary serial case reports (e.g., Mehegan & Dreifuss, 1972) to systematic reports of standardized psychometric, language, and/or reading tests (Cobrinik, 1974; Fontenelle & Alarcon, 1982; Richman & Kitchell, 1981; Silberberg & Silberberg, 1971). Together these studies confirmed the existence of hyperlexic children and began documenting the syndrome's recurrent characteristics.

Experimental Studies

Several groups of investigators not only reported scores on standardized psychometric tests but also began adapting and developing experimental and nonstandardized measures to study this unique condition. Some provided more extensive

TABLE 4-1. Hyperlexia Studies Reviewed

	No. of subjects		Age range	Definition/Criteria for inclusion
	Male	Female		
Case Studies				
Phillips (1930)	1		10 yr	"Conspicuous gift for words"
Scheerer, Rothmann, and Goldstein (1945)	1		Birth to 15 yr	Detailed case history
Silberberg and Silberberg (1968)	2	2	7 yr 10 mo to 8 yr 2 mo	Reading recognition 1 yr above expected level for grades 1–3, and 1.5 yr above for grades 4–6
Cain (1969)	1	2	6 yr 1 mo to 8 yr	Brief case description
Goodman (1972)		1	8 yr	Detailed case description
Elliott and Needleman (1976)		1	5 yr 8 mo	"A remarkably accelerated ability to recognize written words which may or may not occur with truly pathological conditions."
Aram, Rose, and Horwitz (1984)	1		39 yr	Word recognition far in advance of any other cognitive skill; reading onset prior to speech
Descriptive Studies				
Silberberg and Silberberg (1971)	28[a]		Preschool to grade 4.5	Reading recognition level 1.5 grades (grades 1 and 2) or 2.0 grades (3rd grade and up) above expected level
Mehegan and Dreifuss (1972)	11	1	5 to 9 yr	"Unusual and premature talent in reading against a background of generalized failure of development or marked impairment of language functions."

Study	N	Sex[a]	Age range	Description
Cobrinik (1974)	6	0	12 yr 2 mo to 14 yr 9 mo	Unexpected rote reading despite moderate-to-profound intellectual retardation
Richman and Kitchell (1981)	8	2	5 yr 9 mo to 9 yr 7 mo	Word recognition on WRAT more than 2 years above expected level of achievement
Fontenelle and Alarcon (1982)	7	1	4 to 17 yr	Higher rote word recognition than expected from level of cognitive functioning

Experimental Studies

Study	N	Sex[a]	Age range	Description
Huttenlocher and Huttenlocher (1973)	3	0	4 yr 11 mo to 7 yr	Case history description
Healy, Aram, Horwitz, and Kessler (1982)	11	1	5 to 11 yr	1. Early intense reading onset—before 5 yr 2. Superior word recognition 3. Disordered cognitive/linguistic behavior
Cobrinik (1982)	9	0	9 yr 8 mo to 13 yr 2 mo	1. Precocious, self-taught emergence of reading between 3 and 5 yr 2. Context of severe language deviation, impaired comprehension, emotional withdrawal
Aram, Ekelman, and Healy (1984)	12	0	7 yr 8 mo to 13 yr 7 mo	Same as Healy, Aram, Horwitz, and Kessler
Goldberg and Rothermel (1984)	7	1	5 yr 2 mo to 17 yr 8 mo	Case history consistent with previous descriptions

[a] Sex not given.

description of the behaviors associated with hyperlexia (Healy, Aram, Horwitz, & Kessler, 1982; Huttenlocher & Huttenlocher, 1973), while others began to tease apart these children's performance on various visual and linguistic components of reading (Aram, Ekelman, & Healy, 1984; Cobrinik, 1982; Goldberg & Rothermel, 1984).

To date, the literature provides a surprisingly consistent description of hyperlexics' cognitive, linguistic, behavioral, and reading characteristics. Only beginning to be addressed is how and why this exceptional reading skill develops. Before we present a composite picture of the characteristics associated with hyperlexia, we consider the issue of its definition and the criteria for its diagnosis.

Definition of Hyperlexia

As initially used by Silberberg and Silberberg (1967), "hyperlexia" referred to children whose ability to recognize words was significantly higher than either their ability t comprehend the material read or their level of verbal functioning. In addition, these authors observed that over one half of the 28 children composing their initial group had been diagnosed as retarded, autistic, or manifesting behavior suggesting some form of cerebral dysfunction. Five evidenced word recognition as preschoolers. This study outlined three major criteria inconsistently used by later writers to define hyperlexia: (1) discrepancy between word recognition and comprehension, (2) related behavioral disorders, and (3) early onset. Operationalizing these criteria has given rise to three main problems of definition: specifying the nature and degree of discrepancy between word recognition and other aspects of cognitive development, the necessity of having associated developmental disorder, and untutored onset in the preschool years.

Specifying the Discrepancy Between Word Recognition and Other Aspects of Cognitive Development

The one universally recognized indicator of hyperlexia has been exceptional word-recognition skill. Typically, determination of this exceptionality has been based on clinical observation and history rather than on formal criteria, and its application has been reserved for children whose ability to read stands out as an unexpected talent. Notable discrepancies between word-recognition skills and a measure of language or reading comprehension are often evidenced through case descriptions or test results, yet specific criteria for discrepancy are rare.

Thus, though all agree that word recognition is advanced, the questions remain, in comparison to what, and how much discrepancy exists? Silberberg and Silberberg (1967) initially suggested that the comparison be made to word comprehension or verbal functioning level. The following year, they suggested that a comparison be drawn between a child's expected and observed reading level, as calculated by use of the norms provided for reading recognition by the *Wide Range Achievement Test [WRAT] Manual* (Jastak & Jastak, 1965), with children "designated as hyperlexic if their reading score is one year above expected level in the first

three grades and 1.5 years above expected level in the fourth, fifth and sixth grades"
(Silberberg & Silberberg, 1968, p. 4). By 1971, Silberberg and Silberberg had
modified their formula to require 1.5 years' discrepancy in grades one and two, and
2 years' discrepancy thereafter.

It is probable that most children described in the literature as hyperlexic
would meet the Silberbergs' criteria if they were applied. The fact remains that
except for Richman and Kitchell (1981), who adhered to the 2-year discrepancy
between actual and expected word recognition, investigators have not explicitly
employed these criteria.

What appears to have been lost in the Silberbergs' formula is a more direct
comparison to reading comprehension and to verbal skills—a comparison that has
yet to be uniformly operationalized. In part, the failure to agree upon what aspects
of behavior must be discrepant from word recognition and by how much may
simply reflect the early stage of investigation in this area. Moreover, many young
or severely impaired hyperlexics are difficult to test, limiting the usefulness of
standardized results. As we will show later, however, this issue may require some
resolution lest the term "hyperlexia" be overgeneralized.

A final point relevant to discrepancy criteria is the necessity that the gap
between word recognition and other aspects of development be maintained as the
children grow older. Our clinical experience and limited data suggest that not all
hyperlexic preschoolers continue their extraordinary word-recognition skills into
the teen years. Some appear to become uninterested in reading in adolescence, and
a few narrow the gap in reading-skill areas.

The Necessity of Having an Associated Developmental Disorder

While all investigators addressing hyperlexia would agree that word recognition
must be a superior skill, the issue of whether or not hyperlexic children must also
present a significant cognitive and/or behavioral disorder is disputed. At the heart
of the disagreement is a basic difference in how hyperlexia is viewed. Those who
simply require accelerated word-recognition skills typically see hyperlexia as a
normal developmental variant; in contrast are those who see the exaggerated word
recognition as a symptom of a more pervasive developmental disorder.

In the Silberbergs' initial group (1967), over half had been diagnosed as
mentally retarded, autistic, or having a cerebral dysfunction; it is not clear if the
others were unlabeled because they were developing normally otherwise or because
they had not received any special assessments. The authors suggested then that
hyperlexia might be viewed as a "physiological variant" manifested as a specific
talent independent of general intellectual functioning. In articles in 1968 and 1971,
however, they presented hyperlexia as the positive extreme on a normal continuum
of discrepancy between actual and expected word reading. This perspective was
picked up by Niensted (1968), who identified 26 of 45 public school children as
hyperlexic because the level of their word-list reading was at least one year higher
than their silent comprehension level. Hypothesizing that overemphasis on the
teaching of word-calling skills accounted for these results, she "cured" the "hyperlexics" by use of inservice teacher training and remedial instruction. Though we

TABLE 4-2. Developmental Data for Hyperlexic Subjects

	No. of subjects	Onset of word Recognition	Handedness R	L	Both	Disorders reported
		Case Studies				
Phillips (1930)	1					Mongoloid
Scheerer, Rothmann, and Goldstein (1945)	1	Less than 4 yr			1	Idiot savant; mentally deficient; schizophrenic
Silberberg and Silberberg (1968)	4	One at 18 mo 3 unknown	2			One possibly autistic; one retarded
Cain (1969)	3					Psychotic
Goodman (1972)	1	1 yr			1	Autistic savant
Elliott and Needleman (1976)	1	15 mo				Apraxia of speech
Aram, Rose, and Horwitz (1984)	1	$4\frac{1}{2}$ yr		1		Autistic; retarded
		Descriptive Studies				
Silberberg and Silberberg (1971)	28					Anxiety disorders; hyperactive; autistic
Mehegan and Dreifuss (1972)	12	3 to 5 yr	2		10	Two psychotic; five severely mentally retarded; all language disordered
Cobrinik (1974)	6	2 to 5 yr				All severely disturbed; frequent autistic characteristics noted; schizophrenia
Richman and Kitchell (1981)	10					Hyperactive; language delayed; learning disabled; autistic
Fontenelle and Alarcon (1982)	8					Mentally retarded
		Experimental Studies				
Huttenlocher and Huttenlocher (1973)	3	One at less than 4 yr One at less than $2\frac{1}{2}$ yr One unknown	3			Autistic; schizophrenic
Healy, Aram, Horwitz, and Kessler (1982)	12	$2\frac{1}{2}$ to 4 yr	4	2	6	Mentally retarded; language delayed; behavioral disorders
Cobrinik (1982)	9	3 to 5 yr				Schizophrenic; autistic; retarded, early onset psychoses; chronic brain syndrome
Aram, Ekelman, and Healy (1984)	12	2 to $3\frac{1}{2}$ yr				Mentally retarded; autistic; language delayed
Goldberg and Rothermel (1984)	8	Seven at 4 yr One unknown				Retarded; language delayed; hyperactive; autistic

believe this case represents an inappropriate use of the term "hyperlexia," it illustrates the need for a definition that is based on more than superior word recognition alone.

The majority of clinicians and investigators describing hyperlexia are addressing a unique group of children whose reading is remarkable precisely because of significant, and typically pervasive, delays in other aspects of development. Indeed, most investigators have required both advanced word recognition and some type of developmental delay. Summary information on the developmental disorders reported among hyperlexic children is presented in Table 4-2.

In short, although some have maintained that hyperlexia be viewed as the high end of the normal word-recognition continuum, the predominant view has been that hyperlexic children are not otherwise normal. We maintain that abnormal or deficient development in other areas is as much a part of the phenomenon of hyperlexia as is advanced word recognition, and we will limit our discussion to children who demonstrate both.

The Criterion of Early Onset

A final point of dispute concerning criteria for diagnosing hyperlexia is the necessity for precocity in age of onset. As Table 4-2 shows, early word-recognition skills have often appeared in hyperlexic children—early in reference to time and to other developmental skills. Often, but not always, the fact that these children read is established during the preschool years. Reading frequently precedes other developmental milestones, notably speech. Some investigators have required preschool reading recognition for a child's inclusion in a group study (e.g., Aram, Ekelman, & Healy, 1984; Healy *et al.*, 1982), but no consensus exists as to how early reading must emerge to be considered hyperlexic. It may be that we should view age of reading onset as relative to other aspects of cognitive development; for severely impaired children, later occurrence may still be precocious in comparison to other functioning.

Nonreading Characteristics of Hyperlexic Children

The following sections summarize available information on general intellectual development, speech and language abilities, social and psychiatric status, motor skills, other special talents, academic achievement other than reading, handedness, sex, genetic/familial findings, and neurological status.

General Intellectual Development

Most studies addressing hyperlexia have provided some estimate of the children's intellectual level. Some estimates have been based on clinical judgment, for example, functioning as an "imbecile" (Phillips, 1930) or in the moderately to severely retarded range (Mehegan & Dreifuss, 1972). Many report IQs obtained using a variety of instruments, including verbal tools, nonverbal measures, or those

TABLE 4-3. Reports of Hyperlexics' Intellectual Functioning

	Measure used	IQ	Cognitive profile
		Case Studies	
Phillips (1930)	Clinical judgment	"Low grade imbecile"	Deficient in associability; inflexibility of associations
Goodman (1972)	Stanford-Binet Leiter International Performance Scale	37 86	Good visual discrimination and memory; inability to recall simple motor sequences; skill in automatic associations
Aram, Rose, and Horwitz (1984)	WISC WAIS	60s	
		Descriptive Studies	
Silberberg and Silberberg (1971)	Stanford-Binet WISC	Nontestable to 126	
Cobrinik (1974)	WISC	Full scale IQ: 47–71 Verbal IQ: 50–63 Performance IQ: 44–82	Strengths: Block Design, Similarities and Digit Span Weaknesses: Comprehension, Picture Completion, Picture Arrangement, Coding
Richman and Kitchell (1981)	WISC	Full scale IQ: 92–116 M Verbal IQ: 92.60 M Performance IQ: 110.00	Low Verbal/high Performance; all associative reasoning tests significantly lower than memory

Fontenelle and Alarcon (1982)	WISC-R WPPSI	Full Scale IQ: 57–118	For three subjects, Verbal IQ higher than Performance IQ; for four subjects, Performance IQ higher than Verbal IQ; for five subjects, spatial and visual memory higher than sequential and conceptual IQs

Experimental Studies

Huttenlocher and Huttenlocher (1973)	One subject: Stanford-Binet WISC	77	
Healy, Aram, Horwitz, and Kessler (1982)	McCarthy Scales	Verbal IQ: 104 Performance IQ: 85 62 to 91	Scores on tests of organizational relationships significantly lower than scores on repetition memory
Aram, Ekelman, and Healy (1984)	McCarthy Scales WISC-R	68 to 99	
Goldberg and Rothermel (1984)	Four subtests from WPPSI, WISC-R, and WAIS		Of four subtests, best on Block Design; profile similar to that of an autistic

F, Full; $\bar{M}$, Mean.

permitting comparison between verbal and performance abilities. Table 4-3 details the testing of intellectual skills in studies to date. While the scores evidence a considerable range, the majority of children present at least some degree of general intellectual limitation and would be classified as at least borderline or mildly mentally retarded.

Beyond overall IQ level, the available cognitive profiles obtained from IQ tests are of interest and are summarized in Table 4-3. While typically it appears that Performance IQ surpasses Verbal IQ, this has not been an invariable pattern, with reports of Verbal IQ higher than Performance IQ for some hyperlexic children (e.g., Fontenelle & Alarcon, 1982).

Other investigators have examined variability in subtest performance. Three studies looked at performance on subtests of the Wechsler Preschool and Primary Scale of Intelligence (WPPSI), the Wechsler Intelligence Scale for Children (WISC), and the Wechsler Adult Intelligence Scale (WAIS), reporting essentially compatible findings. Richman and Kitchell (1981) found their relatively higher functioning group to perform significantly lower on all categorization, associative, and reasoning subtests than on memory tests. Similarly, Cobrinik's (1974) subjects, functioning in the mentally defective range, were most successful on Block Design and Repetition of Digits and most impaired in Comprehension, Arithmetic, Picture Completion, Picture Arrangement, and Coding. Of the four subtests administered to Goldberg and Rothermel's subjects (1984) (Vocabulary, Digit Span, Sentences, Block Design, Digit Symbol, Coding, Animal House), the hyperlexics performed best on Block Design, though all scores fell below the mean of the standardization sample. These investigators remarked about the similarity to the profile of autistic children.

Finally, Healy *et al.* (1982) found relative strengths in the performance of 12 hyperlexic subjects on the McCarthy Scales of Children's Abilities in Verbal Fluency (e.g., the number of animal names that can be given in 20 seconds) Numerical Memory (digit repetition), Tapping Sequence and Block Building. They found a deficit in Number Questions, Word Knowledge (definitions), Verbal Memory II (retelling a story), Counting and Sorting, and Puzzle Solving. Scores on five repetition memory tests were significantly better than those on five tests requiring knowledge of organizational relationships. These investigators suspected a generalized cognitive deficit in forming superordinate schemata, which was not specific to the visual or auditory modality because difficulty was evidenced on both visual-performance and verbal tasks.

Despite the considerable IQ range of children studied as hyperlexics, a fairly consistent intellectual profile emerges. Strengths lie in tasks requiring perceptual or unanalyzed memory functions, regardless of whether the information is presented orally or visually. Deficits in reasoning or in drawing meaningful relationships are evident in both verbal and performance areas.

Speech and Language Abilities

Hyperlexic children often come to professional attention because of failure to develop speech and language as expected. Throughout the studies reviewed, many

TABLE 4-4. Speech and Oral Language Abilities of Hyperlexic Subjects

| | Language delay | | Reading before or coincident with speaking | Comprehension disorder | Inappropriate oral communication | | | | |
	Delayed onset	Interrupted			Echolalia	Impaired expressive language	Inappropriate personal communication	Impaired articulation	Prosodic irregularities
Case Studies									
Phillips (1930)				+					
Cain (1969)	+		+	+	+	+	+	+	+
Goodman (1972)			+	+	+	+			
Elliot and Needleman (1976)			+	−	−	+		+	
Aram, Rose, and Horowitz (1984)	7½ yr		+	+	+	+	+		+
Descriptive Studies									
Silberberg and Silberberg (1971)		+							
Mehegan and Dreifuss (1972)	+	+	+	+	+	+	+	+	+
Cobrinik (1974)	+	+	+	+	+	+	+	+	+
Richman and Kitchell (1981)				+		+			
Fontenelle and Alarcon (1982)				+	+	+			
Experimental Studies									
Huttenlocher and Huttenlocher (1973)	+	+	+	+	+	+	+	+	+
Healy, Aram, Horwtiz, and Kessler (1982)	1 to 5 yr	+	+	+	+	+	+		+
Cobrinik (1982)					+		+	+	+
Aram, Ekelman, and Healy (1984)	+	+	+	+			+		+
Goldberg and Rothermel (1984)	3 to 6 yr	+	+	+	+	+	+	+	+

Note. + present; − absent.

81

children have been initially diagnosed as language delayed or carry a diagnosis such as autism, in which language delay is one primary characteristic (see Table 4-2).

Except for Silberberg and Silberberg (1967, 1968, 1971), who do not provide information about speech and language skills, and the educators who view hyperlexia as a normal variant, all other investigators thus far have found notable speech and language abnormalities, (see Table 4-4). Repeatedly documented are delayed and interrupted language milestones, severe comprehension disorders, inappropriate oral communication, impaired articulation, and prosodic irregularities. Information pertinent to each abnormality will be reviewed briefly.

DELAYED AND INTERRUPTED LANGUAGE MILESTONES

At least three aspects of language onset are notably abnormal among hyperlexic children: delay in using single words and connected sentences; onset of using several single words, followed by complete stopping of oral language for up to several years; and onset of speech after or coincident with identification of words, spelling of words, or reading aloud.

Virtually all investigators who have reported language milestones have documented delays in using single words and, especially, connected speech (see Table 4-4). None of Goldberg and Rothermel's (1984) eight subjects began speaking before 3 years of age, and one did not begin until age 6. Subject M. D., (Aram, Rose, & Horwitz, 1984) used no speech other than "mama" and "dada," except in reading aloud, until $7\frac{1}{2}$ years. Of Healy et al.'s (1982) 12 subjects, only one developed single words appropriately at 1 year, but this subject did not begin sentences until age $4\frac{1}{2}$. Four of the 12 began using a few single words around 1 year, but then stopped talking altogether until 4 to $5\frac{1}{2}$ years, an observation noted repeatedly in the histories of hyperlexic children.

In striking contrast to normal children, several hyperlexics have demonstrated reading (word recognition) either prior to or coincident with talking. Cobrinik (1974), Goodman (1972), Elliott and Needleman (1976), Aram, Rose and Horwitz (1984), Goldberg and Rothermel (1984), and Healy et al. (1982) have all provided case examples of word recognition preceding oral language.

Even more notable than the late development of single words are the marked delays in use of connected speech. Healy et al. (1982) and Goldberg and Rothermel (1984) have provided the most extensive information regarding the onset of word combinations and sentences. Only 1 child of the 20 described in both studies used sentences before age 4. Even when sentences developed, they were often inappropriate, as detailed below in the section on Inappropriate Oral Communication.

Thus the delay in using single words and sentences, the extended periods during which children stop talking, and the unusual temporal relationship between reading and language onset all suggest an abnormal pattern of language development in hyperlexic children.

SEVERE COMPREHENSION DISORDERS

Several writers have concluded that a significant deficit in aspects of language comprehension underlies the hyperlexic child's failure to understand much of what is read. Except for performance on picture identification tasks involving single-words, all but one set of investigators (Elliott & Needleman, 1976) have found notable deficiencies when examining aural language comprehension (see Table 4-4). For example, M. D. (Aram, Rose, & Horwitz, 1984) evidenced a profound disorder of language comprehension at 39 years of age, performing between a 4- and 6-year level on a range of syntactic and lexical comprehension tasks. Cobrinik (1974) reported deficiencies on the Comprehension subtest of the WISC, as well as on the Auditory Reception subtest of the Illinois Test of Psycholinguistic Abilities (ITPA). Words describing emotional or physical states, comparative words, words requiring generalization from personal experience, or words imply- ing cause–effect relationships seem to be especially perplexing (Goodman, 1972; Healy et al., 1982; Richman & Kitchell, 1981). Richman and Kitchell concluded that hyperlexic children are deficient in their ability to comprehend and integrate language and therefore have difficulty in conceptual mediation of tasks requiring associational ability.

Likewise, Healy et al. (1982) found their subjects to be very poor in carrying out oral instructions, to perform poorly on the Grammatic Understanding subtest of the Test of Language Development (TOLD), and to be unable to extract infor- mation required for retelling a short story. They concluded that the hyperlexic children's more generalized cognitive deficit prevented their comprehension of the syntactic and semantic features of language spoken to them.

Only Elliott and Needleman (1976) have described a child, whom they term "hyperlexic," in whom language comprehension is well developed. Though this mute child clearly reads, it would appear that a significant motor–speech disorder rather than a more typical hyperlexic pattern characterizes her behavior.

In sum, it appears that a significant disorder of language comprehension, which may well reflect a more pervasive cognitive disorder, is fundamentally associated with hyperlexia.

INAPPROPRIATE ORAL COMMUNICATION

When propositional language does emerge, it is typically described as inappro- priate. Echolalia, impaired expressive grammar and use of semantic information, restrictions in initiation of spontaneous language, and limited interpersonal communication are common (Table 4-4).

Echolalia is described as a characteristic of most, but not all, hyperlexic children (see Table 4-4). For some, echolalia persisted for many years, demon- strated most dramatically by M. D., who remained echolalic at age 39 (Aram, Rose, & Horwitz, 1984). For others, echolalia was relatively short-lived or absent (e.g., Elliott & Needleman, 1976) and thus appears to be a variable finding associated with hyperlexia.

Hyperlexics have been found to be inferior in expressive syntax and in the semantic aspects of language, both on a spontaneous basis and in response to formal testing. Cobrinik (1974) and Fontenelle and Alarcon (1982) found performance on Grammatic Closure ("Here is a dress; here are two_____") and Auditory Associa- tion ("A daddy is big, a baby is_____") to be among the most deficient for subtests of the ITPA. Similarly, Healy et al. (1982) found their hyperlexics' performance on Grammatic Completion and Oral Vocabulary to be among the worst for subtests of the TOLD. Finally, Richman and Kitchell (1981) administered the Rey Auditory Verbal Learning Test (AVLT) and a sentence repetition task to their 10 high-level hyperlexics. Although the subjects demonstrated good recall for unrelated words, their pattern of recall was atypical, lacking a primacy or recency effect. In contrast to good recall of word strings, ability to repeat sentences was significantly below age norms. Failure to recall the last segments of sentences suggested to the investigators that the children approached the task as nonmeaningful rote recall, without semantic or syntactic associations to aid memory.

In addition to having a poor command of expressive language, hyperlexic children frequently fail to initiate language. For example, M. D. (Aram, Rose, & Horwitz, 1984) would respond to simple questions or commands, but would rarely initiate speech. When he did, it often related to one of his preoccupations. Similarly, Mehegan and Dreifuss (1972) noted that only 3 of their 12 hyperlexics ever developed the spontaneous use of language. Inappropriate interpersonal communication has been a universal feature among the hyperlexics we have studied and is a typical finding throughout the research.

In summary, frequent echolalia, the failure to initiate speech or to use language as interpersonal communication, and impairments in the use of expressive syntax, semantics, and pragmatics emerge as the picture of oral language among hyperlexic children.

IMPAIRED ARTICULATION

Reports of an articulation disorder are inconsistent in the studies reviewed. For some of the children described, articulation of speech sounds has been an area of relative strength, with a few developing almost overly precise patterns of articulation even after early histories of difficulty. On the other hand, some continue to present severe articulatory disorders, and at least one totally mute, hyperlexic child has been reported (Elliott & Needleman, 1976), although on other than speech grounds, the classification of this child as hyperlexic is somewhat questionable. Some have commented that speech is more precise in reading than when speaking spontaneously (Healy et al., 1982), but a well-documented study of the articulatory abilities of hyperlexic children has not appeared. At present, it appears that while an articulation defect is often found in early speech, it may not be a characteristic fundamentally associated with hyperlexia.

PROSODIC IRREGULARITIES

A range of prosodic irregularities has also been described, although no study has specifically addressed this subject. Mehegan and Dreifuss (1972) described "pallilalia" in their children, which they characterized as an increasing buildup of speech accompanied by a progressive decrease in volume, resulting in a meaningless, unintelligible jumble. Cobrinik (1982), Healy et al. (1982) and Goldberg and Rothermel (1984) likewise have commented upon impaired prosody, notably an abnormal rate of speech and intonation patterns. Some have suggested that these abnormal prosodic characteristics are evidence of a motor–speech disorder (e.g., Mehegan & Dreifuss, 1972), whereas others have suggested that they reflect a failure to comprehend and use syntactic and semantic features appropriately (e.g.,

Aram, Rose, & Horwitz, 1984). It may be that both are true, at least for some hyperlexic children.

SUMMARY

All of the hyperlexic children in the studies reviewed have been found to be aberrant in terms of the onset and development of oral language, and all present severe disorders of both aural language comprehension and oral communication. Most have been found to present prosodic irregularities, many are described as echolalic, and many present significant articulatory disorders, at least during early years. The weight of the data suggests that a significant disorder of language development, comprehension, and use is an intrinsic feature of hyperlexia.

Social and Psychiatric Status

Since Cain's (1969) and Goodman's (1972) initial case reports, studies of hyperlexic children have invariably reported psychotic or lesser degrees of disturbed social and psychiatric behavior. Generally, most disturbed behavior reported in these studies has been labeled autistic or autisticlike, but the frequency of diagnosed psychoses has varied among studies (see Table 4-2).

A variability in the incidence of psychosis reported among hyperlexic children undoubtedly reflects differences in the training and biases of professionals making the diagnoses, as well as differences in the children. There may be reluctance to use the term "autistic" as a diagnosis. Hyperlexics' social behaviors range widely, from frank autism to limited interpersonal perceptiveness and peer problems, yet all hyperlexics appear to present some degree of atypical social behavior. Healy *et al.* (1982) reported that all 12 subjects were described as difficult and puzzling children, all had difficulty in relating to peers, and all were seen as inflexible and intent on activities of their own choice. Even those who are least impaired are interpersonally unusual children, often demonstrating poor eye contact, little awareness of the listener, and limited appreciation for others' perspectives.

Motor Skills

The motor behaviors of hyperlexic children have been notable in the following respects: extremes in degree; occurrence of repetitive, stereotyped motor activity; delays in milestones of motor development; clumsiness; and difficulty in learning motor sequences.

Hyperactivity has often been described, from aimless walking around (Huttenlocher & Huttenlocher, 1973) to excessive movement that interferes with performance in other spheres. Not all hyperlexic children demonstrate excessive motor activity, however. Some have been seen as hypoactive, sitting for prolonged periods of time absorbed in books or TV, while still others seem normal in their activity level. Repetitive, stereotyped motor activities are also frequently reported but not invariably present. A history of head banging is common, as have been hand flapping, spinning, rocking, the opening and closing of doors, the switching on and off of lights, and the fingering of surfaces (Cobrinik, 1982; Healy *et al.*, 1982; Huttenlocher & Huttenlocher, 1973).

Delays in the onset of walking have been reported only for a minority of hyperlexics (Goldberg and Rothermel, 1984; Goodman, 1972; Silberberg & Silberberg, 1968), although rarely have milestones of motor development been systematically recorded. More common are delays in toileting, especially bowel control, as reported by Healy *et al.* (1982) for 10 of 12 subjects.

While the onset of gross motor milestones (other than bowel control) appears to be normal for many hyperlexic children, the inability to learn simple patterned motor sequences has repeatedly been noted (Cobrinik, 1974; Goodman, 1972; Healy *et al.*, 1982). In the Healy *et al.* (1982) study, such patterned actions as tying shoes, buttoning, zippering, and even opening doors were uniformly delayed. Cobrinik (1974) conjectured that hyperlexics' "acute apprehension of visual form emerged within the context of diffuse motor impulse and the absence of any patterned interaction with the apprehended stimuli" (p. 174). Although many hyperlexic children have well-developed fine motor skills, a subgroup who are notably clumsy demonstrate an apraxiclike disorder, which may account both for their difficulty with sequences of movements and for their articulatory disorders.

What generalizations regarding motor functions, then, apply to hyperlexic children? It appears that most, if not all, have difficulty in learning patterned motor sequences such as self-help skills. Most are delayed in toileting, especially bowel control. Beyond these characteristics, findings are variable.

Other Special Talents

Hyperlexics have demonstrated special abilities other than word recognition, yet, for some, that ability appears as the lone talent. Some hyperlexics have been date calculators (Smith, Chapter 2, this volume), whereas others have remarkable memories for specific domains of information, such as birthdays, ages, street names, makes and models of automobiles, and names and dates of Presidents (Aram, Rose, & Horwitz, 1984; Cain, 1969; Goodman, 1972; Mehegan & Dreifuss, 1972). Astonishing recall for places infrequently visited or routes infrequently taken (Cobrinik, 1974; Mehegan & Dreifuss, 1972) and exceptional musical talent in the auditory recognition of passages, sight reading, and the technical aspects of piano playing (Aram, Rose, & Horwitz, 1984) have been infrequently observed. These "special talents" appear mainly to consist of cataloging information in an area of particular interest, or of a relatively automatic, low-level association based upon frequent co-occurrence of two or more words, such as lists of states and capitals, or yellow pages filled with names of automobile dealerships.

Outside of the recognition of numbers, letters, road signs, and piano music, there are no known reports of hyperlexics learning other symbol systems.

Academic Achievement Other Than Reading

Beyond documenting that many young hyperlexics demonstrate as much interest in numbers as in letters during the early years (e.g., Goodman, 1972), few investigators have commented upon the development of mathematical skills in hyperlexic children. The few reports available suggest that simple calculations, especially addition and subtraction, may be computed quite accurately (Healy *et al.*, 1982; Huttenlocher & Huttenlocher, 1973), but that the ability to understand mathematical concepts is inevitably impaired. Both of the cited studies demonstrated the failure of hyperlexic children on Piagetian tasks of number and volume conservation, while Goldberg and Rothermel (1984) found that their hyperlexics had uniform difficulty on the Mathematical Concepts subtest of the Peabody Individual Achievement Test (PIAT). Once more, it appears that hyperlexics master relatively automatic, associational learning processes rather than those requiring relational or abstract reasoning.

Writing and drawing have rarely been mentioned, but they appear to be a variable skill, reflecting in part the inconsistent motor abilities reported. Mehegan and Dreifuss (1972) described a case in which writing was strewn randomly across a page. We have seen hyperlexics whose writing is normal, as well as one whose teacher considers it his "greatest problem." Drawing also appears to be variable. Although Cobrinik (1974) reported that four of six hyperlexics showed disorganization on the Bender-Gestalt Visual Motor Test, two were said to draw accurate, meticulously detailed scenes or copies of things seen. Personal observation suggests that even when copying is adequate, spontaneous drawing is absent; these children tend to reproduce one figure repetitively, such as an automobile or a stereotyped design. Perhaps either the motor planning or the symbolic demands of creative drawing are beyond their abilities.

Spelling has received surprisingly little documentation in these studies. DeHirsch (1971) asserted that most hyperlexics are good spellers, at least during the early school years; Sam (Goodman, 1972) was spelling the months of the year before beginning to talk. Exceptional spelling of words both forward and backward has been noted (Aram, Rose, & Horwitz, 1984), but the only systematic attempt to study the spelling of hyperlexic children is that of Goldberg and Rothermel (1984), who admnistered the Spelling subtest of the PIAT. While the performance of their eight subjects was at a relatively high level, it was restricted to a narrow range. This recognition-level test, however, does not assess the ability to spell spontaneously—an area of potential significance for understanding the reading process in hyperlexics.

Handedness

Comments noting left-handedness or ambidexterity are common in case histories of hyperlexic children, although rarely have handedness tasks been administered. For example, Mehegan and Dreifuss (1972) reported that only 2 of their 12 hyperlexics were definitely right-handed in the absence of familial histories for left-handedness, but they did not state how these observations were obtained. Healy *et al.* (1982) have reported systematically on handedness, which they have determined by using the McCarthy tasks for children and questionnaires they developed for the parents (see Table 4-2). Of their 12 children, 4 were found to be right-handed, 2 were left-handed, and 6 appeared to be ambidextrous. All 12 mothers were right-handed, but 2 fathers were left-handed and 4 were ambidextrous.

Sex

In the studies in which sex has been reported, males far exceed females. Of the 92 cases reported for whom sex has been specified, 81 have been boys and 11 have been girls, yielding a male-to-female ratio of more than 7 to 1 (refer to Table 4-1).

Genetic/Familial Findings

In their initial description, Silberberg and Silberberg (1967) stated that two sets of brothers (one set of twins) were included among their original 20 children. Likewise, Aram, Ekelman, and Healy (1984) included 2 brothers in their group of 12 hyperlexics.

Healy *et al.* (1982) are the only investigators thus far to report hyperlexics' family histories for language or reading disorders. To their surprise, 11 of the 12 presented positive histories for reading disorders on the paternal side, including 8 of 12 fathers who showed clinically significant reading problems, with no mothers reporting reading problems. Finally, 7 of the 12 hyperlexics had male or female siblings with some form of language or learning problems, of whom two were hyperlexic. These investigators concluded that hyperlexia may, in at least some cases, be genetically transmitted and that its expression may be sex-limited. Further, these findings provided additional evidence that hyperlexia may be somehow associated with dyslexia, as had previously been speculated by Benton and Pearl (1978), deHirsch (1971), and Richman and Kitchell (1981).

Neurological Status

While the complex of motor abnormalities, behavioral disorganization, and marked language and learning disorders has suggested to many that hyperlexia must reflect abnormal neurological functioning, no consistent pattern of clinical neurological findings, laboratory findings, or prenatal, perinatal, or postnatal events has thus far been identified among hyperlexic subjects.

Clinical neurological findings (beyond the motor, behavioral, and learning abnormalities we have described) have been highly variable, ranging from overt seizure disorders accompanied by abnormal deep tendon reflexes to completely normal examinations (Goldberg & Rothermel, 1984). Mehegan and Dreifuss (1972), despite documenting a range of abnormal findings, including craniostenosis and mild cranium bifidum, were able to draw site-of-lesion inferences for only one child, who had agenesis of the corpus callosum. Less globally impaired hyperlexics, reflected by IQs within the normal range, have evidenced even fewer localizing or consistent clinical indicators. For example, of the 4 of 10 Richman and Kitchell (1981) subjects referred for neurological examinations, none presented any "hard" findings.

Conventional neurological laboratory findings have been equally unproductive. While some abnormal electroencephalograms (EEGs) have been reported (Elliott & Needleman, 1976; Mehegan & Dreifuss, 1972), no consistent pattern of EEG abnormality arises. Diffuse generalized slowing, diffuse high-voltage slowing (especially in the temporoparietal leads bilaterally; Mehegan & Dreifuss, 1972), and severely abnormal spikes and waves in the left central temporal and occasionally the right temporal area (Elliott & Needleman, 1976) have all been found. Perhaps more puzzling is the fact that normal EEG and other laboratory findings have been reported for severely impaired hyperlexics (Goldberg & Rothermel, 1984), including the individual studies by Aram, Rose, and Horwitz (1984), who, despite significant retardation and autism, had reports of normal EEGs (repeated three times throughout development), a normal pneumoencephalogram, and a normal computed tomography (CT) scan. To date, we know of three CT scans on hyperlexic subjects; all have been read as normal.

Clearly, conventional laboratory findings have not identified the neurological basis for hyperlexia nor contributed much in the way of understanding the neurological mechanisms that give rise to this unusual behavior. Unfortunately, to our knowledge, none of the newer EEG techniques has yet been applied to this study.

Finally, while several authors have reported significant prenatal, perinatal, or postnatal events for hyperlexic children, histories for many are entirely negative. In short, no common picture of findings that could causally explain abnormal neurological functioning has been identified thus far.

Reading

Onset of Reading

The appearance of reading in hyperlexics has been as remarkable as the discrepancy that exists between their word recognition and reading comprehension. The age of onset, the compulsive preoccupation with reading, and the self-taught acquisition all are atypical of normal development.

As previously noted, hyperlexic children begin reading early, particularly in comparison to the onset of other developmental skills, notably speech. The vast majority of hyperlexics first demonstrate word recognition, with a striking uniformity, between $2\frac{1}{2}$ and $3\frac{1}{2}$ years of age. Although it is tempting to relate level of intellectual impairment to age of onset, in our experience the two factors do not appear to be related. A review of the studies in which age of onset has been reported is given in Table 4-2.

A compulsive preoccupation with reading sharply differentiates hyperlexic children from precocious readers who otherwise are developing normally. The total absorption in reading pervades case descriptions. For hyperlexics, reading seems to have replaced other play activities, as noted by Healy et al. (1982).

The predominantly self-taught nature of the reading is evidenced by the abruptness with which the skill seems to emerge and by the parents' surprise at its occurrence. Healy et al. (1982) explored the possibility that early reading was instigated by parents. Quite to the contrary, the desire to read rose entirely from the children. While it is quite possible that, as their children became more accomplished in reading, the parents may have encouraged them, in no case has the onset and early development been found to be related to direct teaching attempts.

How this initial untutored reading occurs is not yet understood. To date, the information available is based on fragmentary, retrospective reports since no study has directly documented the early stages of reading among hyperlexic children. Somewhat more is known about hyperlexics' reading abilities once they have become fluent readers. The following sections summarize this as yet sparse information.

Visual Perception Abilities

Highly developed word-recognition skills combined with the absence of parallel development in language and other cognitive areas have led several writers to presume that a talent in visual skills accounts for hyperlexia. Most have described hyperlexic children's early and unusual visual recognition and recall skills, reporting an unusual memory for routes traveled but once, for product names seen on TV or billboards, for program listings in the newspaper or *TV Guide*, and so forth. Nevertheless, the Silberbergs (1967) cautioned that well-developed visual perception skills seemed inconsistent; whereas some had "extremely well developed skills in visual perception, auditory perception or eidetic word imagery," some possessed "none of these skills, and some even had poorly developed visual and auditory perception" (p. 41). The sparse data available suggest that most, and perhaps all, hyperlexic children are skilled in visual perception tasks requiring visual discrimination and untransformed visual memory, but are impaired when required to make spatial judgments, complete puzzles without a prototype, solve problems, or reason on the basis of visual stimuli. Several studies reporting psychometric findings with hyperlexic children have found strength on block design tests and visual memory tasks, but deficits on picture completion, picture arrangement, coding, picture association, and picture identification tasks. Richman and Kitchell (1981) concluded that hyperlexics' memory skills are among their strongest.

Superior visual discrimination abilities have been reported in several case studies (e.g., Goodman, 1972) and have been substantiated in a recent experimental study described in the next section (Cobrinik, 1982). Healy *et al.* (1982) observed good visual discrimination, but difficulty on tasks requiring organization of patterns for either visually or auditorily presented stimuli. For example, puzzles were assembled "by matching small inner details rather than by forming the broad outline of the figure" (p. 12).

In summary, two generalizations are supported by the present data: Hyperlexics have unusually well-developed visual discrimination skills; on the other hand, their ability to conceptually organize visually derived information may be limited. Whether hyperlexics' good visual discrimination of words arises from a configurational or serial recognition strategy or from a combination of the two is still in question.

Visual Word Analysis

Two studies thus far have directly addressed visual word-analysis skills among hyperlexics. Cobrinik (1982) presented a series of degraded 7- to 9-letter familiar words to nine hyperlexic boys and ten control subjects. Despite having Binet IQs in the 42–70 range and WRAT Word Recognition scores significantly lower than the controls, the hyperlexics deciphered the incomplete words significantly faster and more accurately. The results led this investigator to suggest that configurational judgment and acute pattern recognition are responsible for hyperlexics' remarkable word recognition. Goldberg and Rothermel (1984), however, demonstrate that while pattern recognition may be acute, hyperlexics' visual scheme for orthography is abstract. In perhaps the most exhaustive battery of reading tasks yet administered to hyperlexics, these investigators included a presentation of words made visually deviant through the alteration of case (HOme), orientation $\left(\begin{smallmatrix} c \\ r \\ y \end{smallmatrix}\right)$, linearity $\left(\mathrm{lo}^{\mathrm{n}}{}_{\mathrm{g}}\right)$, and spacing (kit t en), and by the addition of plus signs $(g + o + o + d)$. Only the plus $(+)$ symbols significantly affected hyperlexics' reading speed, suggesting the availability of an abstract orthography not dependent upon any single letter form. The point in development at which an abstract orthography emerges is unknown, yet anecdotal reports frequently comment upon young hyperlexics' skill in reading upside down, backwards, in script, and in print.

Thus, for the present, though visual analysis appears to be acute among hyperlexics, the limited data available suggest that an orthographic system exists beyond simple pattern or configurational analysis.

Oral Reading

ORAL READING OF WORDS

Extraordinary oral word reading has been a key feature associated with hyperlexics. While case studies suggest that these children can read virtually any English word presented, this may not be entirely true; their extraordinary word reading may be influenced by a number of factors, including the regularity of the orthography and the frequency and imagery of the word presented.

The effect of the regularity of orthography has been examined, albeit in a limited manner, in three studies. The 39-year-old subject, M. D., described by Aram, Rose, and Horwitz (1984) was administered the 39 regular and exception words developed by Baron (1977). His few errors suggested that, although M. D. had developed a high degree of competence in following regular grapheme–phoneme correspondence rules, he also had a remarkable store of word-specific print-to-sound associations.

Aram, Ekelman, and Healy (1984) then administered both Baron's and Coltheart's regular-exceptions word lists to a group of 12 hyperlexic children. Significantly fewer errors on the regular word list than on the exceptions list again suggested reliance predominantly on phonemic regularity, with considerable variability in the use of word-specific strategies for exception words.

Finally, Goldberg and Rothermel (1984) included a task presenting ten pairs of words with inconsistent and contrasting pronunciation of identical grapheme clusters (e.g., march, monarch) and a list of 25 exception words (e.g., colonel, yacht). Again, considerable variability was shown among subjects in the ability to use word-specific strategies for exception words. This study also showed that high-frequency and high-imagery words were read most accurately. No difficulty was found in the subjects' reading of number or function words, possibly because of their high frequency.

ORAL READING OF NONWORDS

The evidence available demonstrates that most hyperlexics read nonwords with ease, although some variability is reported. The 12 hyperlexics given the Woodcock Word Attack subtest by Aram, Ekelman, and Healy (1984) fell into two groups, in part distinguished by their ability to read nonwords. Eight were essentially flawless in their reading of the 50 nonword items, all performing at a 12th-grade level, which was at least 5, and usually 7, grade levels higher than their performance on passage comprehension. In contrast, four of the hyperlexics showed an elementary knowledge of phoneme-grapheme correspondence rules, but the decoding of nonwords was more congruent with other areas of reading, and in one case was slightly below passage comprehension. Anecdotal reports have suggested that some hyperlexics have no ability to read nonwords. Clinically, we have observed one such boy, who fit the developmental characteristics of hyperlexia, was able to read a considerable number of single real words, but was completely unable to read nonwords. Since he had never mastered the reading of connected passages, his prowess in reading was much more limited than that of other hyperlexics. It may well be that a range of abilities is present among hyperlexics in their reading of nonwords, yet it appears that the majority are exceptional in this regard, and those who are not may ultimately follow a different developmental course in reading.

ANALYSIS OF ORAL READING ERRORS

While it has been reported that the majority of hyperlexic subjects read connected passages fluently, few investigators have provided specific data. Richman and Kitchell (1981) reported that their subjects' oral reading of stories on the Standard Reading Inventory was above grade level, with at least 80% word accuracy. Healy's (1982) subjects were generally accurate, but were variable in fluency and intonation on the Reading Miscue Inventory. The hyperlexic children tended to self-correct errors immediately after they occurred rather than at the end of a phrase, which is when many normal readers would self-correct, suggesting that the hyperlexics were responding to the perceptual attributes of the text rather than to the meaning. Visual or phonological errors predominated, mainly close graphic or sound substitutions. There were no semantically appropriate substitutions, again evidencing failure to read for meaning. Syntactic substitutions of similar function words did occur occasionally, suggesting at least some degree of rote-level mastery of syntax.

Goldberg and Rothermel (1984) reported an error analysis of data obtained from a variety of reading tasks, the majority involving words or word pairs. Using Patterson's (1981) scheme of error analysis, these investigators reported that nonspecific and inchoate errors were the most frequent. Of the meaningful errors, visual errors predominated when subjects were moderately familiar with the words and had other orthographically similar clusters. There was a trend toward more visual errors in short words, suggesting that direct access may have been attempted,

short-circuiting the phonological route. With exception words, however, phonological errors predominated. Semantic paralexic errors were totally absent.

Aram, Ekelman, and Healy (1984) report oral reading errors only for exception word lists. Consistent with Goldberg and Rothermel (1984), all but 11 of the
errors on exception words involved phonological regularization.

Reading Comprehension

Despite the fact that a defining feature of hyperlexia is word recognition far in
advance of reading comprehension, there is surprisingly little objective documentation of the latter. Most early writers observed that hyperlexics could easily recognize words, yet could not comprehend them (e.g., Silberberg & Silberberg, 1968),
although few provided specific information. Mehegan and Dreifuss (1972) reported
that only 1 of their 12 hyperlexics could paraphrase what was read, thus suggesting
comprehension, and only 2 of the 12 could read and then execute instructions.
Richman and Kitchell (1981) could not obtain an 80% comprehension level on the
Standard Reading Inventory until stories were presented that were considerably
below the children's oral reading level. Healy et al. (1982) reported that subjects'
reading comprehension on the second-grade-level Stanford Diagnostic Reading
Test was below the mean for the test, but within one standard deviation. The
pictures provided with the early items on this test were felt to aid these children's
performance considerably, although the degree to which they appreciate the meaning of pictures has not been examined systematically.

Only Aram, Ekelman, and Healy (1984) and Goldberg and Rothermel (1984)
have provided comparative scores for word recognition and reading comprehension
for groups of hyperlexic children. Quite surprisingly, the latter study found no
significant differences between scores on the Reading Recognition and Reading
Comprehension subtests of the PIAT, but this finding may be partially a function
of the type of test item termed "comprehension" on the PIAT, since the same
children responded correctly to only one third of the comprehension questions on
a Durrell paragraph at the grade level at which they recognized words.

Reading profiles of hyperlexic children reported by Aram, Ekelman, and
Healy (1984) may also help explain the lack of discrepancy between word recognition and comprehension for Goldberg and Rothermel's subjects. Significant differences were found between hyperlexics' performance on the Woodcock subtests
requiring single-word identification or phonetic reading of nonwords and their
ability to comprehend words or passages. As seen previously, however, individuals'
scores fell into two groups, sharply differentiated by word-decoding proficiency. It
may well be that previously, in fact, the four weaker decoders' word recognition
had exceeded their comprehension, but at the ages tested for this study (7 years 8
months to 13 years 7 months), word recognition had slowed down or, conversely,
comprehension had caught up. It may be that Goldberg and Rothermel's hyperlexics were more characteristic of the second than of the first group. In any event these
observations raise a number of questions relating to the natural history of reading
in hyperlexics (once a hyperlexic, always a hyperlexic?) and to the relationship
between their word-attack skills and comprehension. In an unpublished study,

Healy (1984) found some evidence that decoding proficiency was inversely related to hyperlexics' comprehension of an aurally presented story. Further research is needed to clarify the relationship of these abilities.

A final aspect of reading comprehension that has received considerable attention is a comparison of reading and aural comprehension. Goodman (1972) appears to be one of the first to have administered tests in both the printed and oral form with no notable differences in results. Similarly, Huttenlocher and Huttenlocher (1973) compared two hyperlexics' performance on two- and three-part directions presented aurally or printed on cards. Despite the fact that both children read the written commands easily, neither child was able to surpass the score obtained when the instructions were spoken. Aram, Rose, and Horwitz (1984) reported similar findings for the patient M. D. when the Peabody Picture Vocabulary Test was presented in the standard aural form versus via the printed word. Patient M. D.'s performances in response to the aural and written items were virtually identical, despite the fact that trials were separated by more than a month.

Healy et al. (1982) compared aural and reading comprehension for their 12 hyperlexics. Subtests from several standardized instruments were administered first auditorily, followed at least 1 week later by presentation of the identical item in writing. Despite a possible training effect, there were no significant differences except on the Grammatic Completion subtest of the TOLD, on which performance was significantly better for the visual than the auditory presentation. The investigators attributed improvement on this one subtest to the increased attention forced by reading the stimulus item as well as to the additional cues provided for accessing rotely acquired syntactic patterns. Otherwise, the uniform lack of difference between hyperlexics' aural and reading comprehension suggests that a primary language comprehension disorder underlies both.

Metalinguistic Knowledge of Reading

Limited attempts have been made to assess hyperlexics' knowledge of various aspects of the reading process. Aram, Rose, and Horwitz (1984), Aram, Ekelman, and Healy (1984), and Goldberg and Rothermel (1984) have attempted to administer lexical decision tasks. Aram, Ekelman, and Healy (1984) abandoned the attempt after repeated failures to explain the task of sorting words into "real " and "pretend" groups. Despite failures with these younger hyperlexics, Aram, Rose, and Horwitz (1984) were able to teach M. D. the lexical decision task. Of 80 words and 80 nonwords, M. D. successfully categorized 60 as "real" and 60 as "not real," failing to categorize correctly only 20 nonwords and 20 words, of which only 1 was a high-frequency word. Goldberg and Rothermel (1984) reported somewhat better success in teaching a lexical decision task with 25 real words and 25 pronounceable pseudowords. Three subjects could indicate "real" or "not," averaging 45 correct out of 50. Performance was better on high-imagery than on low-imagery words. That five subjects could not be taught the task, however, is notably atypical of children their age.

This study included a further attempt to examine metalinguistic knowledge with the same three children, having them indicate whether a grapheme or graphemic cluster had the same or different pronunciation in two different words. Though they appeared to grasp the nature of the task, a response bias toward "different" suggested that perhaps their understanding was less than perfect. Alternatively, this could suggest that they were focusing on the visual form of the words rather than on pronunciation.

These few attempts suggest either that hyperlexics have very limited metalinguistic knowledge of the processes involved in reading or that this knowledge is carried in some cognitive substrate that defies verbal labels. In many respects their seeming inability to reflect upon or analyze aspects of reading is consistent with the more general cognitive limitations discussed previously.

Explanatory Theories

Explanatory theories of hyperlexia need to address the origin of the condition—that is, what caused a child to be hyperlexic—and the processes by which fluent reading is acquired. While the cause and the process of reading in hyperlexia are certainly interrelated, they would appear to require different levels of explanation and will be treated as separate issues in this discussion.

The Cause of Hyperlexia

At least three views of the cause of hyperlexia have been proposed. Before we present our observations, we will review each of the following: (1) hyperlexia as a normal physiological variant; (2) hyperlexia as arising from aberrant psychodynamic factors; and (3) hyperlexia as a neurologically based disorder reflected in atypical cognitive development.

A NORMAL PHYSIOLOGICAL VARIANT

In Silberberg and Silberberg's initial paper (1967), the view that the hyperlexics' ability to recognize words could be seen as a normal physiological variant was only one of three possible causes outlined. The others involved a specific neurological precocity or a possible familial component. As discussed previously, however, these authors (1968, 1971) eventually came to emphasize an explanation of hyperlexia as the superior end of the normal continuum for word-recognition skills. Especially in educational circles, this view was embraced (e.g., Rawson, 1971; Tien, 1971). Tien remarked that many people can read more than they can comprehend, citing the reading of mathematical formulae or the reading aloud of foreign languages.

As a normal variant, hyperlexia might be exacerbated by the teaching method used for reading, as proposed by Niensted (1968). It is recognized that an unbalanced instructional emphasis on decoding at the expense of linguistic meaning may impede reading comprehension, but the data reviewed here strongly suggest that hyperlexia has a more complex etiology. Until we delineate the upper limits of hyperlexic children's range of functioning, however, it is quite possible that some cases of school failure in reading comprehension should be viewed relative to this syndrome.

PSYCHODYNAMIC FACTORS

Psychodynamic factors such as response to parental pressure (Kanner & Eisenberg, 1955) or reaction to a specific event (Cain, 1969) have occasionally been advanced as causes of special talents such as hyperlexia. Most who draw from psychodynamic explanations, however, also appear to incorporate some degree of acknowledgment that hyperlexic children themselves may be primarily disordered and that their disturbed behavior pattern does not necessarily originate from interpersonal or other external experiences. For example, Cain (1969), in discussing special isolated abilities in autistic children, was influenced considerably by Bergman and Escalona's (1948) views that the primary constituents for some psychotic children are intense sensitivity to and preoccupation with specific sensory stimulation. Similarly, Goodman (1972), in explaining Sam's unusual history, attributes his abnormal mental development at least in part to "a deficient motivational system which in turn may derive from an early disturbance of bodily awareness or 'inner status'" (p. 274).

ATYPICAL COGNITIVE DEVELOPMENT SECONDARY TO A NEUROLOGICAL ABNORMALITY

The majority of investigators have attributed hyperlexia to some form of abnormal neurological functioning. A few suggest that hyperlexia represents a specific "neurological precocity" (Elliott & Needleman, 1976) or a specific "physiognomic gift" (deHirsch, 1971). To most, however, hyperlexia is a cognitive *deficit* in which the few skills available are mainly associated with reading recognition. For example, Huttenlocher and Huttenlocher (1973) suggest that the language disorders and apraxic behavior associated with hyperlexia implicate a parietal lobe disorder and comment that excessive reading development may be one of the few achievements available to hyperlexics.

Mehegan and Dreifuss (1972) compared hyperlexics' behavior to "echopraxia," a condition in which a person automatically imitates another's movements. However, when such behavior was observed in adults with acquired neurological lesions, the investigators were unable to localize a site of abnormality since a range of clinical findings implicated unilateral involvement in some subjects and bilateral in others. Finally, because of the exceptionally acute pattern perception and because of similarities to autism, Cobrinik (1982) has speculated that hyperlexia may arise from right-hemisphere mediation of processes usually served by the left hemisphere.

A DEVELOPMENTAL NEUROPSYCHOLOGICAL DISORDER WITH A GENETIC PREDILECTION

Three observations on causation appear unmistakable: (1) Most, if not all, hyperlexics present an array of generally nonlocalizing symptoms associated with neurological dysfunction. (2) An overwhelming majority are male. (3) When studied, the familial incidence of language learning, and especially of reading disorders, is striking.

Most current investigators agree that hyperlexia is difficult to account for except in reference to an abnormally functioning central nervous system. However, it does not appear likely to us, for a number of reasons, that a hypothesis of right-hemisphere mediation will be borne out. Clinical neurological findings do not implicate focal deficits. Further, most hyperlexics are exceptional at verbal sequential and memory tasks as well as at visual pattern analysis, phonic segmentation, and sequencing, all of which is inconsistent with any simple left-hemisphere dysfunction hypothesis. Moreover, as Dennis, Lovett, and Wiegel-Crump (1981) have suggested in their studies of hemidecorticate children, it appears that automaticity of reading skills is mainly subserved by the left hemisphere. If one wishes to speculate about localized impairment, a more tempting hypothesis might be a deficit in some frontal lobe system, as Denckla (1983) has speculated on the basis of brain electrical activity mapping (BEAM) studies with "pure dyslexic" boys. Likewise, the pervasive finding of behaviors suggestive of attention-deficit disorders among hyperlexic children may well prove to be a significant clue. In short, the state of the art in hyperlexia permits little more than speculation about its neurological basis.

A major limitation to identifying any neurological commonalities among hyperlexics has been the limited number who have actually received neurological examinations—and the still smaller number for whom these findings have been reported in anything more than a very fragmentary manner. An absence of consistent positive findings may simply reflect a lack of looking and reporting. Conventional laboratory tests have been no more productive in identifying neurological dysfunctions among hyperlexics than they have for a variety of other developmental cognitive disorders. Until more sensitive and specialized procedures are employed—for example, measuring cerebral asymmetries on CT scans; using functionally oriented tests such as positron emission tomography (PET) scans, cerebral blood flow, or even nuclear magnetic resonance (NMR); or employing newer EEG techniques (e.g., Dawson, Warrenburg, & Fuller, 1982)—it is doubtful that much more will be learned in this area.

Even if a neurological dysfunction is eventually clarified, however, one still must explain how it occurred. Two mutually compatible possibilities seem reasonable. Some cases may have arisen from any one of a number of prenatal and perinatal events known to affect development of the central nervous system; these cases may represent a minority and may account for hyperlexia in females. For example, a hyperlexic girl with agenesis of the corpus callosum was described by Mehegan and Dreifuss (1972) as was a hyperlexic girl with microcephaly (Lebrun, Van Endert, & Szliwowski, Chapter 12, this volume). For the others, probably the majority, it would appear that genetic factors are implicated, and it may be found that the condition arises predominantly in males with a family history among male members for language learning and especially reading disorders. While these speculations need substantiation from carefully conducted family studies, our reading of the evidence points in this direction and is consistent with recent hypotheses advanced by Geschwind and Galaburda (1985).

How Hyperlexic Reading is Performed

The second question in need of an explanatory theory is how hyperlexics learn to read words in the first place and, once word recognition is mastered, how reading is accomplished thereafter. While it is possible that similar processes underlie both acquisition and accomplished reading among hyperlexics, this is not necessarily the case.

The intellectual and language findings reviewed in this chapter consistently demonstrate a pronounced cognitive deficit in most areas of language comprehension, association, and reasoning skills, as well as a failure to develop superordinate relational schemes, in contrast to relatively or exceptionally well-developed verbal memory, sequential skills, acute visual discrimination, and pattern recognition.

Huttenlocher and Huttenlocher (1973) presented a model for explaining the reading process in hyperlexics. They noted that hyperlexics' primary speech functions are intact, but that they have a marked difficulty in associating the visual and auditory schema of words with the meaningful concept of the word. Fay (1975) likewise has viewed hyperlexia as a short-circuiting of meaningful interpretation, or the "written language analogue" of echolalia.

Aram, Rose, and Horwitz (1984) interpreted M. D.'s reading performance in terms of the reading models of the acquired dyslexics presented by Marshall (1984). The patient M. D.'s pattern of adept grapheme–phoneme correspondences (Route C), combined with lesser, but nevertheless well-developed, specific whole-word print-to-sound associations (Route B) and minimally utilized lexical/semantic representation (Route A) is very similar to the acquired surface dyslexic reported by Bub (1985) and to a patient with a reading disorder secondary to dementia reported by Schwartz, Saffran, and Marin (1980). While many of the hyperlexic children are not as extreme in their abilities as M. D., all appear to underutilize the meaningful route for reading, relying predominantly on phonic or visual–configurational routes.

The relative importance of hyperlexics' use of phonetic versus visual routes for reading remains to be fully investigated. We maintain that the exceptional word-attack skills and the greater facility with regular than with exception word forms show a reliance on phonetic reading strategies. As noted previously, however, all hyperlexics do not demonstrate exceptional word-attack skill, and some may prefer the visual route. It is possible that the alternate use of visual, phonic, and linguistic strategies in reading represents a developmental progression of reading stages that is differentially achieved by hyperlexic as well as normal readers. One means of exploring this issue further might be to investigate hyperlexic's strategies for spelling regular words, exception words, and nonwords.

Returning to the question of how hyperlexics learn to read in the first place, only a few speculations are possible since no study has detailed these early stages. It would appear that, aside from intense preoccupation, the course of hyperlexics' early reading is much like that of other early readers: First, there is predominantly visual iconic processing (labels, signs, etc.) with concrete associations, and, later, repeated association with sound–symbol relationships are generalized into rules for word attack (Durkin, 1980). Considering the amount of time spent fixating on the written word, hyperlexics' automatization of phonic principles may represent paired-association learning rather than rule abstraction and generalization. Our personal observation suggests that most hyperlexics have mastered a range of word-attack strategies, including the visual recognition of common words and word parts as well as auditory segmentation, sequencing, and blending. Continued accomplished word reading, however, seems to require a combination of visual and auditory analysis skills that not all early hyperlexics possess (Healy, 1984).

The question of why these youngsters fixate on reading may be a difficult one to answer. Several investigators have suggested that it is the only skill available to them or, possibly, the only thing that makes sense to a disordered nervous system.

Directions for Further Research

Throughout this chapter we have repeatedly noted the limitations in available data and have suggested areas and ideas for further investigation. Here we will attempt to summarize these areas.

Nature of the Reading Process. First, we would consider the relative use of word-specific versus phonological strategies for lexical access. Basic but disputed is the relative dependence upon visual versus phonological strategies for word recognition. This could be investigated further through a variety of experimental tasks using regular and exception words, nonwords, homophone tasks, and so forth.

A second area of investigation would focus on the limits of meaningful reading comprehension. If most hyperlexics do not read with comprehension at the level of their word recognition, what aspects of, for example, semantic and syntactic features are understood? Nonverbal response modes for assessing comprehension might be explored. While our findings strongly point to a generalized cognitive deficit underlying the failure of meaningful interpretation across both verbal and nonverbal (e.g., Piagetian, mathematical and pragmatic) skills, the interaction of these two domains bears investigation.

Third, we would examine the process by which hyperlexics initially begin to read. While some suggest that acute pattern perception is responsible for the initial word recognition, other anecdotal information suggests incipient hyperlexics also demonstrate a fascination with letters and sound–symbol relationships. A comparison with other early, nonhyperlexic readers might clarify these strategies.

Finally, we would answer these questions: Does spelling among hyperlexics show predominantly visual or phonological strategies? How do spelling strategies parallel those used in word recognition?

Individual Differences Among Hyperlexics. While a continuum of skills may well exist for some aspects of behavior (e.g., intellectual level, social interpersonal behavior), at least two areas evidence potentially quantitative differences among hyperlexics. They are (1) the relative use of visual versus phonological strategies, and (2) the presence or absence of significant motor–speech disorders frequently referred to as apraxic-like. These two areas of differences appear central to an understanding of hyperlexia. If all hyperlexics do not read by the same route, how can these differences be explained, and how do they relate to other aspects of behavior? If significant motor–speech difficulties exist for some but not for others, is the speech delay secondary to motor rather than to language-comprehension factors? Further, how does the presence of a motor–speech disorder relate to the use of a visual versus a phonological word-recognition strategy?

The Natural History of Hyperlexia. Beyond documenting the initial stages of word recognition, several other changes over time warrant investigation. (1) Do initial word-recognition strategies persist for fluent reading? If not, how do they change? (2) Is the relative discrepancy between word recognition and reading comprehension maintained or does it change among hyperlexics, and what factors relate to this change? (3) Are there identifiable stages that are common among hyperlexic readers, and, if so, how are they related to more normal reading development? (4) What interaction, if any, exists between intellectual functioning and the continued course of hyperlexics' reading?

The Familial Incidence and Type of Language Learning and of Reading Disorders. At a minimum, family studies must be undertaken if the mode of genetic transmission is to be better understood.

The Neurological Dysfunction Underlying Hyperlexia. As evidenced in this chapter we know next to nothing about the neurological basis of hyperlexia. At least three approaches seem warranted: (1) Systematic clinical neurological examinations of a group of hyperlexics. (2) Use of more dynamic special laboratory tests, for example, ERP measures of hemispheric activation during reading, PET scans, or possibly even NMR. (3) Measurement of cerebral asymmetries from CT or NMR scans.

The Incidence and Relationship to "Normal" Comprehension Deficits. Hyperlexia research to date presents few conclusions and many questions, one of which is the frequency of the syndrome's occurrence. While it has been assumed to be a relatively rare phenomenon, extension of the upper limits for subject inclusion (e.g., Richman & Kitchell, 1981) may well produce cases of children functioning in public school classrooms without special labels, regarded only as "strange" or "puzzling," or even admired for their oral reading skills. Even if, as we believe, the condition represents an identifiable abnormality rather than an extension of normal abilities, a continuum may still exist, in which the less impaired may represent the greater diagnostic challenge. As yet, the characteristics of reading comprehension disorders have not been quantified, but the study of hyperlexia may contribute significantly to this growing field of interest.

Prognosis for Children Found To Be Hyperlexic. Professionals dealing daily [3] with parents of the "real" children behind these experimental reports need better answers to the inevitable question, "What will happen to my child?" Our clinical experience and the limited long-term perspective available from the literature (Aram, Ekelman, & Healy, 1984) suggest that differential courses may be followed, depending on several factors such as severity of intellectual impairment, quality of cognitive stimulation in the home, educational or therapeutic intervention, and, possibly, profile of cognitive abilities. Longitudinal research may help families and educational professionals as well as clarify the developmental aspects of the syndrome.

Treatment. It is not generally possible to delay a search for effective treatment strategies until a disorder is fully understood. Neuropsychologists are in a position to advise parents and educators, who usually are confounded by the anomalies that hyperlexic children present. For example, Healy (1982) recommended that young children exhibiting hyperlexic behaviors be discouraged, or even prevented, from engaging in obsessional reading by the substitution of play and concept-building activities at an appropriate sensory-motor level. While such redirection requires extensive personal supervision, we are following one case in which it has been accomplished, apparently with positive results. Similar interventions with cognitive modification procedures (e.g., Feuerstein, 1982) may at least be attempted. Further research may reveal whether hyperlexics' reading should be viewed only as a manifestation of pathology or whether this "talent" may also be used as a tool for enhancing their language communication and understanding.

References

Aram, D. M., Ekelman, B. L., & Healy, J. M. (1984, June). *Reading profiles of hyperlexic children*. Paper presented at the meeting of the International Neuropsychology Society, Aachen, West Germany.

Aram, D. M., Rose, D. F., & Horwitz, S. J. (1984). Hyperlexia: Developmental reading without meaning. In R. N. Malatesha & H. A. Whitaker (Eds.), *Dyslexia: A global issue* (pp. 517–531). The Hague: Martinus Nijhoff.

Baron, J. (1977). Mechanisms for pronouncing printed words: Use and acquisition. In D. LaBerge & S. J. Samuels (Eds.), *Basic process in reading: Perception and comprehension* (pp. 175–216) Hillsdale, NJ: Erlbaum.

Benton, A. L., & Pearl, D. P. (Eds.). (1978). *Dyslexia*. New York: Oxford University Press.

Bergman, P., & Escalona, S. K. (1948). Unusual sensitivities in very young children. *The Psychoanalytic Study of the Child, 3,* 333–354.

Bub, D., Cancelliere, A., & Kertesz, A. (1985). *Whole-word and analytic translation of spelling to sound in a non-semantic reader* (pp. 15–34) Hillsdale, NJ: Erlbaum.

Cain, A. C. (1969). Special "isolated" abilities in severely psychotic young children. *Psychiatry, 32,* 137–149.

Cobrinik, L. (1974). Unusual reading ability in severely disturbed children. *Journal of Autism and Childhood Schizophrenia, 4,* 163–175.

Cobrinik, L. (1982). The performance of hyperlexic children on an "incomplete words" task. *Neuropsychologia, 20,* 569–577.

Dawson, G., Warrenburg, S., & Fuller, P. (1982). Cerebral lateralization in individuals diagnosed as autistic in early childhood. *Brain and Language, 15,* 353–368.

deHirsch, K. (1971). Are hyperlexics dyslexics? *Journal of Special Education, 5,* 243–246.

Denckla, M. B. (1983). Learning for language and language for learning. In U. Kirk (Ed.), *Neuropsychology of language, reading, and spelling*. New York: Academic Press.

Dennis, M., Lovett, M. W., & Wiegel-Crump, C. A. (1981). Written language acquisition after left or right hemidecortication in infancy. *Brain and Language, 12,* 54–91.

Durkin, D. (1980). *Teaching young children to read*. Newton, MA: Allyn & Bacon.

Elliott, D. E., & Needleman, R. M. (1976). The syndrome of hyperlexia. *Brain and Language, 3,* 339–349.

Fay, W. H. (1975). Discussion. In L. A. Lockman, K. F. Swain, J. S. Drage, K. G. Nelson, & H. M. Marsden (Eds.), *Workshop on the neurological basis of autism* (NICDS Monograph No. 23). Washington, DC: U.S. Government Printing Office.

Feuerstein, R. (1982). *Instrumental enrichment*. Baltimore: University Park Press.

Fontenelle, S., & Alarcon, M. (1982). Hyperlexia: Precocious word recognition in developmentally delayed children. *Perceptual and Motor Skills, 55,* 247–252.

Geschwind, N., & Galaburda, A. M. (1985). Cerebral lateralization: Biological mechanisms, associations, and pathology: Parts 1, 2, & 3. A hypothesis and a program for research. *Archives of Neurology, 42,* 428–459, 521–552, 634–654.

Goldberg, T. E., & Rothermel, R. D. (1984). Hyperlexic children reading. *Brain, 107,* 757–785.

Goodman, J. (1972). A case study of an "autistic savant": Mental function in the psychotic child with markedly discrepant abilities. *Journal of Child Psychology and Psychiatry, 13,* 267–278.

Healy, J. (1982). The enigma of hyperlexia. *Reading Research Quarterly, 17,* 319–338.

Healy, J. (1984). *Auditory verbal repetition memory as a predictor of nonsense word recognition in hyperlexic children.* Unpublished manuscript.

Healy, J. M., Aram, D. M., Horwitz, S. J., & Kessler, J. W. (1982). A study of hyperlexia. *Brain and Language, 17,* 1–23.

Huttenlocher, P. R., & Huttenlocher, J. (1973). A study of children with hyperlexia. *Neurology, 23,* 1107–1116.

Jastak, J., & Jastak, S. (1965). *Wide range achievement test manual.* Wilmington, DE: Guidance Associates.

Kanner, L., & Eisenberg, L. (1955). Notes on the follow-up studies of autistic children. In P. H. Hock & J. Zubin (Eds.), *Psychopathology of childhood* (pp. 229–239) New York: Grune & Stratton.

Marshall, J. C. (1984). Toward a rational taxonomy of the developmental dyslexias. In R. N. Malatesha & H. A. Whitaker (Eds.), *Dyslexia: A global issue* (pp. 45–58). The Hague: Martinus Nijhoff.

Mehegan, C. C., & Dreifuss, M. B. (1972). Hyperlexia: Exceptional reading ability in brain-damaged children. *Neurology, 22,* 1105–1111.

Niensted, S. M. (1968). Hyperlexia: An educational disease? *Exceptional Children, 35,* 162–163.

Patterson, K. E. (1981). Neuropsychological approaches to the study of reading. *British Journal of Psychology, 72,* 151–174.

Phillips, A. (1930). Talented imbeciles. *Psychology Clinics, 18,* 246–255.

Rawson, M. B. (1971). Let's shoot for eulexia—not at hyperlexia. *Journal of Special Education, 5,* 247–252.

Richman, L. C., & Kitchell, M. D. (1981). Hyperlexia as a variant of developmental language disorder. *Brain and Language, 12,* 203–212.

Scheerer, M., Rothmann, E., & Goldstein, K. (1945). A case of "idiot savant": An experimental study of personality organization. *Psychological Monographs, 58,* 1–63.

Schwartz, M. F., Saffran, E. M., & Marin, O. S. M. (1980). Fractionating the reading process in dementia: Evidence for word-specific print-to-sound associations. In M. Coltheart, K. Patterson, & J. C. Marshall (Eds.), *Deep dyslexia* (pp. 259–269). London: Routledge & Kegan Paul.

Silberberg, N., & Silberberg, M. C. (1967). Hyperlexia: Specific word recognition skills in young children. *Exceptional Children, 34,* 41–42.

Silberberg, N., & Silberberg, M. C. (1968). Case histories in hyperlexia. *Journal of School Psychology, 7,* 3–7.

Silberberg, N. E., & Silberberg, M. C. (1971). Hyperlexia: The other end of the continuum. *Journal of Special Education, 5,* 233–242.

Tien, H. C. (1971). Hyperlexia, hypolexia, or dyslexia. *Journal of Special Education, 5,* 257–259.

5

A Neuropsychological Substrate for Talent in Second-Language Acquisition

ETA I. SCHNEIDERMAN
CHANTAL DESMARAIS

The goal of this chapter is to put forward some testable hypotheses concerning a neuropsychological basis for talent in adult second-language learning. We begin by defining talent for second-language learning and proceed to define the task of language learning within the framework of a linguistic theory of language acquisition (Chomsky, 1975, 1980, 1981). A neuropsychological substrate for talent in second-language learning is then proposed within this theoretical framework. The proposed substrate is described in terms of greater neurocognitive flexibility for talented than for untalented learners. Greater neurocognitive flexibility permits the talented learner to avoid processing second-language input via cognitive pathways that have been established for handling the first language. As a consequence, input in the second language of the talented learner is more likely to interact directly with the language properties inherent in the human mind that have been proposed within Chomsky's framework. Since access to these properties is essential to the process of language acquisition, the talented learner would be in a better position to develop an accurate grammar of the second language.

Evidence in support of the proposed hypotheses is drawn from research on child and adult acquirers and on bilinguals' psychological functioning. We conclude with suggestions for further research to validate the hypotheses.

A Definition of Talent

Truly talented second-language learners are virtually indistinguishable from native speakers of their second (or subsequent) language(s). This talent is thought to be rare in adults who begin acquiring their second language after puberty, although its actual extent is unknown. According to both an estimate by Selinker (1972) and

Eta I. Schneiderman. Department of Linguistics, University of Ottawa, Ottawa, Ontario, Canada.
Chantal Desmarais. School of Human Communication Disorders, McGill University, Montreal, Quebec, Canada.

self-report data from adult immigrants learning second languages in the United States and Israel (Seliger, Krashen, & Ladefoged, 1975), it is represented in roughly 5% of the adult population.

Although the focus of this chapter is on the minority of "talented" adults who achieve nativelike proficiency in their second language, this group likely represents an artificial division of what must essentially be a continuum of ability. Thus we acknowledge that there are probably degrees of talent among "untalented" second-language learners. That is, the attributes of the talented learner may be possessed to greater or lesser degrees by those who are apparently incapable of achieving full, nativelike proficiency in a second language.

The 5% minority who are talented achieve nativelike competence in all aspects of the second language. It is possible, however, that a greater percentage achieve nativelike competence in all the grammatical (i.e., morphological, syntactic, and semantic) aspects of the second language, but not in accent (Scovel, 1969). To date, there has been very little research on the question of whether individuals exhibit varying degrees of talent for the grammatical versus accent components of second languages. The only such study we are aware of is that of Neufeld (1980), which suggests that talent for nativelike pronunciation is separate from talent for the other aspects of language, including what he terms a nativelike appreciation of phonology.

Another rationale for separating talent in producing the phonetic elements of a second language from other aspects of the system is the existence of individuals who are excellent mimics of sound systems, but who do not necessarily show talent for other aspects of the grammar. Comedians such as Danny Kaye and Peter Sellers may be examples of this talent for production (although their language learning accomplishments remain to be researched).

Peter Sellers was well known for his ability to mimic numerous dialects of English and English spoken with various foreign accents. Witness his portrayal of the American president, a mad German scientist, and an upper-crust British officer in the Stanley Kubrick film *Dr. Strangelove or How I Learned to Stop Worrying and Love the Bomb*. Danny Kaye was famous for speaking a kind of gobbledygook or gibberish while delivering a convincing phonological impression of a variety of foreign languages.

A well-known example of someone whose grammatical talent vastly outstrips his talent for accent is Henry Kissinger, the former Secretary of State of the United States. Mr. Kissinger is an extremely accomplished speaker of English who has not shed his German accent.

Given the preceding evidence, it seems reasonable to posit at least two substrates underlying talent in second-language acquisition, one that encompasses semantic, syntactic, morphological, and passive phonological knowledge (henceforth to be referred to as "talent for grammar") and one for phonetic production (henceforth to be referred to as "talent for accent"). The thrust of this chapter will be to account for these two major components of talent in second-language learning.

It is worth noting here that the greater talent for grammar than for accent displayed by Henry Kissinger and Neufeld's subjects is probably much more common than the reverse. However, there has been a bias toward focusing on a native-like accent when discussing talent in second-language learning. This may be partially explained by native speakers' tendency to downgrade judgments of overall performance in the presence of a nonnative accent (Johansson, 1975, 1978a, 1978b, and as cited in Eisenstein, 1983; Piazza, 1980; Tardif & d'Anglejan, 1981; Varonis & Gass, 1982) or to overlook grammatical errors in the presence of a nativelike accent (Varonis & Gass, 1982). These findings concerning the effects of accent on the nativeness of a learner's speech raise the possibility that research on second-language acquisition may fail to consider a large number of individuals who possess talent for grammar but not for accent. There is also a danger of mistakenly ascribing talent for grammar to those possessing only talent for accent.

Assessment of Nativelike Abilities

A major difficulty in carrying out research on talent in second-language learning is identifying truly talented learners. Most of the research on the "good language learner" (e.g., Naiman, Frohlich, Stern, & Todesco, 1978) and on modern language aptitude (see Carroll, 1981; Carroll & Sapon, 1959; Pimsleur, 1966) has focused on successful classroom learners. Scores on classroom tests and/or standardized language achievement tests have traditionally been used to distinguish successful from unsuccessful learners (Carroll, 1981; Naiman *et al.*, 1978). To our knowledge, no research except that of Neufeld has been based on learners whose global grammatical or accent performance is judged to be nativelike. This is probably due to the lack of knowledge concerning the criteria used by native speakers for judging nativeness and fluency and to the expediency of using established testing materials. There is certainly no evidence to suggest a relationship between performance on such tests and native speakers' judgments of nativeness and fluency.

There is also no evidence that ability to do well on classroom tests is related to talent in learning second languages. Such tests are often based on discrete material that was presented in the classroom and not on an assessment of nativeness. Furthermore, some recent research suggests that certain types of instruction, such as inductive or deductive methods, are more suited to the cognitive styles of some individuals than others (see Hartnett, 1975; Krashen, Seliger, & Hartnett, 1975; Stieblich, 1983; Wesche, 1981). These factors make it difficult to assess the results of earlier classroom-based research on modern language aptitude and the qualities of the good language learner, since some instructional settings may have been prejudicial to some learners. There are even some scholars who dismiss the conscious learning of grammatical rules that generally occurs in formal instructional settings as unrepresentative of or unrelated to the unconscious process of language acquisition (see Dulay, Burt, & Krashen, 1982; Krashen, 1981).

For the purpose of this chapter, talented adult learners would be those who could pass a careful screening process in the second language. This would include judgments by native speakers of both accent and grammar, preferably independently. The talented learner's grammatical intuitions in the second language would also be compared with those of native speakers (e.g., see Adjemian & Liceras, 1984; Gass, 1980; Ioup & Kruse, 1977). In addition, second-language speech samples from the talented learner would be examined by linguists for evidence of nonnative constructions or articulatory interference.

Another factor that may be indicative of talent is the ability to acquire a language in a relatively short time. We will argue later that speed of acquisition may be a secondary outcome of talent, although not a fundamental manifestation of it. However, because speed is difficult to define, we do not include it in the screening process for talented learners.

A Necessary But Not a Sufficient Condition

Although we observe relatively few individuals who display exceptional talent in second-language learning, there may be more who possess the requisite neuropsychological substrate but who have not exploited it. One obvious reason for this would be lack of exposure (or adequate exposure) to a second language. The implications of quality and quantity of input for a model of adult talent in second-language learning are discussed later in the chapter.

Other factors that would enhance or inhibit second-language achievement are well documented in the literature on second-language learning. These include attitude, motivation, social distance, and ego-permeability (Clément, 1978; Gardner & Lambert, 1972; Guiora, Beit-Hallahmi, Brannon, Dull, & Scovel, 1972; Guiora, Brannon, & Dull, 1972; Guiora, Buchtel, Herold, Homburg, & Woken, 1983; Schumann, 1976). In a later section of this chapter, we will attempt to integrate this research into our own model of a neuropsychological substrate for second-language talent.

A Theory of Language Acquisition

To speculate on a neuropsychological substrate underlying talent for second-language acquisition, we must first define the task of second-language acquisition within a theoretical framework. The theoretical perspective on language acquisition adopted here is the one developed by Chomsky (1975, 1980, 1981) and currently held by most generative grammarians. Although the theory provides an account of first-language acquisition, cogent arguments have been made for its application to second-language learning (see Cook, 1985).

In brief, Chomsky noted that small children acquire complex grammatical forms within a relatively short time span and with only a limited set of data as input. To account for this, he posited the existence of language properties inherent in the human mind. These language properties make up what is termed "Universal Grammar," a set of general organizational principles of grammar, common to all languages, that are hypothesized to have their basis in human biology. According to Chomsky, Universal Grammar is represented in the brain as a "faculty" and as such is a "mental organ" (Chomsky, 1980).

The implementation of each of the principles of Universal Grammar may vary from language to language. The range of possible implementations of a given principle is termed a "parameter." The parameter choices within Universal Grammar are vast and allow for great variety among human languages. Each "setting" of a parameter (a particular implementation of a principle) will have wide-reaching effects in determining specific aspects of the grammar.

Word order in sentences is an example of a property of grammar likely resulting from the setting of a parameter in Universal Grammar. Although the possibilities for arranging the major lexical elements in a sentence are numerous, languages exhibit three most common, basic word orders. These are subject-verb-object (exemplified by English), subject-object-verb (exemplified by Japanese), and verb-subject-object (exemplified by Classical Arabic). Furthermore, languages place the complements of nouns either immediately before or immediately after them. One does not find languages that permit a noun at the beginning of a sentence, and its complement, such as a relative clause, at the end. Thus English grammar, in conformity with the principles of Universal Grammar, permits sentences such as 1, but rejects 2. (Linguists use an asterisk to denote an ungrammatical sentence, and that convention is adopted here.)

(1) The man who(m) I saw yesterday wore a blue coat.
(2) *The man wore a blue coat who(m) I saw yesterday.

Chomsky's theory represents all languages as having a great degree of commonality in that they are all based upon the organizing principles of Universal Grammar. The distinctions between specific languages are considered to result from differences in the implementation of these principles. Under this characterization, it is the task of the first-language learner to discover which parameter settings derived from Universal Grammar are relevant for a particular language environment. These parameter settings make up what is termed the "core grammar" of a language.

In addition to core grammar, each language contains rules that are more idiosyncratic and less strictly bound by the principles of Universal Grammar. These rules constitute "peripheral grammar." Such structures may evolve as a result of the history of a language and its speakers, through borrowings from other languages, and so forth. Rules that are less in conformity with the principles of Universal Grammar are considered to be "marked." Thus rules of peripheral grammar are generally more marked than rules of core grammar. However, within core grammar, some parameter choices may be less common (i.e., more marked) than others.

The relationship between core and peripheral grammar has not been clearly defined, and the Chomskian theory of acquisition does not yet provide a satisfactory account of the acquisition of peripheral grammar and the theory of markedness.[1]

---

1. Degree of markedness is thought to play a role in determining the order in which parameters are fixed and rules are acquired in the first language. Since unmarked rules do not deviate from the preprogrammed language principles that the child's mind possesses, they will presumably be acquired first. Children tend initially to ignore marked structures, which are, after all, more a part of peripheral grammar. They set these structures aside, presumably until they are "ready." However, order of acquisition cannot always be reliably predicted on the basis of degree of markedness (see Chomsky, 1981).

Given this uncertainty, we must essentially concern ourselves here with the acquisition of core grammar. Nonetheless, it seems plausible to assume that there are universal principles governing the structure of peripheral grammar that have yet to be discovered. Thus much of the ensuing discussion in this chapter may also turn out to be applicable to the acquisition of peripheral grammar.

An important consideration in any theory of language acquisition is the role of cognitive and physical maturation. The effect of maturation on the acquisition process is viewed as follows: The ultimate goal of the Chomskian theory of language is to account for the knowledge that native speakers have of their language. This knowledge must be described in such a way that it is "learnable." That is, an individual possessed of the principles of Universal Grammar and provided with normal language input must be able to correctly set the parameters of a language in conformity with its structure. In theory, this can be described as if it were an instantaneous event. In fact, it takes time for the system to develop. This is because language acquisition is taking place in the context of a developing and growing organism whose initial capacities to store and reproduce input are extremely limited. To cope with these limitations, the child acquirer adopts certain strategies, such as putting some structures aside while focusing on others.

In summary, the theory of first-language acquisition outlined here claims that language acquisition is an automatic process triggered by the confrontation between Universal Grammar and the language input that children receive from their environment. Children take several years to set the basic parameters of their first language because the input can be exploited only as cognitive and physical development permit.

If this theory of acquisition applies to second-language acquisition, then the adult with access to Universal Grammar and exposure to language stimuli should proceed through the acquisition process without the constraints imposed by cognitive and physical immaturity. However, it has been suggested that the adult's cognitive and physical maturity is not necessarily a positive factor in acquisition.

In fact, various explanations centering around neuropsychological or cognitive maturity, to which we will return later, have been offered for the apparent loss of capacity to achieve nativelike competence in second languages after puberty (Krashen, 1973; 1975; Lenneberg, 1967; Penfield, 1965; Scovel, 1969). These tend to account for the 95% of the population who lack exceptional talent, but none is satisfactory with respect to the 5% who are the focus of this chapter. We will endeavor to account for those talented individuals within the framework of the theory of acquisition presented here.

A Neuropsychological Perspective on the Child Acquirer

In this section we will outline those characteristics of children acquiring their first language that could be extended to the neuropsychological profile of talented adult second-language learners. The assumption underlying this approach is that all normal children are talented in learning a first language because all normal children eventually master one.[2]

To accomplish this task, children must select from among an extremely large but finite number of grammars permitted by the principles of Universal Grammar. Because children have no prior knowledge of the specific language they are about to acquire, they are initially open to all the possibilities that Universal Grammar permits. But as they begin fixing parameters, the structures of their developing grammars become increasingly refined, thereby constraining and restricting the selection process.

Another way to view the fixing of parameters is in terms of the fixing of neural pathways that encode and decode language stimuli. Once these pathways are formed, corresponding processing strategies will be adopted. As the child matures, these strategies will be further refined, and the ultimate outcome will be a mature grammar that relies primarily on the shortest and most efficient processing routes. Thus the process of acquisition is one of a reduction of possibilities, both in terms of parameter settings and processing routes as strategies. In the initial stages of acquisition, the child can be viewed as maximally flexible. As the first language develops, flexibility gives way in favor of the fixing of a grammar and the establishment of corresponding processing strategies.

Talent and Flexibility in Second-Language Acquisition

Grammar

The mechanism described in the preceding paragraph is a reasonable, efficient, and economical way to function. It is natural to rely on processing shortcuts in performing recurring cognitive tasks. The major disadvantage of such a strategy lies in not being flexible enough, in a neurocognitive sense, to bypass the established system and its strategies when they are inappropriate to incoming stimuli. We argue that this is the case for most adult second-language learners. That is, they may be tempted to try to process second-language input as if it were part of the first-language system rather than independent of it. This puts them at a tremendous disadvantage since, according to the Chomskian theory of acquisition, the parameters of a grammar can only be set through the direct interaction of relevant language data with unconscious knowledge of the principles of Universal Grammar. If the Chomskian theory of acquisition applies to second languages, then the structures of a first language could not mediate in the process of second-language acquisition (Cook, 1985). For example, if a first language has set a particular

---

2. Above-average intelligence is not required for successful first-language acquisition. Nor is it necessary to be at an advanced level of cognitive development. All normally developing children begin to speak within their first 2 years, and, somewhere between the ages of 3 and 5, they have set almost all the parameters of the grammar of their first language. Many mentally retarded children also acquire language. Therefore, except for the most severely handicapped children, being at one end or the other of the intelligence continuum does not appear to significantly affect the process of acquiring a first language.

parameter such that its sentence word order is subject-object-verb, the first-language grammar could not mediate in the learning of a second language with a verb-subject-object order.

Where parameters in the first and second language are set similarly, it might appear that mediation via the first language is possible. However, certain aspects of the second-language grammar may be virtually impossible to acquire in this manner. Such an outcome is suggested by research on the acquisition of relative clauses by French-speaking learners of Spanish as a second language (Adjemian & Liceras, 1984). Although French and Spanish are very similar with respect to the parameter settings affecting relativization, even advanced French learners of Spanish experienced problems with the selection of certain Spanish relativizers.

We are not arguing here that untalented learners are inherently incapable of resetting parameters in the sense that the principles of Universal Grammar are not available to them. Rather, they lack the neurocognitive flexibility to avoid established pathways early on in the acquisition process. On the other hand, neurocognitively flexible, talented learners have an extraordinary capacity to initiate new strategies or processing pathways when faced with novel cognitive tasks.

This difference between talented and untalented learners may be observable in their second-language acquisition strategies as well as in their performance on a number of first-language-related tasks. For example, untalented learners may commit more interference errors than talented learners. Krashen (1981) suggests that interference errors are more common in the early stages of acquisition, when learners, lacking structures in the second language, resort to first-language structures to express themselves in the second language. This behavior should be more prevalent in, and should last longer for, untalented learners.

Another observable difference between talented and untalented learners that would result from varying degrees of flexibility in dealing with novel language material would be speed of acquisition. The flexible learner would be less likely to head off in an unfruitful direction and would consequently achieve more accurate representation of the second-language grammar in less time. Although there is, as yet, little documented evidence concerning the relative speed of acquisition of talented versus less talented second-language learners, there is abundant anecdotal evidence of talented learners who appear to pick up languages in only a matter of weeks.[3] Furthermore, as a consequence of being "slow," the untalented learner may experience more frustration during the acquisition process, which might negatively influence ultimate second-language achievement by creating attitudinal problems. All the factors cited in the preceding paragraphs may contribute to lack of progress, or "fossilization," which is commonly reported for (untalented) adult second-language learners.

The kinds of differences we would expect between talented and untalented learners in performing certain cognitive tasks in their first language are discussed in later sections of this chapter.

---

3. It is unclear, however, on what these impressions are based. They may, for example, be based on skill in reproducing the second-language accent or in acquiring certain communicatively useful routines (see Dulay *et al.*, 1982). As was noted earlier, there is experimental evidence that a good accent upgrades native speakers' judgments so that syntactic errors are less readily noticed (Varonis & Gass, 1982).

Flexibility in Adults Versus Children

We have argued that the talented second-language acquirer has more of the necessary neurocognitive flexibility than the untalented acquirer to resist the temptation of employing existing strategies for processing the first language and is thus more open to establishing the parameters of the second language. First-language learners have the necessary flexibility almost by default.[4] Child second-language acquirers seem to have more of it than most adults, probably because prepubescent children are still undergoing cognitive changes that will lead to further fixing of the neural pathways that represent the most efficient processing of the first language.

This child–adult difference in flexibility is illustrated by research on phonetic perception indicating that adults and older children are less able to discriminate between speech sounds than infants when these sounds are not distinctive in the older subjects' first language (Trehub, 1976; Werker, Gilbert, Humphrey, & Tees, 1981; Williams, 1979) and that adults discriminate on the basis of the phonetic categories of their first language (Broselow, Hurtig, & Ringen, 1983; Goto, 1971; Horibe & Furuhashi, 1974; Miyawaki, et al., 1975; Scholes, 1968; see Strange & Jenkins, 1978, for a review). Trehub points out that we would normally expect adults to outperform children on perceptual tasks. She suggests that "language-specific experience might provoke the ultimate loss of discriminative capacity with respect to nonfunctional phonetic distinctions" (Trehub, 1976, p. 471). We would predict that the talented second-language acquirer, as a result of neurocognitive flexibility, would maintain a level of discriminative capacity similar to that of young children. Furthermore, although the child–adult differences just cited are restricted to the phonetic aspects of language, it may be possible, in the future, to design studies that deal with other components of the linguistic system.

In comparing the talented adult second-language learner to the child first-language learner, we are assuming that the mechanisms for language acquisition outlined within the Chomskian framework are equally applicable to the adult. We take this to be the most parsimonious position on this issue, since the final product is the same in both cases (see Macnamara, 1976). There are also findings from a number of studies indicating that children and adults go through essentially the same stages in acquiring various linguistic forms (see Dulay et al., 1982, Chapter 6, for a review). Moreover, given that the principles of Universal Grammar apply to all languages and that they are represented in the brain as a mental organ for language, it is difficult to imagine how the

---

4. Flexibility as it is used here is not to be confused with the plasticity of function that permits the young child's brain to compensate for the loss of certain function-specific areas of cortex in the event of brain damage. Such plasticity is believed to account for the absence of permanent aphasia after left-hemisphere damage in children (Basser, 1962; Dennis, 1980; Dennis & Kohn, 1975; Dennis & Whitaker, 1976; Milner, 1974; Rasmussen & Milner, 1977; White, 1961) and for the remarkable linguistic achievements of young hemidecorticates (Dennis, 1980; Dennis & Kohn, 1975; Dennis & Whitaker, 1976).

knowledge of a grammar of a specific language could be arrived at without utilizing these principles.[5]

To reiterate, then, we are claiming that, because of their neurocognitive flexibility, both child and talented adult language learners have direct access to the principles of Universal Grammar and, when provided with adequate language input, can set the parameters of a language. Because they lack the necessary flexibility, untalented adult language learners are less able to set new parameters correctly. This at least partially accounts for the inability of untalented adults to attain nativelike fluency in a second language.

Accent

The neurocognitive flexibility just described is meant to account for grammatical talent in second-language learning. That is, it accounts for the setting of parameters for all aspects of the grammar except phonetic production, or accent, which, we have argued, constitutes a separate component of talent.

A similar case can be made for flexibility as the construct underlying talent for accent. Flexibility for accent would be manifested in terms of the motor pathways or programs that are established to control articulatory movements in the first language. Those with this neuromuscular flexibility would be freer to establish new pathways to control articulation and achieve nativelike production in the sound system of the target language. Those who are less flexible would tend to employ the existing pathways whose output most closely resembles the phonetic forms of the target language. Thus a speaker of English might produce a high back rounded vowel (such as [u] in "boot" or [ʊ] in "put") as the closest approximation to the high front-rounded French vowel [ü] (as in the French pronoun *tu*).

Children are still in the process of forming the neuromuscular pathways for their first language. Consequently, they may be inherently more flexible than adults with respect to articulation in a second language. What we cannot yet explain is why more individuals appear to retain the flexibility necessary for acquiring the grammatical components of a second language than for acquiring the accent.

This difficulty may be partially explained by evidence that the temptation to use existing motor pathways is probably a very strong one. For example, a tendency has been shown for fluent bilinguals to average phonetic production values over their two languages (see Obler, 1982). However, such averaging can only be detected through the use of sophisticated acoustic measurement techniques, and even linguists are otherwise unable to detect it (L. K. Obler, personal communication, October, 1985). Thus fluent bilinguals make a slight accommodation to some

---

5. Some authors have suggested, however, that adults have alternative second-language-learning strategies, such as conscious rule learning, monitor use (Krashen, 1981), and a general problem-solving cognitive system (Felix, 1981, 1985). These strategies involve mechanisms of conscious learning unavailable to children, since they are based on a degree of cognitive maturity normally not arrived at until puberty. Neither Krashen nor Felix equates the product of such learning with the knowledge of grammar described by Chomskian theory. Krashen holds that conscious rule learning is separate and independent from true acquisition, while both Felix and Krashen suggest that adult learners may rely on these conscious mechanisms to the detriment of the unconscious process of acquisition.

principle of economy for the two systems, but not enough of one to compromise the nativeness of their accent in either language.[6]

Alternative Explanations for Talent

Although we have suggested that a type of neurocognitive and neuromuscular flexibility accounts for the difference between talented and untalented adult acquirers, there are, of course, other possible explanations within the framework of the Chomskian theory of acquisition. In the following paragraphs, we argue that the three foremost of these could not adequately account for talent in second-language learning.

One alternative explanation for adult talent in second-language learning is that for most untalented individuals the principles of Universal Grammar are no longer available after the parameters of a first language have been set. In other words, the principles of Universal Grammar become the primary mechanisms of storage and processing for the parameters of the grammar they served to set. This theory is untenable, since it prohibits any language acquisition beyond about age 5, when most parameters of the first language have presumably been set. Thus it would contradict the widely held belief, based on long-standing observation, that most children up until 12 or 14 years of age are talented at second-language acquisition (see Lenneberg, 1967; Penfield, 1965; Scovel, 1969). Furthermore, this explanation puts even the simultaneous acquisition of two first languages into question, since it would be impossible for the principles of Universal Grammar to become the primary mechanisms of storage and processing for two different sets of parameters.

A second, related possibility is that, as they mature, the brains of untalented learners lose access to the underlying principles of Universal Grammar. This would have to be based on some by-product of the maturation process and is akin to the notion of a "critical period" for language acquisition, ending at the onset of puberty (Lenneberg, 1967; Penfield, 1965). We reject this explanation because it implies that talented second-language acquirers never achieve full neural maturity. We would expect this to have far-reaching consequences for cognitive capacity, which seem unreasonable and unnecessary to consider at this point.

Another possible explanation for second-language talent, which was alluded to in an earlier section of this chapter, concerns the quality and quantity of input required by talented individuals. Dulay *et al.* (1982), among others, have argued that adult learners are hampered by inappropriate second-language input. Such input is characterized by a lack of sensitivity to the learner's need for simple, concrete, contextually bound discourse. Children, on the other hand, are generally thought to be provided with good, comprehensible input. This would suggest that talented adult learners may be able to make do with less input than untalented learners. However, there is also ample anecdotal evidence to suggest that years of

---

6. This notion of economy may apply to bilinguals' grammars as well, but as yet there is little research on the grammatical intuitions of bilinguals to support it.

exposure make no difference for the apparently untalented learner. Thus we reject the make-do-with-less explanation as not having sufficient explanatory power to account for talent.

Input, Speed, and Talent

Given the inadequacy of the three alternative explanations just discussed, we maintain that the notion of flexibility proposed in this chapter provides the best account of talent in second-language learning. However, we do not reject the possibility that the ability to make do with less input may be an indirect consequence of language-learning talent in adults.

Within the framework of the Chomskian theory of language acquisition, the language learner requires access to Universal Grammar and exposure to language input to trigger the formation of a specific grammar. As was noted previously, the talented adult learner is not hampered in this process by cognitive and physical immaturity, which undoubtedly places severe limitations on the amount of language input that the young child can process and retain. Consequently, the talented adult learner may be capable of exploiting input more thoroughly than the child and may require less of it.

This child–adult difference in cognitive development may also result in talented adults' being faster language learners than very young children. As tentative support for such a hypothesis, we can again cite anecdotal reports of talented adults who appear to acquire new languages in a matter of weeks. Further support is provided by studies comparing adult and child second-language learners. Although the results of these studies are contradictory, some researchers report that adult (postpubescent) learners are initially faster than children (Ervin-Tripp, 1974; Fathman, 1975; Snow & Hoefnagel, 1978). Others report the reverse (Magiste, 1986; Yamada, Takatsuka, Kotake, & Kurusu, 1980). Unfortunately, most of these studies deal only with the beginning stages of learning and do not relate ultimate attainment to initial speed.

Correlates of Talent in Neurological Organization

In this section we speculate on how the flexibility required for successful learning of a second-language grammar might be manifested in terms of neurological organization in its grossest sense. That is, we explore this issue in terms of degree of left-laterality for language.

It is well known and widely accepted that language, for the majority of right-handed adults, is processed primarily in the left cerebral hemisphere (see Lecours & L'Hermitte, 1979, Chapter 2). The first-language linguistic abilities of the mature right hemisphere are thought to be severely restricted compared to those of the left (see Millar & Whitaker, 1983; Schneiderman, 1986; Searlemann, 1977; E. Zaidel, 1973). However, there is also evidence (cited later) to support a more prominent role for the right hemisphere in the acquisition of language as well as in other complex cognitive systems such as reading and music. This evidence can be viewed in terms of structural differences between the two hemispheres that underlie a right-hemisphere advantage in the apprehension of novel stimuli across various modalities (Goldberg & Costa, 1981). Goldberg and Costa describe the process of learning as being heavily dependent on the right hemisphere's preponderance of interareal connections and on the greater proportion of associative cortex in the right than in the left hemisphere (Polyakov, 1966; cited in Goldberg & Costa, 1981). Within this model, the left hemisphere plays a major role in storing and operating the descriptive systems (or task-specific cognitive strategies) formed during the learning process.

In support of this view, Goldberg and Costa cite studies in which subjects exhibited right-hemisphere dominance during early exposure to novel stimuli and in which increasing familiarity with those stimuli corresponded with a shift to left-hemisphere dominance. These include a face-recognition task (Reynolds & Jeeves, 1978), verbal naming of unfamiliar visual symbols (Gordon & Carmon, 1976), and dichotically presented musical sounds (Kallman & Corballis, 1975) and musical patterns (Spellacy, 1970). There are also studies in which a left-hemisphere advantage for trained musicians contrasted with a right-hemisphere advantage for subjects who were musically naive (Bever & Chiarello, 1974; Johnson, 1977). Similarly, a stronger right-ear advantage for Morse code has been reported for experienced Morse code operators than for naive subjects (Papcun, Krashen, Terbeek, Remington, & Harshman, 1974).

In addition to the studies cited by Goldberg and Costa, there is both clinical and experimental evidence of greater right-hemisphere processsing of language in bilinguals and second-language acquirers than in monolinguals (for reviews see Albert & Obler, 1978; Galloway, 1982; Obler, 1981; Schneiderman, 1986; Vaid, 1983; Vaid & Genesee, 1980). For instance, there are studies where bilinguals were shown to be more left-lateralized in their first language than in their second (Gaziel, Obler, Bentin, & Albert, 1977; Maitre, 1974; Obler, Albert, & Gordon, 1975; Schneiderman & Wesche, 1983; Silverberg, Bentin, Gaziel, Obler, & Albert, 1979; Sussman, Franklin, & Simon, 1982; Sewell & Panou, 1983). Other studies report proficient bilinguals to be more left-lateralized in their second language than were nonproficient bilinguals (Gaziel et al., 1977; Obler et al., 1975; Silverberg et al., 1979; Wesche & Schneiderman, 1982). All of the preceding findings suggest that the right hemisphere plays a major role in the acquisition of various skills and knowledge, including language, which are then organized into left-hemisphere-based descriptive systems.

It is our contention that a descriptive system for language is essentially a set of highly efficient processing strategies based on the neural networks, which are activated when the parameters of a particular language are set. The organization of the left hemisphere may make it particularly well suited for the storage and operation of such processing strategies (Goldberg & Costa, 1981). However, inasmuch as these strategies may generally simplify and possibly speed up the cognitive task of language processing, they may also reduce the average speaker's unconscious tendency to seek out or utilize alternative processing strategies. Only a few, flexible individuals may tend to process in a more open-ended manner. That is, they may be more apt to rely on the right hemisphere to develop apparently unusual or innovative strategies in carrying out various language-related tasks. Such persons would also likely be better second-language learners, since, as was noted previously, an ability to bypass established first-language processing modes may permit second-language input to interact directly with the properties of Universal Grammar. This would result in the correct setting of parameters in the second language.

We have discussed the predominantly left-hemisphere-based descriptive system for language proposed by Goldberg and Costa (1981), which we presume to exist for all speakers of a language. We have also hypothesized additional right-hemisphere-based flexibility for language processing in talented second-language learners. It therefore would seem reasonable to assume that talented learners are utilizing a proportionally greater amount of cortex for language functioning than untalented learners. Since this additional cortex would be located in the right hemisphere, talented learners may appear to be less left-lateralized for language than individuals who are less flexible and consequently less talented for second-language learning. Indirect support for this hypothesis comes from research linking divergent thinking ability and right-hemisphere dominance for language (Tegano, Fu, & Moran, 1983).

There is other, more indirect evidence for the view that talent in second-language learning and a more bilateral pattern of representation for language are related. A number of lay beliefs single out two groups, children and females, as having greater than average talent in second-language learning (see Naiman et al., 1978). Although the research evidence is somewhat contradictory, both these groups are generally believed to be less left-lateralized for language than the "norm" (Bryden, 1979; Segalowitz & Bryden, 1983; Witelson, 1976; 1977). Interestingly, the norm for laterality is based on right-handed, monolingual adult males, who, according to the lay beliefs about second-language learning, are generally thought to be less talented than women.[7] Furthermore, C. J. (the talented learner studied by Novoa, Fein, & Obler, Chapter 15, this volume) is predominantly left-handed, and left-handers as a group have also been shown to be less left-lateralized for language than the norm (Corballis, 1983; Segalowitz & Bryden, 1983; Witelson, 1980).

Cognitive Consequences of Flexibility

Along with its obvious advantages for second-language learning, flexibility may carry with it some less desirable cognitive consequences. We have argued that those who are talented in second-language learning use a greater than average proportion of right cortex for language functions. This may affect performance in tasks normally associated with the right hemisphere, the most predominant of which can be subsumed under the heading of visuo-spatial abilities. Thus the talented second-language learner may exhibit mild to severe visuo-spatial disabilities such as would

---

7. Some indirect evidence in support of the lay belief in female superiority for language learning is found in studies of language aptitude in high school students (Carroll & Sapon, 1959; Naiman et al., 1978; Powell, 1979).

be evidenced in tests of mental rotation of figures, figure–ground relations, and orientation in space. Novoa, Fein, and Obler's (Chapter 15, this volume) subject, C. J., supports this view. He did relatively poorly on tests of visuo-spatial ability and reports himself to be "inadequate in skills relating to directionality and spatial orientation" (Novoa et al., p. 294). These researchers also note that C. J. relies on verbal strategies to perform nonverbal tasks.

Essentially, we are presenting a compensatory model, in which greater abilities in one area could result in weaker abilities in another, or in which a weakness is compensated for elsewhere by a particular strength or talent. Another type of compensatory model as it relates to dyslexia is discussed in a recent article by Geschwind and Galaburda (1985). As noted in the introduction to this volume, Geschwind and Galaburda present a rather complex argument for which there is very little direct experimental support. They suggest that there may be " a 'pathology of superiority,' that is, compensatory growth leading to superior development of some portions of the brain as a result of poorer development of others" (Geschwind & Galaburda, 1985, p. 522).

These compensatory models imply a causal relationship between certain exceptional abilities and disabilities, such as C. J.'s language-learning and visuo-spatial abilities. Clearly, further experimental and clinical results would be required to support such a claim.

Flexibility and Bilingualism in Children

Indirect evidence for the construct of neurocognitive flexibility is provided by research indicating that early childhood bilinguals enjoy certain cognitive advantages over monolingual children (see Bain & Yu, 1978; Balkan, 1970; Cummins, 1978; Feldman & Shen, 1971; Hakuta, 1983; Landry, 1974; McLaughlin, 1978). For example, bilingual children exhibited superior performance over monolingual children on "discover the rule" problems (Bain & Yu, 1978) and on tests of divergent thinking that focused on aspects of cognitive functioning such as fluency, flexibility, and originality (Balkan, 1970; Feldman & Shen, 1971; Landry, 1974).

Landry interpreted his data as evidence that bilingual children, in overcoming the influence of "negative transfer" (or interference) from the first language into the second, had acquired a kind of resistance to negative transfer in general. He concluded that they had a "flexibility set," which is advantageous in divergent thinking tasks where one must be inventive and original.

If we account for language acquisition in terms of parameter theory, we can view the cognitive advantages of childhood bilingualism as resulting from the setting of different parameters in the two languages. When faced at an early age with the necessity of setting up alternative neural pathways and processing strategies for incoming language data, the child may be generally less inclined to rely on more fixed and rigid strategies for a number of cognitive tasks. As a result, the child becomes more flexible. Thus these findings provide some support for the argument linking the setting of parameters with flexibility and further suggest that the effects may be bidirectional. The bidirectionality could also apply to adults, in that the setting of new parameters may result in enhanced flexibility. This would partially account for the lay belief that the more languages one knows, the easier it is to learn new ones (e.g., see Naiman *et al.*, 1978).

The effect of bilingualism on cognitive flexibility in children raises two further questions. The first is whether such flexibility gained in childhood is carried through to maturity. The second concerns the manner in which individuals not exposed to second languages in childhood might cultivate and retain their childhood flexibility into adulthood. Both of these questions could be addressed through empirical investigation.[8]

Affective Factors and Flexibility

In an earlier section of this chapter, affective factors such as attitude, motivation, and ego-permeability were cited as necessary for the exploitation of the neuropsychological substrate for language-learning talent in adults. For example, a positive relationship has been demonstrated between success in second-language learning and the learner's favorable attitude toward the speakers of the second language. This attitude comprises factors such as an integrative motivation toward the group speaking the second language, lack of ethnocentrism, and minimal social distance between the two groups (Clément, 1978; Gardner & Lambert, 1972; Schumann, 1976).

Ego-permeability has been cited more specifically as an important prerequisite for acquiring a nativelike accent in a second language (Guiora, Beit-Hallahmi, Brannon, Dull, & Scovel, 1972; Guiora, Brannon, & Dull, 1972; Guiora *et al.*, 1983). That is, empathic learners are presumably able to extend the boundaries of their egos to include the new identity that is implied by sounding like a native speaker of another language. This view is supported by sociolinguistic research that provides evidence for the relationship between social identity and accent (see Biondi, 1975; Labov, 1972). Conversely, it has been suggested that some learners may choose to retain a foreign accent because of a certain social prestige it accords them (Hill, 1970) or in order to provide themselves with an excuse to fall back on should they make a sociolinguistic (Ervin-Tripp, 1972) or grammatical error (Dulay *et al.*, 1982).

The child in a foreign language environment is more likely than the adult to acquire the second-language grammar and a nativelike accent. The child is also more likely to succeed at social integration. Children are probably under greater social pressure than adults to integrate, and this may partially explain the child's superior success rate (McLaughlin, 1978). In addition, we presume that the child has more of the neuromuscular flexibility necessary for producing a nativelike accent in the second language.

It is also possible that the process of acculturation involves the establishment of neurocognitive structures for sociocultural identity and belief systems. These

---

8. Balkan's (1970) findings with subjects aged 11 through 17 provide some indication that bilingual children do retain their advantage.

neurocognitive structures most likely share universal properties cross-culturally and probably resemble those established for the grammar of a language. Thus it is possible that a type of neurocognitive flexibility underlies exceptional ease at adapting to novel sociocultural and belief systems. Children are still forming the pathways for these systems and would be inherently more flexible in that regard.

Guiora *et al.* (1983) have already suggested that there is a right-hemisphere-based neuropsychological substrate underlying ego-permeability. Future research might provide further links between the right hemisphere and this proposed substrate for positive attitudes and motivation in second-language learning.

Suggestions for Further Research

In this chapter we have argued that the neuropsychological substrate underlying talent for second-language learning manifests itself in terms of several types of flexibility. Neurocognitively flexible individuals do not necessarily rely on a single set of predominant pathways for language-related processing but use, instead, a variety of processing strategies and associated neural pathways. Thus neurocognitive flexibility allows the learner to handle novel input in a way that is free of the grammar of the first language, which was formed based on the parameters of that language. The learner can then directly access Universal Grammar to set the parameters of the second language. The notion of flexibility was also applied to the neuromuscular pathways that are set to govern articulation in the first language and that must be reset for subsequent languages. The positive affective factors that facilitate language learning may also be dependent on a similar type of sociocultural flexibility. When these three types of flexibility converge in an individual who has adequate exposure to a second language, the result is nativelike acquisition of that language.

Although we have not defined the setting of parameters in specific neurophysiological terms, such as the activation of various groups of neurons, future techniques for brain research may eventually allow us to test such a claim and to examine more directly the performance of other cognitive tasks by talented and untalented learners. Until then, our hypotheses concerning flexibility must be tested by using more indirect types of measures.

Supporting our hypotheses concerning the talented learner would involve administering a variety of tests to both talented and untalented second-language learners. These would focus on cognitive and articulatory flexibility with respect to unfamiliar language input as well as to various first-language-related tasks. The battery would include tests of visuo-spatial ability, measures of laterality, tests of phonetic perception, tests of grammatical intuition, and tests of such affective factors as ethnocentrism and ego-permeability. It would also be interesting to examine performance on certain more traditional types of aptitude tests that are reported to be good predictors of second-language accent (see Carroll, 1981). These include tests of phonetic mimicry and phonetic coding ability.

With the exception of visuo-spatial ability, we would generally expect talented learners to outperform untalented learners on the preceding tests. In some cases we may observe other types of differences. For example, in a test of phonetic perception, in addition to finding that talented learners may be unusually sensitive to unfamiliar phonetic distinctions, we would expect them to demonstrate a broader spectral range for a given phoneme in their first language than is normally reported for monolingual speakers (see Obler, 1982).

In evaluating any test results, it would be as important to look at the strategies employed as at the final scores. Rather than adopt conventional strategies in carrying out a variety of tasks, the flexible individual may employ idiosyncratic and possibly less direct processing routes. This could have detrimental effects, such as slower speed on certain tasks and lack of conventionality of responses. Both these factors would tend to lower scores on standardly scored tests (Carroll, 1983). Flexible individuals might also employ a variety of strategies in performing a task but arrive at the same response as those who are less flexible. Furthermore, flexible individuals may be perfectly capable of using, and willing to employ, more conventional strategies in performing various tasks. Thus personality attributes could independently affect results. For example, on several occasions, C. J. (Novoa, Fein, and Obler's subject) reiterated that he has always made an effort to be different and unique in his behavior. It is difficult to judge whether this is an accommodation to his inherent flexibility or an attempt on his part to enhance or emphasize it. We would also expect to find talented learners to exhibit superior memory for unfamiliar items, advantages in verbal over nonverbal or visuo-spatial skills, and a less left-lateralized than normal substrate for language.

Another possible avenue of investigation is to compare the profile of the talented learner with that of the bilingual child in terms of the cognitive flexibility and other advantages that bilingual children exhibit over monolinguals. Additional questions would be whether such flexibility attained in childhood carries over into adulthood and whether there are degrees of flexibility that correlate with degrees of second-language talent.

Acknowledgments

We are grateful to Loraine Obler and Deborah Fein for encouraging us to embark on this project. We would also like to express our appreciation to Patricia Balcom, Christian Adjemian, and Douglas Saddy for their critical comments on an earlier draft of this paper, although the ideas expressed here do not necessarily reflect their own points of view.

References

Adjemian, C., & Liceras, J. (1984). Accounting for adult acquisition of relative clauses: Universal Grammar, L1, and structuring the intake. In F. R. Eckman, L. H. Bell, & D. Nelson (Eds.), *Universals of second language acquisition* (pp. 101–118). Rowley, MA: Newbury House.

Albert, M., & Obler, L. (1978). *The bilingual brain: Neuropsychological and neurolinguistic aspects of bilingualism*. New York: Academic Press.

Bain, B., & Yu, A. (1978). Toward an integration of Piaget and Vygotsky: A cross-cultural replication (France, Germany, Canada) concerning cognitive consequences of bilinguality. In M. Paradis (Ed.), *Aspects of bilingualism* (pp. 113–126). Columbia, SC: Hornbeam Press.

Balkan, L. (1970). *Les effets du bilingualisme français-anglais sur les aptitudes intellectuelles.* Brussels: AIMAV.

Basser, L. S. (1962). Hemiplegia of early onset and the faculty of speech with special reference to the effects of hemispherectomy. *Brain, 85,* 427–460.

Bever, T. G., & Chiarello, K. (1974). Cerebral dominance in musicians and non-musicians. *Science, 185,* 537–539.

Biondi, S. J. (1975). *The Italian-American child: His sociolinguistic acculturation.* Washington, DC: Georgetown University Press.

Broselow, E., Hurtig, R. R., & Ringen, C. (1983, August). *The perception of second language prosody.* Paper presented at the Tenth International Congress of Phonetic Sciences, Utrecht, The Netherlands.

Bryden, M. P. (1979). Evidence for sex-related differences in cerebral organization. In M. Wittig & A. C. Petersen (Eds.), *Sex-related differences in cognitive functioning: Developmental issues* (pp. 121–143). New York: Academic Press.

Carroll, J. B. (1981). Twenty-five years of research on foreign language aptitude. In K. C. Diller (Ed.), *Individual differences & universals in language learning aptitude* (pp. 83–118). Rowley, MA: Newbury House.

Carroll, J. B. (1983). Studying individual differences in cognitive abilities: Through and beyond factor analysis. In R. F. Dillon & F. F. Schmeck (Eds.), *Individual differences in cognition* (Vol. 1, pp. 1–33). New York: Academic Press.

Carroll, J. B., & Sapon, S. M. (1959) *Modern language aptitude test, Form A.* New York: The Psychological Corporation.

Chomsky, N. (1975). *Reflections on language.* London: Temple Smith.

Chomsky, N. (1980). *Rules and representations.* Oxford: Blackwell.

Chomsky, N. (1981). *Lectures on government and binding.* Dordrecht, Holland: Foris Publications.

Clément, R. (1978). *Motivational characteristics of Francophones learning English.* Quebec City: International Centre for Research on Bilingualism, Laval University.

Cook, V. J. (1985). Chomsky's universal grammar and second language learning. *Applied Linguistics, 6*(1), 2–18.

Corballis, M. C. (1983). *Human laterality.* New York: Academic Press.

Cummins, J. (1978). Metalinguistic development of children in bilingual education programs: Data from Irish and Canadian Ukrainian-English programs. In M. Paradis (Ed.), *Aspects of bilingualism* (pp. 127–138). Columbia, SC: Hornbeam Press.

Dennis, M. (1980). Language acquisition in a single hemisphere: Semantic organization. In D. Caplan (Ed.), *Biological studies of mental processes* (pp. 159–186). Cambridge, MA: The MIT Press.

Dennis, M., & Kohn, B. (1975). Comprehension of syntax in infantile hemiplegics after cerebral hemidecortication: Left hemisphere superiority. *Brain and Language, 2,* 472–482.

Dennis, M., & Whitaker, H. A. (1976). Language acquisition following hemidecortication: Linguistic superiority of the left over the right hemisphere. *Brain and Language, 3,* 404–433.

Dulay, H., Burt, M., & Krashen, S. (1982). *Language two.* New York: Oxford University Press.

Eisenstein, M. (1983). Native reactions to non-native speech: A review of empirical research. *Studies in Second Language Acquisition, 5*(2), 160–176.

Ervin-Tripp, S. (1972). On sociolinguistic rules: Alternation and co-occurrence. In J. J. Gumperz & D. Hymes (Eds.), *Directions in socio-linguistics, the ethnography of communication* (pp. 213–250). New York: Holt, Rinehart & Winston.

Ervin-Tripp, S. (1974). Is second language learning like the first? *TESOL Quarterly, 8,* 111–127.

Fathman, A. (1975). Language background, age and the order of acquisition of English structures. In M. Burt & H. Dulay (Eds.), *New directions in second language learning, teaching, and bilingual education* (pp. 33–43). Washington DC: Teachers of English to Speakers of Other Languages

Feldman, C., & Shen, M. (1971). Some language-related cognitive advantages of bilingual 5-year-olds. *Journal of Genetic Psychology, 118,* 235–244.

Felix, S. (1981). *Competing cognitive structures in second language acquisition.* Paper presented at the First European–North American Workshop on Cross-Linguistic Second Language Acquisition Research. Los Angeles.

Felix, S. (1985). More evidence on competing cognitive systems. *Second Language Research, 1,* 47–72.

Galloway, L. M. (1982). Bilingualism: Neuropsychological considerations. *Journal of Research and Development in Education, 15*(3), 12–28.

Gardner, R. C., & Lambert, W. E. (1972). *Attitudes and motivation in second-language learning.* Rowley, MA: Newbury House.

Gass, S. (1980). An investigation of syntactic transfer in adult second language learners. In R. C. Scarcella & S. D. Krashen (Eds.), *Research in second language acquisition: Acquisition research forum* (pp. 132–141). Rowley, MA: Newbury House.

Gaziel, T., Obler, L., Bentin, S., & Albert, M. (1977, October). *The dynamics of lateralization in second language learning: Sex and proficiency effects.* Paper presented at Boston University Conference on Language Development, Boston.

Geschwind, N., & Galaburda, A. M. (1985). Cerebral lateralization: Biological mechanisms, associations, and pathology. 2. A hypothesis and a program for research. *Archives of Neurology, 42,* 521–552.

Goldberg, E., & Costa, L. D. (1981). Hemisphere differences in the acquisition and use of descriptive systems. *Brain and Language, 14,* 144–173.

Gordon, H., & Carmon, A. (1976). Transfer of dominance in speed of verbal response to visually presented stimuli from right to left hemisphere. *Perception and Motor Skills, 42,* 1091–1100.

Goto, H. (1971). Auditory perception by normal Japanese adults of the sounds "L" and "R." *Neuropsychologia, 9,* 317–323.

Guiora, A., Beit-Hallahmi, B., Brannon, R., Dull, C., & Scovel, T. (1972). The effects of experimentally induced changes in ego states on pronunciation ability in a second language: An exploratory study. *Comprehensive Psychiatry, 13,* 421–428.

Guiora, A., Brannon, R., & Dull, C. (1972). Empathy and second language learning. *Language Learning, 22,* 111–130.

Guiora, A., Buchtel, H., Herold, A., Homburg, T., & Woken, M. (1983, March). *Right "hemisphericity" and pronunication in a foreign language.* Paper presented at Teachers of English to Speakers of Other Languages '83, Toronto.

Hakuta, K. (1983). New methodologies for studying the relationship of bilingualism and cognitive flexibility. *TESOL Quarterly, 17,* 679–681.

Hartnett, D. D. (1975). *The relation of cognitive style and hemisphere preference to deductive and inductive second language learning.* Unpublished master's thesis, University of California at Los Angeles, Los Angeles.

Hill, J. H. (1970). Foreign accents, language acquisition, and cerebral dominance revisited. *Language Learning, 20,* 237–248.

Horibe, N., & Furuhashi, S. (1974). Hierarchy of aural perception difficulties at several levels of English teaching. *JACET Bulletin, 5,* 87–106.

Ioup, G., & Kruse, A. (1977). Interference versus structural complexity as a predictor of second language relative clause acquisition. In *Proceedings of the Second Language Acquisition Forum* (pp. 48–60). University of California at Los Angeles, Los Angeles. ERICED 176579.

Johansson, S. (1975). *Papers in contrastive linguistics and language testing*. Lund Studies in English 50.

Johansson, S. (1978a). *Studies of error gravity: Native reactions to errors produced by Swedish learners of English*. Gothenburg Studies in English 44.

Johansson, S. (1978b). Problems in studying the communicative effects of learners' errors. *Studies in Second Language Acquisition, 1,* 41–52.

Johnson, P. R. (1977). Dichotically-stimulated ear differences in musicians and non-musicians. *Cortex, 13,* 385–389.

Kallman, H. W., & Corballis, M. C. (1975). Ear asymmetry in reaction time to musical sounds. *Perception and Psychophysics, 17*(4), 368–370.

Klatzky, R. L. (1975). *Human memory: Structures and processes*. San Francisco: W. H. Freeman.

Krashen, S. (1973). Lateralization, language learning and the critical period: Some new evidence. *Language Learning, 23,* 63–74.

Krashen, S. (1975). The development of cerebral dominance and language learning: More new evidence. In D. Dato (Ed.), *Developmental psycholinguistics: Theory and applications* (pp. 209–233). Washington, DC: Georgetown University Press.

Krashen, S. (1981). *Second language acquisition and second language learning*. Oxford: Pergamon Press.

Krashen, S. D., Seliger, H. W., & Hartnett, D. D. (1975). Two studies in adult second language learning. *Kritikon Litterarum, 3,* 220–227.

Labov, W. (1972). *Sociolinguistic patterns*. Philadelphia: University of Pennsylvania Press.

Landry, R. G. (1974). A comparison of 2nd-language learners and monlinguals on divergent thinking tasks at the elementary school level. *Modern Language Journal, 58,* 10–15.

Lecours, A. R., & L'Hermitte, F. (1979). *L'aphasie*. Paris: Flammarion.

Lenneberg, E. (1967). *Biological foundations of language*. New York: Wiley.

Macnamara, J. (1976). Comparison between first and second language learning. *Die Neueren Sprachen, 25*(2), 175–188.

Magiste, E. (1986). Special issues in second and third language learning. In J. Vaid (Ed.), *Language processing in bilinguals: Psycholinguistic and neuropsychological perspectives* (pp. 97–122). Hillsdale, NJ: Erlbaum.

Maitre, S. (1974). *On the representation of second language in the brain*. Unpublished master's thesis, University of California at Los Angeles, Los Angeles.

McLaughlin, B. (1978). *Second-language acquisition in childhood*. Hillsdale, NJ: Erlbaum.

Millar, J. M., & Whitaker, H. A. (1983). The right hemisphere's contribution to language: A review of the evidence from brain-damaged subjects. In S. J. Segalowitz (Ed.), *Language Functions and Brain Organization* (pp. 87–113). New York: Academic Press.

Milner, B. (1974). Functional recovery after lesions of the nervous system, 3. Developmental processes in neural plasticity. Sparing of language functions after early unilateral brain damage. *Neuroscience Research Program Bulletin, 12,* 213–217.

Miyawaki, K., Strange, W., Verbrugge, R., Liberman, A. M., Jenkins, J. J., & Fujimura, O. (1975). An effect of linguistic experience: The discrimination of [r] and [l] by native speakers of Japanese and English. *Perception & Psychophysics, 18*(5), 331–340.

Naiman, N., Frohlich, M., Stern, H., & Todesco, A. (1978). *The good language learner*. The Ontario Institute for Studies in Education, 7.

Neufeld, G. G., (1980). On the adult's ability to acquire phonology. *TESOL Quarterly, 14,* 285–298.

Obler, L. K. (1981). Right hemisphere participation in second language acquisition. In K. Diller (Ed.), *Individual differences & universals in language learning aptitude* (pp. 53–64). Rowley, MA: Newbury House.

Obler, L. K. (1982). The parsimonious bilingual. In L. K. Obler & L. Menn (Eds.), *Exceptional language and linguistics* (pp. 339–346). New York: Academic Press.

Obler, L. K., Albert, M., & Gordon, H. (1975). *Asymmetry of cerebral dominance in Hebrew-English bilinguals.* Paper presented at the Thirteenth Annual Meeting of the Academy of Aphasia, Victoria, Canada.

Papcun, G., Krashen, S., Terbeek, D., Remington, R., & Harshman, R. (1974). Is the left hemisphere specialized for speech, language and/or something else? *Journal of the Acoustical Society of America, 55,* 319–327.

Penfield, W. (1965). Conditioning the uncommitted cortex for language learning. *Brain, 88*(4), 787–798.

Piazza, L. (1980). French tolerance for grammatical errors made by Americans. *The Modern Language Journal, 64,* 422–427.

Pimsleur, P. (1966). *The Pimsleur language aptitude battery.* New York: Harcourt Brace Jovanovich.

Polyakov, G. (1966). Modern data on the structural organization of the cerebral cortex. In A. R. Luria (Ed.), *Higher cortical functions in man* (pp. 39–69). New York: Basic Books.

Powell, R. C. (1979). Sex differences and language learning: A review of the evidence. *Audio Visual Language Journal, 17,* 19–24.

Rasmussen, T., & Milner, B. (1977). The role of early left-brain injury in determining lateralization of cerebral speech functions. In S .J. Diamond & D. A. Blizard (Eds.), *Evolution and lateralization of the brain. Annals of the New York Academy of Sciences, 229,* 355–369.

Reynolds, D. M., & Jeeves, M. A. (1978). A developmental study of hemisphere specialization for recognition of faces in normal subjects. *Cortex, 14,* 511–520.

Schneiderman, E. I. (1986). Leaning to the right: Some thoughts on hemisphere involvement in language acquisition. In J. Vaid (Ed.), *Language processing in bilinguals: Psycholinguistic and neuropsychological perspectives.* (pp. 233–251). Hillsdale, NJ: Erlbaum.

Schneiderman, E. I., & Wesche, M. B. (1983). The role of the right hemisphere in second language acquisition. In K. M. Bailey, M. H. Long, & S. Peck (Eds.), *Second language acquisition studies* (pp. 162–174). Rowley, MA: Newbury House.

Scholes, R. J. (1968). Phonemic interference as a perceptual phenomenon. *Language and Speech, 11,* 86–103.

Schumann, J. (1976). Social distance as a factor in second language acquisition. *Language Learning, 26,* 135–143.

Scovel, T. (1969). Foreign accents, language acquisition, and cerebral dominance. *Language Learning, 19,* 245–254.

Searlemann, A. (1977). A review of right hemisphere linguistic capabilities. *Psychological Bulletin, 84*(3), 503–528.

Segalowitz, S. J., & Bryden, M. P. (1983). Individual differences in hemispheric representation of language. In S. J. Segalowitz (Ed.), *Language functions and brain organization* (pp. 341–372). New York: Academic Press.

Seliger, H., Krashen, S., & Ladefoged, P. (1975). Maturational constraints in the acquisition of a native-like accent in second language learning. *Language Sciences, 36,* 20–22.

Selinker, L. (1972). Interlanguage. *International Review of Applied Linguistics, 10,* 209–231.

Sewell, D. F., & Panou L. (1983). Visual field asymmetries for verbal and dot localization tasks in monolingual and bilingual subjects. *Brain and Language, 18*(1), 28–34.

Silverberg, R., Bentin, S., Gaziel, T., Obler, L. K., & Albert, M. L. (1979). Shift of visual field preference for English words in native Hebrew speakers. *Brain and Language, 11,* 99–105.

Snow, C., & Hoefnagel-Hohle, M. (1978). Age difference in second language acquisition. In E. Hatch (Ed.), *Second language acquisition* (pp. 333–344). Rowley, MA: Newbury House.

Spellacy, F. (1970). Lateral preferences in the identification of patterned stimuli. *Journal of the Acoustical Society of America, 47*(2), 574–578.

Stieblich, C. (1983). *Language learning: A study on cognitive style, lateral eye-movement and deductive vs. inductive learning of foreign language structures.* Unpublished doctoral dissertation, McGill University, Montreal.

Strange, W., & Jenkins, J. J. (1978). Role of linguistic experience in the perception of speech. In R. D. Walk & H. L. Pick, Jr. (Eds.), *Perception and experience* (pp. 125–169). New York: Plenum.

Sussman, H., Franklin, P., & Simon, T. (1982). Bilingual speech: Bilateral control? *Brain and Language, 15,* 125–142.

Tardif, C., & d'Anglejan, A. (1981). Les erreurs en français langue seconde et leurs effets sur la communication orale. *Canadian Modern Language Review, 37,* 706–723.

Tegano, D. W., Fu, V. R., & Moran, J. D. (1983). Divergent thinking and hemispheric dominance for language function among preschool children. *Perceptual and Motor Skills, 56,* 691–698.

Trehub, S. E. (1976). The discrimination of foreign speech contrasts by infants and adults. *Child Development, 47,* 466–472.

Vaid, J. (1983). Bilingualism and brain lateralization. In S. J. Segalowitz (Ed.), *Language functions and brain organization* (pp. 315–339). New York: Academic Press.

Vaid, J., & Genesee, F. (1980). Neuropsychological approaches to bilingualism: A critical review. *Canadian Journal of Psychology, 34,* 417–445.

Varonis, E. M., & Gass, S. (1982). The comprehensibility of non-native speech. *Studies in Second Language Acquisition, 4*(2), 114–136.

Werker, J. F., Gilbert, J. H. V., Humphrey, K., & Tees, R. C. (1981). Developmental aspects of cross-language speech perception. *Child Development, 52,* 349–355.

Wesche, M. B. (1981). Language aptitude measures in streaming, matching students with methods, and diagnosis of learning problems. In K. C. Diller (Ed.), *Individual differences & universals in language learning aptitude* (pp. 119–154). Rowley, MA: Newbury House.

Wesche, M. B., & Schneiderman, E. I. (1982). Language lateralization in adult bilinguals. *Studies in Second Language Acquisition, 4*(2), 153–169.

White, H. (1961). Cerebral hemispherectomy in the treatment of infantile hemiplegia. *Confinia Neurologica, 21,* 1–50.

Williams, L. (1979). The modification of speech perception and production in second-language learning. *Perception & Psychophysics, 26*(2), 95–104.

Witelson, S. F. (1976). Sex and the single hemisphere: Specialization of the right hemisphere for spatial processing. *Science, 193,* 425–427.

Witelson, S. F. (1977). Early hemisphere specialization and interhemispheric plasticity: An empirical and theoretical review. In S. J. Segalowitz & F. A. Gruber (Eds.), *Language development and neurological theory* (pp. 149–158). New York: Academic Press.

Witelson, S. F. (1980). Neuroanatomical asymmetry in left-handers: A review and implications for functional asymmetry. In J. Herron (Ed.), *Neuropsychology of left-handedness* (pp. 79–113). New York: Academic Press.

Yamada, J., Takatsuka, S., Kotake, N., & Kurusu, J. (1980). On the optimum age for teaching foreign vocabulary to children. *International Review of Applied Linguistics, 28,* 245–247.

Zaidel, E. (1973). *Linguistic competenece and related functions in the right hemisphere of man following commissurotomy and hemispherectomy.* Unpublished doctoral dissertation, California Institute of Technology, Pasadena.

6

The Varieties of Musical Talent

Tedd Judd

Overview of Musical Talent

Lateralization of Music

"What a musician! She must have an exceptional right hemisphere!" This type of remark is being heard with increasing frequency. It reflects a widespread belief that music is a function of the right cerebral hemisphere and that this knowledge is somehow fundamental to our understanding of music and the brain. It seems appropriate, therefore, to begin this chapter with a discussion of the lateralization of musical abilities in the brain.

In 1895 Edgren reviewed 50 cases of amusia, that is, acquired neurological disorders of musical abilities. He compared amusia to aphasia, that is, acquired disorders of language. He concluded that, though amusia and aphasia did not always coincide, amusia, like aphasia, resulted from left-hemisphere damage and that music therefore was a left-hemisphere function. But in 1898 Ludwig Mann published a case of a singer who had suffered a traumatic injury to the posterior, inferior part of the right frontal lobe and who was left unable to sing or whistle accurately. Four similar cases came out of World War I, tempting some investigators to conclude that music was a right-hemisphere function. Then in 1920 Henschen reviewed more than 300 cases in which music had been investigated. Only the 5 already mentioned involved unilateral right-hemisphere damage and no aphasia. He concluded that music was a left-hemisphere function. Consequently, in 1935 Weisenburg and McBride were able to write, "The older supposition that music depended largely on the right hemisphere . . . has been discarded" (p. 117).

In 1962, however, Brenda Milner demonstrated an acquired impairment in tonal memory and timbre discrimination in patients undergoing right, but not left, anterior temporal lobectomy. Around the same time, the dichotic listening technique was developed for the inferential study of brain lateralization in normal individuals. In 1964 in a dichotic listening experiment with normal persons, Doreen Kimura found a left-ear, or presumed right-hemisphere, advantage in identifying excerpts of baroque music. There followed the widespread belief that

Tedd Judd. Department of Psychiatry and Behavioral Medicine, Pacific Medical Center, Seattle, Washington.

music was a right-hemisphere function. Then in 1974 Bever and Chiarello demonstrated a right-ear, or presumed left-hemisphere, advantage on a monotic musical task with trained choirboys, thus shuttling music once again across the corpus callosum into the left hemisphere, at least for "musicians." This result held the promise of resolving the contradictions in the literature to that point. Unfortunately, several subsequent studies failed to replicate this result or replicated it only in part (Reineke, 1982; Zatorre, 1984).

From this brief review it should be clear that the search for the cerebral hemisphere to which music is lateralized is misguided. Similarly, musical talent cannot be accounted for by a presumption of an exceptional cerebral hemisphere, right or left. Rather, it appears likely that the whole brain is involved in music, with different areas making their own characteristic contributions. But to better understand those contributions and their relationships to talent, we need a better understanding of the nature of musical skills and behaviors, and for this we must turn to psychomusicology.

The Psychology of Musical Abilities

Many different skills are involved in musicality. They range from fairly discrete and musically specific skills such as absolute pitch, through more general, but largely musical, skills such as pitch discrimination, melodic memory and harmonic analysis, to skills such as complex motor planning, rhythmic abilities, and social judgment, which are included in musical behaviors but are also involved in many nonmusical activities. But our understanding of musical talent is hindered by the lack of any adequate theory of musical abilities. What might such a theory look like? To begin with, we would want to have a description, catalog, or classification of musical behaviors that would define our domain of interest. We would also need a catalog or classification of musical skills.

We would then need to determine the connections between the skills and the behaviors. Which combinations of skills are necessary and sufficient for accomplishing which behaviors? Which skills are critical and which are peripheral? What are the different ways in which a given musical activity can be carried out? It is especially within this domain of empirical research that neuropsychology can make its distinctive contribution.

Figure 6-1 illustrates, facetiously, one small piece of what such a theory of musical abilities might look like. We can come to understand the problems and complexities involved in constructing such a theory by examining two of the musical activities and their component skills in a little more detail (Table 6-1).

Consider the component tasks involved in playing the lead marimba in an African marimba band.[1] The music comes from an entirely aural (unwritten) tradition. Each section of each piece consists of a short (2–20 seconds) repeated pattern, with each marimba playing a different part. The lead starts with a given melody and

---

1. I chose this example for two reasons. One is that the psychology of music suffers from an overreliance on examples from Western classical music. The other reason is that the example is familiar to me, since I play in an African-style marimba band and studied marimba with Dumi Maraire of Zimbabwe.

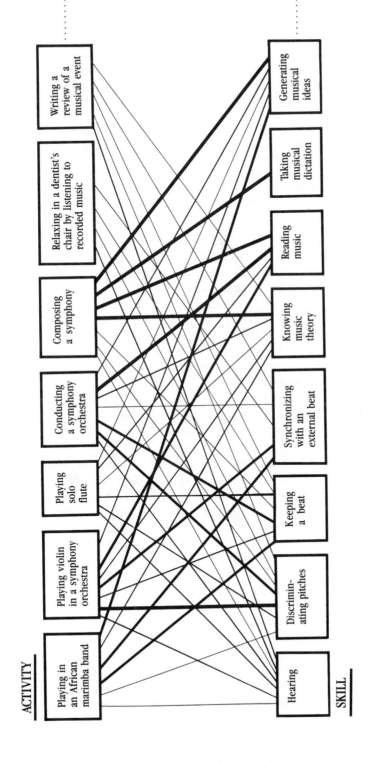

FIGURE 6-1. What a theory of musical behaviors might look like.

ACTIVITY

Writing a review of a musical event

Relaxing in a dentist's chair by listening to recorded music

Composing a symphony

Conducting a symphony orchestra

Playing solo flute

Playing violin in a symphony orchestra

Playing in an African marimba band

SKILL

Generating musical ideas

Taking musical dictation

Reading music

Knowing music theory

Synchronizing with an external beat

Keeping a beat

Discriminating pitches

Hearing

129

TABLE 6-1. Comparison of Skills Involved in Two Musical Activities

Playing lead marimba in an African marimba band	Playing violin in a symphony orchestra
Listen to the band and coordinate with it, especially rhythmically	Listen to the orchestra and coordinate with it, especially on intonation and dynamics
Maintain and manipulate tempo	Follow the conductor
Remember and produce the patterns and structure of the piece	Read the music
Plan and play variations	Minimize variations
Alter the piece according to the performance of the other players and the response of the crowd	Ignore the audience—accept coordination from the conductor and the score
Maintain excitement (much facial expression, body movement, whistling, shouting, singing)	Maintain decorum (modest body language)

plays variations on that melody, making incremental changes with each repetition, developing that melody and moving through several other predetermined melodies involving different pitch ranges of the instrument. The other instruments play variations that respond to the variations of the lead. As part of the development of the piece, the lead plays various musical signals that move the piece from one section to another and then end it. Thus the lead player must listen to the entire band and coordinate with it. The lead is also responsible for maintaining and manipulating the tempo. The lead must remember the patterns and structure of the piece, and plan and play variations in accordance with that structure and the rules of the music. The lead must listen to the band in order to adapt variations to its playing, avoiding cross rhythms when the band is not well coordinated, extending variations to which the band responds well, and so forth. The dancing, clapping, whistling, and other responses of the crowd must also be attended to and responded to by the lead in the development of the piece.

To keep all of this going, the lead might rely on extensive rehearsal in order to establish a fairly fixed development of the piece, with little deviation from one performance to another. Another strategy is to develop a large repertoire of possible variations to chose from. Still another strategy is to be fairly spontaneous, inventing new variations on the spot. The structure can be remembered with varying degrees of help from auditory, kinesthetic, visual, and verbal memory. Listening to the rest of the band requires a periodic allocation of attention away from the task of playing and planning, along with a certain ability to be distracted by deviations from the expected. Maintaining tempo would appear to involve kinesthetic and/or auditory memory in addition to sensitivity to change in tempo.

By contrast, a violinist playing in a symphony orchestra need not give much attention to remembering a piece or its structure, since it is all written down. The demands on maintaining tempo and rhythmic coordination with the rest of the orchestra are much lower than for the lead marimba player, since the conductor and the score are doing much of that work. The violinist must, however, maintain a visual-motor or visual-auditory coordination. The violinist must also work constantly at staying in tune, which is not necessary for the marimba player because the marimba is a fixed-pitch instrument. Reading the music from the page is also required (although some apparently make up for poor reading skills by memorizing the music). In reading the music, a wide array of strategies is possible. A given note might be read more or less directly—this visual display corresponds to this hand action—or it might go through any of the following intermediate internal representations: the note might be thought of as part of a larger pattern, such as a run or a chord; it might be read by its letter name and then played; it might be read in terms of its harmonic function; or it might be read as an auditory image of the note. It might also be read in terms of its position relative to neighboring notes (Judd, 1979; Judd, Gardner, & Geschwind, 1980, 1983; Sloboda, 1978).

We can see from these two examples that what appear superficially to be similar activities—playing a marimba and playing a violin in an ensemble—actually involve very different skills, which depend upon the musical culture, the instrument, and the individual. Each of these behaviors, then, involves a vast array of component skills and alternative strategies. When we consider the variety of behaviors to be accounted for, the enormousness of the task of developing a theory of musical talent becomes more understandable.

So far, most research on musical abilities has focused on efforts to determine what are basic musical skills—those that can be reliably defined, tested, and distinguished from one another. The usual experimental approach to this task involves giving a large variety of musical ability tests to a population of subjects and performing a factor analysis on the results. There have been several attempts to do this, which have primarily emphasized auditory receptive abilities and the more specifically musical skills (see Shuter-Dyson & Gabriel, 1981, for a review). The results are not entirely consistent, but they point toward separate factors involving pitch discrimination, tonal memory, rhythmic abilities, and comprehension of such complex relationships as harmony and form.

The Neuropsychology of Musical Abilities

Neuropsychology, as Obler and Fein (Chapter 1, this volume) assert, is good at telling us about dissociations—what skills are not necessary to carrying out a given activity. Through experiments of nature in cases of brain damage and other conditions, we can hope to discover dissociations among musical skills that can tell us some things about how those skills and activities are organized in the brain. One way in which such a program can be carried out is illustrated in the case study that follows (Judd, 1979; Judd, Arslanian, Davidson, Locke, & Mickel, 1979).

A CASE STUDY

The patient was a 51-year-old, right-handed male university professor of music and a composer who, 10 years prior to our investigation, suffered an innominate artery occlusion as a complication of surgery for an aneurism in the subclavian artery. He showed a left hemiplegia, which soon resolved except for the arm; a left hemisensory deficit, and a left visual neglect, although visual fields were full. A CT scan obtained 8 years after his stroke revealed a large right frontoparietal lesion and a separate right posterior temporal lesion. Despite some lethargy, he resumed teaching music 3 months after the stroke, and in a year he took up conducting an orchestra again. Over the next several years, he spent three summers in Europe and learned two foreign languages while he was there. In the few years preceding our investigation, he wrote a music theory textbook containing many original musical examples.

Despite these accomplishments, he complained to his neurologist of a variety of problems. He had trouble following the logic of conversations. Using a dictionary had become a slow, letter-by-letter process. He got lost in oral foreign language drills because he could not tell which small grammatical part of the teacher's repeated questions had been changed. He failed at attempts to draw in perspective. He frequently got lost, sometimes even in his hometown. He had difficulty figuring out what mathematical operations were needed to deal with everyday situations such as making change or leaving a tip in a restaurant.

In the musical realm, his piano playing was severely handicapped because of his hemiplegia, although his right hand could play as well as ever. His conducting was less inspired, and he found that he had particular difficulty conducting music with shifting meters, such as the finale of Stravinsky's *The Firebird*, where there are seven beats to a measure with irregular subdivisions. Such music had previously presented no problems for him.

He complained of drastic changes in perceiving and recognizing played notes, giving him total insecurity in taking musical dictation. He also complained of difficulty in writing music, which is best described in his own words:

> The bane of my classroom existence for the past 10 years has been an inability to write freely in a given time signature without making any errors in reckoning the prescribed number of beats per measure. The heretofore automatic process of measuring has been supplanted by a tendency to measure in terms of phrase length. Currently I have been reduced to digital computation to check the accuracy of my music on the board.

In addition, he said that he frequently failed to space notes on the page appropriately, in accordance with their relative durations.

He did not listen to music for enjoyment as frequently as he used to, and he said that he no longer had significant emotional experiences from listening to music, although he had no difficulty remembering the emotional meanings that he had attached to particular pieces in the past. Finally, his musical composition since the stroke was very limited, despite efforts to continue with it. One reason he cited was that he was no longer able to create the appropriate emotional milieu or atmosphere that he felt to be a prerequisite to composing. This appeared to be a very important factor for him, but it is difficult to define or describe. It involves the ability to recall vividly a series of scenes, situations, or moods and then to use those recollections to generate a coherent piece of music.

He experienced another difficulty with composition as well, which is best expressed his own words:

> I seem to be very aware of an inability to synthesize information and to then draw conclusions based upon the interaction of the factors involved. This particular manifestation of insecurity I consider to be a lack of ability to create a Gestalt. It is in this

TABLE 6-2. Summary of Difficulties Observed in a Composer with a Right Hemisphere Stroke

Difficulty	Nonmusical Complaints	Nonmusical Tests	Musical Complaints	Musical Tests
Left hemiplegia	Weakness	Neurological exam	Playing piano, bass conducting	Piano playing
Left hemisensory deficit	Decreased sensation	Neurological exam	Loss of keyboard sense	Piano playing
Left visual neglect	Fails to notice things	Neurological exam, Digit Symbol		
Impaired singing			Decreased range, quality, and power	Singing
Auditory temporal resolution impairment	Hearing change	Counting short trains of rapid clicks	Difficulty with dictation and hearing rhythms	Duration discrimination, rhythm reproduction, and dictation
Memory impairment	Difficulty with word finding and arithmetic	Naming, Calculations, Wechsler Memory Scale	Dictation and theory	Dictation, theory, and melody recall
Motor perseveration		Writing "MN" repeatedly in cursive	Rhythm errors in playing and conducting	Rhythm reproduction
Set-shifting difficulties	Difficulty with conversation, following directions, language drills, dictionary use, and calculations	Test directions, Wisconsin Card Sort Test, Digits Backwards, Shipley Institute of Living Scale Abstractions subtest, Raven's Progressive Matrices, The Visual-Verbal test, arithmetic test	Mixed-meter conducting and composing	Rhythm reproduction, melody reproduction, meter determination, and rhythm reading
Impaired gestalt formation	Difficulty with drawing, finding his way, conversation, arithmetic, and learning the Russian alphabet	Block Design, Picture Arrangement, Object Assembly, Shipley Institute of Living Scale Abstractions subtest; Hooper Visual Organization Test, drawings, stick patterns, 3D blocks, Raven's Progressive Matrices, The Visual-Verbal test, Porteus Mazes, Wisconsin Card Sort Test	Difficulty with writing the correct number of beats per bar, spacing notes on the page, and composing, (especially counterpoint)	Writing, meter determination, excerpt identification, analysis, composing counterpoint, pitch stream segregation
Decreased affective involvement with music	Lethargy		Less involved, listens less	

sense I shall use the term. The compositional process for me at this time seems to lack a Gestalt. Notes are correct, orchestration skills are very much intact and show no diminution. Content, however, is dull, lifeless (soulless). Since the compositional process has for me been one of working at several levels of the on-goingness of the melodic, harmonic, rhythmic flow simultaneously and keeping track of the various factors, I find that I am not able to maintain a thread of continuity and must work in small segments which, while, appropriate and significant in themselves do not inter-relate with each other. Interestingly enough, I have little difficulty writing in a serial technique. I find it relatively simple, but I have never been overawed by the musical content of this style of composition. The manipulation and the various row manifestations present no problem.

His introspections were generated essentially independently of any knowledge of current theorizing about brain function.

Table 6-2 summarizes his condition as determined by his reports and our testing. This table lists ten deficits, with their musical and nonmusical components and their subjective and objective manifestations. For example, he complained of difficulty with gestalt formation, as noted previously. His complaints encompassed both musical and nonmusical activities, including problems with composing, writing notes on the page, drawing, finding his way, and calculating a tip in a restaurant. On testing we found that he did show the difficulties mentioned and that he was also impaired on musical analysis, identifying written musical excerpts out of context, determining appropriate meters for sequences of notes written without bar lines, visual construction tasks and verbal and nonverbal concept formation tasks. This category of difficulties clearly could be subdivided, and other interpretations of our findings are possible. Nevertheless, this case study demonstates some of the right hemisphere's distinct contributions to musical behaviors, even in an individual whose musical abilities are largely intact.

In the sections that follow I elaborate on points raised by this case, discussing, first, relationships between musical and some nonmusical skills and second, relationships among musical skills as they are dissociated by a variety of neuropsychological variables and by general and personal observations. My intention is to give a broad survey of the field so as to stimulate interest in neglected areas, such as music in the congenitally deaf, musical idiot savants, and musical learning disabilities, rather than giving an exhaustive review of a few overworked topics, such as dichotic listening and measures of cerebral dominance.

Relationships Between Music and Other Skills

Hearing

Acquired Deafness. Music is often regarded as an exclusively auditory phenomenon, yet the musical abilities of the deaf demonstrate that it is not so simple. Beethoven, Fauré, Franz, Smetana, and Vaughan Williams all became deaf in their later years, yet continued to produce mature compositions with no sign of diminished composing ability (Hood, 1977). On the contrary, their auditory and social isolation may have allowed for greater productivity through lessened distractions.

Smetana claimed, "I have completed in these three years of deafness more than I had otherwise done in ten" (p. 266, Large, 1970). Clearly, hearing is not critical to the composing process for some individuals. Although composing may be developmentally founded upon hearing, it appears that it can become a purely cognitive process which transcends hearing. The talented composer is capable of realizing what a piece of music will sound like through auditory imagery. The abilities to "hear out" a score when reading it and to write down what one creates can be as automatic (with the proper training in solfeggio and dictation) as knowing what a text will sound like without reading it aloud and writing a message without speaking it. It is no more surprising that these composers were able to continue their work when deaf than that they were able to read and write language.

Performance on the piano remains possible for some after acquired deafness (Hood, 1977; Knight, 1924). Gates and Bradshaw (1974) found that switching off the sound on an electric keyboard barely affected performance for keyboard players with normal hearing, although delayed auditory feedback was very disruptive to performance. Variable-pitch instruments, high-pitch instruments, and those that allow greater manipulation of timbre present relatively greater difficulties for the accomplished performer who becomes deaf (Hood, 1977). Distortion of hearing through sensorineural hearing loss is especially troublesome to the performer. It appears that distortion of auditory feedback—whether through sensorineural hearing loss or delayed auditory feedback—is more likely to disrupt musical performance than lack of auditory feedback.

Among those with acquired deafness, some continue to enjoy attending live musical performances (Knight, 1924). Clearly, sound is not the only thing musical performance is about. The contemporary composer John Cage has made this point in another way by giving entire concerts (for the hearing) consisting of silence.

Congenital Deafness. The musical abilities of the congenitally deaf are even more instructive. Schools for the deaf have been training bands since the turn of the century (Edwards, 1974). One such band was described as being in great demand for playing dances for the hearing because of its excellent rhythm. Singing has been taught, and there have been some successful choirs.

The congenitally deaf generally appreciate loud and strongly rhythmic music most easily. Some of their music appreciation is truly auditory. Atkins and Donovan (1984) have demonstrated that hearing aids bring most of the sounds of the music classroom within the range of hearing for even some of the profoundly hearing impaired. Yet much of the music appears to be perceived and learned through visual and tactile modalities (Cleall, 1983). Harmony, timbre, the upper range of pitch, and the lower levels of loudness are among the more difficult aspects of music for the deaf to appreciate, aspects that require finer auditory discrimination.

These observations suggest transmodal appreciation of certain aspects of music, especially rhythm and social exchange. This converges with some evidence from experimental psychology. Miner (1903) used flashing lights to demonstrate that many of the basic phenomena of rhythmic grouping observed in the auditory modality are present in vision as well. Transmodal appreciation of cognitive structures relevant to music, particularly temporal patterns, is currently being investigated in people with normal hearing (cf. Martin, 1972; Povel, 1981; Restle, 1970).

Inasmuch as some of the congenitally deaf musical groups appear to have achieved a proficiency that has been seriously regarded by the hearing as enjoyable (and not just sympathetically tolerated as an indulgence or a curiosity), it can be said that some congenitally deaf display musical talent. Unfortunately, there seems to be only one detailed psychological study of musical ability in a congenitally deaf individual (Révész, 1954). That study demonstrated the importance of rhythm and nonauditory vibration sense in music appreciation, but the subject was not a performer. Cleall (1983) described a 17-year-old profoundly deaf piano and percussion student at the Royal Academy of Music in Great Britain who began to lose her hearing at age 8, the same age at which she began music lessons. More case studies of music learning in the deaf would clearly be of interest, especially of performers. This could help us understand in more detail which aspects of music are specifically auditory and which are based on more general properties of the nervous system. For example, the auditory system is exquisitely sensitive to temporal recurrence or periodicity in the range of pitch perception. Is this sensitivity an auditory specialization that also extends to lower frequencies and provides the basis for musical rhythmic phenomena, or is musical rhythm founded on more general periodicity sensitivities in the nervous system that can be as easily accessed via other modalities? What are the other cognitive strengths of successful congenitally deaf musicians? Do they have superior musical auditory memory? Kinesthetic sequencing skills? Do they have an unusual reliance on mathematical or spatial skills to accomplish their musical achievements?

Little mention has been made to date of creative musicality among the congenitally deaf. This void should not be construed as an indication that they are incapable of significant musical creativity. Like women, the congenitally deaf have, until relatively recently, been restricted in partaking of the musical education and encouragement necessary to compose, for example. It is too soon to judge their capacities in this regard. Just as a color-blind person could have difficulty with oil paints but produce good charcoal sketches, so could the congenitally deaf come to produce a valid and interesting, but possibly restricted, genre of music.

Vision

A number of interesting neuropsychological questions can be asked about blind musicians. Do the blind develop superior auditory abilities, or do they simply use available information more fully? Do blind musicians working within a written musical culture but using an aural approach have a different conceptualization of the music? Does the use of braille music notation influence the blind musicians' conceptualization of the music? Unfortunately, the systematic study of musical abilities in blind versus sighted populations has so far yielded inconclusive results (see Shuter-Dyson & Gabriel, 1981, and Stankov & Spilsbury, 1978, for reviews).

Intelligence(s)[2]

Musical Idiot Savants. The phenomenon of musical idiot savants, mentally retarded individuals with normal or superior musical skills, is frequently mentioned, but there are only 18 cases in the English literature with any specificity at all in their descriptions. Major characteristics of these cases are summarized in Table 6-3 (and discussed by Charness, Clifton, and MacDonald, Chapter 14, this volume).

Those subjects who are truly exceptionally talented musically and in some cases seriously involved in music making with normal musicians tend to be only borderline or mildly mentally retarded (Anastasi & Levee, 1960; Scheerer, Rothmann, & Goldstein, 1945; Viscott, 1970). They tend to show prominent emotional disturbances and to have unusual family dynamics, which contribute significantly to the maintenance of musical skills. These individuals are also the most musically flexible and creative among the idiot savants, showing sensitivity to musical interpretation and some ability to improvise. Exceptional creative musicality among the mentally retarded has not been reported. Even these higher level idiot savants display some of the characteristics of cognitive rigidity, lack of abstract reasoning skills, and exceptional focus on mechanical skill and rote memorization typical of idiot savants (Hill, 1978).

Moderately to severely retarded musical idiot savants generally show musical performance abilities that are comparable to those of many normal individuals in technique and sometimes in music reading (Judd & Judd,[3] cited in Charness, Clifton, & MacDonald, Chapter 14, this volume; Minogue, 1923; Owens & Grimm, 1941; Rife & Snyder, 1931). Creativity and musical interpretation are usually lacking, and the performances are described as mechanical or lacking in feeling. Their performances are typically solo or leadership (e.g., playing piano while others sing along), because their cognitive rigidity makes it difficult for them to adapt to making music with others.

Though some of the idiot savants receive social reinforcement for their music, most of them clearly get intrinsic reinforcement and spend long hours playing alone for their own enjoyment. For example, Scheerer *et al*'s (1945) subject mostly played "monotonous sequences of his own fancy" (p. 8) and was obsessed with a few classical records. This would help to explain why all but two are pianists, since the piano is especially suitable for solo playing.

Ten of the subjects are blind, lending support to the sensory deprivation and compensation theories of idiot savants (Hill, 1978). All play by ear, and only four can read music. Fifteen are reported to have exceptional musical memories, although what this means is not always clear. In some cases (e.g., Corner, 1985) it may simply refer to a large repertoire. More commonly, it is said that the subject can repeat a piece accurately after a single hearing. Formal testing is uncommon, however, and when done, may sometimes yield a different result (Charness,

---

2. Gardner's (1983) book, *Frames of Mind: The Theory of Multiple Intelligences,* has revived interest in multifactorial theories of intelligence. This section discusses the dissociation of musical abilities from other forms of intelligence, be they single or multiple.

3. This previously unpublished case study was conducted in 1978.

TABLE 6-3. Summary of Cases of Musical Idiot Savants

Case	Sex/IQ	Etiology	Blind	Emotionally disturbed	Family musical history	Plays piano	Sings	Has absolute pitch	Plays by ear	Reads music	Exceptional Memory Musical	Exceptional Memory Nonmusical	Calendar calculator
Anastasi and Levee (1960)	M/Verbal IQ 92 Performance IQ 52	Encephalitis		*		*		*	*?	*	?	*	
Charness, Clifton, and MacDonald (Chapter 14, this volume)	M/severely retarded	Premature birth, right hemiplegia, epilepsy	*		*	*	*	*	*		*?		
Corner (1985)	M	Movement disorder	*			* and accordian			*		*?		
Judd and Judd (cited in Charness, Clifton, and MacDonald, Chapter 14, this volume)	M/47	Anoxia at birth	*	*	*	*		*	*	–			*
LaFontaine (1968)	1 F/41	Premature birth	*	*	*	*	*	*	*	*?	*?		
	2 M/16	Down syndrome			*	*	*?		*		*?		
	3 M/69	Petit mal seizures?			*	*		*?	*	–	*?		
Minogue (1923)	M/46	Meningitis		*		*	*		*	*	*	*	
Monty (1981)	M/"Retarded"	Premature birth, cerebral palsy	*		foster	*	*		*		*		
Owens and Grimm (1941)	F/20				*	*			*		*?		
Rife and Snyder (1931)	1 F/"Imbecile"		*				*		*		*?		
	2 F/"Imbecile"		*		*	*			*		*		
	3 F/"Idiot"				*	*			*		*?		
	4 M/"Idiot"		*		*	*			*		*?		
Scheerer, Rothmann, and Goldstein (1945)	M/50	Schizophrenia ?		*		*	*	*	*		*	*	*
Seguin (1866)	M/"Idiot"	Microcephaly	*			*			*		*		
Tredgold (1922)	F/"Imbecile"		*			*	*		*		*?		
Viscott (1970)	F/Verbal IQ 65 Performance IQ 87			*	*	*	*	*	*	*	*	*	*

Note: Symbols: *, feature is present; –, feature is absent; ?, feature is poorly described or difficult to determine; blank cells, feature was not mentioned.

Clifton, & MacDonald, Chapter 14, this volume) Other evidence suggestive of exceptional musical memory in many of these individuals is the presence of absolute pitch in seven of them.

Beyond these generalizations, however, there are many eccentricities, peculiarities, and differences among the cases, suggesting multiple causes. Viscott's (1970) subject, for example, never practiced but played only for pleasure. Her Performance IQ exceeded her Verbal IQ by 22 points, she was an avid concertgoer, and her family was very emotionally expressive. By contrast, Anastasi and Levee's (1960) subject never played for pleasure but practiced 9 hours a day. His Verbal IQ exceeded his Performance IQ by 40 points, he rarely went to concerts, and he and his family were emotionally cool and distant.

A number of hypotheses have been advanced to explain idiot savants including concrete thinking, sensory deprivation, compensation, genetics, and exceptional memory or concentration, but no single explanation has been adequate in accounting for all reported phenomena.[4] (Hill, 1978). From the available reports, it is clear that musical idiot savants devote enormous efforts to their musical pursuits. Most of their musical achievements do not appear to be exceptional for those who have given that much effort. But the memorization skills of many of them are clearly out of the ordinary, even for skilled musicians. Thus the literature clearly supports the rare emergence of musical skill markedly out of proportion to other intellectual abilities, but offers no conclusive evidence other than unusual memorization skills as to why this occurs.

Future studies of idiot savants might explore their musical memories in more detail. Some questions of interest would be the following: Is the extraordinary memory confined by musical style? Is nonmusical auditory memory also exceptional? Is nonauditory memory also exceptional, including procedural memory (see the Memory section of this chapter)? If errors or peculiarities of interpretation are intentionally introduced in the presentation of a piece of conventional music, will the subject reproduce the performance slavishly, including the errors, or will some judgment and abstraction enter in? What are the limitations to their musical talents?

Musical Learning Disability. The reverse of idiot savants—highly intelligent individuals lacking musical skills—has not been systematically studied, but it is probably quite common. The first national assessment of musical performance in the United States (National Assessment of Educational Progress, 1974) reported that no greater than 90% of its subjects in any age group, including adults, could give an acceptable performance on fairly rudimentary musical tasks, such as singing a well-known song or tapping the beat to a piece of music. Studies of "monotones," also known as "tone-deaf" persons, "uncertain singers," or "poor-pitch singers," estimate a prevalence of 5% or greater of the population (Shuter-Dyson & Gabriel, 1981).

The failure to develop music has not been given the attention that has been lavished on the failure to develop language, for example. It has been demonstrated that most who have been considered "monotones" actually produce tones

---

4. Hill (1978) argues from the assumption that any explanation proposed ought to be able to account for all idiot savants, a peculiar position given the variety of skills exhibited by idiot savants.

of varying pitches. They can be trained to sing accurately, which also brings about an improvement in their low performance on tests of pitch discrimination (Welch, 1979). But the complex factors that might contribute to the failure to develop musically remain largely unexplored. I predict that such investigations will find that some individuals fail to develop musical abilities because of lack of instruction or encouragement, some because of early frustrating or traumatic experiences with music, and some because of auditory or motor impairments. When these causes have been excluded, there may remain a group of individuals who could be considered learning disabled in music. The characteristics of such a group would be likely to tell us much about the nature of musical development and about other learning disabilities. For example, there is likely to be a group of developmental dyslexics whose language-reading difficulties are primarily visually based and thus who may also have difficulty learning to read music. Other dyslexics whose problem is more linguistic and/or semantic may not have musical difficulties. Some may have difficulty with auditory and/or sequential processing that is evident both in language and in music, and so forth. Poor-pitch singers are known to perform poorly on tests of pitch discrimination, tonal memory, and vocal range (Welch, 1979). Among these may be some who have a specific musical learning disability. The relationships between poor-pitch singing and other musical and nonmusical abilities remain to be explored. In my experience poor-pitch singers are not at all uncommon among intelligent and well-educated persons and even among instrumental musicians.

Interestingly, among poor-pitch singers males apparently outnumber females, possibly by as much as 7 to 1 (Shuter-Dyson & Gabriel, 1981). This is similar to the preponderance of males among developmental dyslexics. Although Hill (1978) reported a preponderance of males to females of greater than 5 to 1 in idiot savants generally, there is a sex ratio of 11 males to 7 females in the small collection of musical idiot savants reviewed here.

Language

Music has frequently been called a language (Dupré & Nathan, 1911; Henson, 1977), even the universal language. Within the past decade there have been several attempts to take this metaphor seriously and to apply linguistic analysis, particularly generative grammars, to musical structures.[5] Successes such as those of Lerdahl and Jackendoff (1983) have led to speculations as to whether generative grammar represents an underlying neurological stratum common to many modes of thought.

Neuropsychology tells a different story. There are now several reports of patients who had strokes in the posterior half of the left cerebral hemisphere but who continue to read, write, compose, conduct, and perform music with little apparent impairment, in spite of sometimes severe aphasias, or language disorders (Assal, 1973; Basso & Capitani, 1985; Bouillaud, 1865; Judd et al., 1983; Lamy,

---

5. This idea actually goes back many centuries, and the attempts have been well reviewed by Powers (1980).

1907; Luria, Tsvetkova, & Futer, 1965). These patients were, of course, impaired in their ability to talk about music. Our patient described below in the Musical Memory and Procedural Memory section had pure alexia (a language reading disorder) with relatively preserved music reading, although the more usual pattern is for musical alexia to accompany linguistic alexia (Judd, 1979; Judd et al., 1980, 1983). An analysis of this case indicated that several of the differences between the phonetic system for writing English and the staff music notation system are neurologically significant. These include nominal versus ordinal and intervalic representation of information, and phonetic versus idiographic representation of information.

Likewise, a number of patients with right frontal lobe lesions show disturbances of musical expression without appreciable language disorders, except, in some instances, disturbance of speech prosody, or the "melody" of speech (Botez & Wertheim, 1959; Mann, 1898; Würtzen, 1903).

But the more usual pattern is for musical disorders (amusias) to accompany aphasias. For example, Henschen (1920), in an exhaustive review of the literature to that date, found 314 cases of amusia, all but 13 of whom were also aphasic.

There is as yet no satisfactory explanation for these findings, although it is evident that there must be considerable individual variation in the cortical representation of music (Benton, 1977). Additionally, more recent investigations using primarily the dichotic listening technique suggest that the skills and strategies available and the demands of the task (but not the nature of the stimulus) influence which cerebral hemisphere best processes both musiclike and languagelike stimuli (Gates & Bradshaw, 1977). It may well be that the areas of the brain especially involved in music for any individual depend not only on what musical activities that individual usually engages in but also on the approaches or strategies typically employed (Goldstein, 1948). This possibility is depressingly difficult to investigate clinically and even experimentally. In any case it is clear that music and language can each be carried on independently of the other. Composers, in particular, can carry on their work in spite of aphasia. Therefore, what distinguishes language areas of the brain would appear likely to be something other than their capacity to process generative grammars.

Memory

Musical Memory in Amnesics. The importance of different types of musical memory varies considerably from culture to culture and from activity to activity. This is amply demonstrated by a number of patients that I and others have seen.

Two amnesics that I have seen had an interesting preservation of musical skills. Both were middle-aged men who suffered ruptures of aneurisms in the anterior communicating artery, with damage to the frontal lobes and subcortical structures involved in memory. Both were seen years after the damage had occurred, and both had severe to profound anterograde amnesia (the inability to retain new material in memory for longer than a minute or so) and moderate frontal lobe syndrome (social disinhibition, difficulty in planning, lack of awareness of, and concern about, deficits). Both had normal language and low-normal IQs, but both were so severely impaired cognitively with their amnesia and frontal lobe syndrome that they required nursing home care.

The subject W. A. M. was an amateur singer who spent most of his time on the hospital ward singing unaccompanied songs in a clear and beautiful voice. He had a large repertoire but usually sang only one or a few verses, and he often sang the same song all day long, apparently unaware that he was repeating himself. Although his repertoire became frozen at the time of his injury, his amnesia did not stop him from producing beautiful music.

My second musical amnesic patient, G. M., had been a high school music teacher. He was still able to sight sing well, sight read in playing the piano, and play from memory pieces he had known prior to his hemorrhage. In fact, he sang regularly in a church choir. When I tested him, he initially made some reasonable errors in sight singing some unfamiliar material but corrected himself and improved his performance with repetition. When he came back to the selection later, he was able to sing it correctly, although he claimed not to recognize it. Consistent with his teaching background, he was able to correct my errors in sight singing and make appropriate suggestions for rehearsal. As is typical of anterograde amnesics, his immediate memory was intact. He was able to repeat seven digits forward and five digits backward as well as short melodies sung to him, and he could also tap back short rhythms.

Starr and Phillips (1970) have described a patient who had a profound anterograde amnesia resulting from a surgical lesion but who nevertheless was able to learn new pieces on the piano. Like G. M., he denied any knowledge of the piece, but given the opening bars, he played it through without difficulty. Gardner (1975) described a similar case of an amnesic patient who was also able to learn some rhyming lyrics to the piano piece he had mastered. These last two subjects were also shown to have preserved learning of simple motor skills, such as mirror writing and doing simple mazes.

These four cases illustrate that many aspects of musical performance are still possible even in the almost complete absence of major memory mechanisms. Indeed, it appears that even music learning can take place in the face of amnesia. Music learning is part of a cluster of special learning abilities that are spared in the amesic syndrome.

What are these special learning abilities? They include classical and operant conditioning; motor skills, such as rotor pursuit tasks and mirror writing; perceptual learning, such as identifying incomplete pictures of objects; and complex learning, such as the learning of musical pieces or mathematical procedures (Parkin, 1982). These special skills have been described as "semantic," "procedural," or "habit" memory, or "knowing how" as contrasted with "knowing that" (Parkin, 1982).

Musical Memory and Procedural Memory If the medial temporal lobe, so consistently implicated in the amnesic syndrome, is not critical to this other type of learning, what other area is ? The first clue comes from animal studies. Baker and Thomas (1965) reported that rats with cingulum lesions failed to learn an alternation task and concluded that for the rats the cingulum was important for temporal integration of sequential behavior. The cingulum is an area of cortex just above the corpus callosum with strong connections to the frontal cortex and the limbic system, including the hippocampus and other areas involved in memory. A series of studies of various species with lesions in the frontal cortex has revealed a variety of related deficits in the regulation and sequencing of responses. In a review of these studies, Nauta (1971) concluded, "It could even be suggested that the [animal with a frontal lobe lesion] has suffered a memory impairment after all, even though this loss affects the storage of its action plans rather than that of its external-perceptual images" (p. 184).

Bancaud *et al.* (1976) found that stimulation of the cingulate cortex in humans during surgery for epilepsy produced complex coordinated movements involving, especially, the hands and mouth. They concluded that the cingulate cortex "seems to have a major role in inciting to action and in coordination of highly complex movements" (p. 724). Faillace, Allen, McQueen, and Northrup (1971) studied four patients before and after bilateral cingulotomies for intractable pain. Cingulotomy is essentially a refinement of the frontal lobotomy procedure and involves discrete lesions to the cingulate bundle, a main connection between the cingulate cortex, the hippocampus, and the frontal cortex. All four patients showed major postsurgical impairments in learning a complex tapping sequence. The test consisted of tapping four geometric figures in a row in a specified, demonstrated order. The most complex of these sequences was 1 2 3 4 3 2 1 2 3 4 2 3 1 2 3 4 3 2 1. This sequence is quite long but has considerable structure, which makes it possible for normal persons to learn it relatively easily. That structure is not unlike many musical structures—one might call it an ABA, or theme and variation.

I had the opportunity to examine a musician, K. M., 3 years after bilateral cingulotomy for pain and depression (Teuber, Corkin, & Twitchell, 1977). She came to me complaining of difficulty in learning, remembering, responding to, composing, reading, improvising, and performing music. She claimed that component skills were intact but that she had difficulty in putting them all together to play and sing a song and in maintaining the flow of the music. She also complained of difficulty in following the logic of a conversation or story, in remembering appointments and where she had put things, and in playing chess and gin rummy.

An extensive battery of neuropsychological tests a few months after the surgery (Teuber *et al.*, 1977) and a Halstead-Reitan Neuropsychological Test Battery 2 years after surgery had been normal except for mild memory impairment, which was attributed to electroconvulsive shock prior to surgery. However, she was markedly impaired on my replication of Faillace *et al.*'s (1971) sequential tapping task (described above). On each sequence she performed less than one-half the number of repetitions that each of my five controls produced.

She was able to play guitar and sing, with only a few hesitations, an over-learned song she had composed 5 years earlier. This song demonstrated that she had a high level of proficiency in singing, chording, and finger-picking, and that she had been proficient at composing. She was able to name and imitate chords, play named chords, match pitches, and identify musical symbols and their significance. However, she was very deficient in learning new chord sequences, melodies, and rhythms, and had difficulty with simple rhythmic tasks. Her sight reading was very hesitant and unmusical, but this had never been a well-practiced skill for her.

This case presents a striking double dissociation with the cases of amnesia described previously. Whereas the other subjects were amnesic for most material and showed some sparing of Nauta's "action plan" learning, including music, K. M. showed only mild impairments on most memory tasks but had marked difficulty on complex motor sequence learning, particularly for music. Her impairment appears to be primarily in learning "action plans" and in prospective memory (remembering to do something at the right time; Meacham & Leiman, 1982) rather than in the retrospective memory (cued recall of past events or stimuli) most often tapped by conventional memory tests.

This conclusion must be tentative, however. The tasks given to K. M. were not strictly comparable to those on which amnesics showed preserved learning. Furthermore, the results are culture bound. K. M.'s impairments reflect her style of doing music, but another of Teuber *et al.*'s (1977) subjects, C. E., resumed her work as a church organist after two bilateral cingulotomies. Presumably, her habitual use of sight-reading skills and of a familiar repertoire allowed C. E. to overcome any problems she may have had in complex motor sequence learning, just as K. M. was able to perform when new music learning was not required. Replication of my findings in other cingulotomy patients, especially musicians, is needed. Also, the Faillace *et al.* task and music learning tasks should be given to amnesics to see if learning is preserved.

In this context it is interesting to consider the case of the composer with alexia but without agraphia described in the Language section of this chapter. He had a moderate anterograde amnesia, especially for verbal material. When a short melody was played for him to learn, he had a great deal of difficulty with the task that was comparable to his difficulty in learning new verbal material. Even when the melody was mastered, his ability to recall it after a delay of 5 minutes was flawed. However, when he was asked to generate a new melody, he produced one that was much longer than the melody he had been taught, and he had no difficulty recalling it after a comparable delay. This relative preservation of memory for self-generated material did not extend to verbal material. Paragraphs he attempted to write were filled with half-completed and improperly completed sentences—he was able to write down his thoughts, yet could neither read nor remember what he had written in order to complete the sentence properly.

His differentiated memory skills were also reflected in his song-composing process. He had his text tape-recorded and listened to it many times trying to learn it, doing so only with great effort. By contrast, he had little difficulty remembering his plan for composing and what he had actually composed until he got around to dictating it or writing it down. As had been the case before his stroke, it made little difference to him whether or not he used the piano when composing. I speculate that his relatively well preserved memory for self-generated musical material was due to intact frontal lobes and "action plan" memory mechanisms. Since he did not need to play his compositions in order to remember them, I suspect that the composing process involved a planning or arranging of musical ideas or images that might be considered covert or implicit motor sequencing or planning. This idea could be tested by asking amnesics to generate and remember new material of various kinds.

The Varieties of Musical Memory. One other area of musical memory touched by neuropsychology is immediate melodic memory. Milner (1962) gave the Seashore Measures of Musical Talents to patients undergoing unilateral anterior temporal lobectomy for epilepsy and found that those with right temporal lobe surgery had deficits on the Tonal Memory subtest, which involves immediate melodic memory. These patients were unselected for musical talent, but James Carlsen (personal communication, 1979) has told me of his extensive and unsuccessful attempts to rehabilitate a talented musician with traumatic right temporal lobe damage who had a persistent, severe impairment in immediate melodic memory. Thus the right temporal lobe appears important in immediate musical memory just as the left temporal lobe is important in immediate verbal memory.

Moreover, it has been my experience that there are considerable individual differences in music-learning styles. In my marimba band, for example, some people learn new parts primarily by melodic memory, then pick them out "by ear" on the instrument. Others rely heavily on the visual position of the notes, rather like one would learn Faillace *et al.*'s (1971) sequential tapping task. Some use counting, musical theory concepts, or other verbal mnemonics. Some are dependent upon hearing the other parts in the piece in order to remember their own, whereas others prefer to learn their parts alone and then may have difficulty fitting them in with the others. After learning a part the first time, some people will rely on motor memory and sticking patterns (which hand strikes which note) in order to remember the part at the next rehearsal. Actually, everyone uses all of these strategies at one time or another, but individual preferences are clearly—sometimes maddeningly—identifiable.

Factor analytic studies of musical abilities have confirmed that musical memory is complex and multifaceted (Shuter-Dyson & Gabriel, 1981). This is true even though most of the memory tests and the well-researched tests of musical abilities look primarily at immediate auditory memory. Recent studies in cognitive psychology have likewise suggested that even immediate auditory memory for simple melodies involves somewhat different processes for contour, interval, and rhythm (Shuter-Dyson & Gabriel, 1981).

In a recent validation study of the Seashore Measures of Musical Talents, Tonal Memory, in which the subject is asked to indicate which note is changed in the second playing of a short pitch sequence, was the only subtest of six on which professional orchestral musicians clearly showed superior performance (Henson & Wyke, 1982). Tonal memory, even more than pitch discrimination, is the area most often impaired in poor-pitch singers (Welch, 1979). Moreover, tonal memory improves when these individuals are given appropriate vocal training.

Excellent musical memory is often mentioned in descriptions of musical prodigies. Mozart's skills in this area are perhaps the most remarkable on record. He reportedly "stole" an important and complex choral work of his day by hearing it once in performance and then writing it down with only a few errors. Exceptional musical memory is most often described as the ability to play a piece of music upon hearing it a very few times. This most likely involves not just "action plan" memory but also auditory memory, at least in the short term, since the piece must be remembered in some form long enough to play it. Doubtless, in the very talented musician these different types of memory are highly developed and well integrated. In the case of at least some idiot savants exceptional musical memory appears to accompany exceptional memory in other limited realms, such as the verbal and the mathematical.

In aural musical cultures the "folk process" involving forgetting can be important to musical development (Seeger, 1977). The development of music notation systems can diminish the importance of music memorization in culture (Kaufmann, 1972). We have seen in the example of amnesics that new learning ability can be unnecessary for some forms of musical expression. In the case of idiot savants we have seen that exceptional musical memory can be part of a performer's strength without necessarily resulting in creativity. In spite of these exceptions, however, musical memory in its many forms appears to be central to many aspects of musical talent.

Future studies could look at the nature of music learning in amnesics and at the relationships between musical memory and other forms of memory in normal persons, mnemonists, idiot savants, and musicians. Further differentation of the components of music learning is called for, and studies of individual differences are also needed. Such studies, along with developmental studies of musical memory and the effects of training on musical memory, would be especially important for music education. Finally, examining the process of musical forgetting would be helpful in understanding the folk process and the evolution of musical cultures.

Relationships Among Musical Skills

In spite of more than a century of observations, neuropsychology has been able to demonstrate only the crudest of reliable dissociations within the realm of musical skills.

Expressive Versus Receptive Skills

The dissociation between expressive and receptive musical skills is often seen in normal persons as a consequence of their development. Some poor-pitch singers and noninstrumentalists nevertheless are music lovers with acute perceptions and knowledge of music, and some deaf individuals can perform musically (as described above).

This dissociation is well supported in the clinical literature, with impairments in musical expression being associated with lesions in either frontal lobe, and impairments in musical reception being associated with lesions in either or both temporal lobes (for reviews, see Benton, 1977; Dorgeuille, 1966; Gates & Bradshaw, 1977; Marin, 1982; Wertheim, 1969). Expressive amusics are typically well aware of their musical errors and are able to demonstrate intact musical perceptions. Expressive aphasia and/or disorders of speech prosody are sometimes also present. In the case of receptive amusia, sound perception is frequently distorted, making expression difficult because of distorted feedback. This is similar to the music performance difficulties in individuals with sensorineural hearing loss. In addition, there is a resemblance to aphasias in that the so-called receptive aphasias also include a related expressive language disorder.

Rhythm Versus Pitch

Entire genres of music exist that are primarily rhythmic, with very little melodic or harmonic structure; thus the dissociation between rhythm and pitch occurs naturally (e.g., West African drumming ensembles, the drum cadences of North American marching bands). The opposite phenomenon, a rhythmless music, is hard to imagine, though some musical cultures certainly have limited rhythmic variations (e.g., Gregorian chant) or development (e.g., much of Western tonal music when compared to classical Indian or sub-Saharan African music).

A trade-off between pitch and rhythm is often available to musicians practicing alone: They can take the extra time needed to get the pitches right, thereby distorting the rhythm, or they can get the rhythm right and sacrifice the pitches. This trade-off was described in Mann's (1898) case of a singer with impaired pitch control resulting from a right frontal lesion.

The clearest dissociations of pitch from rhythm are in cases like Mann's, in which pitch control is lost. In these instances rhythm is often preserved. Similarly, reports of singing with intracarotid amytal injections (which paralyze one cerebral hemisphere at a time—a presurgical procedure to determine language laterality) note preserved rhythm with both left and right injections, although pitch is disturbed with right injection (Borchgrevink, 1982; Gordon & Bogen, 1974).

Difficulty in repeating tapped rhythms can be associated with apraxia and/or a more general amusia. When this impairment accompanies intact singing, the rhythm of the singing itself is often intact (Ustvedt, 1937). Rhythmic abilities appear to depend upon the type of activity examined and may not be unitary. Rhythm and pitch are less clearly dissociated in the receptive amusias.

Synchronization

The ability to coordinate one's music making rhythmically with another is a skill that is distinct from the mere perception, production, or reproduction of rhythms. It appears to have a separate stage of development (Shuter-Dyson & Gabriel, 1981). This characteristic of music is one of its most significant social features. It distinguishes much of music making from much of language behavior. Among mammals, the ability appears to be unique to humans, and among all animals, only humans appear to perform the feat at a variety of tempos spanning several octaves. Nevertheless, it has received relatively little attention in neuromusicology and psychomusicology.

Among normal individuals, some musicians manage to advance fairly far on their instruments through solo practice, but have considerable difficulty in achieving ensemble coordination. Others, by contrast, may be rhythmically imprecise when playing alone but will play well in ensemble. I have observed a few brain-damaged patients who can give passable performances of pieces alone but who cannot coordinate with, and especially, follow, others. This is particularly true of those with right brain damage or Wernicke aphasia (Walthard, 1927) and an impaired awareness of their own errors. On the other hand, many Broca aphasics cannot imitate or maintain singing alone, yet can sing accurately (though perhaps without words) with the facilitating presence of another singing voice. This phenomenon is one of the aspects of music exploited by melodic intonation therapy for aphasics (Sparks, Helm, & Albert, 1974).

There is a need for further investigation of this neglected skill in normal persons as well as in the brain damaged. It would be a necessary component of an analysis-by-synthesis model of music perception.

Other Musical Skills

Music Reading and Writing. Unlike the case with language, convincing cases of isolated musical alexia or agraphia have not been reported. They frequently accompany a more general amusia. Musical alexia can but need not accompany language alexia in the absence of amusia (see Judd, 1979, and Judd, Gardner, & Geschwind, 1980, 1983, for reviews).

Playing an Instrument. Instrumental amusia, a specific loss in the ability to play a musical instrument, has not been specifically described very often, perhaps because hemiplegia frequently confounds the situation. It most often accompanies apraxia and/or expressive amusia for singing (Botez & Wertheim, 1959).

Summary

In this very brief review of dissociations within the realm of musical skills, which mostly summarizes the conclusions of other reviewers (Benton, 1977; Dorgeuille, 1966; Edgren, 1895; Gates & Bradshaw, 1977; Henschen, 1920; Marin, 1982; Ustvedt, 1937; Wertheim, 1969), we can see that such skills are usually not impaired in isolation but rather are impaired as part of more general deficits that are not specifically musical.

Future Directions

Case Studies

The clinical case study as a means of demonstrating dissociations of skills will lie at the heart of the neuropsychological study of musical talent. This method must be applied not only to the clinical populations discussed in this chapter, but also to a wide variety of clinically normal but musically exceptional individuals. Such work would be of little value without adequate methodology. Several authors (Dorgeuille, 1966; Jellinek, 1956; Ustvedt, 1937; Wertheim, 1969) have outlined the components of a thorough neuromusicological examination, but neither standardized materials and methods nor normative data are yet available. Educational and research tests of musical abilities, such as those by Bently, Colwell, Drake, Gaston, Gordon, Kwalwasser, Seashore, and Wing (see Shuter-Dyson & Gabriel,

1981, for a review), fill some of this gap but by no means all of it. Moreover, a thorough neuromusicological examination must be integrated with a thorough neuropsychological examination surveying perceptual, cognitive, and motor skills. Refinement of techniques for taking musical histories is also needed (Grison, 1972).

Such an approach is likely to reveal dissociations and clusterings of skills, giving us insight especially into the higher levels of musical functions involved in talent. It would also be useful in moving toward a theory of musical abilities as discussed previously, in providing control data for clinical neuropsychological case studies, and in providing validation of tests of musical abilities for educational purposes.

Comparative Psychomusicology

Another source of individual differences in musical skills to which this case study method can be applied is cultural variations. We have seen from several examples that different musical genres and cultures require or encourage quite different constellations of musical skills, with different neuromusicological consequences. A thorough understanding of musical abilities from a brain perspective requires that we explore a broad sampling of cultures. Such a collaboration with ethnomusicologists is likely to reveal dissociations not otherwise available. The invariants, or musical universals (Harwood, 1976; Lerdahl & Jackendoff, 1983)[6] thus discovered are likely to have even more profound implications for psychomusicology theory and brain theory, just as the study of linguistic universals has contributed to the development of general theory in linguistics.

Developmental Psychomusicology

A complete theory of musical abilities must also be a developmental theory. A theory that purports to describe the structure of musical skills must conform to the sequence(s) in which those skills were acquired. Thus children constitute another group of exceptional individuals who can be studied for dissociations of musical skills.

One group clearly well suited to the case study method is musical child prodigies. This field is still in its infancy. There is a mere handful of directly observed cases (see Feldman, 1980, and Scott & Moffett, 1977, for reviews), and all are prodigies of Western classical music. Feldman (1980) argues convincingly that child prodigies result not from genetics or special circumstances alone but from a rare coincidence of gifts and opportunities. He further asserts that prodigies usually go through the normal sequence of learning in their chosen fields but at an accelerated rate. Some further trends can be gleaned from retrospective biographical studies. Scott and Moffett (1977) have found that early skills within the field are more consistently found in successful musicians, especially composers, than in high achievers in other fields. Musical child prodigies are also very likely to come from musical families.

6. *Ethnomusicology*, Volume 15 (1971), and *The World of Music*, Volume 19 (1977) and Volume 26 (1984), contain issues dedicated to the question of universals in music.

Much work is required to fully substantiate these preliminary observations. Beyond this, many important questions remain. For example, what exactly do the musical child prodigies' gifts consist of? Are the special skills sensory, motor, conceptual, mnemonic, a combination, or something else? How specific are the gifts to music? How specific are the gifts within music? How idiosyncratic are the gifts? In what ways are musical child prodigies similar to and different from child prodigies in other fields?

In the realm of development we are not, however, confined to observing natural experiments and case studies. We can test theories of musical abilities through experimental attempts to train those abilities. For example, can intensive and specific training in tonal memory improve that skill? Will that result in improved singing or improved potential for learning to sing? Can the ability to keep a steady beat be improved though training? Will that result in improved memory for or execution of complex rhythms? More generally, what are the most common, the easiest, and the possible routes of acquisition for the various musical skills?

Are there critical periods for learning various musical skills? The tremendous individual variation in musical skills and training makes it likely that we can address the critical period question much more directly for music than for, say, language (Lenneberg, 1967). This can be approached by comparing the process and speed of musical skill acquisition in children (Gardner, 1982) and adults (Holt, 1978; Sudnow, 1978). An experimental design could match groups of children and adults for performance on carefully selected musical ability tests and compare their performance on commercially available computerized training modules.

Cognitive Psychomusicology

The case study methods provide one type of information for a theory of musical abilities. A second source of such information is perceptual and cognitive studies of the processes involved in musical behaviors and experiences. Although the language used in these fine-grained analyses is somewhat different from the language used to discuss musical abilities, with some effort translations can be made and methodologies adapted. For instance, there has been much work demonstrating different processing channels within the auditory modality (Reineke, 1982). Deutsch (1970), for example, has demonstrated that if one hears a short string of spoken digits followed by a short string of tones or vice versa, one can recall both, whereas two strings of digits (or of tones) cannot be recalled accurately. Such a dissociation between immediate tonal and verbal memory is also evident with brain damage (Milner, 1962). Since talented musicians appear to be consistently superior in immediate tonal memory (Henson & Wyke, 1982), it would be interesting to know whether or not they are also consistently superior in immediate verbal memory.

The models of perceptual and cognitive psychologists often involve a series of processing stages or functions. If these functions can be operationalized as skills that can be tested, then the method of dissociations through case studies of exceptional individuals can be used as a partial test of the models. If these endeavors are successful, then the models can be used to help construct a theory of musical abilities.

Conclusions

Musical abilities, and therefore musical talents, are not unitary but take many forms. It appears quite likely that most, if not all, areas of the brain contribute to the many activities we call musical, although different areas make their characteristic contributions.

If any cluster of skills is central to musical talent it is musical memory. A strong melodic memory appears to be a consistent trait of orchestral musicians and musical idiot savants. It is, by inference, a large part of what accounts for the accomplishments of composers with acquired deafness, and it is a fairly reliable marker of musical prodigies. Deficient melodic memory is characteristic of poor-pitch singers, and it improves when their singing improves. The capacity to remember musical material and to think musically appears to be a consistent companion to the successful development of many types of musical talent. The particular form that one's musical achievements might take—performer, composer, analyst, critic, leader—and the instruments and genres of achievement may be further determined by other capacities—sensory, motor, mathematical, linguistic, reading, spatial, sequential, and social skills.

Yet even musical memory is not a unitary skill. It is not simply the capacity to maintain and call up auditory images of musical sounds. It involves a rich set of associations of musical sounds with ideas and images in other modes and modalities of thought. Musical talent, then, may involve not just a superior capacity for auditory imagery coupled with adequate or strong skills in a few other areas but the successful integration of musical memory with many other skills—many brain areas—to achieve a musical end. The talented musician may be the person who has developed many redundant ways to accomplish musical tasks in order to be able to choose the most efficient for any specific task. That person may show little loss of musical ability in the face of aphasia, alexia, deafness, blindness, some forms of amnesia, or even a major right-hemisphere stroke, because alternate strategies may be available for most musical activities.

Viewed in this way, neuropsychology can help us to see the varieties of musical talent more clearly. It can begin to provide some answers and not just questions. And it can help us find ways to ferret out hidden talents and to make music more accessible to all.

Acknowledgments

I would like to thank Thomas Judd for help in examining the male musical idiot savant described in Table 6-3; Kate Greishaber, Dumi Maraire, Toni Reineke, Mary Smith, Betsy Walker, and the editors for comments on drafts; and Melodee Singh, Raj Singh, and Barbara Rigsby for help in preparing the manuscript.

References

Anastasi, A., & Levee, R. F. (1960). Intellectual defect and musical talent: A case report. *American Journal of Mental Deficiency, 64,* 695–703.

Assal, G. (1973). Aphasie de Wernicke sans amusie chez un pianiste. *Revue Neurologique*, *129*, 251–255.

Atkins, W., & Donovan, M. (1984). A workable music education program for the hearing impaired. *Volta Review*, *86*, 41–44.

Baker, D. J., & Thomas, G. J. (1965). Ablation of cingulate cortex in rats impairs alternation learning and retention. *Journal of Comparative and Physiological Psychology*, *60*, 353–359.

Bancaud, J., Talairach, J., Geier, S., Bonis, A., Trottier, S., & Manrique, M. (1976). Manifestations comportementales induites par la stimulation electrique du gyrus cingulaire anterieur chez l'homme. *Revue Neurologique*, *132*, 705–724.

Basso, A., & Capitani, E. (1985). Spared musical abilities in a conductor with global aphasia and ideomotor apraxia. *Journal of Neurology, Neurosurgery, and Psychiatry*, *48*, 407–412.

Benton, A. L. (1977). The amusias. In M. Critchley & R. A. Henson (Eds.), *Music and the brain* (pp. 378–397). Springfield, IL: Charles C. Thomas.

Bever, T. G., & Chiarello, R. J. (1974). Cerebral dominance in musicians and non-musicians. *Science*, *185*, 137–139.

Borchgrevink, H. M. (1982). Prosody and musical rhythm are controlled by the speech hemisphere. In M. Clynes (Ed.), *Music, mind and brain* (pp. 151–158) New York: Plenum.

Botez, M. I., & Wertheim, N. (1959). Expressive aphasia and amusia following right frontal lesion in a right-handed man. *Brain*, *82*, 186–202.

Bouillaud, J. B. (1865). Sur la faculté du langage articulé. *Bulletin de l'Academie de Medicine*, *30*, 752–755.

Cleall, C. (1983). Notes on a young deaf musician. *The Psychology of Music*, *11*, 101–102.

Corner, V. (1985, May 16). Musical talent brightens life of blind, severely retarded man. *The Toronto Star*.

Deutsch, D. (1970). Tones and numbers: Specificity of interference in short-term memory. *Science*, *168*, 1604–1605.

Dorgeuille, C. (1966). *Introduction a l'étude des amusies*. Paris: Thèse.

Dupré, E., & Nathan, M. (1911). *Le langage musical: Etude medico-psychologique*. Paris: Alcan.

Edgren, I. (1885). Amusie (Musikalische Aphasie). *Deutsche Zeitschrift für Nervenheilung*, *6*, 1–64.

Edwards, E. M. (1974). *Music education for the deaf*. South Waterford, ME: Merriam-Eddy.

Faillace, L. A., Allen, R. P., McQueen, J. D., & Northrup, B. (1971). Cognitive deficits from bilateral cingulotomy for intractable pain in man. *Diseases of the Nervous System*, *32*, 171–175.

Feldman, D. H. (1980). *Beyond universals in cognitive development*. Norwood, NJ: Ablex.

Gardner, H. (1975). *The shattered mind*. New York: Alfred A. Knopf.

Gardner, H. (1982). *Art, mind, and brain: A cognitive approach to creativity*. New York: Basic Books.

Gardner, H. (1983). *Frames of mind: The theory of multiple intelligences*. New York: Basic Books.

Gates, A., & Bradshaw, J. L. (1974). Effects of auditory feedback on a musical performance task. *Perception and Psychophysics*, *16*, 105–109.

Gates, A., & Bradshaw, J. L. (1977). The role of the cerebral hemispheres in music. *Brain and Language*, *4*, 403–431.

Goldstein, K. (1948). *Language and language disturbances*. New York: Grune & Stratton.

Gordon, H. W., & Bogen, J. E. (1974). Hemispheric lateralization of singing after intra-carotid sodium amylobarbitone. *Journal of Neurology, Neurosurgery, and Psychiatry, 37,* 727–738.

Grison, B. (1972). *Une etude sur les alternations musicales au cours des lésions hemispheriques.* Paris: Thèse.

Harwood, D. L. (1976). Universals in music: A perspective from cognitive psychology, *Ethnomusicology, 20,* 521–533.

Henschen, S. E. (1920). *Klinische und anatomische Beitrage zur Pathologie des Gehirns, Vol. 5,* Stockholm: Nordische Bokhandeln.

Henson, R. A. (1977). The language of music. In M. Critchley & R. A. Henson (Eds.), *Music and the brain* (pp. 233–254). Springfield, IL: Charles C. Thomas.

Henson, R. A., & Wyke, M. A. (1982). The performance of professional musicians on the Seashore Measures of Musical Talent: An unexpected finding. *Cortex, 18,* 153–158.

Hill, A. L. (1978). Savants: Mentally retarded individuals with special skills. *International Review of Research in Mental Retardation, 9,* 277–298.

Holt, J. (1978). *Never too late: My musical life story.* New York: Delacorte Press.

Hood, J. D. (1977). Deafness and music appreciation. In M. Critchley & R. A. Henson (Eds.), *Music and the brain* (pp. 323–343). Springfield, IL: Charles C. Thomas.

Jellinek, A. (1956). Amusia. *Folia Phoniatrica, 8,* 124–149.

Judd, T. (1979). *Towards a neuromusicology: The effects of brain damage on music reading and musical creativity.* Unpublished doctoral dissertation, Cornell University, Ithaca, NY.

Judd, T., Arslanian, A., Davidson, L., Locke, S., & Mickel, H. (1979, February). *A right hemisphere stroke in a composer.* Paper presented at the meeting of the International Neuropsychological Society, New York.

Judd, T., Gardner, H., & Geschwind, N. (1980). *Alexia without agraphia in a composer* (Technical Report No. 15). Cambridge, MA: Harvard Project Zero.

Judd, T., Gardner, H., & Geschwind, N. (1983). Alexia without agraphia in a composer. *Brain, 106,* 435–457.

Kaufmann, W. (1972). *Musical notations of the orient.* Magnolia, MA: Peter Smith.

Kimura, D. (1964). Left–right differences in the perception of melodies. *Quarterly Journal of Experimental Psychology, 16,* 355–358.

Knight, A. C. (1924). Why give up your music? *Volta Review, 26,* 297–298.

LaFontaine, L. (1968). *The idiot-savant: Ten case studies.* Unpublished master's thesis, Boston University, Boston.

Lamy, M. H. (1907). Amnesie musicale chez un aphasique sensoriel, ancien professeur de musique, conservation de l'execution, de la lecture, de l'improvisation et de la composition. *Revue Neurologique, 63,* 688–693.

Large, B. (1970). *Smetana.* London: Duckworth.

Lenneberg, E. H. (1967). *Biological foundations of language.* New York: Wiley.

Lerdahl, F., & Jackendoff, R. (1983). *A generative theory of tonal music.* Cambridge, MA: The MIT Press.

Luria, A. R., Tsvetkova, L. S., & Futer, D. S. (1965). Aphasia in a composer. *Journal of the Neurological Sciences, 1,* 288–292.

Mann, L. (1898). Casuistische Beitrage zur Hirnchirurgie und Himlokalisation. *Monatschrift fur Psychiatrie und Neurologie, 4,* 369–378.

Marin, O. (1982). Neurological aspects of music perception and performance. In D. Deutsch (Ed.), *The psychology of music* (pp. 453–477). New York: Academic Press.

Martin, J. (1972). Rhythmic (hierarchical) vs. serial structure in speech and other behavior. *Psychological Review, 79,* 487–509.

Meacham, J. A., & Leiman, B. (1982). Remembering to perform future actions. In U. Neisser (Ed.), *Memory observed* (pp. 327–336). San Francisco: W. H. Freeman.

Milner, B. (1962). Laterality effects in audition. In V. B. Mountcastle (Ed.), *Interhemispheric relations and cerebral dominance* (pp. 177–195). Baltimore: The Johns Hopkins University Press.

Miner, J. B. (1903). Motor, visual and applied rhythms. *Monograph Supplement, Psychological Review, 5,* 1–106.

Minogue, B. M. (1923). A case of secondary mental deficiency with musical talent. *Journal of Applied Psychology, 7,* 349–352.

Monty, S. (1981). *May's boy: An incredible story of love.* Nashville: Nelson.

National Assessment of Educational Progress. (1974). *The first national assessment of musical performance* Report 03-MU-01 Washington, DC: U.S. Government Printing Office.

Nauta, W. J. H. (1971). The problem of the frontal lobe: A reinterpretation. *Journal of Psychiatric Research, 8,* 167–187.

Owens, W. A., & Grimm, W. (1941). A note regarding exceptional musical ability in a lowgrade imbecile. *Journal of Educational Psychology, 32,* 636–637.

Parkin, A. J. (1982). Residual learning capability in organic amnesia. *Cortex, 18,* 417–440.

Povel, D. J. (1981). Internal representation of simple temporal patterns. *Journal of Experimental Psychology: Human Perception and Performance, 7,* 3–18.

Powers, H. S. (1980). Language models and musical analysis. *Ethnomusicology, 24,* 1–60.

Reineke, T. (1982). Simultaneous processing of music and speech. *Psychomusicology, 1,* 58–77.

Restle, F. (1970). Theories of serial pattern learning: Structural trees. *Psychological Review, 77,* 481–495.

Révész, G. (1954). *Introduction to the psychology of music.* Norman, OK: University of Oklahoma Press.

Rife, D. C., & Snyder, L. (1931). Studies in human inheritance. 6: A genetic refutation of the principles of "behavioristic" psychology. *Human Biology, 3,* 547–559.

Scheerer, M., Rothmann, E., & Goldstein, K. (1945). A case of "idiot savant": An experimental study of personality organization. *Psychological Monographs, 58,* 1–63.

Scott, D. F., & Moffett, A. (1977). The development of early musical talent in famous composers: A biographical review. In M. Critchley & R. A. Henson (Eds.), *Music and the brain* (pp. 378–397). Springfield, IL: Charles C. Thomas.

Seeger, C. (1977). *Studies in musicology 1935–1975.* Berkeley: University of California Press.

Seguin, E. (1866). *Idiocy and its treatment by the physiological method.* New York: Wood.

Shuter-Dyson, R., & Gabriel, C. (1981). *The psychology of musical ability* (2nd ed.). London and New York: Methuen.

Sloboda, J. (1978). The psychology of music reading. *The Psychology of Music, 9,* 1–27.

Sparks, R., Helm, N., & Albert, M. (1974). Aphasia rehabilitation resulting from melodic intonation therapy. *Cortex, 10,* 347–359.

Stankov, L., & Spilsbury, G. (1978). The measurement of auditory abilities of blind, partially sighted, and sighted children. *Applied Psychological Measurement, 2,* 491–503.

Starr, A., & Phillips, L. (1970). Verbal and motor memory in the amnestic syndrome. *Neuropsychologia, 8,* 75–88.

Sudnow, D. (1978). *Ways of the hand: The organization of improvised conduct.* Cambridge, MA: Harvard University Press.

Teuber, H. L., Corkin, S., & Twitchell, T. E. (1977). A study of cingulotomy in man. In *Appendix: Psychosurgery* (DHEW Publication No. OS 77-0002). Washington, DC: U.S. Government Printing Office, pp. IIIi-III115.

Tredgold, A. F. (1922). *Mental deficiency (amentia)* (4th ed.). New York: Wood.

Ustvedt, H. J. (1937). Uber die Untersuchung der musikalischen Functionen bei Patienten mit Aphasie. *Acta Medica Scandinavica, 86,* (Suppl. 86, 1-737).

Viscott, D. S. (1970). A musical idiot savant: A psychodynamic study, and some speculations on the creative process. *Psychiatry, 33,* 494–515.

Walthard, L. (1927). Bemerkungen zum Amusie-Problem. *Schweizer Archiv für Neurologie und Psychiatrie, 20,* 295–315.

Weisenburg, T., & McBride, K. E. (1935). *Aphasia: A clinical and psychological study.* Brattleboro, Vt: Hildred and Co.

Welch, G. F. (1979). Poor pitch singing: A review of the literature. *The Psychology of Music, 7,* 50–58.

Wertheim, N. (1969). The amusias. In P. J. Vinken & G. W. Bruyn (Eds), *Handbook of clinical neurology* (Vol. 4). Amsterdam: North-Holland.

Würtzen, C. H. (1903). Einzelne Formen von Amusie, durch Beispiele beleuchtet. *Deutsche Zeitschrift für Nervenheilkunde, 24,* 465–473.

Zatorre, R. J. (1984). Musical perception and cerebral function: A critical review. *Music Perception, 2,* 196–221.

7

The Chess Mind

LEE D. CRANBERG
MARTIN L. ALBERT

> *There must have been a time when men were demigods or they could not have invented chess.—Gustav Schenk (cited in Reider, 1959, p. 320)*

First appearing in approximately A.D. 600 in India and developed to its present form over several centuries and continents, the game of chess has an abiding history. Through the ages it has continued to evoke something akin to "autistic passion"[1] in its serious devotees, who are willing to sit hours on end, one day and the next, in youth and old age, endeavoring to unravel its mysteries. The number of books written about chess exceeds the number written about all other games combined (Fine, 1967), a testimony, no doubt, to the persistent intrigue of a game that has virtually limitless possibilities. To play through all permutations of the first ten moves alone, each move played at a rate of one per second, would engage the day and night energies of every man, woman, and child on earth for the next 217 billion years.

Since it is impossible to calculate all the exponential consequences of a move through this maze of innumerable possibilities, a player must rely on uncertain assessments. In the course of a game, the player must make uncertain decision after uncertain decision, move after move, and whether those decisions tend in a superior direction is only determined objectively if they culminate in a win.

Hence chess has the curious quality of being simultaneously unfathomable yet fathomable. As Newell, Shaw, and Simon state, "It pits two intellects against each other in a situation so complex that neither can hope to understand it completely, but sufficiently amenable to analysis that each can hope to outthink his opponent" (Newell, Shaw, & Simon, 1963, p. 39). It is no wonder that former world champion A. Anderssen dubbed the game the "gymnasium of the mind" (Mengarini, 1963, p. 64) or that Goethe called it "the touchstone of the intellect" (Johnson-Laird & Wason, 1977, p. 531).

---

1. A phrase coined by George Steiner (1973).

Lee D. Cranberg and Martin L. Albert. Section of Behavioral Neuroscience, Department of Neurology, Boston University Medical School, Boston, Massachusetts; and Section of Behavioral Neuroscience, Department of Neurology, Boston Veterans Administration Medical Center, Boston, Massachusetts.

It is no wonder also that cognitive psychologists have used the game as a model for how humans solve problems. The pieces are in full view for both sides, and results are based strictly on intellectual prowess. No element of hidden resources, feinting, or luck intrudes. Furthermore, the culmination of each game in a win, loss, or draw allows a ready ranking of players on the basis of playing results. An international rating system, in fact, assigns a numerical index, ranging roughly from 500 to 3000, to one's ability based on one's tournament results.[2] Cognitive psychologists have used the rating system to divide players along skill lines in a series of experiments that have done much to elucidate the cognitive elements of chess mastery.

Following the lead of the cognitive psychologists, brain scientists also ought to focus attention on the game. The human brain can so master the staggering complexities of chess that it consistently beats the most advanced computers, and the neurology underlying that amazing feat deserves study. A model of how the brain achieves prowess in chess could then be developed to further our understanding of other behavioral realms. For example, later in this chapter we indicate how such a model can be applicable to the study of cerebral dominance and handedness.

In this chapter we review what is known about the brain mechanisms required to play skillful chess, and then we elaborate our theory on the subject. In I. The Chess Players, we look at who plays chess, paying particular attention to those biological traits that may bear on the structure and function of the brain. Among those biological traits is nonchess intelligence, which is dealt with separately in II. Intelligence in Chess Players. In III. Proficiency at Chess, we review the cognitive psychology of chess—that is, the analysis of the thinking strategies employed to produce good moves. In IV. The Neurology of Chess, we speculate on the brain mechanisms that might underlie those strategies or that might be necessary to explain other known phenomena. We develop a theory of the neurology of chess, which we then check against the available physiological data, handedness data, and brain lesion data. In V. Conclusion, we evaluate the success and applicability of the proposed theory.

I. The Chess Players

Chess is a game that can be assayed and enjoyed by nearly everyone, regardless of background. But as we shall see, the top players in the world are overrepresented by youthful men—many of them from the Soviet Union, many of them Jewish, and more than a few of them mathematicians. Cultural factors, and perhaps some biological ones as well, conspire to yield this curious demography of chess talent.

---

2. Most beginners would be at the 500 to 1000 level. Among the 30,000 rated members of the United States Chess Federation (the major, mass-membership chess organization in the country), the median rating is approximately 1600, consistent with a strong amateur's level of play. Those having a minimum rating of 2200 are designated "chess masters" and constitute the upper 3% of all rated U.S. players (*Chess Life*, 1985). The world's highest rated player is world champion Gari Kasparov, with a rating of 2715 (*Chess Informant*, 1985).

After originating in the East, chess spread throughout the world and is now truly an international game. Today many countries, from Iceland to the Philippines, from Argentina to Denmark, can claim at least one grandmaster. For historical reasons, however, chess is most popular in the West—in Europe and especially in the Soviet Union. Approximately 5 million Soviets are regular players. The genuine national enthusiasm for the game and an elaborate state-sponsored system of identifying, training, and supporting promising players have given the Soviets—with the brief exception of the Fischer comet—a monopoly on the world chess championship since the end of World War II.

The Soviet emphasis on identifying talent early is appropriate, since in the history of chess most world-caliber players showed impressive flair for the game in childhood. Samuel Reshevsky, later the U.S. champion for many years, was conducting simultaneous exhibitions at age 6, when he could barely see the board over the top of the table. After learning the game at age 5, future world champion José Raul Capablanca displayed remarkable precocity in becoming the Cuban national champion by age 12. Similarly, after learning the moves at age 6, Bobby Fischer advanced rapidly to become the U.S. champion at age 14.

The real zenith comes a bit later. The age at which the 15 world champions from 1851 to the present each ascended to the throne ranges between 21 and 37 years and averages 29 years. Playing strength usually peaks sometime in the fourth decade (Buttenwieser, 1935; Elo, 1965; Lehman, 1953) before starting to undergo a very slow decline (Buttenwieser, 1935; Elo, 1965). Nonetheless, Alekhine was still world champion when he died at age 54, and Lasker placed third in the prestigious international tournament in Moscow in 1935 at age 67, indicating that one can remain highly competitive even into the senium.

Another noteworthy phenomenon about top chess players is that many of them have been Jewish. Of the 15 world champions since 1851, seven (Steinitz, Botvinnik, Smyslov, Tal, Spassky, Fischer, and Kasparov) can claim Jewish ancestry. In the famous U.S.–U.S.S.R. radio match after World War II, the Soviet team of ten included five Jews, and the U.S. team included seven. And in a later match the British included five Jews on their team. Although vague "racial"/genetic explanations have been advanced (Binet, 1966/1893; Spanier, 1984), most likely the success of Jews in chess is attributable to a variety of cultural factors (e.g., a Jewish tradition that encourages intellectual achievement; the historical fact that, unlike some other competitive activities, chess was not prohibited to Jews; and the fact that Jews often committed themselves only to portable activities in the event of evictions and enforced relocations).

Any genetic theory of chess skill, moreover, would have to deal with the troublesome fact that in chess, unlike music or scholarship, there are hardly any instances of great skill running in families (Bakwin, 1973; Binet, 1966/1893). Binet's (1966/1893) observation that the greatest players of the 1800s "have not passed their talent on to their descendants" applies to modern-day grandmasters as well.

Curiously, although the links between genetics and chess skill are murky, interest in the game along gender lines is blatantly obvious. The game seems to appeal almost exclusively to men. Among its amateur enthusiasts, men outnumber women by approximately 4 to 1. And at the higher levels, women are even less well represented. None of the top 135 players in the United States is a woman, and a similar pattern of male dominance is obvious in the Soviet Union and elsewhere.[3]

Other games such as bridge—where many women play well and where women have been members of world championship teams—do not share this male bias in so striking a degree. What makes chess different? Several explanations have been offered. The arcane psychoanalytic explanation is that male Oedipal desires are aroused by a game promoting murder of a king (Coriat, 1941, as discussed in Smith, 1975; Jones, 1931) and that therefore only males have strong psychic motivation to excel at chess. A biological explanation cites a large body of controversial data attributing an advantage to males in dealing with visuo-spatial material (Harris, 1978; Maccoby & Jacklin, 1974) and concludes that male superiority for the nonverbal, visuo-spatial game of chess is due to sex-determined brain differences.[4] Finally, because chess is a schematized representation of two armies at war, one must acknowledge the cultural bias that encourages boys but not girls to command armies, to participate in war, and to take up an interest in the game. When it comes to explaining male preeminence in chess, it may well be that as with Jews in chess, cultural factors are at least as important as biological ones.

Another noteworthy aspect about top chess players is that many of them have been very adept mathematicians (Binet, 1966/1893; de Groot, 1965), which may not be surprising if one assumes that both disciplines draw on similar reservoirs of nonverbal, visuo-spatial skills. Former world champions A. Anderssen and Max Euwe were both professional academic mathematicians, and a third world champion, Emanuel Lasker, had a doctorate in mathematics and was friendly with Albert Einstein, with whom he had long arguments about the theory of relativity (Fine, 1967). In de Groot's (1965) survey of 55 grandmasters selected over a 200-year period, 13 had careers in either mathematics or the exact sciences.

Most of the other grandmasters in de Groot's survey held professional positions in culturally prestigious fields, such as medicine, law, psychoanalysis, and music. Other authors have also noted the high intellectual achievements of chess masters outside of chess (Bakwin, 1973; Binet, 1966/1893), which raises the question whether chess masters owe their superior skill at the game in part to a generous endowment of overall intellectual capability. Are chess masters "smarter" than the average man on the street? We examine general intelligence of chess masters in the next section.

II. Intelligence in Chess Players

> To play chess requires no intelligence at all.—José Raul Capablanca (cited in Gardner, 1983, p. 170)

---

3. These gender data are largely derived from the survey reported below on pages 174–177.

4. In this volume and elsewhere, Benbow and co-workers make a similar argument for male superiority in mathematics (Benbow, 1986; Benbow & Benbow, 1984; Benbow & Stanley, 1983).

An illiterate serf on the Indian estate of Sultan Khan was a skilled chess player and an international competitor in the 1930s. Perhaps he was a model for Stefan Zweig's world champion Mirko Centovic in *The Royal Game* (1944), who is depicted as a kind of idiot savant. Turn-of-the-century grandmaster Henry Nelson Pillsbury, on the other hand, was renowned for his prodigious memory in many realms beyond chess. During 10 minutes of intermission between blindfold games, he entertained audiences by memorizing 30 words in a row and then reciting back either the word or its ordinal number (Cleveland, 1907). No less impressive, Bobby Fischer has been rumored to have an IQ in the 180s (Bakwin, 1973). These anecdotes are intriguing, and they highlight the need for careful studies of the intelligence or nonchess intellectual capabilities of top-flight chess players. Lamentably, only a few scientific studies address these issues.

Mental measurement pioneer Alfred Binet was one of the first to theorize about the intellectual capabilities of successful players. He speculated that their ability in chess rested on, among other things, superior imagination and memory. Unfortunately, his studies of grandmasters did not include attempts to demonstrate such supposed superiority in nonchess realms (Binet, 1966/1893).

In 1925 three Russian psychologists invited 12 participants in the international chess tournament in Moscow to serve as subjects for a series of neuropsychological tests (Djakow, Petrowski, & Rudik, 1927, as discussed in de Groot, 1965, and in Fine, 1967). Not surprisingly, the masters performed better than control subjects (not further described) on several tests that involved manipulating chess pieces or that otherwise directly drew on one's fund of chess knowledge.

Various other tests were devoid of chess content. Although the testing techniques that were used are considered unsophisticated by today's standards, areas covered included memory (for numbers and for geometric designs), attention, speed of intellectual processes, and the ability to detect logical patterns (e.g., in a number series). On these tests the masters usually performed no better than the control subjects. Although serious methodological weaknesses undermine the validity of the study, the idea that chess masters have higher intelligence with superior memory and better capacities of concentration was not substantiated.

At age 8 chess prodigy Samuel Reshevsky submitted to several psychometric tests administered by the Swiss psychologist Franziska Baumgarten (Baumgarten, 1930, as discussed in de Groot, 1965, and in Fine, 1967). He did exceptionally well on a task requiring memorization of matrices of single-digit numbers, but on most other tasks, including visual memory tasks for less abstract material, he actually performed below average. His verbal development was markedly delayed and was in fact below the norm for 5-year-old Berlin boys. Baumgarten's conclusion that chess skill is thus separate from prowess in other intellectual realms agrees with that of the Russian psychologists. The validity of Baumgarten's data, however, is clouded by the fact that Reshevsky's early chess successes interfered with his regular attendance at school. Furthermore, his upbringing in an Orthodox Jewish household, with its scholastic emphasis on Hebrew and the Talmud, made it difficult to compare his lower verbal scores (tested in German) with scores of the non-Jewish Berlin boys who formed her normative population.

Finally, Lane and Robertson (1979) conducted several investigations on the thinking processes of novice and strong amateur chess players (maximum rating: 2050). Although they chose to confine their published remarks to the performance of the subjects on specific chess-related tasks, an unpublished investigation (D. Lane, personal communication with N. Charness, 1980) failed to reveal any correlation between chess ability (as measured by chess rating) and performance on a nonchess, visuo-spatial task (the Guilford-Zimmerman Spatial Visualization Subtest, Form B; Guilford & Zimmerman, 1953). Since no masters were included among their subjects, the study reveals nothing about the visuo-spatial abilities of highly skilled players.

Aside from the Russian study and Baumgarten's case report, each over 50 years old, and Lane and Robertson's unpublished investigation of amateur players, we could find no other studies of the intellectual capacities of chess players. Those capacities could be gauged in strong players with many of the newer psychometric instruments now available. Until modern-day studies take advantage of these improved techniques, the extent of nonchess intelligence among chess masters will remain in doubt.

The limited evidence outlined in this section suggests that remarkable chess skill can exist in isolation, unaccompanied by other noteworthy intellectual abilities. The functional elements that constitute specialized chess expertise are outlined in the next section.

III. Proficiency at Chess

> As genetics needs its model organisms, its *Drosophila* and *Neurospora*, so psychology needs [chess].—Herbert A. Simon and William G. Chase (Simon & Chase, 1973, p. 394)

Pattern Recognition in Chess

The seminal investigations on the cognitive psychology of chess were performed by the Dutch psychologist and chess master Adriaan D. de Groot (1965). He examined the common sense assumption that players excel at the game if, compared to their opponents, they can see a greater number of moves ahead. By asking subjects to think out loud as they studied selected positions, he was able to chart the reported thinking processes of players of different strengths.

He discovered that on the average, grandmasters searched no further than their weaker counterparts. (On the average, grandmasters and strong amateurs each searched to a maximum depth of six or seven moves.) Instead, the superior play of the grandmasters rested on their prompt ability to size up the demands of the position, identify plausible moves, and conduct their subsequent search along profitable lines. While grandmasters were heading down the right path, weaker players were less adept at thinking up good moves and instead ventured down many blind alleys. Both groups of players searched equally far and with equal fervor, but only the strong players reached their target of confirming a satisfactory move because only they began their search with a satisfactory move.

Hence, as de Groot observed, the searching process for the grandmaster was mostly a *post hoc* justification for good moves that had come to mind almost instantly. The grandmaster's superior chess ability had been demonstrated during the initial rapid assessment of the position prior to the need for calculation.

Intrigued, de Groot wondered if a test measuring one's ability to assimilate a position rapidly would alone be enough to distinguish masters from lesser players. His suspicions were confirmed when he presented a game position for no more than a few seconds and then had his subjects reconstruct the position from memory. The masters demonstrated rapid absorption of the position by reconstructing it flawlessly, whereas weaker players made many errors. Chase and Simon (1973a) later replicated de Groot's experiment with the added control condition that nongame positions created through random placement of the pieces were also used. The failure of grandmasters to reconstruct random positions any better than novices demonstrated that grandmaster superiority with game positions rested on a repertoire of chess knowledge built up through their actual play rather than on any detached superior visual memory *per se*. Game positions were perceived quickly because they had familiar components. Random positions were not amenable to decomposition into familiar components and therefore were not amenable to rapid memorization.

In a model worked out by Simon, Chase, and others, the familiar components in a grandmaster's memory are primarily patterns of specific piece configurations, or "chunks" (Chase & Simon, 1973a, 1973b). Each familiar chunk may contain up to five or more pieces, and each chunk is remembered as a single unit. Hence, depending on the extent of a player's catalog of such chunks, a crowded game position with 20 to 25 pieces could be decomposed and remembered efficiently as a mere handful of familiar chunks. Commonly occurring chunks, such as a fianchettoed bishop in front of a castled king position, are learned early and are familiar even to novices. Less common patterns may arise only once in a thousand games, so that only those players with much practice and study of the game would be likely to be acquainted with them. Simon and Gilmartin (1973) have estimated that a grandmaster, through vast experience with the game, has built up a storehouse of 50,000 patterns of unique piece configurations, a storehouse comparable in size and in facility of access/manipulation to the established vocabulary of a native-language speaker. The grandmaster has attained fluency in chess.

The patterns of piece configurations are each linked in memory with certain strategies or tactics, so that once a position is conceived in terms of its component patterns, plausible moves spring to mind out of those patterns. Just as one fluent in a language generally does not need to stop and think before starting a sentence, so one fluent in the patterns of chess pieces does not need to engage in much conscious thought before generating a plausible move. The larger the storehouse of patterned piece configurations and the more that subtle differences among patterns are all included, the more likely the storehouse can be called upon to describe precisely a position at hand, and the more likely the moves it suggests will be appropriate to that specific position. Thus the large storehouse of patterns enables not only efficient memorization but also strong play.

Now we see why de Groot's grandmasters had discovered strong moves even before beginning to calculate the possibilities. The moves had come to them out of their large, refined storehouse of patterns. As Newell and Simon (1972, p. 783) state: "Thus, the chessmaster's ability to designate large configurations of relations enables him to evaluate certain situations without much detailed sequential calculation. With each familiar feature there can be stored in memory appropriate move generators. . . . It is as 'automatic' as 'A headache? Take aspirin'." Contrary to popular opinion, chess players need not be deep thinkers.

Accordingly, chess players can maintain high performance even when they have scarcely any time available for calculations. Former U.S. champion Walter Browne is known for his ability to get out of time pressure with a string of effective moves made in a matter of seconds. In an experimental setting Dreyfus tried to eliminate the luxury of chess calculation altogether by making his master subjects concentrate on a mathematics calculation task while they were simultaneously playing speed chess. They still beat their lesser opponents not similarly handicapped (S. Dreyfus, personal communication, 1984).

To reiterate what has been discussed thus far and to begin an enumeration of three ways in which pattern recognition is necessary in chess play, we can say, first, that pattern recognition often minimizes or even obviates the need for subsequent analysis/calculation/searching ahead. As Bronstein and Smolyan state, "A strong player requires only a few minutes of thought to get to the heart of the conflict. You see a solution immediately, and half an hour later merely convinces yourself that your intuition has not deceived you" (Spanier, 1984, p. 194). Petrosian used to say he knew he was out of form when his calculations did not confirm the validity of his first impressions (Hearst, 1967).

The second useful function of pattern recognition in chess is that it steers calculations down the right paths in those positions where detailed calculations are unavoidable. Let us say that in a certain position a daring knight sacrifice is contemplated. A careful player must examine all lines of play stemming from the sacrifice in order to be certain that each results in adequate compensation; otherwise, the whole sacrifice idea would be unsound. In other words, the appeal of the sacrifice must be demonstrated. Hence skillful chess playing at times calls for an interplay of move proposals with subsequent investigatory calculation—i.e., hypothesis generation with hypothesis testing.

As it turns out, accurate investigatory calculations are themselves highly dependent on one's skills at pattern recognition. In any investigatory search, the exponential possibilities of an opponent's reply, followed by one's counterreply, and so forth, need to be pruned to a manageable number by restricting one's search to plausible moves for each side. These plausible moves themselves are suggested by the recognition of patterns inherent in projected evolving game positions. Hence in a grand recursive process, a proposed move such as a knight sacrifice is validated by calculations which are no more than a series of other, later proposed moves, each requiring validating calculation, and so forth. The driving force behind this process is the recognition of patterns. The more refined one's storehouse of patterns and the more surefooted its move generators, the greater the validity of the whole "move proposal–calculation verification" scheme (Charness, 1981b).

Hence we see that pattern recognition is at the root of a player's ability both to find moves quickly "without thinking" and to think through, efficiently and productively, the consequences of those moves that do require more deliberation. Pattern recognition also facilitates a third ability critical to any superior chess player—the ability to plan ahead. Especially in quiet positions devoid of ongoing exchanges or other immediate tactical demands, it is necessary to formulate an overall strategy for the future. Pattern recognition has the versatile quality of suggesting not just solitary moves but also general plans that are implemented in a string of moves. Noticing the pattern of a queenside pawn majority, for instance, could lead to the idea of creating a passed pawn, which in turn could suggest the need for supporting that pawn with a rook. Thus a player would search for the most efficient means to maneuver a rook behind his queenside pawns. The point here is that perception of a queenside pawn majority did not *ipso facto* suggest the rook move that followed, but rather it suggested a plan which included the rook move. As Church and Church (1977, pp. 136–137) explain, "[Pattern recognition] will normally be associated with goals and plans rather than specific moves. The treatment of the legal move as the elementary unit of chess thinking is concrete but undoubtedly misguided".

Having established at least three indispensable functions of pattern recognition in chess, we can now return to the paradox presented at the start of the chapter—that humans can excel at a game of unfathomable dimensions. With a finite storehouse of patterned piece configurations in memory, limitless game positions can be construed as certain arrangements of familiar patterns—patterns which in turn suggest strong moves, selected calculations, or appropriate plans for that position. Even though the storehouse contains only familiar patterns, novel arrangements of those patterns can describe novel positions. Thus the pattern-recognition strategy is well suited to dealing with the full proliferation of possibilities that may arise in chess.

The parallels to language are striking. Just as a finite vocabulary can be arranged in varying sequences to convey a nearly infinite number of thoughts, so a finite inner storehouse of patterned piece configurations can be arranged in varying juxtapositions to describe a nearly infinite number of possible chess positions. And just as an enlarged vocabulary enhances precision of expression, so an extensive chess storehouse enhances precision of play.

The prime importance of pattern recognition in the mastery of chess was worked out in the 1930s and in the postwar years by de Groot (1965, 1966) and in the 1960s and 1970s by a team at Carnegie-Mellon University that included Nobel prize winner Herbert Simon, William Chase, and others (Chase & Simon, 1973a, 1973b; Simon, 1979; Simon & Chase, 1973). Because chess has been used by cognitive psychologists as a model for how humans solve problems, it received further attention from a host of later investigators whose contributions replicated, extended, and appropriately modified the work of their predecessors (Charness, 1976, 1977, 1981a, 1981b, 1981c; Church & Church, 1977; Fine, 1965; Frey & Adesman, 1976; Goldin, 1978a, 1978b, 1979; Holding, 1979; Holding & Reynolds, 1982; Lane & Robertson, 1979; Scurrah & Wagner, 1970; Tikhomirov & Poznyanskaya, 1966-1967, winter; Wagner & Scurrah, 1971). The notion that pattern recognition is at the center of chess skill and that calculation is only at its periphery—a notion that struck de Groot with all the force of a counterintuitive revelation—remains accepted today. In fact, the capacity for pattern recognition, as uncovered in chess, has been shown to be necessary for proficiency in many other problem-solving domains, ranging from bridge to physics (Chase & Chi, 1979).

Humans versus Computers

The efficacy of human pattern recognition is highlighted when comparing human strategy at chess with the strategy of a computer. A human can rely on pattern recognition to generate either plausible individual moves or overarching plans (that can be implemented in a string of moves). Chess-playing computers, as they are programmed today, do not operate from a storehouse of patterns. Instead they play at the concrete level of one move at a time, examining every legal move to a depth limited by finite computing time,[5] analyzing the resultant positions according to an elaborate evaluation equation, and then tracing back up the move tree to choose the move that led to the best set of evaluation scores (Dembart, 1984; R. Hyatt, personal communication, 1984). In the course of considering every legal move, the computer inadvertently matches the human feat of finding plausible individual moves. Likewise, by examining all legal moves to a certain depth (up to about four moves for each side by the most sophisticated computers today), the computer can provide a naive observer with the appearance of engaging in short-range planning (assuming that the number of moves required to consummate the "plan" falls within the limited depth of the exhaustive computer search). For example, Hans Berliner (1978, p. 747) writes that Chess 4.6 "has to date made several well known manoeuvres without having the slightest knowledge of the manoeuvre, the conditions for its application, and so on; but only knowing [through brute force calculation] that the end result of the manoeuvre was good".

This is truly *artificial* intelligence. Humans rely on their ability to recognize patterns and apply appropriate strategic thinking to make such maneuvers. The machine, on the other hand, mechanically applies its brute-force calculations and unthinkingly comes up with an identical, "intelligent" short-range maneuver. To paraphrase Hans Berliner (1978), machines do not mimic human thought but rather have their own unique "cognitive" style.

The reason good human players continue to beat the best chess-playing computers is that the exponential possibilities in chess eventually overwhelm a cognitive style based on analyzing all variations. Since even the most technically sophisticated computers can analyze all variations to a maximum depth of only about four moves for each side, any long-range plans requiring more than four moves to unfold would be beyond the computer's horizon. Through the use of pattern recognition, strong human players have no trouble developing plans that

---

5. Some cutoff depth is necessary, since not even the most sophisticated computer can calculate all variations in chess. If a computer attempted to analyze all first moves to their legal conclusions (i.e., win, loss, or draw) at a rate of a thousand billion billion variations a second, the task would require more than 10^{91} years—considerably longer than the current age of the universe (Hearst, 1967).

often exceed that depth. In the example given earlier of a rook supporting a queen-side pawn majority, it may take two or three moves to bring the rook into position, another four or five pawn pushes to force the creation of a passed pawn, and then another two or three pawn advances before promotion. Hence the plan, which is quite elementary from a pattern-recognition point of view, will not bear fruit until at least eight moves have been played by each side. It is thus quite beyond the vision of a computer. Through the use of long-range plans, humans can consistently outplay computers. For chess, the human cognitive style remains superior to that of a computer.[6]

Computer programmers who wish to upgrade the playing strength of their machines have been tempted to adopt the human cognitive style, and in fact some attempts have been made to provide a computer with a storehouse of chess patterns and with heuristic instructions on how to employ those patterns in the successful manipulation of novel positions (Berliner, 1978). But progress has been difficult. As computer programmers listen expectantly in order to relay the know-how to their machines, human masters have been hard pressed to articulate their great skill. The human storehouse of patterns, each linked to certain moves or plans, has been assembled and operates in a nonverbal, visuo-spatial, chess-specific realm, which is difficult to describe to a computer (Hearst, 1977).

The Acquisition of Chess Skill

In fact, chess expertise is hardly any easier to describe in English than in Fortran. All the books written about chess and the numerous magazines and journals devoted to the game can only but crudely sketch the nonverbal essence of the game. Independent of authors or columnists, one grasps the subtleties of the game by oneself. The acquisition of a highly refined storehouse of piece configurations is a lonely, personal achievement.

The achievement does not come overnight. Obviously, practice and much playing of the game are necessary to build up such a storehouse, and Simon and Chase (1973; Chase & Simon, 1973b) estimate that the effort takes thousands of hours. It seems that all players, even the most precocious, must make the necessary investment of time and develop through stages of beginner, intermediate, and merely strong before they become masters. No exception seems to exist in chess history, although Morphy is often touted as someone whose chess talent sprang forth, *de novo*, fully developed, since his first formal competitions earned him recognition as the best player in the world. Even in Morphy's case, however, a careful review of the historical record reveals a preliminary period of much private home practice and protracted cultivation of ability before he emerged so brilliantly on the public chess scene (de Groot, 1965).

An investment of time alone does not guarantee masterhood. A refined repertoire of chess patterns cannot be acquired passively, through mere exposure to the

---

6. The world's best computer, Cray Blitz, plays at a weak master level (current rating: approximately 2200) — that is, below the current level of skill of several hundred U.S. players. In 1978 and again in 1984 Scottish national champion David Levy collected several thousand British pounds in a series of well-publicized wagers by beating the world's best computer in lopsided matches.

game and rote practice. The individual must actively build that repertoire and then rebuild it as necessary. The successful individual must forever be an iconoclast. A remembered general pattern that has been retained to characterize a number of similar, yet slightly different, positions must be destroyed and replaced in memory by a series of well-differentiated specific patterns, each best suited to characterize specific differences amongst those positions. As the player builds an ever-enlarging storehouse of patterns, the right questions must be asked, and the player's skepticism must allow him or her to transform one early conception into several refined versions (Auble, 1982; Bransford, Nitsch, & Franks, 1977, as discussed in Auble, 1982).

Given enough opportunity and effort, can anyone assemble a storehouse of sufficient scope and refinement to be a chess master? Reuben Fine (1967) notes that many enthusiastic players tend to reach a plateau at an amateur's level of ability and are unable to advance further, implying that sustained effort alone may not be sufficient. Out of thousands of chess enthusiasts, only a few emerge to become masters. In addition to practice and effort, masterhood may also be predicated on a superior neurological endowment. Do special qualities of mind allow some players to jump over barriers with seeming ease, to zero in on the right questions, to destroy old patterns and create new ones with an alacrity that may result in a master's grasp of the game within the first decade of life? The innate brain mechanisms required to play skillful chess are discussed in the next section.

IV. The Neurology of Chess

A Speculative Hypothesis

Noting that chess may be mastered at a very young age, George Steiner (1973) pointed to two other fields in which creative results have been achieved before the age of puberty—music and mathematics. As Steiner pointed out, other fields, such as art, may have precocious imitators, such as the young Picasso who exactly mimicked his father's drawings. But only in chess, music, and mathematics have profound, original insights been contributed by preadolescents. Reshevsky and Capablanca were executing highly original combinations before their ninth birthdays. Mozart and Rossini composed unprecedented music during their preteen years. And Gauss saw deep into prime number theory and algebraic series by age 10.

The association between mathematics and chess was mentioned earlier. As was pointed out, many top chess players are also adept mathematicians. Both fields are dominated by men (Benbow & Benbow, 1984; Benbow & Stanley, 1983; Kolata, 1983). Both fields involve highly developed nonverbal capacities, and both rely on specialized visuo-spatial skills. Music composition, too, can take its place alongside mathematics and chess as a nonverbal endeavor, overrepresented by men, where the physical arrangement of abstract dynamic relationships exploits spatial skills (Harris, 1978). As George Steiner (1973, p. 52) explained, "the solution of a mathematical problem, the resolution of a musical discord or conclusion of a contrapuntal development, the generation of a winning chess position can be envisaged as [spatial] regroupings" that have their own abstract internal logic. If a regrouping is successful, the end result is a release "of tension between energy

levels so as to achieve a harmoniously efficient posture or configuration", aesthetically affirming the validity of the internal logic.

In neurophysiological terms, Steiner wondered whether

> all three [fields] involve enormously powerful but narrowly specialized areas of the
> cortex. These areas can somehow be triggered into life in a very young child and can
> develop in isolation from the rest of his psyche. Sexually and socially unformed, very
> possibly backward in every general respect, the child virtuoso or pre-teen-age chess
> master draws on formidable but wholly localized synapses in the brain.[7]

For three reasons we propose the right hemisphere as the site of those
localized synapses responsible for proficient chess play.[8] First, the nonverbal,
visuo-spatial skills that the game of chess demands are best realized by the
right hemisphere. Second, pattern recognition—the key element of proficiency
at chess—is also best accomplished by the right hemisphere. And third, the
gender differences in proficiency at chess can be interpreted to suggest right-
hemisphere competence for chess. Each of these three reasons will be discussed in
some detail.

First, since chess cognition is nonverbal, it does not depend on the proven
superiority of the left hemisphere in verbal matters. Yet, as an activity with an
inherent spatial logic, it may very well depend on the proven superiority of the right
hemisphere in spatial reasoning (Benton, 1985; Hécaen & Albert, 1978). It is
known, for instance, that lesions of the right hemisphere result in derangements of
spatial perception. For example, patients with right-hemisphere lesions may have
difficulty in establishing an internal representation of the layout of their hospital
ward or in orienting themselves with respect to its external representation on a
map. Although they may remember landmarks to guide themselves from one room
to another, they lack an internal geographic schema that would allow them to
navigate the same route with their eyes closed. Since the adroit navigation of chess
pieces probably depends on an intact set of similar internal spatial schemata, chess
talent probably relies on the right hemisphere.

The second reason we cite to justify a theory of chess proficiency residing in
right-hemisphere structures relates to how the brain processes and recognizes patterns. As we have seen in the previous section, chess skill is based on the ability to
perceive familiar patterns in a game position and to recognize appropriate moves
and strategies inherent in those patterns. Pattern recognition often proceeds
rapidly, as, for instance, when de Groot's grandmaster subjects memorized a complex position in a matter of seconds, or when Walter Browne scrambled out of time
pressure with a series of rapid-fire moves. In these top players, each grouping of
pieces is recognized instantaneously and remembered as a whole chunked unit
because it is matched with appropriate piece configuration patterns in their

---

7. The quoted material is from page 52 of *Sporting Scene: White Knights of Reykjavik* by G. Steiner,
1973. London: Faber and Faber. Copyright 1972, 1973 by George Steiner. Reprinted by permission.

8. Although we will restrict our comments to why we believe that specialized mechanisms underlying
chess ability may be preferentially localized in the right hemisphere, much of our rationale is undoubtedly applicable to music and mathematics, which have also been ascribed at times to the right hemisphere (Gardner, 1983).

memory. Beginners who have no such storehouse of patterns must laboriously register each arrangement one piece at a time. Roland Puccetti (1974) argued that the piece-by-piece approach is a left-hemisphere function, whereas masterful gestalt pattern recognition is possible only in the right hemisphere. Various experiments demonstrate that holistic thinking—including the ability to recognize a pattern *in toto*—is most efficiently performed by the right hemisphere (Bever, 1975). Accordingly, skillful chess play may rely most heavily on the right hemisphere.

Third, and finally, the sex data mentioned elsewhere in this chapter (cf. pages 158–159 and 175–176) could be interpreted to suggest right-hemisphere proficiency for chess. Almost all Federation International des Echecs (the international chess federation) grandmasters are males. Few women excel at the game. Perhaps cultural or psychoanalytic variables are in part to blame. But as with sex differences in mathematics ability (see Footnote 4), the possibility of an underlying biological explanation cannot be readily dismissed.

According to a theory propounded by Norman Geschwind, the presence of intrauterine testosterone produced by the developing male fetus slows development of its own left hemisphere, which leads to compensatory enhanced development of its right hemisphere. In female brains, influenced by less testosterone, the left hemisphere develops apace, and there is no need for compensatory right-hemisphere overdevelopment (Geschwind & Behan, 1982; Geschwind & Galaburda, 1985). The comparative male-female result is a male brain with a right-hemisphere advantage. Geschwind's theory would thus explain male superiority for chess if one assumes that chess skill resides in the right hemisphere.

The converging evidence from these three different sources lends credence to our speculative hypothesis. The nonverbal, visuo-spatial nature of chess and its reliance on gestalt pattern recognition could imply that chess skill is primarily dependent on right-hemisphere mechanisms. Furthermore, such a theory of the neurology of chess, when combined with Geschwind's hormonal theory of hemispheric development, could lead to a plausible explanation for why men seem to enjoy an advantage at the game. The pertinent brain structures would include the right parietal, right temporal, and perhaps right frontal regions.

We are now ready to extend into neurological realms the analogy we developed earlier between language and chess. Just as the left hemisphere is the preferred neurological substrate for the organization of language, we argue that the right hemisphere has a complementary responsibility as the preferred substrate for the organization of chess talent. Specifically, just as the left hemisphere has evolved a specialized role in the capacity to store, retrieve, and manipulate the tens of thousands of words necessary to use language skillfully, so the right hemisphere has a specialized role in performing a conceptually similar task that uses different operands, the operands of chess patterns. Specifically, the right hemisphere is responsible for storing, retrieving, and manipulating the tens of thousands of piece configuration patterns necessary to play chess skillfully.

Does our theory of right-hemisphere localization of chess talent jibe with the available biological data? In the remainder of this section we check our theory against the available data relating chess and the brain. First, we discuss the physiological correlates of chess play, dwelling primarily on brain electrical activity in chess players (pp. 170–174). Next, we report on our own study of the handedness of chess players (pp. 174–177). We then conclude the section with a review of known instances of chess players who have suffered strokes or other brain lesions (pp. 177–185).

The Physiology of Chess

White opposes black, and each side tries to defeat the other. Chess is a fiercely competitive game, where the victories are sought with enthusiasm and the defeats are often extremely disheartening (Menninger, 1942). The emotional involvement of the players is reflected in a variety of physiological parameters (galvanic skin response, breathing rate, blood pressure, and pulse rate) that tend to peak dramatically at critical junctures in the game (Leedy & Dubeck, 1971; Pfleger, Stocker, Pabst, & Haralambie, 1980; Tikhomirov & Vinogradov, 1970). While on the surface the chess player may appear unperturbed as he quietly concentrates on a game, in fact he is tolerating a series of marked physiological gyrations such as are depicted in Figure 7-1. The stress of this physiological maelstrom, repeated game after game, may contribute to the documented decreased longevity of chess masters (Barry, 1969).

Although changes in pulse rate, galvanic skin response, blood pressure, and breathing rate can be pronounced during a game, they reveal little about where in the brain chess thinking occurs. Charting a different physiological index—brain electrical activity as measured by an EEG—holds more promise for localizing chess talent. An EEG machine registers the sum of electrical activity from numerous individual neurons located within a particular area of the brain. It is unable to tell us what each individual neuron is doing, but it does reflect the total electrical activity of large sections of the brain and is thus well suited to detect gross asymmetries in electrical function when comparing one hemisphere to the other.

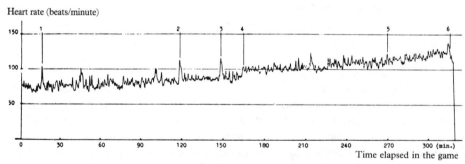

FIGURE 7-1. Sharp accelerations in a grandmaster's pulse rate occurred at critical moments in a tournament game: (1) after a novel opening had been played; (2) prior to an important decision with lasting consequences; (3) while awaiting his opponent's move, the player spotted a weakness in his own position; (4) at the beginning of a wild skirmish; (5) when both players were beginning to get into time pressure; and (6) upon relaxation after winning the game. Adapted from "Sportmedizinische Untersuchung an Schachspielern der Spitzenklasse [Sports Medical Examination of Top Class Chess Players]" by H. Pfleger, K. Stocker, H. Pabst, and G. Haralambie, 1980. *Münchener Medizinische Wochenschrift, 122* (Nr. 28), p. 1043. Copyright 1980 by the editors of *Münchener Medizinische Wochenschrift*. Reprinted by permission.

Studies using EEGs have investigated a variety of chess-playing subjects. Two studies describe certain rare players with preexisting epilepsy whose seizures can be triggered by playing chess (Forster, Richards, Panitch, Huisman, & Paulsen, 1975; Han-pai, Chen, & Chih-p'ing, 1965). A generalized convulsion was observed in one player immediately after he had excitedly discovered a winning escape from a difficult position (Han-pai, Chen, & Chih-p'ing, 1965, Case 4).[9] Another epileptic player attempted to make an illegal move and was corrected. Frustrated, he suffered seven seizures while delaying inordinately over an alternate move (Forster, Richards, Panitch, Huisman, & Paulsen, 1975). Earlier in the game, when this same player made routine opening moves, and later when he was winning comfortably, no seizures occurred, which led Forster and his colleagues to theorize that an emotional element such as tension or being on the defensive was a necessary trigger for such seizures. Although seizures could be evoked in this patient when he chose from a menu or on other occasions of forced decision-making, chess was a particularly reliable epileptogenic stimulus because of the stress associated with the need to juggle numerous interdependent variables in complex positions. In general, the EEGs of these players did not show any asymmetries of brain electrical activity, either in the baseline record or after exposure to chess had evoked diffuse disruption of electrical activity (generalized dysrhythmia; Forster, Richards, Panitch, Huisman, & Paulsen, 1975; Han-pai, Chen, & Chih-p'ing, 1965).

Perhaps more applicable as a test of our theory are the EEG studies on healthy, nonepileptic players. During an international tournament, V. Malkin (1982) had an opportunity to record EEGs on 26 world-class chess players, including such luminaries as Bronstein, Geller, Polugaevsky, Tukmakov, and former world champion Tal. Routine EEGs performed prior to their games were in general normal and indistinguishable from those of the general population (see Figure 7-2), although it was noteworthy that many players had an alpha frequency within the lower ranges of normal, at 8–9 hertz. Malkin interpreted these low-normal alpha frequencies as a manifestation of the players' abilities to relax before a game.

The EEGs obtained on a few of the players while they were pondering the position of an interrupted (i.e., adjourned) game with their eyes closed revealed underlying eye movements. In fact, the EEG reader was able to tell when these players were thinking about their game, based on the presence of the underlying eye movements. He surmised that they were scanning the mental visual image of the position. Other players were able to mull over their adjourned positions without the telltale eye movements, which led Malkin to conclude that the latter group analyzed positions with less reliance on visual imagination and more reliance on abstract spatial perception. Although Malkin reported in detail on the eye movements of his subjects, he unfortunately neglected to say anything about the electrical activity going on in the brain itself. It thus seems that Malkin overlooked a good opportunity to report on the electrophysiological correlates of chess thinking in some of the world's best players.

---

9. It is unclear from the English translation of this article whether the subject was playing chess as we know it in the West or instead Chinese chess (hsiang ch'i), a similar game with a similar origin but with slightly different rules.

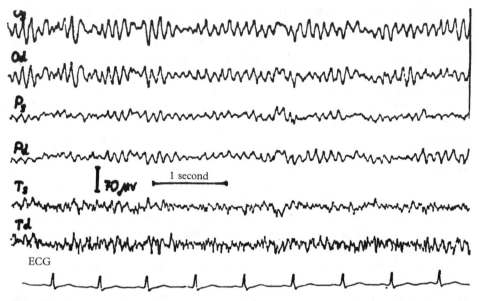

FIGURE 7-2. Routine EEG of former world chess champion Mikhail Tal. The EEG is normal. Adapted from "[The electroencephalography of chess players]" by V. Malkin, 1982. *Shakhmatnyi Byulleten, 8*, p. 14. Copyright 1982 by the editors of *Shakhmatnyi Byulleten*. Reprinted by permission.

A different EEG study does comment on brain electrical activity as it evolved during the course of an entire game. Chess master Errol Liebowitz, ranking in the top 100 U.S. chess players, submitted to a continuous EEG recording while he played a game of chess with his eyes closed (E. Liebowitz, personal communication, 1984). Once he decided on a move, he said it to his opponent and coinvestigator. In general, throughout the game there was a high degree of right-hemisphere activity (with background frequencies often in the fast, beta range), while left-hemisphere activity was usually less rapid (with background frequencies usually only in the slower, alpha range). As an example, the tracing depicted in Figure 7-3, obtained prior to Liebowitz's move in a "quiet" position with few immediate tactical demands, shows significantly faster right-hemisphere background activity compared to the left hemisphere. Only at tactical junctures in the game, where careful sequential calculations were necessary and where Liebowitz believed that much of the analysis occurred within a subvocalized verbal framework (e.g., thinking to himself, "If I go here, then he goes there, and I reply . . ."), did left-hemisphere activity match right-hemisphere activity.

One must be unusually cautious about interpreting these EEG results. The implication could be drawn that Liebowitz's right hemisphere had the major responsibility for determining chess strategy and selecting the appropriate moves, while his left hemisphere played a secondary, supplementary role. Such an implication is surely overdrawn, however, since sheer volumes of electrical activity do not necessarily point to hierarchies of brain function.

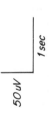

Left hemisphere

Right hemisphere

FIGURE 7-3. An EEG tracing for U.S. chess master Errol Liebowitz, obtained while he was playing a game of chess. As he ponders a "quiet" position with few immediate tactical demands, right-hemisphere activity is faster than left-hemisphere activity (monopolar lead placement at C_3 and C_4). Reproduced by permission of Errol Liebowitz.

Furthermore, using one of us (L. D. C.) as a subject, we were unsuccessful in our attempts to duplicate Liebowitz's findings. The subject was a 33-year-old, right-handed, strong amateur player with a rating in the 1800s. Initially, a standard 16-channel baseline EEG was recorded with eyes closed, and the results were normal, with no hemispheric asymmetries. The recording was continued while the subject then played a game of blindfold chess with his eyes closed. His moves and his opponent's responses were announced orally. No discernible changes from the baseline EEG recording could be detected, and no hemispheric asymmetries emerged.

Taken all together, the EEG studies discussed in this section render limited judgment on our theory and point to the need for further studies using systematic, reliable methodologies that control for subjects' preexisting epilepsy, playing strength, and other variables. Although not corroborated by our own particular study, the suggestion arising from Liebowitz's work that chess thinking is associated with preponderant right-hemisphere electrical activity is one finding which could cautiously be used to support our theory and which definitely merits further investigation.

We move now from an examination of an individual player's particular physiological or brain electrical behavior during an individual game to a look at certain traits of a large number of chess players. Are there any telltale biological traits identifying enhanced right-hemisphere development that chess players possess in superabundance? The results of a survey of the rates of left-handedness in chess players are discussed next.

The Handedness of Chess Players

Left-handers are overrepresented among talented mathematicians (Annett & Kilshaw, 1982; Benbow, 1986; Benbow & Benbow, 1984; Kolata, 1983) and perhaps also among talented artists, engineers, and music composers (Marx, 1982). Since few of these activities have a significant manual component, it is not readily apparent why one's success at them should be linked in any way to one's hand preference.

Indeed, the answer is not known, but certain speculations have attempted to link hand preference with an underlying brain organization that could be advantageous for developing proficiency in certain cognitive fields. A number of neuroanatomical studies that have compared the brains of right- and left-handed individuals do, in fact, uncover persistent brain differences between the two groups. Although brain measurement techniques have varied, including CT scanning (LeMay, 1976), pneumoencephalography (McRae, Branch, & Milner, 1968), and cerebral angiography (LeMay & Culebras, 1972), the consistent conclusion among these various studies has been that right-handers have more markedly asymmetrical brains, usually reflecting a greater volume of tissue in the left hemisphere. Left-handers, on the other hand, tend to have more symmetric brains, so that the left-hemisphere bias is either attenuated or mildly reversed (Galaburda, LeMay, Kemper, & Geschwind, 1978; LeMay & Geschwind, 1975, as discussed in Galaburda, LeMay, Kemper, & Geschwind, 1978).

Though purely speculative, it is possible that the attenuation of the anatomical asymmetry that favored the left hemisphere could be associated with relative enhancement of the right hemisphere and relative increased proficiency in right-hemisphere cognitive tasks. We have already alluded to the nonverbal, visuo-spatial nature of mathematics and music and to attempts to link those skills to right-hemisphere function (Gardner, 1983). Art and engineering are equally nonverbal, no less reliant on visuo-spatial talent, and perhaps equally likely to depend on right-hemisphere proficiency. Pushing speculation to its logical conclusion, we might theorize that left-handers would be overrepresented among talented mathematicians, music composers, artists, and engineers because of a greater statistical likelihood of having a brain organization favoring proficiency in those fields.

Pursuing the notion that left-handedness could be linked with right-hemisphere talents and pursuing the theory that chess proficiency depends on right-hemisphere abilities, we sought to determine the rates of left-handedness among chess players. Our subjects were drawn from the 30,000 rated members of the United States Chess Federation (USCF). Each subject had played at least 20 tournament games and had thereby acquired a numerical rating of his or her ability (see Footnote 2 for a brief description of the rating system). We speculated that these chess enthusiasts might have a higher rate of left-handedness than does the general population.

Questionnaires were sent to a total of 396 players, who were divided into a master group and an amateur group. The master group consisted of the top 200 rated players in the USCF. They had a minimum rating of 2252 and included the U.S. champion, his major competitors, and all other top players in the country. The amateur group consisted of 196 players sampled from the bottom 20% of all rated players in the USCF. They had a maximum rating of 1274, which is indicative of mediocre playing strength. A game between an individual in the master group and an individual in the amateur group should result in a win for the former at least 999 times out of 1,000 (Elo, 1978).

Subjects were asked to identify their handedness according to one of four categories: (1) right-handed, (2) left-handed, (3) ambidextrous, or (4) left-handed as a child and later switched to right-handed (i.e., converted left-hander). Sex and age data were also collected.

A total of 266 players responded to the questionnaire, for a response rate of 67%. Self-reported handedness rates for players of each sex are recorded in Table 7-1. Male chess players were almost twice as likely to be non-right-handed (18.6%) than are males in the general population (10% to 13.5%; Bryden, 1982; Geschwind, 1983; Porac & Coren, 1981), a statistically significant difference, even assuming the maximum 13.5% rate in the general male population ($\chi^2 = 4.92$; $p < .05$). Female chess players had a rate of non-right-handedness (3.3%) not significantly different from that of the general female population (6% to 9.9%; Bryden, 1982; Geschwind; 1983, Porac & Coren, 1981).

The number of female chess players was so small ($N = 30$) that significant handedness differences from the male chess players were difficult to document. The trend falls short of statistical significance ($\chi^2 = 3.42$; $.05 < p < .10$) but does parallel sex differences in the general population: chess-playing males had a higher rate of non-right-handedness than did chess-playing females (18.6% vs. 3.3%).

TABLE 7-1. Handedness of Chess Players

	Males ($N = 236$)	Females ($N = 30$)
Right-handed	192 (81.4%)	29 (96.7%)[b]
Non-right-handed	44 (18.6%)[a]	1 (3.3%)[c]

[a]Of the 44 non-right-handed males, 31 were left-handed, 8 were ambidextrous, 3 were converted left-handers, 1 described himself as both left-handed and ambidextrous, and 1 described himself as both a converted left-hander and right-handed.
[b]The right-handed females included 28 amateurs and 1 master.
[c]The sole non-right-handed female was a left-handed amateur.

Controlling for gender, we examined the data to determine if the rates of non-right-handedness differed between the master and amateur groups. The male master and male amateur groups had comparable rates of non-right-handedness (18.1% vs. 19.4%; see Table 7-2), whereas no valid group comparisons could be made for the female players since they had only one master representative (see Table 7-1, notes b and c).

We can see from the data that rates of non-right-handedness can distinguish male chess players from the general male population but cannot distinguish masters from amateurs. We assume that the master and amateur groups that we studied were not sufficiently distinct to harbor differences in handedness rates. It must be remembered that both groups consisted of individuals enthusiastic enough about chess to have joined the USCF and to have played in multiple tournaments. Furthermore, the amateur group may have included some young individuals with superior chess aptitude. An examination of the age data revealed that the master and amateur groups dissociated almost as much on the basis of age as they did on the basis of ability. The median age of the male masters was between 30 and 31 years, whereas that of the male amateur players was between 13 and 14 years. Most of the male amateur players (i.e., 55%, or 53 out of 97 reporting their age) were under 15 years of age, but none of the male masters was that young. Hence the master group consisted of mature individuals who had developed their chess potential to the point that they were the best players in the country, whereas the amateur group consisted largely of novice youngsters who had not yet had a chance to demonstrate the extent of their chess potential. Perhaps in another 15 years some of the youngsters will have advanced to the master group.

TABLE 7-2. Handedness of Male Chess Players

	Masters ($N = 138$)	Amateurs ($N = 98$)
Right-handed	113(81.9%)	79(80.6%)
Non-right-handed	25(18.1%)	19(19.4%)

How do we assess the results of this handedness survey? As with other data presented in this chapter, caution is once again warranted. Although self-report is not the most rigorous means of assessing handedness, at least it is a ready means for acquiring some useful information. No doubt the ease of answering a one-question, self-report item contributed to the high response rate that the survey enjoyed. In view of the lopsided statistical result, it seems unlikely that the alternate use of a more refined handedness measure would have materially altered the major finding gleaned from this survey: namely, that male chess players have a higher rate of non-right-handedness than do males in general.

This is not to imply that the survey found that proclivity for chess is restricted to non-right-handed individuals. (Indeed, the vast preponderance of chess players—like the vast preponderance of humans—was actually right-handed.) What the survey does point out is that a rare trait has emerged as somewhat less rare in a select population, and this statistical phenomenon may shed some light on the nature of that select population.

What light might it shed? We reiterate the line of speculative reasoning developed earlier. Like mathematics, chess is not a manual skill where one's hand preference should have any bearing on ability. But if we trace back to underlying brain structure, we may cite absence of right-hand preference as a motor marker for an enhanced right-hemisphere prowess that may be operative in cognitive realms as well. Seen in this light, the high rates of non-right-handedness among chess enthusiasts may reflect an enhanced degree of right-hemisphere competence among chess players and could lend support to the notion outlined earlier that chess skill is linked to the right hemisphere. A derivative conclusion drawn from this study is that since handedness is determined at birth (or at least before chess play begins), and since this study establishes a link, however fragile, between handedness and chess, perhaps proclivity for chess rests in part on predetermined, innate neurological structure.

Most discussion to this point has centered on normal, neurologically intact individuals. But much information can also be gained from careful study of individuals with brain lesions. For instance, a stroke causing destruction of a specific area of the brain may or may not derange one's chess-playing ability, depending on whether that area of the brain contributed to one's ability. The chess consequences of such experiments of nature are discussed next.

Brain Lesions in Chess Players

We searched the chess and medical literature for reports of the effects of brain lesions on chess-playing ability. We found published case reports pertaining to seven players. Furthermore, through announcements in selected local and national chess tournaments and chess magazines (including *Chess Life*, which is the official publication of the USCF and which has a circulation of 35,000), we located three additional players with brain lesions for whom we were able to gather detailed medical and chess-skill information. The findings for the seven subjects in the published cases and for the three subjects we contacted directly are outlined in

Table 7-3.[10] Subjects 1 through 8 had acquired their neurological lesions after they had learned how to play chess, whereas Subjects 9 and 10 suffered congenital lesions.

In addition to uncovering the case reports listed in Table 7-3, we found earlier authors who made general comments about the preservation of chess skill in aphasics. In his 1926 volume on aphasia, Henry Head (1926) mentioned that he often inquired about chess ability in his aphasic patients. He searched for preserved thinking processes that might be demonstrable over the chess board. Taylor (1962) also cited chess play as a source of intellectual achievement for aphasic individuals isolated from the speaking world by virtue of their brain lesions.

The accounts of two players not listed in Table 7-3 because of incomplete historical information illustrate how chess may remain as one of few available social and intellectual outlets following traumatic aphasia. (We are indebted to chess and professional colleagues for sharing these cases with us.) A 55-year-old, right-handed former dentist who suffered global aphasia and right hemiparesis from a head injury sustained in a motor vehicle collision has CT scan evidence of extensive tissue loss in the left frontal, parietal, and temporal lobes. He avidly enjoys playing chess. Similarly, a 37-year-old man who also suffered aphasia and right hemiparesis following a motor vehicle collision displays such an intense interest in the game and such a careful, thoughtful demeanor over the board that his therapists decided to use chess as a focus for his rehabilitation program. He displays clear evidence of learning in the chess realm when, for example, he avoids opening sequences that had previously led to disaster.

Sparing of chess ability in aphasic patients with acquired left-hemisphere lesions is, in fact, predicted by our hypothesis that chess proficiency is primarily attributable to right-hemisphere structures. Included in Table 7-3 are three well-documented instances of right-handed, strong amateur players, each of whom suffered a sizable aphasia-producing left-hemisphere lesion that had little or no effect on chess-playing ability (Subject 1 is described in Head, 1926; Subject 2 is described in Tonkonogy, 1986; Subject 3 is described in Sevush, Roeltgen, Campanella, & Heilman, 1983).

Subject 1 was a 30-year-old, right-handed, "highly intelligent" staff officer of the British army who sustained a compound depressed skull fracture over the left parietooccipital area as a result of a kick from a horse (Head, 1926, case 2). The lesion extent was estimated at the time of surgery to include cortical tissue of the left angular gyrus, superior parietal region, and parietooccipital area. Consistent with

---

10. Several well-known chess players are not included in Table 7-3 for various reasons. International grandmaster Isaac Kashdan lived for three years with various neurological deficits following a left thalamic intraparenchymal hemorrhage, but the effects on his chess ability are unknown since he never attempted to resume playing the game. The Russian politician and chess master A. F. Ilyin-Genevsky is well known in chess lore for having to relearn the game from scratch following a wartime disability. We discovered that the temporary disability was not the neurological disorder of head injury as is widely believed but rather the psychiatric syndrome of "shell shock" (Ilyin-Genevsky, 1985). Finally, four prominent historical figures—Zuckertort and world champions Morphy, Capablanca, and Alekhine—all suffered strokes before age 54 (Binet, 1966/1893; Fine, 1967). (Interestingly, Zuckertort's stroke occurred in the midst of a game (Binet, 1966/1893).) None of these four players is listed in Table 7-3 since either their stroke was immediately fatal or its effect on chess play was not documented.

TABLE 7-3. Chess Players with Brain Lesions

Subject	Type of lesion	Lesion site	Premorbid chess ability	Effect of lesion on chess ability
1	Depressed skull fracture	Left posterior parietal and parietooccipital cortices	"Above average"	No change
2	Infarct	Extensive portions of the left hemisphere (additional small right parasagittal lesion)	Good amateur	No change
3	Infarct	Left hemisphere (insula; superior temporal gyrus, including Wernicke's area; and supramarginal gyrus)	Good amateur (rating = 1793)	No major change (rating = 1539)
4	Lacunar infarct	Small lesion in the right internal capsular area	International Grandmaster (rating > 2400)	No change (rating > 2400)
5	Uncertain (venous infarct vs. contusion)	Right parasagittal frontoparietal area	Good amateur (rating in 1800s)	No change (rating in 1800s)
6	Infarct	Right hemisphere	Casual player	No change
7	Infarct	Right parietooccipital area	Casual player	Contralateral neglect of the chessboard and pieces
8	Infarct	Left parietooccipital area	Casual player	Contralateral neglect of the chessboard and pieces
9	Unknown congenital	Unknown	Does not apply	Lesion before chess was learned; now mediocre amateur
10	Neonatal hypoglycemic seizures	Left-hemisphere dysfunction (relatively preserved right-hemisphere function)	Does not apply	Lesion before chess was learned; now mediocre amateur (rating = 1336)

his posterior left-hemisphere lesion, he had, on examination 28 weeks later, loss of vision in the right visual field without accompanying motor or sensory deficits. Also consistent with his posterior left-hemisphere lesion, he had a fluent aphasia characterized by word-finding difficulties (i.e., anomia), minimal auditory comprehension deficits, inability to read, and inability to write (alexia with agraphia). Consistent with preservation of right-hemisphere visuo-spatial abilities, his production and appreciation of drawings was generally intact as was his sense of geographic orientation. Although we have no account of the subject's premorbid chess abilities, we are told that following his injury "he was able to play chess well" (Head, 1926,

Vol. 2, p. 41) and that his ability was "above the normal average" (Head, 1926, Vol. 1, p. 256).

Likewise, Subject 2 continued to play well following a left-hemisphere lesion (Tonkonogy, 1986, case 17; J. Tonkonogy, personal communication, 1986). He was a 53-year-old, right-handed full professor of literature in the Soviet Union when he was devastated by a very large cerebral infarction. Complete thrombotic/atherosclerotic occlusion of the left internal carotid artery and extensive atherosclerosis of the right internal carotid artery and of multiple cerebral arteries were revealed at autopsy 18 months later. Also revealed at autopsy was extensive destruction of the left hemisphere corresponding to the distribution of the left internal carotid artery and including the supplementary motor area, Broca's area, the lower half of the motor and sensory strips, the insula, the anterior part of the superior temporal gyrus, the rolandic operculum, and the inferior parietal lobule. (Also present was a small infarct in the right parasagittal

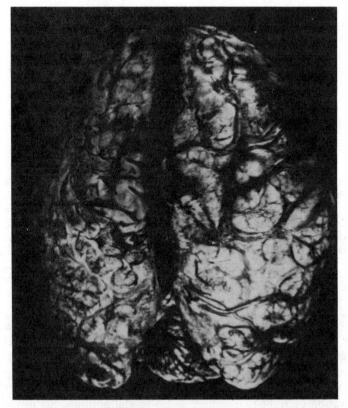

FIGURE 7-4. Autopsy specimen of Subject 2 (Table 7-3). Note the diminished volume of the left hemisphere. From *Vascular Aphasia* (p. 141) by J. Tonkonogy, 1986. Cambridge, MA: Bradford Books/The M.I.T. Press. Copyright 1986 by The Massachusetts Institute of Technology. Reprinted by permission.

portion of the corpus callosum lying medial to the anterior limb of the internal capsule.) Figure 7-4 is a photograph of the gross autopsy specimen, and Figures 7-5 and 7-6 are drawings of the lesion location on the mesial and lateral surfaces of the left hemisphere.

His large left-hemisphere lesion was responsible for a number of deficits, including apparent loss of vision in the right visual field, right-sided weakness (worse in the arm than in the leg), and decreased sensation of pinprick on the right. Also, he had a severe global aphasia with speech output reduced to virtually a solitary nonsense syllable and with severe impairment of comprehension of even simple linguistic material. Furthermore, he was apraxic for both limb and buccal-facial commands. Finally, reading, writing, and calculation were all impossible. On the other hand, skills dependent on the right hemisphere, such as spatial orientation and ability to find his way on the ward, were preserved.

Also preserved was his chess ability. Like many Russian male intellectuals, he had been an avid player and had achieved a strong amateur's level. After his stroke, his enthusiasm and apparent success at the game did not wane. While in the hospital, he achieved much satisfaction from spending a good portion of each day playing chess. For instance, his contests with the senior ward physician—an acknowledged accomplished player—often ended in hard-fought draws. (It is possible that modest declines in his ability were overlooked since his chess skill was never studied in a systematic way, and no numerical ratings of his skill were ever documented.)

A similar set of circumstances surrounds Subject 3, also a right-handed, well-educated polyglot and strong amateur chess player who also suffered a left-hemisphere ischemic infarction at age 53 (Sevush, Roeltgen, Campanella, & Heilman, 1983, patient 1). A head CT scan performed one month after his

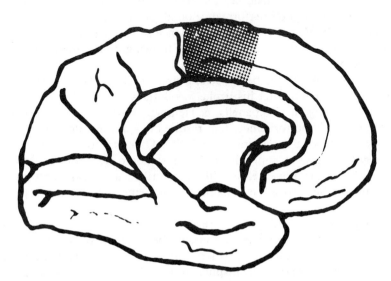

FIGURE 7-5. Diagram of lesion extent on the mesial surface of the left hemisphere, Subject 2 (Table 7-3). The supplementary motor area is involved. Reprinted by permission of Dr. J. Tonkonogy.

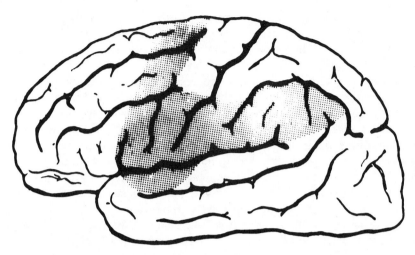

FIGURE 7-6. Diagram of lesion extent on the lateral surface of the left hemisphere, Subject 2 (Table 7-3). Broca's area, the lower half of the motor and sensory strips, the insula, the anterior part of the superior temporal gyrus, the rolandic operculum, and the inferior parietal lobule are all involved. Reprinted by permission of Dr. J. Tonkonogy.

stroke revealed attenuation in the left insula, left superior temporal gyrus (including Wernicke's area), and left supramarginal gyrus, with no other lesions seen (see Figure 7-7). He had no lasting visual or motor impairments. Findings on his language examination were consistent with Wernicke's aphasia and included fluent paraphasic speech, limited auditory comprehension, and the production of paraphasic errors on oral repetition and on object naming. Visuo-spatial and visuo-motor abilities, generally dependent on right-hemisphere structures, were preserved, as evidenced in part by good performance on all of the following tasks: the Block Design subtest of the Wechsler Adult Intelligence Scale (Wechsler, 1958), Raven's Progressive Matrices (Raven, 1956), executing drawings to command, and copying complex figures.

Prior to his stroke he had been a strong amateur chess player, with a rating of 1793. His playing strength after his stroke was initially estimated in the 1500–1600 range (Sevush, Roeltgen, Campanella, & Heilman, 1983), an estimate later confirmed by tournament performances that resulted in a documented stable rating of 1539 (S. Sevush, personal communication, 1985). Though a drop of some 200 rating points represents a loss of approximately one standard deviation of competitive ability, the subject can nonetheless still be described as a reasonably proficient player. In spite of his stroke, he remains a strong amateur with much preserved ability.

Our hypothesis would predict relative preservation of chess ability in players with large left-hemisphere lesions, a phenomenon we see in Subjects 1 through 3, and the hypothesis also predicts significant derangement of chess ability in other players with large right-hemisphere lesions. But our series is inadequate for use in testing the latter prediction since our series contains no players with documented large right-hemisphere lesions. Subjects 4 through 6 (Table 7-3) do have

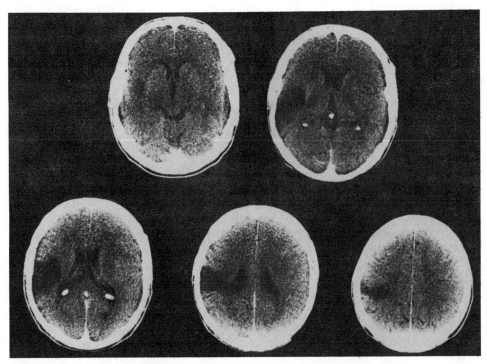

FIGURE 7-7. CT scan demonstrating a left-hemisphere lesion involving the insula, superior temporal gyrus (including Wernicke's area), and supramarginal gyrus, Subject 3 (Table 7-3). From "Preserved oral reading in Wernicke's aphasia" by S. Sevush, D. P. Roeltgen, D. J. Campanella, and K. M. Heilman, 1983. *Neurology, 33*, p. 917. Copyright 1983 by the editors of *Neurology*. Reprinted by permission.

right-hemisphere lesions, but in each instance the lesion is either small or indeterminate. Arthur Bisguier (Subject 4) is a 57-year-old, right-handed International Grandmaster, one of the top handful of players in the country, whose lacunar (hemorrhagic) infarct four years ago in the region of the right internal capsule was so small and its effects so transient that all significant neurological signs had resolved within a matter of days, and his chess ability was unimpaired. Likewise, a 43-year-old, right-handed strong amateur player (Subject 5) had a right parasagittal hemorrhagic lesion three years ago that was so delimited and clinically benign that it resulted in little lasting neurological impairment (except for minimal residual spasticity in the left lower extremity, which causes a slight limp) and no change in his chess ability (premorbid rating = 1800; postmorbid rating = 1844).

Finally, Eric Hodgins (Subject 6), a converted left-hander and former general manager of *Time* magazine who wrote an autobiographical account of his stroke, also had a right-hemisphere lesion and no reported change in his chess ability (Hodgins, 1964). For various reasons, his case is also inadequate as a test of our hypothesis. First, although the stroke left residual left-sided weakness, left-sided sensory deficits (including diminished proprioception and diminished light-touch sensation), and a curious fluent aphasia that caused him to commit many spelling and writing errors, the extent of his lesion is unknown since CT scans were not then available and no postmortem information was ever documented. Second, he had been only a very casual chess player (a self-described "wood-pusher") and had not participated in tournaments where an objective rating of his ability would have been recorded. Hence the inadequate knowledge of lesion extent and his very poor premorbid ability conspire to deprive his case of exemplary value when inquiring into the effects of a large right-hemisphere lesion on chess ability.

Two other subjects included in Table 7-3 were casual chess players who displayed contralateral visual neglect over the chessboard following parietooccipital infarction (Subject 7 is described in Cherington, 1974; Subject 8 is described in Cherington & Yarnell, 1975). They are included in the table for the sake of completeness, in order to present all published cases of chess players with brain lesions, but in actuality their premorbid chess ability is not strong enough for their experiences to serve as any test of our hypothesis of the neurology of chess.

In reviewing the acquired-lesion data (Subjects 1 through 8), one finds several well-documented instances of established players with large left-hemisphere lesions and relatively preserved chess ability (Subjects 1 through 3) but no complementary instances of established players with large right-hemisphere lesions. We assert that these findings support a hypothesis such as ours which predicts little perturbation of chess ability when the left hemisphere is significantly disrupted. Since our hypothesis would predict major disruption of chess ability when a large right-hemisphere lesion occurs, perhaps our failure to find chess players with large right-hemisphere lesions has been owing, in part, to the fact that our search beyond the literature had been restricted to still-active tournament players and USCF members. We are continuing our efforts to locate players—whether active or retired—with large right-hemisphere lesions.

The final two subjects in Table 7-3 (Subjects 9 and 10) both had congenital brain lesions with subsequent lifelong intellectual deficits, and yet each learned to play a reasonably fair game of chess. Their experiences may give us insight into the minimum neurological substrate necessary to develop talent at the game. At least for Subject 10, that minimum substrate appears to be a relatively intact right hemisphere.

A 54-year-old man (Subject 9) reported by Cleveland (1907) eighty years ago, described simply as a "congenital idiot," could neither read nor write and could not report or remember the current month or his age. He often spent his time playing with toys or picture books, and he seemed to be readily pulled to various tactile or visual stimuli. Although he had been institutionalized nearly all his life, it was uncertain when or how he had learned to play chess. He played the game very quickly and often recognized important patterns (e.g., a bishop fork) instantaneously. Although his level of play was strictly amateurish, his degree of success at the game far exceeded his achievement in other intellectual realms.

A 16-year-old, left-handed boy (Subject 10) was the product of an uncomplicated pregnancy and delivery, but he had seizures attributed to hypoglycemia on the second day of life. With appropriate glucose treatment, the seizures ceased and never recurred, but his EEGs over the ensuing months showed impressive slow waves of only $1\frac{1}{2}$ hertz in the left temporooccipital region and multifocal spike and sharp waves predominantly in the right hemisphere. These EEG findings are consistent with underlying neurological damage, particularly in the left hemisphere. Developmental delay, especially in linguistic areas, soon became evident. At two years of age he had only a two-word vocabulary, and by four years it had increased to only about 20 words. In school he had much difficulty learning to read and has always required special English classes. Mathematics, on the other hand, has been his strong subject at school, and he is an average or better-than-average mathematics student. He also has no trouble localizing himself in space, even when the family goes out, for instance, on a long and convoluted drive. Motor deficits include a marked squint (left exotropia) and decreased gross and fine motor control, especially in right-sided extremities. In summary, his neurological profile is primarily one of left-hemisphere dysfunction (left-hemisphere slow waves on EEG, developmental language disorders, motor deficits primarily involving right-sided extremities) and relatively preserved right-hemisphere function (left-handedness, intact spatial abilities).

He was first introduced to chess at age five but did not begin playing seriously until age 15. During the last year, he has played at least an hour a day and has participated in many tournaments. Like Subject 9, he plays very quickly and has attained a weak but credible level of skill. His current chess rating is 1336.

In summary our theory is supported by the lesion data compiled in Table 7-3. Chess skill can exist independent of language problems (Subjects 1, 2, 3, 6, 9, and 10) and independent of left-hemisphere dysfunction (Subjects 1, 2, 3, and 10). Safely ensconced presumably in the right hemisphere, chess talent is little perturbed by derangements elsewhere in the brain.

V. Conclusion

We hold that our theory of right-hemispheric specialization for chess has been consistent with and occasionally even directly bolstered by the various data reviewed above—the physiological data (pp. 170–174), the handedness data (pp. 174–177), and the brain lesion data (pp. 177–185). Now we can confront the question posed earlier—whether chess mastery requires a special neurological endowment. One may speculate that individuals with larger or better developed right hemispheres might have a crucial advantage at the highly competitive game. Norman Geschwind's theory of the biological basis of cerebral dominance suggests one prenatal mechanism by which the right hemisphere might acquire that superior development. And as we discussed earlier, high rates of left-handedness may be a marker indicating that serious chess players possess a high incidence of enhanced right-hemisphere development. Thus proclivity for chess, including the talent necessary to become a master, may be linked—at least as a statistical phenomenon—to innate, specially developed right-hemisphere capabilities.

Subject 10 (Table 7-3) may be an instructive example. Prenatal or perinatal factors had skewed his brain development toward an asymmetry of hemispheric competence favoring the right hemisphere. The result was a pattern of intellectual weaknesses (e.g., in language) and strengths (e.g., in geographic orientation) that mirrored his asymmetry of hemispheric competence. We attribute his enthusiasm and proclivity for chess to the competence of his favored right hemisphere. Just as biological endowment has "predetermined" the chess and other intellectual achievements of Subject 10, we assume that it also determines, at least in part, the superior chess talent present in the masters of the game.

In summary, we propose for future study the following speculative hypothesis regarding brain-chess relationships: The capacity to play superior chess is neurologically determined. It is a capacity that develops more commonly in males and in left-handers. The primary locus of this capacity is in the right hemisphere. Consequently, individuals with enhanced right-hemisphere development may have an advantage at chess, while individuals with even large lesions elsewhere in the brain may be at no particular disadvantage. Fundamental to excellence in chess is the ability to learn and retain a vast chess "vocabulary" of piece position patterns, and the right hemisphere mediates this ability in a manner analogous to the way in which the left hemisphere mediates one's facility with words.

Acknowledgments

Preparation of this chapter was supported by the Veterans Administration Medical Research Service and N.I.H. Grant NS07239A. The authors would like to thank Mildred Beck, Dale Brandreth, Hiram Brownell, Casey Bush, Neil Charness, Chris Chase, Jon Frankle, William Gittleson, Beat Hiltbrunner, Randall Hough, Tedd Judd, Elena Kamenetsky, Suzanne Ruscitti, Anthony Saidy, Steven Sevush, Claire Sybertz, and Joseph Tonkonogy for their assistance in the preparation of this chapter. We also gratefully acknowledge the contributions of Arthur Bisguier, Isaac Kashdan (deceased), and the many other chess players who shared their medical histories with us.

References

Annett, M., & Kilshaw, D. (1982). Mathematical ability and lateral asymmetry. *Cortex, 18,* 547–568.

Auble, P. (1982). *An examination of expertise.* Unpublished manuscript, Vanderbilt University (Department of Psychology), Nashville.

Bakwin, H. (1973). The chess prodigy. *Clinical Pediatrics, 12,* 575–576.

Barry, H. (1969). Longevity of outstanding chess players. *Journal of Genetic Psychology, 115,* 143–148.

Baumgarten, F. (1930). Wunderkinder. *Psychologische Untersuchungen, 8,* 184.

Benbow, C. P. (1986). Physiological correlates of extreme intellectual precocity. *Neuropsychologia, 24,* 719–725.

Benbow, C. P., & Benbow, R. M. (1984). Biological correlates of high mathematical reasoning ability. In G. J. De Vries, J. P. C. De Bruin, H. B. M. Uylings, & M. A. Corner (Eds.), *Progress in brain research* (Vol. 61, pp. 469–490). Amsterdam: Elsevier Science Publishers.

Benbow, C. P., & Stanley, J. C. (1983). Sex differences in mathematical reasoning ability: More facts. *Science, 222,* 1029–1031.

Benton, A. (1985). Visuoperceptual, visuospatial, and visuoconstructive disorders. In K. M. Heilman & E. Valenstein (Eds.), *Clinical neuropsychology*. New York: Oxford University Press.

Berliner, H. (1978). Computer chess. *Nature, 274,* 745–748.

Bever, T. R. (1975). Cerebral asymmetries in humans are due to the differentiation of two incompatible processes: Holistic and analytic. In D. Aaronson & R. W. Rieber (Eds.), *Developmental psycholinguistics and communication disorders* (pp. 251–262). New York: New York Academy of Sciences.

Binet, A. (1966). Mnemonic virtuosity: A study of chess players. *Genetic Psychology Monographs, 74,* 127–162. (Translated by M. L. Simmell and S. B. Barren from *Revue des Deux Mondes,* 1893, *117,* 826–859.

Bransford, J., Nitsch, K., & Franks, J. (1977). Schooling and the facilitation of knowing. In R. Anderson, R. Spiro, & W. Montague (Eds.), *Schooling and the acquisition of knowledge.* Hillsdale, NJ: Erlbaum.

Bryden, M. P. (1982). *Laterality: Functional asymmetry in the intact brain.* New York: Academic Press.

Buttenwieser, P. (1935). The relation of age to skill of expert chess players. Unpublished doctoral dissertation, Stanford University, Stanford, CA. (Abstract in *Psychological Bulletin,* 1935, *32,* 529.)

Charness, N. (1976). Memory for chess positions: Resistance to interference. *Journal of Experimental Psychology: Human Learning and Memory, 2,* 641–653.

Charness, N. (1977). Human chess skill. In P. W. Frey (Ed.), *Chess skill in man and machine* (pp. 34–53). New York: Springer-Verlag.

Charness, N. (1981a). Aging and skilled problem solving. *Journal of Experimental Psychology: General, 110,* 21–38.

Charness, N. (1981b). Search in chess: Age and skill differences. *Journal of Experimental Psychology: Human Perception and Performance, 7,* 467–476.

Charness, N. (1981c). Visual short-term memory and aging in chess players. *Journal of Gerontology, 36,* 615–619.

Chase, W. G., & Chi, M. T. H. (1979). *Cognitive skill: Implications for spatial skill in large-scale environments.* (Technical Rep. No. 1). Pittsburgh: University of Pittsburgh, Learning Research and Development Center.

Chase, W. G., & Simon, H. A. (1973a). Perception in chess. *Cognitive Psychology, 4,* 55–81.

Chase, W. G., & Simon, H. A. (1973b). The mind's eye in chess. In W. G. Chase (Ed.), *Visual information processing* (pp. 215–281). New York: Academic Press.

Cherington, M. (1974). Visual neglect in a chess player. *Journal of Nervous and Mental Disease, 159,* 145–147.

Cherington, M., & Yarnell, P. (1975). Amorphosynthesis on the chess board. *Scandinavian Journal of Rehabilitation Medicine, 7,* 176–178.

Chess Informant (1985). *38,* p. 410.

Chess Life. (1985, January). *40* (1), p. 35.

Church, R. M., & Church, K. W. (1977). Plans, goals, and search strategies for the selection of a move in chess. In P. W. Frey (Ed.), *Chess skill in man and machine* (pp. 131–156). New York: Springer-Verlag.

Cleveland, A. A. (1907). The psychology of chess and of learning to play it. *American Journal of Psychology, 18,* 269–308.

Coriat, I. H. (1941). The unconscious motives of interest in chess. *Psychoanalytic Review, 28,* 30–36.

de Groot, A. D. (1965). *Thought and choice in chess.* The Hague: Mouton.

de Groot, A. D. (1966). Perception and memory versus thought: Some old ideas and recent findings. In B. Kleinmutz (Ed.), *Problem solving: Research, method, and theory* (pp. 19–50). New York: John Wiley & Sons.

Dembart, L. (1984, May 12). King of chess computers humbled by wily human. *The Los Angeles Times,* pp. 1, 25.

Djakow, J. N., Petrowski, N. V., & Rudik, P. A. (1927). *Psychologie des Schachspiels.* Berlin: Walter deGruyter.

Elo, A. E. (1965). Age changes in master chessperformance. *Journal of Gerontology, 20,* 289–299.

Elo, A. E. (1978). *The rating of chessplayers past and present.* New York: Arco.

Fine, R. (1965). The psychology of blindfold chess: An introspective account. *Acta Psychologica, 24,* 352–370.

Fine, R. (1967). *The psychology of the chess player.* New York: Dover Publications.

Forster, F. M., Richards, J. F., Panitch, H. S., Huisman, R. E., & Paulsen, R. E. (1975). Reflex epilepsy evoked by decision making. *Archives of Neurology, 32,* 54–56.

Frey, P. W., & Adesman, P. (1976). Recall memory for visually presented chess positions. *Memory and Cognition, 4,* 541–547.

Galaburda, A. M., LeMay, M., Kemper, T. L., & Geschwind, N. (1978). Right-left asymmetries in the brain: Structural differences between the hemispheres may underlie cerebral dominance. *Science, 199,* 852–856.

Gardner, H. (1983). *Frames of mind: The theory of multiple intelligences.* New York: Basic Books.

Geschwind, N. (1983). The riddle of the left hand. In E. Bernstein (Ed.), *1984 Medical and Health Annual* (pp. 38–51). Chicago: Encyclopaedia Britannica, Inc.

Geschwind, N., & Behan, P. (1982). Left-handedness: Association with immune disease, migraine, and developmental learning disorder. *Proceedings of the National Academy of Sciences U.S.A., 79,* 5097–5100.

Geschwind, N., & Galaburda, A. M. (1985). Cerebral lateralization. *Archives of Neurology, 42,* 428–459, 521–552, 634–654.

Goldin, S. E. (1978a). Effects of orienting tasks on recognition of chess positions. *American Journal of Psychology, 91,* 659–671.

Goldin, S. E. (1978b). Memory for the ordinary: Typicality effects in chess memory. *Journal of Experimental Psychology: Human Learning and Memory, 4,* 605–616.

Goldin, S. E. (1979). Recognition memory for chess positions: Some preliminary research. *American Journal of Psychology, 92,* 19–31.

Guilford, J. P., & Zimmerman, W. S. (1953). *Guilford-Zimmerman Aptitude Survey.* Orange, CA: Sheriden Psychological Services.

Han-pai, C., Chen, C., & Chih-p'ing, C. (1965, July). Chess epilepsy and card epilepsy: Two new patterns of reflex epilepsy. *Chinese Medical Journal, 84,* 470-474.

Harris, L. J. (1978). Sex differences in spatial ability: Possible environmental, genetic and neurologic factors. In M. Kinsbourne (Ed.), *Asymmetrical function of the brain* (pp. 405–522). Cambridge, England: Cambridge University Press.

Head, H. (1926). *Aphasia and kindred disorders of speech* (Vols. 1 & 2). New York: MacMillan.

Hearst, E. (1967, June). Psychology across the chessboard. *Psychology Today, 1,* 28–37.

Hearst, E. (1977). Man and machine: Chess achievements and chess thinking. In P. W. Frey (Ed.), *Chess skill in man and machine* (pp. 167–211). New York: Springer-Verlag.

Hécaen, H., & Albert, M. L. (1978). *Human Neuropsychology.* New York: Wiley.

Hodgins, E. (1964). *Episode: Report on the accident inside my skull.* New York: Atheneum.

Holding, D. H. (1979). The evaluation of chess positions. *Simulation & Games, 10,* 207–221.

Holding, D. H., & Reynolds, R. I. (1982). Recall or evaluation of chess positions as determinants of chess skill. *Memory and Cognition, 10,* 237–242.

Ilyin-Genevsky, A. (1986). *Notes of a Soviet master* (D. Brandreth, Ed.). Yorklyn, DE: Caissa Editions.

Johnson-Laird, P. N., & Wason, P. C. (1977). Imagery and internal representation: Introduction. In P. N. Johnson-Laird & P. C. Wason (Eds.), *Thinking: Readings in cognitive science* (pp. 523–531). Cambridge, England: Cambridge University Press.

Jones, E. (1931). The problem of Paul Morphy: A contribution to the psycho-analysis of chess. *International Journal of Psychoanalysis, 12,* 1–23.

Kolata, G. (1983). Math genius may have hormonal basis. *Science, 222,* 1312.

Lane, D. M., & Robertson, L. (1979). The generality of levels of processing hypothesis: An application to memory for chess positions. *Memory and Cognition, 7,* 253–256.

Leedy, C. & Dubeck, L. (1971, December). Physiological changes during tournament chess. *Chess Life and Review, 26,* 708.

Lehman, H. C. (1953). *Age and achievement.* Princeton, NJ: Princeton University Press.

LeMay, M. (1976). Morphological cerebral asymmetries of modern man, fossil man, and nonhuman primate. In S. R. Harnad, H. D. Steklis, & J. Lancaster (Eds.), *Origins and evolution of language and speech* (pp. 349–366). New York: New York Academy of Sciences.

LeMay, M., & Culebras, A. (1972). Human brain: Morphologic differences in the hemispheres demonstrable by carotid arteriography. *New England Journal of Medicine, 287,* 168–170.

LeMay, M., & Geschwind, N. (1975). Hemispheric differences in the brains of great apes. *Brain, Behavior and Evolution, 11,* 48–52.

Maccoby, E. C., & Jacklin, C. N. (1974). *The psychology of sex differences.* Stanford, CA: Stanford University Press.

Malkin, V. (1982). [The electroencephalography of chess players.] *Shakhmatnyi Byulleten, 8,* 12–14.

Marx, J. L. (1982). Research news: Autoimmunity in left-handers. *Science, 217,* 141–144.

McRae, D. L., Branch, C. L., & Milner, B. (1968). The occipital horns and cerebral dominance. *Neurology, 18,* 95–98.

Mengarini, A. (1963, March). Chess: Some philosophical considerations. *Chess Life, 18,* 64–65.

Menninger, K. (1942). Chess. *Menninger Clinic Bulletin, 6,* 80–83.

Newell, A., Shaw, J. C., & Simon, H. A. (1963). Chess-playing programs and the problem of complexity. In E. A. Feigenbaum & J. Feldman (Eds.), *Computers and thought* (pp. 39–70). New York: McGraw-Hill.

Newell, A., & Simon, H. A. (1972). *Human problem solving.* Englewood Cliffs, NJ: Prentice-Hall.

Pfleger, H., Stocker, K., Pabst, H., Haralambie, G. (1980). Sportmedizinische Untersuchung an Schachspielern der Spitzenklasse. [Sports Medical Examination of Top Class Chess Players] *Münchener Medizinische Wochenschrift, 122,* (Nr. 28), 1041–1044.

Porac, C., & Coren, S. (1981). *Lateral preferences and human behavior.* New York: Springer.

Puccetti, R. (1974). Pattern recognition in computers and the human brain: With special application to chess playing machines. *British Journal for the Philosophy of Science, 25,* 137–154.

Raven, J. C. (1956). *Raven's progressive matrices.* London: H. K. Lewis.

Reider, N. (1959). Chess, Oedipus, and the Mater Dolorosa. *International Journal of Psychoanalysis, 40,* 320–333.

Scurrah, M. J., & Wagner, D. A. (1970). Cognitive model of problem-solving in chess. *Science, 169*, 209–211.

Sevush, S., Roeltgen, D. P., Campanella, D. J., & Heilman, K. M. (1983). Preserved oral reading in Wernicke's aphasia. *Neurology, 33*, 916–920.

Simon, H. A. (1979). *Models of thought*. New Haven, CT: Yale University Press.

Simon, H. A., & Chase, W. G. (1973). Skill in chess. *American Scientist, 61*, 394–403.

Simon, H. A., & Gilmartin, K. J. (1973). A simulation of memory for chess positions. *Cognitive Psychology, 5*, 29–46.

Smith, W. H. (1975). An approach to the analysis of activities: The game of chess. *Menninger Clinic Bulletin, 39*, 93–100.

Spanier, D. (1984). *Total chess*. New York: E. P. Dutton.

Steiner, G. (1973). *Sporting scene: White knights of Reykjavik*. London: Faber and Faber.

Taylor, M. L. (1962). Linguistic considerations of verbal behavior in the brain-damaged adult. Unpublished manuscript. (Reviewed in Hodgins, 1964, pp. 95–98.)

Tikhomirov, O. K., & Poznyanskaya, E. D. (1966-67, winter). An investigation of visual search as a means of analyzing heuristics. *Soviet Psychology, 5*, 3–15.

Tikhomirov, O. K., & Vinogradov, Ye. E. (1970, spring–summer). Emotions in the function of heuristics. *Soviet Psychology, 8*, 198–223.

Tonkonogy, J. (1986). *Vascular aphasia*. Cambridge, MA: Bradford Books/The M.I.T. Press.

Wagner, D. A., & Scurrah, M. J. (1971). Some characteristics of human problem-solving in chess. *Cognitive Psychology, 2*, 454–478.

Wechsler, D. (1958). *The measurement and appraisal of adult intelligence* (4th ed.). Baltimore: Williams & Wilkins.

Zweig, S. (1944). *The royal game*. New York: Viking Press.

8

Superior Memory Performance and Mnemonic Encoding

EVAN BROWN
KENNETH DEFFENBACHER

Ancedotes abound of persons supposedly superior at various memory tasks (see, e.g., Barlow, 1952, for a collection), and popular interest has at times been sufficient to allow some such persons to join magicians and mental calculators in making a living by exhibiting their prowess. This interest seems generally to focus on the superior performance of memory tasks that most persons can and often do acomplish, if not so well. Beyond this, the range of memory feats is fairly broad, including some that involve the recall of previously learned material and others where the material is learned at the time, the recall of scenes and other nonverbal material, as well as recall of words or numbers. Assuming that there is any basis at all to these claims of superior memory performance, there would appear to be several reasons why they should be investigated. A person who is unusually good at some memorial task may shed light on more usual functioning and test theories of memory as well as the limits of human performance. Furthermore, from a practical standpoint, cases of superior memory may suggest methods of memory improvement for more "normal" persons or aid us in assessing methods already proposed or in use.

Despite the apparent interest and the potentially useful results, however, careful studies of superior memory performance have been relatively few. Some of these have involved tasks unlike those in which most persons engage (e.g., a musician's recognition of tones as opposed to tunes, a chess player's recall of chess positions) or have examined the recall of material learned prior to the particular study, but most have presented either verbal or nonverbal material and have examined speed of learning, speed of recall, and/or amount recalled.

In this chapter we review experimental studies of persons who were superior at memorizing numbers and other sorts of verbal material. Persons who have demonstrated superior memory for pictorial information were included in our review only if they were also able to use their imagery in the service of remembering verbal items. Following our review, we consider the possible generalizations one might make about our superior memorizers, including, particularly, the roles of

Evan Brown and Kenneth Deffenbacher. Department of Psychology, University of Nebraska, Omaha, Nebraska.

specific techniques, of practice, and of general knowledge and intelligence. We open with a discussion of classical mnemonic techniques, since several of our subjects used them or more modern variations and extensions of them.

Mnemonic Techniques

In the classical mnemonic systems, one would rely on previously memorized visual images of places, or "loci", along paths within or between buildings. In the memory for things, or *memoria rerum*, one would create additional images to represent the major topics one wished to address. Then, in memorizing a speech, for example, one would place the images representing the topics in order along the imaginary paths. In the memory for words, or *memoria verborum*, images representing the exact words would similarly be placed in order along the paths. The latter is clearly the more difficult technique. It requires not only more memorization of paths in order to provide places for the individual words of a speech or other passage to be memorized, but also the creation of images for words or portions of words that lack concrete referents.

In more modern mnemonic systems the methods of loci, particularly the *memoria rerum*, are still preeminent, but changes and additions have occurred, the most important for our purpose being ways of remembering numbers. Here several techniques were originated in (or perhaps before) the 17th century using number–letter substitutions. In what became the most popular variant of these techniques, one would learn the following set of digit–consonant correspondences: $1 = t$, d, th; $2 = n$; $3 = m$; $4 = r$; $5 = l$; $6 = j$, sh, ch, "soft" g; $7 = k$, "hard" c, q, "hard" g, ng; $8 = f$, v, ph; $9 = p$, b; $0 = z$, s, "soft" c. When memorizing a series of numbers, one then converts the digits into corresponding consonants, adds vowels as needed to make words, and places images to represent the words along one's imaginary paths following the technique of the *memoria verborum*. Thus 3.14159 could be remembered by an image of a testing area for angry rodents (a mad rat lab), an image of an insect with mechanized stinger (a motor-tail bee), or any other images that encode the appropriate consonants.

Binet's Studies of Superior Memory

The experimental study of memory performance appears to have begun as an aside to the study of mental calculation. In 1892 the French Academy of Sciences appointed a commission to study the mental calculator Inaudi. Binet, who performed the experiments for the commission, studied Inaudi and another calculator, Diamandi, on memory tasks as well as calculation, and he added the stage mnemonist Arnould by way of comparison. Presumably because mental calculation was the main concern, the memory research focused primarily on number memory and was less detailed than in some of the later studies.

Inaudi

Though the information available is more limited than we might wish, it would appear from Binet's remarks that Inaudi's nonnumerical memory was not unusual (Binet, 1894). His letter span, at six letters, was well within the normal range, while his error-free span for poetry or prose was two lines. Despite his apparent use of auditory imagery in digit memorization, his memory for music was reported to be undistinguished. Perhaps of relevance here is that although he seemed reasonably intelligent, Inaudi had little formal education and lacked intellectual interests outside arithmetic. Anecdotes also suggest that he was somewhat absentminded with respect to events in his everyday life. But where numbers and calculations involving them were concerned, the situation was otherwise. Here, though the exact strength of Inaudi's memory may be open to debate, it is clear that it was at least abnormally good. Binet gives 42 as his estimate of Inaudi's memory limit for recall of digits heard once in series. This estimate can be criticized (Smith, 1983), however, and one can make a case for other values, since it was based on the number correctly recalled on one trial in which 51 digits were presented. Thus, for example, for an error-free recall of all of the digits presented, 36 seems to have been Inaudi's maximum series length, though if one were to insist on a memorization rate of a digit per second, 25 would appear to have been the limit with auditory presentation. Because Inaudi relied on auditory presentation of problems and numbers (and his auditory imagery of them) in his stage performances, it may not be surprising that he was slower to learn digit strings that he had to read. Thus his visual learning of a 25-digit string took 45 seconds in contrast to the 25 seconds required when he heard the string.

In addition to testing Inaudi's learning and recall of digit strings specifically presented for memorization, Binet considered his memory for numbers encountered during calculation. In a sample performance reported by Binet, Inaudi took a total of 10 minutes to calculate mentally without error the subtraction of two 21-digit numbers, the addition of five 6-digit numbers, the square of a 4-digit number, the division of two 4-digit numbers, the cube root of a 9-digit number, and the fifth root of a 12-digit number (the last two being integral roots). Binet estimated that Inaudi had to keep track of more than 200 digits in his head during the interval. Similarly, Inaudi was able to repeat without error some 230 digits dealt with during a performance even when he was tested 12 hours later, provided that no other performance intervened.

Diamandi

Binet's second subject, Diamandi, though another mental calculator, was otherwise different from Inaudi in several ways. Coming from a commercial (export–import) family, as opposed to having a peasant background, he had some knowledge of five languages, much more formal education, and more intellectual interests. In addition, where Inaudi had been a calculator from childhood, Diamandi first developed his abilities apparently in his late teens in connection with the family business. As was the case with Inaudi, Diamandi claimed to use no mnemonic systems. But where Inaudi appeared to rely in part on auditory imagery, Diamandi was a visualizer. When he was given numbers for calculation or memorization, visual digits appeared for Diamandi in his own handwriting (though often with the colors of the original). These visual images were apparently fairly vivid. However, from his performance on a prose-learning task used for testing the visual imagery of French schoolchildren, Binet concluded that Diamandi's imagery was not "photographic."

Though Diamandi's prose memorization was slightly superior to Inaudi's, his digit memorization was not. Not only were Inaudi's mental calculations faster than Diamandi's by factors from six to eight, but Inaudi was also able to learn visually presented digits four times as swiftly, and auditorily presented ones more than eight times as fast. The one digit-memory task in which Diamandi was superior to Inaudi was in speed of recall of information from a previously memorized 5×5 array, particularly when the recall had to be in a different order than by the rows, for instance, up or down the columns, around in a spiral, or along the diagonals. Nevertheless, Diamandi's digit-memorization abilities should probably be regarded as above average in that he was reported to be about twice as fast as Binet, who also was a visualizer.

Arnould

In constrast to Inaudi, Diamandi, and (presumably) Binet, Arnould used an artificial mnemonic system of the digit–consonant sort described earlier. In fact, his digit–consonant pairings were precisely the ones given as examples. Arnould seems to have been an open and cooperative subject of apparently above–average intelligence. Unfortunately, he was neither tested nor discussed in as great detail as were the calculators, since he was brought in essentially as an example of a mnemotechnician to compare with them. Thus what we largely have is his performance on some of the number memory tasks used with Diamandi. Although his unaided digit span was only seven, when he used his system, Arnould was almost as fast as Diamandi in learning visually presented strings of fewer than 25 digits, and with longer strings (up to 200, the longest tested) he was faster. In recall of strings, Arnould was somewhat slower than Diamandi, though he could typically exceed one digit per second.

Studies by Müller and Hegge

Rückle

When professor Georg Müller learned that there was a mathematics student, a Dr. Rückle, with quite unusual memory abilities studying at Göttingen, he considered it his duty to study this memory more closely. He was able to do so in two series of studies, completed in 1906 and 1912. Although Rückle's memory constituted the occasion for the studies, Müller extended them to include as well parallel investigations of persons with memories in the more normal range, not just to provide a quantitative basis for evaluating Rückle's performance but to compare the methods of learning and recall and to consider points pertaining to a general theory of memory and memory imagery. Though Müller's main concern was with memory, he also briefly examined Rückle's abilities as a mental calculator and compared them with Inaudi's. Müller's results on Rückle, together with the results of the parallel studies, the comparisons, and the theoretical implications, ultimately appeared in three massive volumes and a major article (Müller, 1911, 1913a, 1913b, 1917), perhaps the most extensive study of memory ever undertaken by a single investigator.

Despite Müller's research and Thorleif Hegge's brief study (Hegge, 1929), relatively little is known of Rückle's life outside the laboratory. He received his PhD in mathematics from Göttingen in 1901 (Smith, 1983) and went from there to Cassel in 1902, where he was based during the main series of studies, completed in 1906. At Cassel, Rückle may well have had an academic appointment, since Müller speaks of him engaging in scientific or professional work between experiments and notes that he had not practiced memorization of number series for a long time, in contrast to Inaudi and Diamandi who were professional, continually practicing number learners at the time of Binet's testing (Müller, 1911). Later, however, between 1906 and 1912, Rückle did appear in stage performances as a calculator and number memorizer and did practice memorization—as well as study number theory—with the intent and result of improving his performance (Müller, 1913a). As with Inaudi and Diamandi, Rückle did not rely on an artificial mnemonic system; he relied, rather, on concrete and detailed visual imagery and, where numbers were concerned, on an extensive and flexible knowledge of their characteristics and relationships.

Rückle was clearly superior to Binet's (1984) subjects in his digit-memorization capabilities, particularly during the later (1912) testing after his work on the stage. When originally tested in the experiments of 1902–1906, his digit span was at least as good as Inaudi's: To match Binet's somewhat suspect claim of 42 for Inaudi, Rückle needed to see all of the digits simultaneously for a period of time corresponding to a little over a second per digit (Müller, 1911). With the (for him) less preferred mode of auditory presentation, the span depended upon whether and how the digits were grouped when presented to him as well as upon the rate of presentation and the amount of practice. In the earliest testing, when 25 digits were read to him as five 5-digit numbers, or when 24 were read as four 6-digit numbers, he could repeat them without error when the reading rate was about one digit per second. Ungrouped numbers required either a reduction to about 18 digits or a slower reading rate. Somewhat later within the 1902-1906 research, after some practice on other memory tasks, Rückle had one series correct, one with one error, and one in which the trial was apparently aborted in three attempts to memorize 36-digit strings read to him (ungrouped) at about a second per digit (39, 40, and 34 seconds, respectively; Müller, 1911).

In 1912 Müller tested Rückle with four series of 60 digits read to him at about a second per digit, using a similar procedure but requiring the numbers to be repeated backward as well as forward in at least one case, and permitting prompts. One series was repeated without error backward and then forward, whereas the other three required one, two, and four prompts, where Rückle asked Müller for a digit (Müller, 1913a) Although none of these tasks correspond precisely to those currently used to estimate digit span, they would seem to suggest an auditory span (the usual digit-span tests are auditory) of *at least* 18 in the earliest testing, increasing to about twice that with practice on related tasks, and reaching about 60 much later, after stage work that apparently included the recall of auditorially presented digits as part of the performance.

With visual presentation Rückle's performance at learning digits was markedly faster than that of Binet's subjects. As mentioned previously, Binet compared learning and recall speeds of Inaudi and Diamandi with a 5 × 5 digit square, finding Inaudi to be faster in the learning, but Diamandi generally faster in the recall. When tested earlier, in the 1902–1906 experiments, Rückle learned such an array in a mean time of 20.2 seconds, as compared to 45 seconds for Inaudi and 180 seconds for Diamandi. In 1912 Rückle's learning time averaged 12.7 seconds for the 25 digits (Müller, 1913a). Recall and recitation times for Rückle in the earlier testing were generally similar to, if slightly faster than, those for Diamandi. By 1912 they differed mainly in that Rückle had become much faster at reporting the digits in unconventional orders, "reading" them off along the diagonals or in a spiral in somewhat less time than the 19 seconds it took Inaudi to retrieve and repeat them in rows from left to right.

Further examples of digit-memory superiority would include performance with longer strings: To learn 102 digits, Rückle took from 3 to 6 minutes in the earlier tests and between 2 and 3 minutes in 1912 (Müller, 1913a), whereas to learn 100 digits, Inaudi took 12 minutes, and the others, about twice that much time. Similarly, it took Rückle about 18 minutes to learn 204 digits before his stage experiences and about half that much time in 1912, whereas Diamandi required 75 minutes and Arnould 45 minutes for 200 digits—Inaudi not having been tested at this string length. Finally, in what seems to have been his longest string, Rückle memorized 408 digits in 1912, taking somewhat less than 27 minutes for the project. We should, of course, note that these memorization performances were not always completely error free. In Rückle's case, the majority were, but in some strings he had as many as four errors, where an error might be a mistake made but corrected by Rückle, a mistake not corrected, or a request by him for a digit as a prompt. Recitation of the string of 408 digits, for example, involved two mistakes that Rückle himself corrected and one request for a prompt from Müller.

Though Müller's greater concern was with number memory, he also examined Rückle on several nonnumerical tasks in 1902–1906 (Müller, 1911), finding his memory to be strongly supranormal there as well. In one set of experiments Müller followed Ebbinghaus's (1885) procedure, presenting the syllables of a given nonsense-syllable series simultaneously on a single piece of paper for Rückle to memorize. Learning times here averaged 36, 96, and 117.5 seconds for 12-, 18-, and 24-syllable strings, respectively. By way of comparison, Müller notes that Ebbinghaus needed more than 400 seconds to learn a 24-syllable series and that Steffens' (1900) significantly above average subject, Mrs. Schmidt, required about 200 seconds for a 16-syllable series. With the Müller and Schumann (1984) procedure of serial presentation of syllables one at a time on a rotating memory drum, Rückle required six trials with the series (six rotations of the drum) t 9 seconds per trial in order to learn a 12-syllable series, where, according to Müller, a learner of average ability and some practice with the task requires about 13–14 trials.

In the 1902–1906 studies involving consonant memorization (Müller, 1911), the comparison group—which Rückle outperformed—seems to have consisted of several of the Göttingen lab's professional inhabitants. For a simultaneously exposed series of 20 consonants, Rückle required an average of 43.5 seconds of learning time, whereas the best of the other subjects, Dr. David Katz, required 97 seconds. Similarly, mean learning time for 25 consonants arrayed in a square was 75 seconds for Rückle versus 151 seconds for Katz. With auditory presentation of consonants rhythmically grouped in threes, Rückle required three 16-second presentations, or 48 seconds total, to learn a series of 18 consonants; the nine other subjects required from 100 to 380 seconds each.

Other, miscellaneous tasks considered in the initial work (Müller, 1913a) included memorization of a series of 12 color names, a series of 12 nonsense figures, and a passage from Byron's *Childe Harold* (in translation). Simultaneous exposure was used for the elements of each series; for the color series Rückle averaged 30 seconds and for the nonsense figures, 23 seconds, while the comparison subjects required between 129 and 232 seconds. An array of 25 nonsense figures took Rückle 286 seconds. For the Byron passage, the comparison subject was Mrs. Schmidt, mentioned previously; she took 110 seconds to learn it, while he took 70.

In 1912 Müller returned to some of these tasks, finding, in contrast to the results with numbers, that Rückle's nonnumerical memory performance had, if anything, declined in the interim, though it was still superior to that of the earlier comparison subjects. Color names went from 30 to 33.5 seconds, 20-consonant series from 43.5 to 69 seconds, 25-consonant arrays from 75 to 87 seconds, and 24-syllable series from 117.5 to 222.5 seconds average time for memorization (Müller, 1913a). Accounting for this decline is problematic, but Müller notes Rückle's extreme concentration on mathematical work in the immediately prior years, when he often devoted 8 hours a day to exploring the properties of numbers, with particular concern for aspects and relationships of relevance to mental calculation and number memorization. These concerns then came to occupy him to the relative exclusion of other aspects. For example, even in the number memorization, no longer would "birthdate of Plato" likely have come forth as an aid for "427" as it once did. Rather, presumably, the preeminent aspect of 427 for Rückle in 1912 would have been its quality of being "61×7."

Though Müller apparently did not test Rückle with strings of concrete nouns, Thorleif Hegge (1929) did. Hegge tested Rückle four times with serial lists of 100 concrete nouns presented auditorily at 7–10 seconds per noun. His best score was 71 correct on a second, corrected recall. Under the same conditions, Bergh, another subject studied by Hegge (see next section) scored 94 correct. As usual for Rückle, simultaneous visual presentation brought better results. Even with this procedure, however, it required almost 32 minutes for him to match Bergh's score. According to Hegge, since the nature of the task precluded the use of Rückle's special knowledge of numbers, and since he reported that each concrete noun aroused detailed images from different periods of his life (which only confused him), Rückle was forced to rely on rote memory. The result in the auditory presentations was a breakdown in memorizing part way through the list.

Bergh

As indicated, Hegge studied, in addition to Rückle, the Norwegian philologist and amateur mnemonist Paula Bergh (Hegge, 1918–1919a, 1918–1919b, 1929). Bergh employed a version of the classical mnemonic system of loci. When memorizing concrete nouns, she visualized the referent of each noun and placed the resulting images in order on a mental landscape. Insofar as possible she arranged the images as a connected chain of natural causes and effects. Digits were handled similarly, except that she first had the extra task of converting them to objects or persons. Hegge is not clear as to how the conversion was accomplished, but the imagery was apparently not derived from a digit–consonant encoding. Not surprisingly, her memory for long serial lists of concrete nouns was exceptional; after one study trial—evidently self-paced—she gave 77% of a 350-item list correctly, and a year later she could still give 17% correctly. Since she did not possess Rückle's special knowledge of numbers, and since her mnemonic system required more time and effort for digits than for words, her digit-memorization times were clearly inferior to his, 104 minutes as compared to 27 for learning a 408-digit string, for example, though with such long strings she was faster than Diamandi.

Other Earlier Studies

Isihara

The stage mnemonist Sigeyuki Isihara was studied by Tokasa Susukita (1933, 1934). Apart from the fact that Isihara may have been the most powerful user of a mnemonic system ever to be studied, this work is especially interesting because of Susukita's comparisons with Binet's and Müller's subjects and results on similar tasks and because of his curve-fitting and mathematical analyses. From Susukita's comments it is apparent that Isihara was of at least average academic ability. He was transferred from an agricultural school to a more academic one as a result of school performance, and he acquitted himself successfully. Isihara originally began travelling as a professional mnemonist in order to obtain money to continue his education. He had become aware of mnemonics while in school and had read books on psychology, particularly regarding memory. When studied, he was 26 and had been a professional mnemonist for several years.

In the memorization of numbers and nonsense syllables—to the extent that the latter can be compared in different languages—Isihara was at least as fast as Rückle. His learning times were shorter for digit strings of all lengths than were Rückle's in the 1902–1906 experiments. With the improved number performance of 1912, Rückle's times were similar to Isihara's for shorter strings, but Isihara was faster with longer ones. In addition, Isihara memorized longer number lists than the 408-digit list that Rückle is recorded to have attempted, including one memorization of 2,400 digits that was accomplished with 99.7% accuracy in 4 hours.

Isihara's methods were similar to those advocated in the number–consonant modifications of the classical art of memory used by Arnould. However, he made one major change. Instead of converting digits into consonants and adding vowels, he converted them directly into syllables, with a choice of about five alternate syllables for each digit. He would group the syllables into words and then recode them as visual images on a mental landscape. (The morphophonemics of Japanese, with its smaller number of possible syllables, makes this process both simpler and more efficient than it would be in an Indo-European language.) Susukita notes the similarity of the visual encoding to that reported for Bergh but seems unaware of its classical antecedents. Although Susukita did not include any task precisely the same as those used by Hegge with Bergh, Isihara was able to learn a list of 50 first names and 50 last names in less time than Hegge provided Bergh to memorize 100 concrete nouns. Thus it appears likely that Isihara may have been at least her equal—and Rückle's superior—in learning such verbal lists.

As with Müller, though to a lesser extent, there is much of Susukita's work that we cannot present, work concerned more with mnemonic process than with result. He did some curve fitting for learning time as a function of amount of material, for instance, finding that with digits, nonsense syllables, and names the learning time required tripled (approximately) for each doubling in the amount of material. He noted that the same relationship held for digits for Rückle as well, but noted that with Inaudi the learning time quadrupled for each doubling of material to be learned. Finally, he examined in some detail Isihara's long-term memory for digits, analyzing for reminiscence, the causes of retrieval failures and errors, and so forth.

Finkelstein

We have been able to examine three investigations of the Polish government clerk, mental calculator, and number memorizer Salo Finkelstein (Bousfield & Barry, 1933; Sándor, 1932; Weinland, 1948). Though Finkelstein did not have a university education, he was widely traveled and read, and seemed possessed of at least average intelligence.

According to Finkelstein's self-report, he used no mnemonic system to aid his digit memorizations but rather relied on familiarity with the properties of numbers and on quite vivid visual imagery. Whether digits were spoken or written, they appeared in Finkelstein's own hand on a mental "blackboard," six at a time in a horizontal row. Bousfield and Barry (1933) concluded after their testing of him that his imagery was eidetic. This point seems debatable, since there is at least some documentation of his various memory capabilities that seems at odds with an eidetic interpretation. His letter span was only average, and his memory for visual forms, if anything, was below average (Sándor, 1932). On the other hand, while 20 might be a fairly optimistic estimate of his auditory digit span, his visual span has been reported to have been as high as 39, even with a 4-second presentation, provided that the digits were in his preferred form, a straight horizontal line (Weinland, 1948). However this may be, his digit memorization times for longer lists were clearly inferior to those of Rückle and of Isihara, being virtually the same as those of Inaudi for lists in excess of 60 digits and slightly better for shorter lists (Sándor, 1932).

More Recent Studies of Superior Memory

S. (S. V. Shereshevskii)

This sometime musician, vaudeville actor, efficiency expert, newspaper reporter, and stage mnemonist is almost certainly the best known of the mnemonists that have been at all systematically studied, a fact stemming in part from a fairly general ignorance among psychologists of the earlier studies (see Brown & Deffenbacher, 1975). Also contributing to S.'s notoriety have been the ready accessibility of Aleksandr Luria's (1968) small book about him and the fascination with Luria's clinical claims for a "psychological syndrome" caused by S.'s having an exceptional memory.

According to Luria (1968, p. 8), S. was from a rather large family of rather "conventional, well balanced" individuals, some of them "gifted." His mother was "well read," and his father operated a bookstore in a small Jewish community. Though he was nearly 30 years old before Luria's investigations made him realize that his memory abilities were at all unusual, he had apparently had extraordinarily detailed, concrete visual memories even in childhood and had long been able to adapt his vivid visual images for memorization, encoding nonvisual information in largely visual form. For the most part he seems simply to have used the classical methods of loci (without the more modern number–letter encodings), though Luria appears to have been unaware of the parallel. In addition, he apparently made some use of synesthesia, particularly in the form of visual experiences (sometimes ones of flavor or touch) provoked by nonverbal stimuli or unfamiliar words. These synesthetic responses, however, seem to have been as much a hindrance as a help, where the sound of Luria's voice, for example, might have produced a visual image that interfered with the ones S. was attempting to report from memory.

Luria does not give much quantitative information regarding S.'s memory despite an association of almost 30 years. Early on he had become convinced that S.'s memory had little limitation, provided that there was enough time to encode the material, generally about 3–4 seconds per item. Measured with the more rapid presentation rate of standard digit-span procedures, S.'s memory would presumably not have seemed supranormal. When the encoding time was sufficient, however, he learned a matrix of 50 random digits in 180 seconds and then repeated the entire matrix by rows from top to bottom without error in 40 seconds. Without giving details, Luria (1968) indicates that a random array of letters took "roughly the same amount of time" (p. 19).

While Rückle or Isihara would have learned the digits about four times as rapidly—comparable data are lacking for consonant–vowel mixtures of letters—these are clearly extremely good performances. What is more striking, though, is Luria's claim for the durability of S.'s memory traces. Again without giving details, Luria indicates that S. could repeat such an array with complete accuracy after a delay of several months. Further, S. seems to have been able to retrieve materials even after a delay of several years. Though a multiyear test of the 50-digit matrix was not reported, S., with a nonsensical mathematical "formula" having close to 50 elements, took 7 minutes for learning (and initial recall?) and was still able to "trace his pattern of recall in precise detail" (p. 51) after 15 years when asked without warning for the information. Though the data on their long-term memory storage of nonsense materials are sparse, we doubt that any of the other mnemonists we have reviewed would have done this. Without an intention to retain the material, it is clear that at least Rückle and Isihara would not have, since both showed loss in recall of digits over time. Memorization of pi to a large number of digits, as practiced by Aitken (discussed next) and others, differs in that a single string is being selected for attention and periodic rehearsal, with the intent of committing it to permanent storage. Whether S. intended it or not, he appears to have committed to permanent store the accumulated nonsense of a life as a memorizer.

Aitken

The case of Professor Alexander Aitken is frustrating but tantalizing. It is frustrating, on the one hand, because there is a wealth of anecdotal material surrounding his abilities that is hard to evaluate and summarize. Likewise frustrating is that his abilities were little subjected to experimental tests. It is tantalizing because both the anecdotes and the firmer facts show him to have been extremely able in several different ways. Ian Hunter discussed Aitken's abilities with him and examined available materials from several sources in addition to persuading him to take part in some experimental tests. Hunter (1977) describes Aitken as a man of generally outstanding intellect, a brilliant mathematician, and an accomplished violinist in addition to being a mental calculator and being possessed of an exceptional memory. As noted near the beginning of Hunter's memorial review, apart from any other consideration, Aitken's case must dispell any impression that one might get from Luria's (1968) report on S. that memory for detail precludes creative work with general ideas.

As indicated, the direct experimental tests of Aitken's memory that have been recorded are relatively few. According to Hunter (1977), when Aitken was tested in 1932 with a presentation rate of two items per second, he had an auditory digit span of 13, a visual digit span of 15, and an auditory letter span of 10. When Hunter did the testing for an auditory digit span in 1961 (reported in Hunter, 1977), Aitken got two out of three correct spans of 12 digits with a slow rate of 1.5 second per digit, and 15 digits correct when they were read in the manner he preferred, in rapid groups of 5 digits per second, separated by 1-second pauses between groups. No other spans were attempted, nor were there additional trials at these lengths and rates.

The other two experimental tests reported were of very long term memory abilities, using materials Aitken had memorized in 1932. One set of materials was a list of 16 randomly selected 3-digit numbers presented visually at 2 seconds per digit group. The numbers were learned in four trials, for a learning time of 128 seconds. When tested later, he got 15 groups correct after 2 days, 12 groups after

4 years, and 9 groups after 28 years. The other materials were better retained. They consisted of a list of 25 words that we would describe as high in imagery-eliciting value. Presented auditorily at one word per second, the list was learned in four trials (100 seconds total time). Later testing resulted in Aitken's giving all words correctly after a week, 22 words correctly after 3 months, all correctly except for a displacement of one word after another 15 months, and all correctly and in order after an additional 27 years.

Aitken reported little difficulty in learning and remembering material he found interesting, material that was not too "repellant." As a result, over the years he developed a vast, finely articulated cognitive system with respect to many areas of knowledge but particularly with respect to mathematics and music. When confronted with material to be memorized, his approach was to become quite still and relaxed, refraining from deliberate interpretation of the material, preferring to clear his mind and let properties of the material reveal themselves. The result was the integration within his very large knowledge base of a number of subtle as well as not-so-subtle aspects of the information being memorized (Hunter, 1968).

In any event, he did not appear to use any standard mnemonic devices, unless imposing a particular rhythm and tempo in learning and recitation be considered a mnemonic. There was no visual or auditory imagery evident in his number memorizing. His memory coding for numbers, at least, would seem to have been more like that of someone committing a musical score to memory.

An example should suffice to make this point. At one time in his life, Aitken decided it would be interesting to learn pi to 1,000 places. In accomplishing this feat, he arranged the digits in groups (measures or bars?) of 50, consisting of 10 subgroups of 5 digits each. Reading over a row with a particular rhythm and tempo, he found that learning 50 digits was easy: "The learning was rather like learning a Bach fugue" (Hunter, 1962, p. 257). His recitation of pi to 1,000 places was paced in similar fashion, 5 digits per second, with a 0.5-second pause between groups of 5.

V. P.

Shortly after the appearance of Luria's (1968) account of S.'s mnemonic capabilities, two American experimental psychologists published the results of their systematic study of another mnemonist, V. P. (Hunt & Love, 1972). Interestingly, V. P. grew up in a Latvian city close to where S. had been raised. An only child of an intellectual family, V. P. was precocious. He began reading at $3\frac{1}{2}$ years, had memorized the street map of a city of 500,000 by age 5, and had memorized 150 poems for a contest by age 10.

He is the only one of the subjects reviewed for whom an IQ score has been made available—136 on the WAIS. Though this is fairly high, it may well have been an underestimate, since English was not V. P.'s native language. In addition, he had a very high score on a test designed to measure Guilford's (1967) perceptual speed factor. Finally, he was multilingual and well read, and therefore had a rather large supply of verbal associations available for building distinctive stimulus codes. Thus, confronted with a list of verbal materials to learn, he rapidly formed rather idiosyncratic verbal associations. For instance, his associations to individual items in a list of nonsense syllables presented by Hunt and Love (1972) included a Latin proverb, the name of an American political scientist, and the Hebrew word for Gentile. With strings of numbers, he instead associated ages, dates, distances, and arithmetic relationships to groups of digits three to five in length.

How these associations were then stored is not clear, though he denied use of the method of loci, and Hunt and Love found no evidence of synesthesia or of unusually vivid visual imagery, much less eidetic imagery. In their view V. P. appeared to employ semantic encodings rather than imaginal ones.

His caliber of mnemonic performance has been well documented by Hunt and Love through extensive testing with modern as well as traditional tasks used by experimental psychologists. On the task with which he can be most readily compared with S., V. P. required 390 seconds to learn a matrix of 50 random digits, and 42 seconds to recall the entire matrix. Times for S. to learn and recall a 50-digit matrix were 180 seconds and 40 seconds, respectively. Since V. P.'s encoding speed was apparently greater than S.'s, he was able to have his digit span assessed at the usual 1-digit-per-second rate. Initially, his span was a not unusually large 8 or 9; with minimal practice he was able to increase it to 17.

Though not as impressive as S. at retaining prose for lengthy periods, V. P. was far superior to the best of the university subjects available to Hunt and Love (1972) at accuracy of recalling brief stories such as Bartlett's (1932) "The War of the Ghosts." Indeed, whereas the students' memories for particular nouns and verbs in the original stories showed a very definite decline over time, V. P.'s memory, though not verbatim, was little changed over retention intervals ranging from an hour to a year.

He was likewise vastly superior to University of Washington students at keeping track of arbitrary verbal information in the shorter term. With Sternberg's (1966) task involving search of short-term memory, V. P. was apparently able to process as many as six items in parallel, whereas the students presumably had to engage in an exhaustive serial search of items in short-term memory in order to determine whether a currently presented item was presented moments before.[1] When V. P.'s auditory short-term memory was assessed by the procedure of Peterson and Peterson (1959), he did not show the usual decline in recall accuracy over a period of up to 18 seconds after item presentation. His forgetting curve remained essentially flat, at about 80% correct recall. Apparently he was able to eliminate, by

---

1. Here the subject is read or shown a string of items, perhaps letters or digits, that typically varies in length from one to six. When satisfied that these items are in short-term memory, he or she presses a button that initiates presentation of a single test item. The experimenter measures the subject's reaction time in order to determine whether the test item was or was not a member of the set in memory. Presumably, a person must compare the test item with each of the just-stored items. For persons who have not had extensive practice at this task with a given type of memory item, there is a linear increase in reaction time with increases in memory-set size, indicating a serial search of items in short-term memory. A parallel search process would be indicated by a reaction-time function that remained flat across increases in memory-set size. Those having extensive practice with items of a particular sort show reaction-time curves that approximate the flat function exhibited by V. P. Of course, V. P. had had no prior experience with the Sternberg task.

means of his distinctive encodings, the usual interference effects engendered by having been presented with similar verbal items on previous testing trials. Because of these proactive interference effects, typical learners, such as the student control subjects of Hunt and Love (1972), likewise show about 80% correct recall after a 3-second delay but then exhibit a decline in accuracy to just 50% correct recall after an elapse of 15–18 seconds.

S. F. and D. D.

These two gentlemen are of interest primarily because they are, as far as we know, the only two mnemonist subjects to have been studied throughout the period of their acquisition of mnemonic superiority. As reported in several published sources (Chase & Ericsson, 1981, 1982; Ericsson & Chase, 1982; Ericsson, Chase, & Faloon, 1980), both received extensive training and practice (200–300 hours) on a standard digit-span testing procedure, with auditory presentation at the rate of one digit per second. They moved from essentially normal performance to digit spans that were clearly supranormal, as high as 82 in the case of S. F., and 75 in the case of D. D. For S. F. at least, this training also resulted in learning speeds for visually presented matrices of 25 or 50 digits that were superior to those reported for Inaudi, Diamandi, S., and V. P., though slower than Rückle's and Isihara's on comparable tasks. Transfer of training to a nonnumerical task did not occur, with S. F.'s letter span remaining a prosaic six. Presentation of the digits at a faster rate than that used in training also prevented much transfer: With a rate of 3 per second, the span was increased only from 9 digits to 11.

The technique used by these number mnemonists was worked out by S. F. during his digit-span training. An undergraduate at Carnegie-Mellon University, S. F. was a talented amateur runner and tended to encode groups of 3 to 4 digits as actual or plausible running times. Less frequently, he encoded number groups as ages or dates. As training progressed, both subjects found or created additional times, ages, or dates, increasing their store of possible encodings. To get beyond a span of about 18 digits, however, this technique had to be supplemented by formation of what Chase and Ericsson call "supergroups," a hierarchial arrangement of groups of groups. For further details on the organization of material in memory and its encoding and retrieval, see, particularly, Chase and Ericsson (1982) and the discussion by Ericsson and Faivre in Chapter 24 of this volume.

T. E.

Of all the mnemonists, T. E. is the most recently studied (Gordon, Valentine, & Wilding, 1984). He is the scion of a middle-class British family who now works as a civil servant. Though he eventually earned a first-class honors degree in philosophy from the University of London, he had not shown any particularly unusual memorial or other intellectual talents as a child or adolescent. In fact, his talents as a memorizer only really began to develop after age 15, when he purchased a book offering to develop a "super power memory."

His primary mnemonic technique for remembering number strings and arrays is that of the digit–consonant substitution scheme discussed earlier in this chapter and used also by Arnould. When attempting to memorize a matrix of numbers, however, T. E. supplements it with an additional mnemonic device, a peg system of his own invention. To index each row of a matrix, he uses a mental image that has been previously associated with a particular digit. Thus, having previously learned 1 = eat, 2 = inn, and so forth images connected with words representing numbers in the second row of a matrix would be located within the confines of his image of an inn with which he is familiar. In attempting to remember nonsense syllables consisting only of consonants, he inserts vowels, as needed, to make words, a skill he has practiced in connection with the digit–consonant technique. With other verbal materials, he simply tries to link items in a chain of interacting visual images suggested by the items to be learned. Though T. E.'s mnemonic techniques clearly require visual imagery, Gordon et al. (1984) have experimentally ruled out the possibility of his having either eidetic or highly detailed visual imagery.

Gordon et al. (1984) tested T. E. on many of the same tasks that Hunt and Love (1972) used with V. P. The former subject's best digit span achieved was 15, which is supranormal and very close to the span of 17 representing V. P.'s best when digits were visually presented at a rate of 1 per second.

Times required for T. E. to learn and to recall simultaneously presented arrays of digits can be compared directly with those of at least three of the other mnemonists studied. To learn and to recite Luria's (1968) 50-digit matrix, T. E. needed 144 seconds and 54 seconds, respectively. As we noted earlier, V. P. required 390 seconds and 42 seconds, S. F. required 81 seconds and 57 seconds, and S. needed 180 seconds and 40 seconds for learning and recall, respectively. Again, however, Rückle and Isihara would appear to be superior to this group of mnemonists. With arrays of 48 digits, Rückle averaged 52.4 seconds and Isihara 39.6 seconds for learning, while recitation took them 19 seconds and 39.3 seconds, respectively (Müller, 1911; Susukita, 1933). In addition, Aitken took only 128 seconds to learn 48 digits presented in 3-digit groups on a memory drum, and it seems likely that he would have been at least this fast when self-paced.

Finally, as was the case in Hunt and Love's (1972) testing of V. P.'s short-term memory limits, Gordon et al. (1984) found that experimental tasks that make long-term memory coding difficult for typical laboratory subjects and that force them to rely heavily on limited short-term memory capacity did not similarly affect T. E. Gordon et al. (1984) argued that both V. P. and T. E. were able very quickly to give a highly distinctive encoding to the items presented in these so-called short-term memory tasks and to place them in long-term memory, where capacity was not a problem. Except for V. P.'s average 80% accuracy on the task of Peterson and Peterson (1959), both V. P. and T. E. showed near-perfect (96%–100%) accuracy on the various tasks. According to Gordon et al. (1984), in neither case was it evident that T. E. or V. P. had an unusually large short-term memory—they were simply more adept at preventing short-term capacity limitations from being a problem.

Discussion and Conclusions

At first blush the disparities among the various memorizers would seem to prevent any general conclusions. A little reflection, however, does at least suggest some negative ones. First, visual imagery may predominate in our sample, but it does not appear to be necessary. Indeed, in at least the case of Aitken, imagery of whatever modality may not have been important. Second, the intellectual pathology attributed to S.—difficulty with abstract thought, uncontrollable synesthesia responses interfering with attempts to report from memory, difficulty in preventing the retention of useless information—seems to be unique to him. With the others there seems to be no reason to suspect such difficulties and, especially where the two mathematicians are concerned, much reason to suppose the converse. Similarly, the popular view that many, or even all, superior memorizers are somehow idiot savants is clearly false; the memorizers we have considered are not even mildly retarded savants. Rather, they all seem to be of at least average intelligence, and several are clearly well above average. Though an IQ score is available only for V. P., some academic information is available regarding most of the others that can be used to get some idea of general intelligence. Recipients of advanced degrees include Aitken, Bergh, and Rückle; S. F., D. D., and T. E. completed good university programs. Moreover, though Diamandi and Isihara do not seem to have completed their education, there is evidence that each was doing well while enrolled.

The question of memorizer intelligence bears as well on some other issues. Gordon *et al.* (1984) clearly believe that many people could be trained with T. E.'s mnemonic techniques to exhibit the kind of memory performance reported in the literature, and Ericsson and Chase (Chapter 24, this volume) express a similar view with regard to the possibilities for training "all adults" (see also their 1982 article, p. 608). Their respective studies do show, of course, that some persons can achieve striking memorization abilities for some kinds of material with the aid of mnemonic practice. The accomplishments of Arnould, Bergh, Isihara, and S. also support such a claim. However, insofar as the subjects involved may have been of above-average intelligence, and it seems likely that all or almost all were, the possibility exists that some degree of intellectual superiority is necessary for the training to be very successful. Apart from this, with results available for only a small number of subjects, and generally just for the successful learners, there is also the possibility that some more specific quality of mnemonic élan is necessary for success rather than or in addition to general intelligence. Indeed, within the results reported by Chase and Ericsson (1982), there is some suggestion of individual differences. Though D. D. did eventually come close to S. F. in his digit spans, he required almost twice as much training to get there. Further, the experimenters had a third subject who was unable to exceed a digit span of 18 using similar encodings and who quit after being trained for 100 hours, an amount of practice that yielded spans more than twice that large in both S. F. and D. D. Thus it might be for example, that some sort of genetic predisposition—or one based on early childhood experiences—is prerequisite for the efficient formation of the Chase and Ericsson "supergroups."

Gordon *et al.* (1984), after mentioning T. E.'s techniques, make the summary claim that "previous mnemonists who have been studied by psychologists have used very similar techniques" (p. 1). Their list of "mnemonists" includes Aitken as well as S. and V. P., but their comparisons are with V. P. and, occasionally, S.—perhaps Aitken is there by oversight. With V. P. the evidence for the claim is essentially that T. E. and V. P. behave similarly on various tasks, a similarity we have summarized previously. However, use of this similarity in performance to support a claim for similarity in technique is vitiated by some other results. Though T. E.'s average digit span may have been similar to V. P.'s, V. P. started out with a span of 8 or 9 and improved steadily to 17 in the course of five trials. In T. E., on the other hand, we saw little consistent change across trials. The dramatic improvement of V. P. may demonstrate the importance of learning to organize material for memory, but it hardly supports the idea that he was using something similar to T. E.'s digit–consonant encodings or peg words. Furthermore, while T. E.'s technique did not help him on the Sternberg (1966) task of short-term memory search but rather interfered with performance, V. P. was superior both to normals and to T. E. and seemed to be processing in parallel. By his own account, V. P. was using mnemonics of various sorts on some of the tasks, but they do not appear to have been the prelearned, standardized visual encodings of T. E.'s mnemonic system. The subject S. seems to have been more like T. E. in that visual images were involved and stored in a manner resembling the method of loci. Again, however, there appears to have been little reliance on standardized encodings and more on spontaneous associations.

Ericsson and Chase (1982) conclude with a claim that "in every recorded feat of exceptional memory we have identified the same components: the importance of prior experience and practice, the availability of meaningful associations, storage in a long-term memory, and efficient retrieval of information from long-term memory" (p. 615). That storage of some memorial information occurs in long-term memory should come as no surprise. Presumably, their concern is with the more interesting point that information in what at first may appear to be short-term memory, such as digit-span measurement, may instead be long-term memory. Thus what may appear to be a supranormal short-term memory capacity may in fact represent use of long-term memory storage. Certainly there is evidence that material may get into long-term memory in such tasks. And there is further evidence that S. F. improved his digit span markedly without apparently improving his short-term memory. What is not established, though it may be true, is that no cases of supranormal memory performance involve short-term memories of supranormal capacity. Unfortunately, the issue is not an easy one to resolve, particularly with subjects that are not available for retesting.

Prior experience and practice may be important for all persons with superior memories, as Ericsson and Chase (1982) suggest. However, the nature, amount, and role of such practice and experience seem to have varied greatly from subject to subject and even within a subject from task to task. We seem to have one extreme in the users of systems of mnemonics, whether they be users of systems restricted to numbers, such as S. F. and D. D., or users of the more inclusive systems, such as Arnould, Bergh, Isihara, and T. E. Here the relevant practice is with precisely the sorts of materials that are to be memorized and with the specific encoding conversions to be used with them. The amount of time spent in drilling on these skills is not known for the others, but the 200–300 hours for S. F. and D. D. may well be representative.

With S. the relevant practice was also with imagery encodings; however, insofar as images of the numbers themselves were used, practice producing the images may not have been needed. Apart from some minor changes in technique—developing some simpler images for commonly memorized items and learning not to place images in poorly lit places in his mental landscape—S. showed little change during almost 30 years of study.

In V. P.'s case, there would seem to have been extensive practice on memorization as well, quite likely more practice than engaged in by the system users. More important, it would seem that the nature and role of practice was different for him than for the others just considered. The material and tasks in the drills of V. P.'s childhood were not so similar to the material and tasks used in the tests of his memory. Further, he seems not to have drilled on specific encodings. Rather, what he seems to have learned in his prior experience and practice were more general approaches to memorization.

When mental calculators memorize numbers, they would seem to be relying on prior experience and practice. Their practice of digit memorization would be incidental to practice of calculation, but it would still occur. It may well also be that familiarity with the properties and relations of numbers is providing a system of numerical encoding even when the calculator does not report one or denies its use. Thus, when calculators such as Inaudi and Diamandi exhibit strongly superior memories for numbers but not for other materials, there may be little reason to inquire further. But what of Aitken and Rückle? As we have indicated, Rückle was not only among the very best memorizers of numbers but also among the very best memorizers of a wide variety of verbal materials as well as of nonsense drawings. Experimental tests of Aitken were few, but those that were done confirm superiority in letter span and on a word list as well as with numbers. Anecdotes add music and literary materials as objects of memorization for Aitken.

We know little of Rückle's life outside the laboratory, so that we can perhaps imagine him spending all his time before Müller tested him immersed in monkish memorization, preparing for their eventual encounter. With Aitken more biographical information is known that is of relevance to our concerns, and though there is evidence of practice of a sort in what he called his period of "mental yoga" (Hunter, 1962, p. 253), it was not primarily or even secondarily practice at memorization—let alone practice with the specific encodings of a mnemonic system. Rather, what Aitken practiced seems to have been an attempt to make sense of the world, a search for meaningful relationships, particularly in mathematics, music, languages, and literature. Thus in mathematics his early concern was with the properties of numbers and the relationships among them. Knowledge of numerical properties and relationships was acquired for its own sake. It was incidental to Aitken that such knowledge may have conferred on him an advantage in the memorization of numbers.

Practice would seem to have been involved in developing superior memorization abilities, though by no means always practice at that task or directed to that end. Does that mean practice is sufficient, or is some other predisposing factor or constellation of factors necessary? Unfortunately, we lack information here on such conceivable correlates as handedness, cerebral dominance, the possibility of damage to various brain areas, and so forth, and have something of a psychometric workup only on V. P. That the subjects are almost all male is probably not a coincidence but seems more likely to have resulted, at least primarily, from the predispositions of societal expectation and pressure than from ones of chromosomes or androgenization. A tendency for subjects to live near active researchers seems unedifying as well.

As we noted before, however, there is evidence, particularly from academic achievement, that all or almost all of the memorizers were probably at least above average in general intelligence. If we consider the nature of their mnemonic accomplishments in this context, a further pattern emerges. Among the people who memorize specific kinds of materials by using encoding techniques especially practiced for the purpose, three—S. F., D. D., and T. E.—are described by their researchers as having an average or normal intelligence and indeed may well be fairly normal among college graduates. Arnould and Isihara came from times and places where college attendance was less frequent, as did the two calculators, Inaudi and Diamandi, whose memorization superiority was restricted to numbers. Descriptions of them are sparse, but the information available is not inconsistent with their intelligence being similar to the others mentioned. Thus, while superior memorization performance with these techniques may require more intelligence than average, it may not demand an outstanding intellect.

The more general approaches and accomplishments of V. P., Aitken, and Rückle would seem to be more demanding in their prerequisites, and the subjects in question seem to be of superior or even outstanding intellect as well. Is this a coincidence? We doubt it very much, particularly where Aitken is concerned. Even if intelligence were only a matter of speed of learning and not of something more fundamental, one would have to have a goodly measure of it to match the prior experience, practice, and wealth of association that he could bring to bear.

For the purpose of some mnemonists, then, prior practice with specific encodings for a specific domain is sufficient. For others, it is necessary to memorize digits based on associations developed and practiced in mental calculation. Still others must employ more general approaches requiring more general knowledge or more general techniques, together with the greater general intelligence necessary to pull it off.

References

Barlow, F. (1952). *Mental prodigies*. New York: Philosophical Library.

Barlett, F. C. (1932). *Remembering: A study in experimental and social psychology*. Cambridge: Cambridge University Press.

Binet, A. (1894). *Psychologie des grands calculateurs et jouers d'échecs*. Paris: Librairie Hachette.

Bousfield, W., & Barry, H. (1983). The visual imagery of a lightning calculator. *American Journal of Psychology, 45*, 353–358.

Brown, E., & Deffenbacher, K. (1975). Forgotten mnemonists. *Journal of the History of the Behavioral Sciences, 11,* 342–349.

Chase, W. G., & Ericsson, K. A. (1981). Skilled memory. In J. R. Anderson (Ed.), *Cognitive skills and their acquisition* (pp. 59–117). Hillsdale, NJ: Erlbaum.

Chase, W. G., & Ericsson, K. A. (1982). Skill and working memory. In G. H. Bower (Ed.), *The psychology of learning and motivation* (Vol. 16, pp. 1-58). New York: Academic Press.

Ebbinghaus, H. (1885). Über das Gedächtnis. Leipzig: Duncker.

Ericsson, K. A., & Chase, W. G. (1982). Exceptional memory. *American Scientist, 70,* 607–615.

Ericsson, K. A., Chase, W. G., & Faloon, S. (1980). Acquisition of a memory skill. *Science, 208,* 1181–1182.

Gordon, P., Valentine, E., & Wilding, J. (1984). One man's memory: A study of a mnemonist. *British Journal of Psychology, 75,* 1–14.

Guilford, J. P. (1967). *The nature of human intelligence.* New York: McGraw-Hill.

Hegge, T. (1918–1919a). Beiträge zur Analyse der Gedächtnistätigkeit, Über ungewöhnliche und illustrierende und lokalisierende Einprägung. *Zeitschrift für Psychologie, 84,* 349–352.

Hegge, T. (1918–1919b). Die grossen Gedächtniskünstler. *Zeitschrift für Psychologie, 84,* 353–354.

Hegge, T. (1929). Some incidental memory experiments with the memory prodigy, Dr. Rückle. *Michigan Academy of Sciences, Arts, and Letters, 10,* 389–396.

Hunt, E., & Love, T. (1972). How good can memory be? In A. Melton & E. Martin (Eds.), *Coding processes in human memory* (pp. 237–260). Washington, DC: Winston.

Hunter, I. M. L. (1962). An exceptional talent for calculative thinking. *British Journal of Psychology, 53,* 243–258.

Hunter, I. M. L. (1968). Mental calculation. In P. C. Wason & P. N. Johnson-Laird (Eds.), *Thinking and reasoning* (pp. 35–45). Harmondsworth: Penguin.

Hunter, I. M. L. (1977). An exceptional memory. *British Journal of Psychology, 68,* 155–164.

Luria, A. (1968). *The mind of a mnemonist.* New York: Basic Books.

Müller, G. (1911). Zur Analyse der Gedächtnistätigkeit und des Vorstellungsverlaufes, 1. *Zeitschrift für Psychologie,* Erganzungsband 5, pp. 1-403.

Müller, G. (1913a). Neue Versuche mit Rückle. *Zeitschrift für Psychologie, 67,* 193–213.

Müller, G. (1913b). Zur Analyse der Gedächtnistätigkeit und des Vorstellungsverlaufes, 3 (sic). *Zeitschrift für Psychologie,* Erganzungsband 8, pp. 1-567.

Müller, G. (1917). Zur Analyse der Gedächtnistätigkeit und des Vorstellungsverlaufes, 2 (sic). *Zeitschrift für Psychologie,* Erganzungsband 9, pp. 1-682.

Müller, G., & Schumann, F. (1894). Experimentelle Beiträge zur Untersuchung des Gedächtnisses. *Zeitschrift für Psychologie, 6,* 81–190; 257–339.

Peterson, L. R., & Peterson, M. J. (1959). Short term retention of individual items. *Journal of Experimental Psychology, 58,* 193–198.

Sándor, B. (1932). Die Gedächtnistätigkeit und Arbeitsweise von Rechenkünstlern. *Charakter, 1,* 47–50.

Smith, S. (1983). *The great mental calculators: The psychology, methods, and lives of calculating prodigies, past and present.* New York: Columbia University Press.

Steffens, L. (1900). Experimentelle Beiträge zur Lehre vom ökonomischen Lernen. *Zeitschrift für Psychologie, 22,* 321–382.

Sternberg, S. (1966). High speed scanning in human memory. *Science, 153,* 652–654.

Susukita, T. (1933). Untersuchung eines ausserordentlichen Gedächtnisses in Japan, 1. *Tohoku Psychologia Folia, 1,* 111–134.

Susukita, T. (1934). Untersuchung eines ausserordentlichen Gedächtnisses in Japan, 2. *Tohoku Psychologia Folia, 2,* 15–42.

Weinland, J. (1948). The memory of Salo Finkelstein. *Journal of General Psychology, 39,* 243–257.

9

Superior Memory: Perspective from the Neuropsychology of Memory Disorders

MARLENE OSCAR-BERMAN

It is likely that the brains of individuals with superior memory (as described by Brown and Deffenbacher, Chapter 8, this volume) have some unique biological characteristics. These characteristics may be inherited; they may develop with training; and/or they may reflect some other internal or external influences. Whatever the etiology, however, I find it intriguing to speculate about the underlying neuropsychological mechanisms. One logical anatomical place to start is somewhere within the same neuronal substrates as those responsible for normal memory storage and retrieval. Since knowledge about neuroanatomical loci in normal memory is derived in part from inferences based on lost function in damaged brains, the study of amnesia will provide the framework within which to explore possible mechanisms for superior memory. Although my argument concentrates on the temporal lobes, I shall touch upon biochemical processes that likely involve the entire brain.

Studies of Anterograde Amnesias and Neurological Patients

In the 1950s and 1960s, the careful scientific study of human anterograde amnesias was beginning to take on considerable momentum. Scoville and Milner (1957) published a detailed description of memory loss in a patient (H. M.) following surgery for the relief of severe epileptic seizures. The lesions involved medial temporal lobe structures bilaterally, and the resulting anterograde amnesia in H. M.—his inability to retain new information—remains unabated today (Corkin *et al.*, 1985). In 1965 Talland's book *Deranged Memory* provided a comprehensive analysis of anterograde amnesia accompanying another neurological disorder, Korsakoff syndrome (Victor & Yakovlev, 1955). The amnesia of Korsakoff syndrome

Marlene Oscar-Berman. Psychology Service, Boston Veterans Administration Medical Center, Boston, Massachusetts; and Department of Neurology and Division of Psychiatry, Boston University School of Medicine, Boston, Massachusetts.

was associated with chronic alcoholism, stroke, toxemia, and other problems involving bilateral damage to some portion of the limbic system, presumed to be connected anatomically with medial temporal lobe structures (Lindquist & Norlen, 1966; Whitty & Zangwill, 1966, 1977). Whatever the etiology, the severe anterograde amnesia characteristic of patients with medial temporal lobe resection and those with Korsakoff syndrome is accompanied by a relatively intact long-term memory and the ability to acquire certain skills. Research on preserved mnemonic capacities in amnesic patients has received considerable attention recently and has detailed aspects of preserved incidental, semantic, or procedural memory abilities compared, respectively, to defective intentional, episodic, or declarative memory (Cohen, 1984; Graf, Squire, & Mandler, 1984; Jacoby, 1984; Kinsbourne & Wood, 1982; Olton, Gamzu, & Corkin, 1985; Oscar-Berman, 1984b).

In contrast to anterograde amnesia, Penfield (summarized by Penfield & Roberts, 1966) described the remarkable recall of past events by awake patients whose brains were being stimulated electrically during routine probing prior to surgical removal of tissue for relief from epilepsy. Patients recounted the experience of having vivid memories for events that had occurred years before, many of which had been forgotten. Penfield reported that in a series of 190 cases of craniotomies where stimulation was applied anywhere on the accessible cortex, "psychical responses" (distinct from sensory or motor responses) "were produced only by stimulation of the temporal lobe" (Penfield & Roberts, 1966, p. 34).

Penfield divided psychical responses into two groups: interpretive and experiential. Interpretive responses were *déjà vu* phenomena, for example, a false sense of general familiarity about a situation. In contrast, experiential responses were more concrete and specific; they were "flash-backs" to an earlier time. It should be noted that experiential responses also were reported by patients during partial epileptic seizures produced by spontaneous discharges in the temporal regions. The excess stimulation that produces seizures may be acting in a manner similar to that of external electrical stimulation imposed by Penfield's probing. Experiential responses involved memory for many details of the previous experience, indeed, for all detail to which the patient "had paid attention" (Penfield & Roberts, 1966, p. 45) or that had "seemed important at the time" (p. 46). For that reason, stimulation-induced experiential responses, more than interpretive responses, resemble those reported in supranormal memories as described by Brown and Deffenbacher in Chapter 8 of this volume. Using more modern terminology, experiential responses likely would be considered in the category of intentional, episodic, and declarative memories mentioned earlier in context of amnesia.

Penfield and Roberts (1966) specifically stressed the importance of the hippocampus for producing these responses:

> When this stimulation of hippocampal gyrus was carried out, the hippocampal formation and amygdaloid nucleus were still intact. But the rest of the anterior half of the temporal lobe had been removed. The fact that stimulation . . . . could still produce a flash-back of former experience would support the suggestion that comes from other evidence (Milner and Penfield, 1955) that the hippocampus of the two sides is, in fact,

the repository of ganglionic patterns that preserve the record of the stream of consciousness. If not the repository, then each hippocampus plays an important role in the mechanism of reactivation of that record. (p. 47)

A Mechanism for Memory Storage

What might be the mechanism by which "reactivation" occurs? Might injury to this mechanism lead to profound amnesia? Might disinhibition or overstimulation of this mechanism allow superior memory performance? In the last decade the search for an understanding of the neuropsychology of human memory has relied more and more upon progress in neurochemistry and neurophysiology. Bliss and his colleagues (Bliss & Gardner-Medwin, 1973; Bliss & Lømo, 1973) noted that repeated electrical stimulation of cells entering rabbit hippocampus would potentiate for weeks the effects of subsequent stimulation. This hypersensitivity could be elicited even by brief, widely spaced intervals of electrical stimulation; it was accompanied by structural changes in dendritic spines and by increased numbers of synapses with other cells. Thus, neuronal events lasting only less than a second could have demonstrable long-term effects on the structure and function of the cell itself and on other cells with which it communicates.

Dendritic receptors of a neuron respond to neurotransmitters released from axonal terminals of other neurons, causing changes in electrical potentials across their membranes. Lynch (1985) has summarized beautifully a convincing body of information suggesting that memories are mediated by a biochemical process triggered by transient physiological events that cause permanent changes in neuronal synapses. The mechanism described by Lynch involves events occurring intracellularly and along the cell membrane.

Neurons maintain low levels of intracellular calcium despite high calcium levels in the blood and cerebrospinal fluid. With stimulation, voltage changes occur across neuronal membranes such that porelike channels allow calcium to rush in. High levels of calcium in the cell activate enzymes and also release chemicals such as neurotransmitters. Thus calcium-related changes are important for normal intracellular functions and for intercellular communication. In the synaptic membranes of the hippocampus, the region studied by Lynch (1985), an important neurotransmitter is glutamate. Lynch found that by adding calcium to hippocampal cells, there is an increase in the number of receptor sites that bind glutamate in this region (just as there is in long-term potentiation). More important, however, Lynch found that the increased number of hippocampal glutamate receptor sites persisted after the excess calcium was removed. Thus calcium appears to play an important role in activating long-lasting chemical changes in neurons, whether the changes are experimentally induced or are the consequence of naturally occurring long-term potentiation.

These observations led Lynch to postulate a mechanism by which memory storage may occur: (1) Neuronal activity increases calcium levels in dendritic spines and neighboring regions; (2) the calcium then activates enzymes that break down their substrate proteins; (3) the degraded proteins can no longer maintain their previous connection between the neuron's cytoskeleton (supporting filaments) and its membrane; (4) an ensuing reorganization of the synapse takes place, including an increase in glutamate receptors; and (5) calcium is pumped out of the dendrite, and the dendrite now is more sensitive to incoming stimulation than it had been before.

This model can account for the basic requirements of normal human memory—its flexibility, durability, and capacity. Might it account for deranged memory or supranormal memory? It is not unlikely that biochemical abnormalities in a mechanism such as that proposed by Lynch would result in cognitive abnormalities. Damage to the brain regions involved in such a process could produce the type of anterograde amnesia described earlier. (We already know that damage to other neurotransmitter systems is associated with severe memory disorders. For example, pathology in the nucleus basalis of Meynert, a major source of cholinergic input to the hippocampus and neocortex, has been documented in Korsakoff patients and in patients with Alzheimer disease; (Arendt, Bigl, Arendt, & Tennstedt, 1983.) It does not seem unreasonable to imagine that *overstimulation* of some cholinergic, glutaminergic, or other neurotransmitter system in the brain (or hypersensitivity of neuronal membranes) might play a role in recalling "experiential responses" as described by Penfield and Roberts (1966) or in facilitating superior mnemonic encoding as described by Brown and Deffenbacher (Chapter 8, this volume).

Where in the brain might such processes occur? On the basis of results of the past 30 years of work in behavioral neurology, one might hypothesize the following: Individuals with special visual memory skills (such as the visual calculators described by Smith in Chapter 2 of this volume) would have "special neurotransmitter activity" involving visual-association cortex; for auditory calculators with poor visuo-spatial skills (such as Fuller and Mondeux), the mechanism might involve areas devoted to the elaboration of auditory input (e.g., the posterior left temporal lobe), with perhaps a de-emphasis on activity in visual-association cortex; in mnemonists who develop verbal systems for recall, the classical language areas may be most important; and for those with strictly numerical talents (such as the case described by Ericsson and Faivre in Chapter 24 of this volume), the left posterior temporal association areas may be suspect. However, the entire cortical mantle cannot be excluded from consideration in each and every case of superior memory (for a discussion of brain areas involved in one form of human amnesia and related cognitive impairments, see Oscar-Berman, 1984a, 1984b). The cerebral cortex contains billions of neurons; it communicates directly or indirectly with all other parts of the brain; it makes functional connections among all incoming sensory modalities; and it plays a role in the execution of complex responses. Subareas of the cortex have their various specialties for visual, verbal, or mathematical processing. These combined characteristics make the cerebral cortex a uniquely well suited candidate for human memory functions. Of course, the speculations made here remain to be tested in the decades to come, in the study of the biological components of normal, subnormal, and supranormal memory processing.

Acknowledgments

Support for the writing of this chapter came from the Medical Research Service of the Veterans Administration and from the following USDHHS grants: NIAAA AA07112 and RSDA AA00061; NINCDS NS07615 and NS06209. I would like to thank Dr. Fred Gault and Ron Ellis for their helpful comments.

References

Arendt, T., Bigl, V., Arendt, A., & Tennstedt, A. (1983). Loss of neurons in the nucleus basalis of Meynert in Alzheimer's disease. *Acta neurologica, 61,* 101–108.

Bliss, T. V. P., & Gardner-Medwin, A. R. (1973). Long-lasting potentiation of synaptic transmission in the dentate area of the unanesthetized rabbit following stimulation of the perforant path. *Journal of Neurophysiology, 232,* 357–374.

Bliss, T. V. P., & Lømo, T. (1973). Long-lasting potentiation of synaptic transmission in the dentate area of the anesthetized rabbit following stimulation of the perforant path. *Journal of Neurophysiology, 232,* 331–356.

Cohen, N. J. (1984). Preserved learning capacity in amnesia: Evidence for multiple memory systems. In L. R. Squire & N. Butters (Eds.), *The neuropsychology of memory* (pp. 83–103). New York: Guilford Press.

Corkin, S., Cohen, N. J., Sullivan, E. V., Clegg, R. A., Rosen, T. J., & Ackerman, R. H. (1985). Analyses of global memory impairments of different etiologies. In D. S. Olton, E. Gamzu, & S. Corkin (Eds.), *Memory dysfunction: An integration of animal and human research from preclinical and clinical perspectives. Annals of the New York Academy of Sciences, 444,* 10–40.

Graf, P., Squire, L. R., & Mandler, G. (1984). The information that amnesic patients do not forget. *Journal of Experimental Psychology: Learning, Memory and Cognition, 10,* 164–178.

Jacoby, L. L. (1984). Incidental vs. intentional retrieval: Remembering and awareness as separate issues. In L. R. Squire & N. Butters, (Eds.), *The neuropsychology of memory* (pp. 145–156). New York: Guilford Press.

Kinsbourne, M., & Wood, F. (1982). Theoretical considerations regarding the episodic-semantic memory distinction. In L. S. Cermak (Ed.), *Human memory and amnesia* (pp. 195–217). Hillsdale, NJ: Erlbaum.

Lindquist, G., & Norlen, G. (1966). Korsakoff's syndrome after operation on ruptured aneurysm of the anterior communicating artery. *Acta Psychiatrica Scandinavia, 42,* 24–34.

Lynch, G. (1985). What memories are made of. *The Sciences, 25,* 38–43.

Milner, B., & Penfield, W. (1955). The effect of hippocampal lesions on recent memory. *Transactions of the American Neurological Association, 80,* 42–48.

Olton, D. S., Gamzu, E., & Corkin, S. (Eds.) (1985). *Memory dysfunctions: An integration of animal and human research from preclinical and clinical perspectives. Annals of the New York Academy of Sciences, 444,* 553.

Oscar-Berman, M. (1984a). Brain. In R. J. Corsini (Ed.), *Encyclopedia of psychology* (pp. 164–167). New York: Wiley.

Oscar-Berman, M. (1984b) Comparative neuropsychology and alcoholic Korsakoff's disease. In L. R. Squire & N. Butters (Eds.), *Neuropsychology of memory* (pp. 194–202). New York: Guilford Press.

Penfield, W., & Roberts, L. (1966). *Speech and brain mechanisms.* New York: Atheneum.

Scoville, W. B., & Milner, B. (1957). Loss of recent memory after bilateral hippocampal lesions. *Journal of Neurology, Neurosurgery and Psychiatry, 20,* 11–21.

Talland, G. A. (1965). *Deranged memory.* New York: Academic Press.

Victor, M., & Yakovlev, P. I. (1955). S. S. Korsakoff's psychic disorder in conjunction with peripheral neuritis. A translation of Korsakoff's original article with brief comments on the author and his contribution to clinical medicine. *Neurology, 5,* 394–406.

Whitty, C. W. M., & Zangwill, O. L. (Eds.) (1966). *Amnesia.* London: Butterworths.

Whitty, C. W. M., & Zangwill, O. L. (Eds.) (1977). *Amnesia* (2nd ed.). London: Butterworths.

10

The Characteristics of Eidetic Imagery

Ralph Norman Haber
Lyn R. Haber

A child is shown an 8-inch × 10-inch picture on an easel and is asked to examine it completely for 30 seconds. The experimenter begins questioning the child as soon as the picture is removed from sight. The following is a transcript of what one 10-year-old boy said after he had looked at Figure 10-1 (see Leask, Haber, & Haber, 1969, for further information and details on the testing procedure). The duration of this report is 5.9 minutes.

> EXPERIMENTER: Can you see anything?
> SUBJECT: Yes, I can see the white and blue sky, and the ground has two different shades of green in it with some blue on it . . . and I can see two different squirrels, one is gray and the Indian's holding him in his hand and eating a nut. There are three birds in the air—they're green, orange—they've got some red on them.
> EXPERIMENTER: Can you see the birds' mouths?
> SUBJECT: No—I can see the deer and the cloth on the Indian's belt, it has many colors on it, yellow is the biggest color—and I can see his bow he's holding, it's got zigzag red on it.
> EXPERIMENTER: Anything else—any other animals?
> SUBJECT: There's three rabbits—two of them are brown and one of them is white—the one brown and white one are next to each other and there's another brown one in the right-hand corner.
> EXPERIMENTER: What are they doing?
> SUBJECT: One over in the right-hand corner is jumping, and the other two are just standing around.
> EXPERIMENTER: Tell me more about the Indian.
> SUBJECT: Well—
> EXPERIMENTER: Start at the top and move down.
> SUBJECT: Well, he's got a headband on—he doesn't have a shirt on, he's got a belt on with a cloth hanging out which is red, yellow. He's got Indian moccasins on—I think they're brown.

Ralph Norman Haber and Lyn R. Haber. Department of Psychology, University of Illinois at Chicago, Chicago, Illinois.

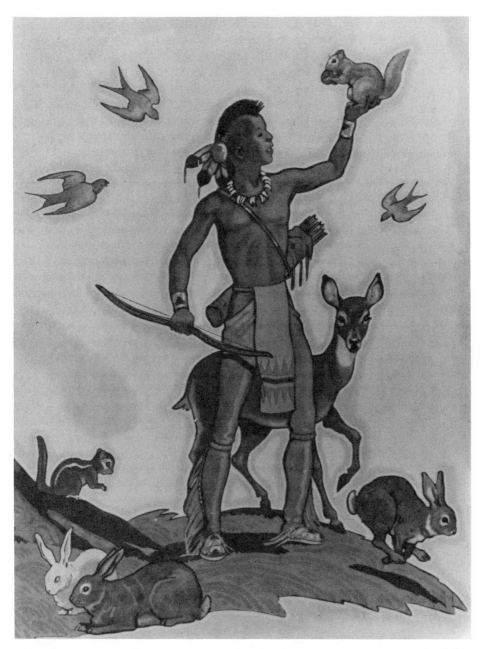

FIGURE 10-1. Black-and-white reproduction of a color picture shown to a 10-year-old boy being tested for eidetic imagery.

EXPERIMENTER: Has he got anything else on?

SUBJECT: No.

EXPERIMENTER: Anything else you can tell me—and tell me if any of the parts go away.

SUBJECT: The rabbits and birds are going away (pause) and the sky (pause) that's it—it's all gone.

Here is a second example, taken from an 11-year-old girl after she had looked at Figure 10-2. The duration of the report is nearly 8 minutes. Again, the experimenter begins questioning after the picture has been removed from sight.

EXPERIMENTER: Do you see anything?

SUBJECT: Yes.

EXPERIMENTER: Start at the left and tell me about it.

SUBJECT: He looks sort of like an elf. He's got a yellow hat and it goes up to a yellow globe—it looks like a sun and the trees behind are sort of bubbly looking—dark green. Ground is dark greenish brown, then there's a momma and a little leopard and there's a native sitting against him. Then there's a pool with a crab on it—coming to it—with a fish in it, and I think there are turtles walking in front and a porcupine down near the right-hand corner of the pool. Then back on the right, there's a tree that separates a cow in half—the cow's brown and white, and there's something up in the tree—I can't see the bottom right-hand corner—there's a sun with a lot of rays on it near the top on the right.

EXPERIMENTER: Can you count the rays?

SUBJECT: About eight . . . (pause) There's a lot in that one.

EXPERIMENTER: Can you see anything else?

SUBJECT: No, (pause) there's something red in the tree around where the cow is.

EXPERIMENTER: Any other animals or people?

SUBJECT: No more people—can't see the right-hand corner. The porcupine has a lot of bristles on it—oh, there's a little something down away from him to the right—it's black and white (pause). That's about all.

EXPERIMENTER: Can you still see it?

SUBJECT: Most of it.

EXPERIMENTER: Tell me if it begins to go away or if you see anything else. (long pause) Still seeing something?

SUBJECT: Yes, but not the sky above the trees. I can't see what's in front of the native anymore—it's sort of going, there's something in the left-hand corner like a clump of bushes—dark, it's fading.

EXPERIMENTER: Tell me what parts fade.

SUBJECT: The right is disappearing—I can still see that cow that's divided by the tree. (pause) Oh! There's a crocodile or alligator in the right-hand corner. You can't see all of him.

EXPERIMENTER: Can you see the right-hand side better now?

SUBJECT: No—that's all I see from it.

EXPERIMENTER: Anything else in the middle?

SUBJECT: Well, there's the fish in the pool and the pool is sort of odd-shaped, there might be something in back of it.

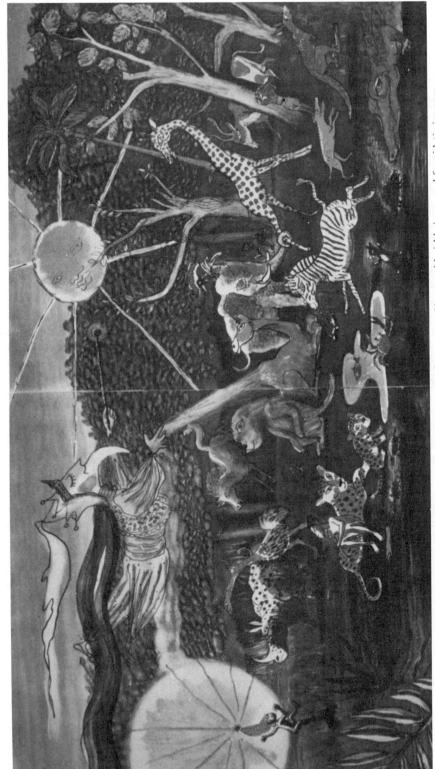

FIGURE 10-2. Black-and-white reporduction of a color picture shown to an 11-year-old girl being tested for eidetic imagery.

EXPERIMENTER: Is there any left now?

SUBJECT: It's very faint—only the bright yellow of the man's hat—that's about all.

EXPERIMENTER: Tell me when it goes away.

SUBJECT: (pause) It's gone.

What is Eidetic Imagery?

Both of these examples illustrate reports given by children of eidetic images. The critical feature is that the children say they can still see a previously viewed stimulus, which in fact has been removed from their view, and they act as if they can examine and describe that stimulus, almost as if it were still in sight.

The ability to have eidetic images—to continue to see a visual representation of prior, but no longer present, visual stimulation—is possessed by only a small percentage of children and by even fewer adults. It does not appear to be either an abnormal or a developmentally immature ability.

The study of eidetic imagery has had a very checkered course during the past century of research effort. Research flourished for 50 years, totally ceased for the next 30, and has been broadly revived for the past 20. As with many abilities that are both unusual in terms of the normal range of cognitive skills and possessed by only a small handful of people, the easiest interpretation of demonstrations of eidetic imagery, such as the two just described, has been that the phenemenon does not exist at all. To account for the data, appeals were made to poor experimental control, to inappropriate demand characteristics of the testing, to the failure or inability of the subjects to understand the task, or to some kind of hypothetical chicanery, benevolent or otherwise, on the part of the researcher.

In the 1960s, after three decades during which no empirical work was done on eidetic imagery, and during which the topic was virtually ignored by theoretical psychology, research and theoretical work in the area began again, primarily as a result of the introduction of a suitable methodology that permitted some confidence in the data and made it much more difficult to dismiss the reported examples simply as error, confusion, or distortion. Since 1964, massive and diversified research programs, located across five continents, operated out of 15 independent laboratories, and based on the screening of samples of subjects approaching 10,000 in number, have independently identified hundreds of eidetic subjects using this methodology (see Haber, 1979a, 1979b, for reviews).

Historically, the research on eidetic imagery has depended on two quite different methods, and within each, on varying degrees of experimental rigor and sophistication. Both methods were used by researchers in the decades prior to the 1930s, though in most cases neither was pursued with sufficient rigor and care. The structural method (see Ahsen, 1977, for descriptions and a review) typically depends on a verbal instruction to evoke a past memory. The subject is then asked if any images are elicited by that memory, and if so, to describe them. This method has been used more recently in the context of clinical and therapeutic programs, because it depends on imagery drawn from personal memories. However, relatively little of the recent work using this method has focused on empirical questions.

The picture elicitation method, which was used in the two examples presented earlier, is more restrictive than the structural method. The subject examines a picture presented on an easel for a period of time; after the picture is removed from sight, the subject is asked to report anything that can still be seen of the picture. This procedure, in contrast to the structural method, permits precise control over the content of the eliciting stimulus, over its exposure duration and conditions, and over the poststimulus duration as well as the conditions of response (see Haber, 1979a, and Leask et al., 1969, for details of this procedure, exact instructions given to subjects, and further examples of testing sessions).

The more recent period of intense research, beginning in the 1960s, has used almost exclusively the picture elicitation method, which was reintroduced and standardized in 1964 (Haber & Haber, 1964). This has resulted in far better control and more consistent results. These results have shown that (1) eidetic imagery can be measured precisely, so that people possessing such imagery can be reliably identified and studied; (2) eidetic imagery can be differentiated from hallucinations, afterimages, nonvisual memory, and visual imagery in general; (3) the characteristics of eidetic imagery can be described and analyzed; (4) while it is easier to find child than adult eidetics, there is neither a necessary negative correlation with age nor any evidence that eidetic subjects are less cognitively developed than noneidetics; and (5) eidetic imagery appears to be qualitatively different from other kinds of visual images.

Measurement Procedures and Identification of Eidetic Subjects

A typical experiment undertaken to identify some eidetic subjects using the picture elicitation method requires that a fairly large sample of subjects be screened, usually individually. The following procedures and instructions are adapted from Haber and Haber (1964) and have been used in this or a closely related form in virtually all of the studies published since 1964.

In most studies the subjects are elementary school children; they are sampled randomly from some or all of the grades, or often the entire student body is used. Some studies have used adults, usually college students, and in a few cases, special populations have been sampled. The research conducted in other cultures has often sampled an entire village.

Such a vast variety of pictures has been used that no claim could be made that the kind of picture matters. Most of the cross-cultural work has used the same "Western" pictures, even though some of them would have been close to meaningless to the population being studied. Typically, a picture is mounted on cardboard and displayed on an easel or other neutral surface larger than the picture. Illumination is normal for the room (though some studies did the testing in natural sunlight outdoors). Generally, a tape recording is made of both the subject's and the experimenter's voices.

The testing typically begins with four brightly colored square patches, to assess afterimages and to accustom the subject to reporting an image after the stimulus has been removed. The experimenter places a square on the easel, leaves it there for 10 seconds, tells the subject to stare at the center of it as hard as possible, and not to move his or her eyes at all as long as the square is there. When the square is taken away, the subject is to continue to stare as hard as possible, looking where the square was. Subjects are told that if they stare hard enough, they will still be able to see something there—very much like when they stare hard at a light bulb and then look away; they can still see something out there in front of their eyes. As soon as the color is taken away, the subject is to tell the experimenter if anything can still be seen on the easel where the color had been.

The experimenter watches carefully during the exposure to be sure the subject's eyes do not move. If the subject reports seeing nothing at all after the square is removed, encouragement is given by assuring the subject that it is all right to see things after the color is removed. If the subject still says nothing is seen, the instructions are repeated to stare hard and fixedly. Then the experimenter presents the next square, increasing the duration by an additional 10 seconds over the previous exposure.

If the subject reports seeing something, that report is allowed to continue spontaneously. When the subject stops, the experimenter asks questions about whichever of the following items that have not been reported: Is the image still visible? What is its color and shape? Do the color and shape change, and if so, how? In what direction does the image move? How does it disappear? The subject is instructed to try to move his or her eyes to the top of the easel and is then asked if the image moves or stays in the same place. The same procedure is followed for the four squares, after which the experimenter starts with the first picture.

The instructions for the pictures are slightly different. The subject is told not to stare in one place, but to move his or her eyes around so as to see all of the details of the picture. Also, when the picture is taken away, the subject is told to continue looking at the easel where the picture was but that he or she is allowed to make eye movements while reporting to the experimenter what is being seen after the picture has been taken away.

The pictures are usually presented for 30 seconds each. The experimenter watches closely to be sure the pictures are scanned and not fixated on. After the first picture is removed, the subject is told to continue to look at the easel and to describe whatever can be seen. The subject is continually reminded to make eye movements. The experimenter notes the relation between direction of gaze and details of report. If the subject reports seeing something, the experimenter asks if it is actually being seen now or is being remembered from when the picture was still on the easel. The experimenter asks frequently if the subject is still seeing something, since subjects often do not report the fading of the image but continue reporting it from memory. If the subject stops talking, the experimenter asks if anything else can be seen. If the subject says yes, the experimenter asks for its description. The experimenter probes for further description and attributes of all objects still visible in the images. This process is repeated for all four pictures. The average time for testing ranges from 4 to 5 minutes for a subject who reports no visual imagery to more than 30 minutes for one with extensive imagery.

This description applies to the procedures used in nearly all experiments reported since 1964. A few have not preceded the eidetic imagery testing with the afterimage induction, and a few other variations have been employed. This procedure allows highly replicable sequences of testing, can be used for longitudinal testing with the same children, and can serve as a base for controlled variations in procedure, such as the kinds of pictures used, the duration of presentation, the pattern of eye movements permitted, the kinds of probe questions asked, and the kinds of actions requested during report. Most of these variations are discussed later, as ways to test particular hypotheses about the properties of eidetic images.

With this picture elicitation method, reported eidetic imagery among Western elementary-school-aged children range from less than 2% to about 15%. No sex differences have ever been reported. One longitudinal study followed the same sample of 12 eidetic children over 7 years and found only one child who failed to remain eidetic over that time. Several studies have been done in non-Western cultures, with subjects selected who presumably have far less exposure to literacy training. These studies report frequencies in the same range or slightly higher. A few studies have used clinically impaired subjects, especially mentally retarded or brain-damaged children and young adults. The results are less consistent, though most of them find percentages in the same range as with normal subjects. Several studies have sampled adult subjects, finding frequencies near zero, except in the non-Western samples. Finally, there are a number of published reports of individual adult eidetic subjects who have been studied and described in great detail (see Haber, 1979b, for a bibliography). However, since the sampling distribution of these case studies cannot be determined, nor can the characteristics of the populations from which they are drawn, the mere popularity of such descriptions tells us little about the likelihood of there being substantial numbers of adult eidetics. Further, a careful reading of these case studies shows that many of the subjects do not meet the basic criteria of eidetic imagery and that many of them show substantial symptoms of hallucinatory or confabulatory activity.

Validating a Reported Image as Eidetic

The most distinctive characteristic of the report of subjects classified as eidetic is that they say they can "see" a stimulus that is not physically present. The image cited by these subjects has most of the properties of a percept of the stimulus itself, as if they were still looking at it. This section examines the criteria that must be applied to these kinds of reports to determine if they should be classified as eidetic images. The criteria focus on differentiating eidetic imagery from four possible alternatives: hallucinations, afterimages, nonvisual remembering, and other kinds of visual imagery.

Differentiating Hallucinations and Afterimages

A report of "I see an Indian on the easel" would be classified as a hallucination if the subject acted as though the stimulus picture were still on the easel, even though the experimenter had removed it. This is an important distinction, because except for this, the most striking characteristic of eidetic images is that the eidetic subjects treat them as similar to their percepts of stimuli currently being viewed. All of the subjects tested by Leask *et al.* (1969) could properly distinguish between seeing the picture and seeing an image of the picture. We never found any confusion between perception and imagination. As long as the subject can make this distinction, then reporting "I see an Indian" is not a hallucination. As noted earlier, some of the case studies of adult eidetic subjects contain just this kind of confusion, suggesting that some qualification should be made in classifying their reports as eidetic.

To differentiate afterimages from eidetic images, the effects of eye movements are noted. It is necessary to maintain a steady fixation on a stimulus to form an afterimage. Further, once an afterimage is formed, subsequent eye movements cause the image to shift with the movements, so that the image itself cannot be scanned. In contrast, all eidetic subjects can move their eyes while looking at the stimulus (which should prevent the formation of an adequate afterimage) and can move their eyes to different locations on the easel when reporting the content that had originally been in those locations. Further, it is unlikely that afterimages last as long as most of the images reported by these subjects.

In our experiments many subjects (subsequently classified as noneidetic) report relatively brief negatively colored afterimages. When such subjects are asked to move their eyes around the easel, without exception they report that the image moves as well. Therefore afterimages do not seem to be related to or responsible for eidetic images. These criteria also have an important bearing on the question of the demand characteristics of the task, since presumably children do not know what kinds of movements they ought to report in order to differentiate the two kinds of images.

Haber and Haber (1964) suggested assessing eye movements only to avoid confounding eidetic images with afterimages and not as a necessary feature of eidetic imagery itself. There is no reason why an eidetic child cannot maintain fixation on one part of an image while reporting another part, or shift eye position around while continuing to describe a small area. Both of these take place while stimuli are actually being viewed, so in theory they can also occur while one is looking at images of such stimuli. Hence eye movement scanning should not be used as a defining characteristic of eidetic imagery, but only to differentiate it from afterimages.

Differentiating Nonvisual Memory and Other Kinds of Visual Images

Differentiating a report based on an eidetic image from one based on some kind of nonvisual memory is more complicated. Failure to properly make this distinction probably accounts for many of the incorrect classifications and inflated estimates of eidetic imagery in the past. The concern is the following: When the young boy in the example given earlier says, "I see the Indian on the easel," could he mean that he remembers, as a result of some kind of verbal encoding, that there was an Indian in the picture that had just been shown on the easel, yet for some reason he chose to describe his nonvisual memory in visual terms—using "see" instead of "remember"?

Much of the research contained in the large monograph by Leask *et al.* (1969) was designed to examine operations converging around the meaning of the subjects'

phenomenological report. The following is a brief summary of the kinds of observations or experimental results that provide converging evidence that permit us to
take at face value children's reports of an image they are currently looking at when
they say they can see it in front of their eyes. These kinds of evidence are relevant
to distinguishing eidetic imagery both from verbally encoded nonvisual memory
and from other kinds of visual images.

1. When an eidetic child reports an image, all of the tenses used in the report
are present—"I see," not "I saw." Conversely, after the child reports that the
image has faded, but is asked to continue reporting a description of the stimulus,
a report presumably based on a verbally encoded nonvisual memory, we find only
past tenses, recounting what is remembered of the stimulus that was seen earlier.
The tense-differentiation criterion has been tested by a number of experimenters,
all with comparable results.

2. When eidetic children describe their images, they do so with fluency and
confidence, as if they were looking at something while reporting it. This fluency
lasts however long the image lasts, which may be a number of minutes in duration.
In contrast, after they report that their images have completely faded, they can still
describe the picture from some kind of nonvisual memory, but they do so with less
confidence and with more hesitations, giving the impression that they are "searching their memory." Further, when eidetic children are shown a picture that does
not lead to an eidetic image, they remember the picture after it is removed, in the
same way as do noneidetic children who never have had an eidetic image. Their
reports sound like attempts to retrieve from a nonvisual memory: After the first few
items, they are filled with hesitations and searching.

3. The duration of exposure of the stimulus picture determines the probability of an image appearing for eidetic children. This happens even for a fully familiar
picture that the eidetic child has seen many times. Further, even when eidetic
children are familiar with a picture, they report they can see an image of only those
parts of the picture they had just looked at. Conversely, they report they can
remember parts that they cannot see in their image. Each of these comparisons
shows that what eidetic children remember about the pictures and what they can
see in an image of it at the moment are independent and are due to different
cognitive operations.

4. If eidetic children look at a picture with one eye covered, an eidetic image
is generally restricted to the open eye. Closing the exposed eye and opening
the other eye (that had been closed during exposure of the picture) destroys the
image. While this may be due to erasure through blinking (see item 7 following),
it suggests that the child must be reporting what is being seen. There are no cases
(at least in normal subjects with their two cerebral hemispheres connected) in
which other forms of visual memory are limited to the eye that originally saw the
stimulus.

5. Eidetic children report that their images disappear by fading, part by part.
The nature of this fading process seems to be the same for all eidetic children, even
those in non-Western cultures. In nearly all cases the fading process is involuntary:
The child cannot control which parts remain visible and which parts fade. Descriptions of the fading of one part of an image while another part is still visible are

difficult to reconcile with reports from verbally encoded memory, in which related and especially adjacent parts tend to be grouped together.

6. Eidetic children report that their image "falls off" the edge and disappears when they attempt to move it from its original surface to another one, very much as would a projected picture fall off the projection screen if the projector was moved. Further, when viewing single letters that slide into place one by one when seen through a window, eidetic children report that they form an image of each letter next to the previous ones by moving their image of each previously seen letter along the surface until they "fall off" at the edge. The number of items that they can maintain in their image depends on the width of the easel surface, not on a fixed memory span. These observations can only be explained by assuming that the child is seeing an image rather than depending on some kind of verbally encoded nonvisual memory.

7. Eidetic children can terminate an image voluntarily by simply blinking their eyes. This in no way interferes with their ability to recall the picture from their verbally encoded nonvisual memory; they simply can no longer see it while they are recalling it.

8. Some, though not all, eidetic children are able to visually combine successively formed images to create a composite image. Several sets of materials have been used in which the composite image contained information that could not be seen or predicted from looking at either stimulus alone. This test is more difficult because it requires the child to be able to form relatively complete images, to have them last a long time, not to have the first fade when the second picture is presented, and to be able to align or overlay them correctly. Control tests showed that children or adults cannot do this task from memory, or from reasoning.

While not every item on the list was tested on every child classified as eidetic, taken together the properties included on the list lend substantial credence to the conclusion that when children classified as eidetic say they see something on an easel after the inducing stimulus has been removed, their report should be taken at face value: they are seeing it and not simply reporting it from a verbally encoded nonvisual memory. The report should be accepted in the same way that a report of seeing something is accepted when the stimulus is actually present on the easel.

The final alternative to be evaluated is that the child's report of seeing something that is no longer present on the easel might be based on some other kind of visual image, not an eidetic image. If the critical feature of an eidetic image is its similarity to actual percepts, then most common visual imagery is not eidetic. Consider, for example, asking subjects to form a visual image of their home for the purpose of counting the number of windows. Most people can do this, and after going through an internal counting process that seems to involve scanning their image, they arrive at the correct number of windows (or close to it). That image is visual, so it shares some of the properties of eidetic images: It is reported in the present tense, it depends on prior seeing of the stimulus, and it is described with fluency (sometimes). But for most of us, that image is not perceptlike: It is not limited to the eye that viewed the stimulus, it does not fade involuntarily and by parts, it does not fall off the surface on which it is projected, it is not terminated by blinking, and it does not visually superimpose to combine with other images. Hence eidetic imagery is a small subclass of visual imagery, with much more restrictive properties.

The tests just described are required whenever it is important to classify correctly a phenomenological report of seeing. Some of these tests involve manipulations or instructions that are time consuming or complicated. Others are easy to check. Failure to perform these tests can result in misclassifications.

Many children sometimes say they see something on the easel after the picture is removed but fail to meet most, if not all, of the criteria just discussed. Most such reports are of afterimages and are easily differentiated from eidetic images by the eye movement criteria. A few children do genuinely confuse seeing with remembering, but their confusions become apparent when their tenses are analyzed, when the hesitant quality of their reports becomes evident, or when they are reviewed based on the other comparisons just noted. A few other children do have the ability to form good visual images, but ones that are not perceptlike, and then they fail the last group of tests just mentioned (e.g., duration of exposure determines probability of an image; imagery is monocularly restricted; images disappear involuntarily by fading; images are restricted to projection surface; images can be blinked away; and images can be superimposed).

One of the most striking features of the data from all experimenters who have sampled subjects with eidetic imagery is that though a number of children meet one or two of the tests while failing the rest, those children who end up being classified as eidetic pass all of the tests without exception. This kind of consistent finding suggests that people possessing eidetic imagery are different from everyone else rather than simply more extreme than the rest of us. We will return to the question of discontinuity with respect to the definition of eidetic imagery.

The Characteristics of Eidetic Images

There is a wealth of data in the recent literature (see Haber, 1979a 1979b) concerning the contents and characteristics of eidetic images. Some of these characteristics have already been covered in the preceding section. But there are other properties that, while not criteria that distinguish eidetic images from other kinds of imagery or from nonvisual memory, provide important information about what eidetic images are like.

The most important characteristic is negative: Eidetic imagery is not photographic. The expectation that eidetic images photographically resemble the stimulus is an old one, and it is often cited in the earlier literature as being critical. Historically, the accuracy criterion for the presence of eidetic imagery was based upon the assumption that such images were faithful reproductions of the inducing picture and would therefore be perfectly accurate—a kind of photographic memory. This expectation that images will be photographically realistic is probably the same one that leads most of us (including specialists who should know better) to think of the perceptual apparatus as being like a camera, the retinal image like a picture, and perceiving like taking a picture. The eye–camera metaphor has been most mischievous in perceptual theories (see Braunstein, 1976, for the best treatment of the history and misuses of this metaphor) and accounts for the mistaken expectation of fidelity in imagery, too. There has been relatively little research on photographic memory *per se* (see Klatzky, 1984, for a summary). What has been done provides scarcely any support for a general concept of photographic memory as the ability to create or maintain visual images or other kinds of visual memories of complex pictorial stimuli in a faithful fashion.

Leask *et al.* (1969) report a number of experiments and demonstrations to show that accuracy cannot be used as a criterion. Some eidetic children can report highly detailed images, whereas others report quite sketchy and fragmentary ones. Several of the experiments involve comparing the accuracy of eidetic children's imagery, evoked by a picture, with the accuracy of control subjects in reporting a picture from memory. No significant differences in accuracy were found in any of these tests. Virtually every investigation of eidetic imagery since 1964, regardless of laboratory, has shown that using accuracy as a criterion is wrong. The reports of eidetic images not only are often fragmentary but also frequently contain details or arrangements not present in the stimulus. Apparently, eidetic images are constructed or organized in the same way in which any memorial representation is organized, so that some visual details are omitted, others moved around, and some added. Thus the content of imagery is also organized and not simply an internal template or photograph of the stimulus. Eidetic images, like perception in general, are constructive and not reproductive (see Haber, 1978, and Haber & Hershenson, 1980 for further details).

Whether or not an object appears in an eidetic image depends on whether that area of the stimulus picture is looked at for at least 3 to 5 seconds. Shorter glances usually fail to produce images of a particular part, even though the child can remember those details when asked about them. The only way to generate a complete eidetic image of a picture is to look at each part of it for enough time. If the picture is quite large, this requires a substantial inspection time. Parts omitted do not appear in an image, even though they are usually remembered. Consequently, an eidetic image may often contain less information than the child's subsequent verbal description based on nonvisual memory for the picture that evoked the image.

On the other hand, as noted before, eidetic children's reports of their images are made fluently and with confidence, as if they are actually looking at what they are describing. However, when they describe the stimulus from their nonvisual memory after their eidetic image has faded, or when noneidetic children describe their memory of a previous stimulus after the first few items are reported, the verbalizations become hesitant, as if they are searching an imperfectly stored and organized memory.

When eidetic children report one eidetic image from a picture, they are likely to report such images for all of the stimuli shown to them.

Most eidetic images last more than a half minute, with the average well over several minutes. (Some investigators have used the duration as a criterion, rejecting any report lasting less than a half minute.)

Several techniques are used by eidetic children to prevent images from forming. The main prevention technique described by nearly all eidetic children is active, cognitive, verbal rehearsal of the stimulus. If, while looking at the stimulus picture on the easel, the child names each of the items in it, no visual image develops. Thus it appears as if eidetic children have two modes of processing visual stimuli: an active visual exploration mode, which leads to a visual image; and a verbal rehearsal mode, which blocks the image, though it may facilitate verbal memory.

The opposition of these two modes probably also accounts for the difficulty eidetic children have in achieving images of print or highly informative or detailed stimuli that they expect to be questioned about. Presented with print, they tend to read it; this, by the very nature of the naming process, prevents an image from forming. The only recent evidence of good memories for print were reported by Leask *et al.* (1969) when the print was nonsense words or when the child was asked to scan or read it backwards. The older reports of exceptional "eidetic images" of print would seem to be due to confoundings created by the elicitation procedures.

Nearly all eidetic children say they can terminate an image by blinking their eyes, looking away, or shifting their gaze to a new stimulus. This apparently helps them control unwanted images and prevents images from overlapping when they scan the world with their eyes or turn pages.

Nearly all eidetic children report the same pattern of fading for their images; this fading is due to a combination of purely visual factors (such as loss of clarity, contrast, color, and distinctiveness) and organizational or meaningful factors that cause whole items to fade out together. Because the descriptions of the images are verbal, the latter factors are probably exaggerated, since it is much easier to say, for example, that the tree is fading than that the left side of the bark is now harder to see.

Only one eidetic child (described in Leask *et al.* 1969) reported that she could make her images last as long as she wanted. If she was not trying, however, the content of her imagery also followed the typical pattern of fading just discussed. Thus, at least when using the picture elicitation method, the fading of the parts of the image is characteristic of eidetic images.

Eidetic children say that they see their images projected onto the surfaces that contain the stimulus. A few, however, report that they can sometimes see an image inside their head. The latter is a much more typical report from some of the eidetic subjects in the African societies studied by Doob (e.g., 1964). It is possible that using the picture elicitation procedure with an easel increases the number of "projected" images compared to what we might have found with a more neutral instruction procedure. However, Doob and others who did find more "inside head" locations also used the picture elicitation procedure with an easel. Therefore it is not known how flexible eidetic subjects can be about where they see their images or whether the location affects the nature of the imagery. In any event, the location of the image—projected in space or inside the head—should not be considered a criterion for eidetic imagery. Presumably, eidetic images can be seen out in space, against a projection surface, inside the head, or even behind the eyelids.

Most eidetic children can move their images around on the surface but not beyond the obvious boundaries of that surface. We do not know much about how they do this, except that it is not necessarily by making an eye movement. We have seen eidetic children scan (move their eyes over) their images while reporting that the images themselves do not move. Presumably, they can also move their images around on the projection surface by some kind of mental effort that is not triggered directly by comparable movements of the eye.

Only a few eidetic children seem to be able to shift their images to another coplanar surface, and fewer still can move them to any surface at will. Why this is more difficult is not known.

If a picture produces an image that is still visible when a second picture is presented, some eidetic children report a composite image of the two pictures. They can describe which parts of the image came from which picture, but they are still seeing a single image of two stimuli. This does not happen to all children, because for some, presenting the new picture terminates the image of the first (presumably because they blink their eyes or glance away).

A few examples of three-dimensional images have been reported, and some children can develop such images with appropriate stimuli easily. A two-dimensional drawing of a Necker cube produces reversals of three-dimensional orientations in images, further supporting the three-dimensionality of eidetic images, at least for some children.

Most eidetic children have no difficulty in getting an eidetic image in one eye alone when they have looked at the stimulus picture with only one eye. However, transferring a monocular image to the other eye is difficult because of the inevitable opening and closing of eyes, which routinely terminates images. Leask et al., 1969 reported that every child who could get a monocular image in one eye could do so for the other eye as well, which is contrary to what Freides and Hayden (1966) reported—that at least some of their eidetic children were unilaterally monocular (though not always the same eye from child to child).

The interviews with parents of eidetic children (reported in Leask et al., 1969) suggested that a few parents were aware of their children focusing on games that could be facilitated by good imagery. The one game specifically mentioned was Concentration, a card game requiring a good spatial memory for the location of briefly glimpsed cards that are otherwise kept hidden from view. Unfortunately, we never tested eidetic children directly on this game. A few children, when specifically questioned, mentioned that their imagery helped them in their schoolwork. However, most denied that this was true, usually claiming that it interfered unless blocked. We had no indication that the eidetic children were more interested or talented in art, drawing, or photography—three activities that might benefit from access to visual memory. On the other hand, our data suggest that eidetic imagery is not helpful at all with reading tasks or with any kind of rote memorization task.

Although most experimenters have demanded that a subject meet all of the kinds of criteria described above before being classified as eidetic, Paivio and Cohen (1977) provided several analyses of the interrelationships among the various criteria themselves. One was a factor analysis of the correlation matrix among the various criterion scores they collected on a sample of 242 second- and third-grade children in London, Ontario. The procedures were modeled closely after those of Haber and Haber (1964). They classified 21 children (8.6% of the sample) as eidetic based upon these criteria and found that two factors accounted for most of the variance among the criterion score correlations. The strongest factor, accounting for 81% of the variance, loaded highly on all of the nonmemory items, such as reported imagery, duration of more than 40 seconds, projection of the image in front of the eyes, being able to scan both the stimulus and the image, and the use of the present tense. These criteria relate to or describe the phenomenological characteristics of the imagery. The second factor was clearly a verbal memory factor, with loadings on the criteria concerned with accuracy of recall of detail and color.

Paivio and Cohen (1977) also provide some data relevant to the discontinuity question. In addition to testing for the presence of eidetic imagery in their sample of 242 children, they administered four tests of spatial abilities, one self-report test of vividness of visual imagery, and two tests of verbal ability. When all the intercorrelations were factor analyzed, these investigators still found the same phenomenological eidetic factor described earlier. This factor had no loadings in common with factors reflecting spatial relations, vividness of imagery, and verbal ability. Therefore, the possession of eidetic imagery is different from either spatial or verbal abilities, and even from self-report measures of the vividness of imagery in everyday life.

Eidetic Imagery and Age

Earlier, we described the consistent finding that eidetic imagery tends to be confined primarily to children and is rarely found in adults. This result permeates the earlier research literature and has been reported several times in the more recent research as well. More often, it is simply taken for granted and not tested further. New experiments are now designed to discover the reason for the apparent negative relationship between frequency of incidence and age. Perhaps the oldest and most important hypothesis concerning the origins and functional significance of eidetic imagery grows out of this supposed relationship: Eidetic imagery is relatively typical or common in very young children and disappears as more advanced cognitive and perceptual processes develop, especially those associated with abstract thought and reading. Nearly every recent investigator has pursued aspects of this developmental hypothesis in one form or another, and a number of tests of its implications have been made.

These experiments are important because they have provided positive and negative information about some of the characteristics of subjects who possess eidetic imagery. However, most of them rest on an initial faulty premise—the assumption of a negative correlation between eidetic imagery and age is probably incorrect. This undoubtedly accounts for the uniform failure to find support for the developmental hypothesis.

Consider, first, whether there is a negative correlation between eidetic imagery and age. It is true that most eidetic subjects found are children, and attempts to find adults by sampling adult populations rarely turn up any eidetic subjects. However, in the only long-term longitudinal study on eidetic imagery, Leask et al. (1969) followed the 12 eidetic children identified by Haber and Haber (1964) for a

7-year period. The age range of the children initially was from 7 to 12 years. We found that 11 of the original 12 eidetic children were still just as eidetic 7 years later. Hence there is no evidence that eidetic children lose their eidetic abilities as they grow older and develop more abstract cognitive skills.

Further, if there is a negative correlation, the greatest number of eidetic subjects should be found in the very youngest age groups. Within the elementary school ages, there is no correlation with age—just as many eidetic subjects are found at age 12 as at age 7. It is of course possible that children younger than 6 or 7 would be more likely to be eidetic and that most would have lost the ability by the first or second grade. Giray, Altkin, Vaught, and Roodin (1976) have reported data on children of 5 and 6. They found higher percentages at these ages than at ages 7–18, though not nearly high enough to lend support to a negative age effect. In contrast, Haber and Haber (1964) were unable to find any eidetics among 5- and 6-year-olds, perhaps because the testing procedures were not well adapted to such young children. If so, then a few may possibly have been eidetic. However, even with these caveats, the prevalence of eidetic children is not overwhelming at younger ages.

In contrast, one study has used the picture elicitation procedure with a geriatric population and found nearly 25% of 90-year-olds meeting the criteria for eidetic imagery (Giray, Altkin, Roodin, Yoon, & Flagg, 1978).

Although the research undertaken with subjects from non-Western cultures was designed to explore the developmental hypothesis (as will be soon described), the results also cast doubt upon the assumption of a negative correlation of eidetic imagery with age. Most of those studies (see Haber, 1979b, for a review) tested adults, and all found some eidetic subjects among them, with higher percentages than have been found in comparable sampling studies carried out in America.

Finally, the highly variable data reported on individual clinical case studies of eidetic imagery come primarily from adults. While such data are undoubtedly contaminated with hallucinatory reports, it is unlikely that this accounts for all of them.

The preceding pattern of findings does not permit any simple conclusions about the relation between eidetic imagery and age. On the one hand, trying to find eidetic subjects by sampling populations is likely to be successful among children but not among adults. On the other hand, child eidetic subjects do not seem to become less eidetic as they grow up, and adult eidetics do exist.

The Developmental Hypothesis

The developmental hypothesis, based on an assumed preponderance of younger eidetic subjects, still might provide a reasonable explanation for why someone is eidetic, regardless of chronological age. This hypothesis has been tested in three different ways: (1) Are eidetics poorer than noneidetics in their abstract skills? (2) Are eidetics more prevalent in less literate societies? (3) Are eidetics more prevalent among the mentally retarded or brain damaged?

The first test of this form of the developmental hypothesis is the prediction that children with eidetic imagery are delayed or retarded on abstract tasks, on the assumption that such tasks interfere with, replace, or overlay eidetic imagery. No experiment since 1964 (and virtually none prior to the 1930s) has reported any significant correlation between the presence or absence of eidetic imagery (or even the degree of eidetic imagery) and intellectual ability, skill at abstract reasoning, school achievement, or reading ability. Eidetic subjects are neither better nor worse on any of these skills or abilities than noneidetic controls at any age (see Haber, 1979a, for a review of these findings). The lack of any such differences between eidetic and noneidetic subjects casts strong doubt on the developmental hypothesis.

Another corollary of the developmental hypothesis was initially explored by Doob (1964) in several African societies and then followed up by a number of others (see Haber, 1979b, for a review). Doob argued that if eidetic imagery was cognitively more concrete, then subjects who never developed complex abstract skills such as reading or who were less exposed to Western-style educational systems should show a higher prevalence of eidetic imagery. Following this reasoning, he contrasted groups of adults that differed in exposure to education or Western culture. In Doob's work, and in the many subsequent studies using African, Brazilian, or Australian subjects contrasted for literacy or formal education, though the incidence of eidetic imagery is more variable, ranging from 0% to 20%, there is no consistent pattern of differences between samples contrasting more with less literate backgrounds.

The cross-cultural research has used the more controlled picture elicitation procedure, but even so, the experimenters have encountered greater difficulties in experimental control than has typically been the case in the Western laboratories, where most of the testing has been done in school, university, or clinic settings. Each of the cross-cultural studies describes the problems in maintaining consistent testing procedures, particularly in assuring that the instructions about what to report mean the same to the subjects as they do to the testers. These difficulties probably account for the greater variability in incidence. Despite these problems, the results do not help the developmental hypothesis.

A third version of the developmental hypothesis was explored by Siipola and Hayden (1965; see also Giray, Altkin, & Barclay, 1976; Giray et al., 1978; Giray, Altkin, Vaught, & Roodin, 1976). They argued that subjects with either mental deficiencies or neurological deficits that interfere with abstract thought processes should be able to maintain access to their eidetic abilities because high levels of cognitive abilities did not develop to replace or interfere with the eidetic skills.

Siipola and Hayden tested 16 brain-injured retardates and found 8 of them eidetic, using the Haber and Haber (1964) procedures and criteria. This high percentage has never been found again. Subsequent studies by Richardson and Cant (1970), Symmes (1971), Gummerman, Gray, and Wilson (1972), and Giray, Altkin, and Barclay (1976) found, respectively, 2%, 19% 0%, and 10% eidetic subjects among brain-injured retardates. Among retardates without obvious evidence of brain injury, Siipola and Hayden (1965), Symmes (1971), Gummerman et al. (1972), and Giray, Altkin, and Barclay (1976), found, respectively, 6%, 13%, 11%, and 4% to be eidetic. The two exceptions to these low numbers are the original finding by Siipola and Hayden (1965) of 50% among 16 brain-injured subjects and a more recent finding by Giray and Barclay (1977) of 78% eidetic persons among 14 hydrocephalic subjects. It is difficult to know how to interpret a few positive findings among a larger number of negative ones, especially since the procedures seem adequate. But with this variable pattern of results, the evidence does little to sustain the neurological deficit version of the developmental hypothesis.

Finally, even given the general low incidence of eidetic imagery, it is still relatively easy to find a few eidetic children in any classroom of a North American elementary school. None of the children so far found by such sampling procedures has had any obvious signs of neurological pathology. Even handedness appears to be appropriately distributed (Leask *et al.*, 1969). Therefore, any link between neurological deficits and eidetic abilities is yet to be demonstrated.

Consequently, regardless of the relation between eidetic imagery and age, the developmental hypothesis, linking eidetic imagery to immature abstract abilities, has not survived any of the tests made of it. There is no hint that eidetic children are less cognitively developed than noneidetic subjects.

An Alternative Hypothesis

Leask *et al.* (1969) offered an alternative hypothesis to account for why some children possessed eidetic imagery but fewer adults did, even without assuming any necessary link between age and incidence of eidetic imagery. Rather, they noted their repeated finding that verbalization during the inspection of a stimulus picture interferes with eidetic imagery. There is already evidence that visualizing and verbalizing are two naturally interfering ways of representing stimulation or memory at all ages and that the degree of interference does not change much with age or cognitive style. The interference of the two modes has been amply demonstrated in adults by Allport, Antonitis, and Reynolds (1972) and by Brooks (1967) for several kinds of simultaneously performed tasks, and it appears as a basic opposition in the literature on lateralization of cerebral hemispheric function (see, especially, Kinsbourne, 1978).

If simultaneous visual and verbal encoding of the same stimulus is very difficult, it might be that only a few children try to focus on visualizing alone or are able to do so. If most children use verbal encoding strategies, eidetic imagery would be blocked. Further, if younger children are better at, or more likely to use, visual strategies, whereas older children and adults rely more upon verbal encoding, then this would account for the greater ease of finding child rather than adult eidetics, without in any way assuming that eidetic children are less cognitively or intellectually developed. This hypothesis has not been specifically tested, so its validity remains to be demonstrated.

Definition of Eidetic Imagery

In earlier sections of this chapter we have provided operational definitions of eidetic imagery. These specific operations are applied to a subject's response, so that the response can be labeled "eidetic" or classified as something else. In this final section these operations are used to provide a theoretical definition of visual imagery by contrasting visual imagery with visual percepts on the one hand and with various forms of nonvisual memory on the other, and then to identify eidetic imagery as a more restrictive case of visual imagery.

Two related questions are considered: (1) What is the difference between a visual image and other ways of perceiving and remembering? (2) What is the difference between an eidetic image and any other kind of visual image?

1. The first question concerns how a visual image differs from visual perception, from visual hallucinations, and from nonvisual memory. The image–percept difference concerns the interpretation of a statement such as "I see a tree right now." A visual percept occurs when I am looking at a tree in front of me that is actually providing stimulation to my visual receptors. The same statement, "I see a tree right now," refers to a visual image or a visual hallucination when there is no tree currently present in my visual field. The critical test between percept versus image or hallucination depends on the presence or absence of the relevant visual stimulation. If the stimulus is present, then this is perception; if not, then it is imagery or hallucination. The critical test between image and hallucination depends on whether the person thinks, in the absence of the stimulus, that it is actually present—if yes, then the statement refers to hallucination; if not, then it refers to a visual image.

The visual image–nonvisual memory difference depends on what I say and on the way I say it. If I say, "I can see the tree now" (in the absence of the tree), and if I act as if I can see it now, then I am referring to a visual image. If I say that I remember seeing the tree before (when it was actually present) but cannot visualize the tree now, then even if I can still describe that tree in some other way, I am referring to some other kind of memory, one different from visual imagery. I may remember how the tree looked, and I may be able to describe what I saw before. The critical test concerns whether I say and act as if I am seeing the tree now. If so, then I am referring to a visual image, and otherwise, to some kind of nonvisual memory. Notice that both of these circumstances refer to a memory—the question is only whether it is a visual memory that can be seen or some other kind of memory that is not visual but that might be verbal, abstract, propositional, or any form not anchored in the visual modality, or some combination of these.

2. How does eidetic imagery differ from other kinds of visual imagery? Are there visual images that would not be called "eidetic," or are the words "eidetic image" and "visual image" synonymous? The research on eidetic imagery, regardless of laboratory, has shown a critical difference, with eidetic imagery being a particular kind of visual imagery, one quite rare. Visual imagery in general, while having the quality of being seen, usually does not have the quality of being akin to looking at the stimulus itself. When it has that latter quality, then it is eidetic. The perceptlike character of the image distinguishes eidetic imagery from other kinds of visual imagery.

Visual imagery in general is described in the present tense because it is being seen right now. Thus the subject says, "I can visualize the tree in my mind's eye. I can see long needles and branches reaching to the ground." Further, it can be described fluently and confidently because it is visually available while the description is being given. Neither of these operations distinguishes the subclass of eidetic imagery from the more general class of visual imagery. Further, their distinction does not hinge on vividness. To say that I "see" my image involves no claim that my image is vivid, only that it is visible. Some visual images may be very vivid and others pale. We need to study this dimension of vividness in eidetic imagery as we do in other forms of imagery, but vividness is not by itself a part of the definition of imagery, eidetic or otherwise.

However, eidetic images do differ from visual imagery in general in that they do not seem to be under complete voluntary control but are determined or influenced by the actual viewing conditions. Six of the eight tests described earlier to differentiate eidetic imagery from nonvisual memory are sufficiently powerful to differentiate it from other kinds of visual imagery. These tests include the following: (1) Whether an image of a particular part of a stimulus appears or not depends on whether that part has just been visually examined; (2) whether that image of a part appears depends on whether that part has been visually examined by the eye that is currently open; (3) whether a part remains visible in the image depends on whether it has yet faded, something that cannot be prevented by the subject; (4) whether a part remains visible depends on whether there is a projection surface against which to see it; (5) whether an image remains visible requires the subject to inhibit eye blinks; and (6) whether an image remains coherent depends on whether subsequent images are present that superimpose and combine together.

These observations suggest that eidetic images resemble percepts much more closely than they resemble more general visual images—they represent an extreme case of being able to visualize in the absence of the stimulus. These six characteristics are rarely present when a person is asked to form and describe a visual image of some previous stimulation. When these characteristics are present, then the image can be called "eidetic"; otherwise, the report that "I see the tree right now" can only be labeled as the much more general class of visual imagery. Only a small handful of people, mostly children, seem able to have eidetic images with these much more restrictive properties.

This definition of eidetic imagery, as more perceptlike than visual imagery in general, is close to the prevailing kinds of definitions offered in the early years of research on this topic. It set eidetic imagery apart as a more extreme form of imagery. In contrast, some of the more recent attempts to understand eidetic imagery have treated it as being more akin to visual imagery in general, as if the two terms were synonymous. Gray and Gummerman (1975) and Roberts-Gray (1979) have argued that eidetic images are merely the more vivid end of a continuum of visual imagery, a position that fails in the light of most of the tests described here. Ahsen (1977, 1979) has taken an even more extreme position, suggesting that the term "imagery" be used for virtually any vivid recall from memory; he makes no demand in his definition that imagery be anchored in particular sensory modalities or that the subject make verifiable statements such as "I am currently seeing my image." While theoreticians are free to define terms to meet their needs, we have tried to be particularly careful to anchor our definitions not only in useful operations but in relation to other constructs and theories that will allow further theoretical advance.

Given this distinction between general visual imagery and more specific eidetic imagery, what can we learn from the impressive evidence that subjects exist who are presumably without eidetic imagery yet are superior in their ability to visualize? Unfortunately, in most of the earlier research and in the newer and growing literature on the functional role of visual imagery in memory (e.g., Shepard, 1978) and in general cognitive processes (e.g., Brooks, 1967; Kosslyn, 1980; Paivio, 1971; Perky, 1910; Sheehan, 1966), the subjects are never asked to describe the modality, the vividness, or the content of their images directly. Rather, that the subject used visual imagery is inferred from the nature of the stimulus material, from the instructions to the subject, or from a postsession questionnaire. For example, Paivio (1971) inferred that his subjects were using visual imagery because (1) he found differences in the memorability of words whose meanings had been previously rated as easy or difficult to visualize; (2) this difference between types of words increased when subjects were instructed to form visual images of the words while trying to remember them; and (3) this difference was larger in those subjects who rated themselves as good at forming visual images in general. Nearly all of the other research on imagery has been based on similarly indirect manipulations.

Therefore, in spite of the success of these kinds of experiments, they tell us little about the nature of visual imagery itself or of possible differences among different kinds of visual imagery. From these results it cannot be established how visual the subject's images are, how long the images last, how complete the details of the images are, and, particularly, whether the subjects "see" the objects being imaged in the same sense that eidetic subjects say they do. Most important in this context, we cannot tell if those subjects were using eidetic imagery or some other kind of visual imagery, or even if there is any other kind of visual imagery. We cannot tell whether in noneidetic subjects visual imagery combines with other kinds of imagery in these tasks. We badly need data on the similarities of these different kinds of visualizing tasks, just as we need to know whether the picture-induction and the instruction-to-visualize procedures produce comparable results.

Eidetic imagery is almost invariably defined in the experimental literature as a form of visual imagery, as distinct from auditory, olfactory, or other modality-specific forms. Thus, we describe eidetic responses as reported visual images of visual stimuli that are not currently in the visual field of view. Does this mean that there are no auditory eidetic images? We see no reason why this should be the case. Although we have implicitly restricted eidetic imagery to the visual modality in our own research, there is no theoretical reason to do so; it should be possible to demonstrate such imagery in other modalities. All that is required is careful attention to definitions and operations. If such imagery is found in other modalities, it is then an empirical matter to determine the relationships among the different kinds of imagery within the same subjects.

Is eidetic imagery, as defined here, the extreme on some continuum, or a discrete ability possessed by only a few? In both Haber and Haber (1964) and Leask et al. (1969) we provided evidence of a discontinuity between the few children classified as eidetic and most of the rest of the children sampled. When the criteria are used separately to classify children, some of them individually produce discontinuous distributions in which there is no overlap between the classifications.

This is true for the eye-scanning measures and the tense switching especially, and to only a slightly lesser degree for the percentage and duration of images. When the several criteria are combined together, however, the discontinuity becomes overwhelming. The occasional child who has a very long afterimage, for example (and who would be classified as eidetic on the duration criterion alone), fails to meet any of the other criteria, so is classified as noneidetic with great confidence. The discontinuity is restricted to eidetic abilities, however, at least based on current data. Neither Paivio and Cohen (1977) nor Leask *et al.* (1969) found any correlation between possession of eidetic imagery and differences in visual, verbal, or abstract cognitive abilities.

The discontinuity in classification strongly suggests that eidetic imagery is a kind of visual representation qualitatively different from any other kind and distinct from normal perception as well. Apparently, a few children have this ability, and only a rare adult does, at least in America. It is this quality of having percept-like visual images that most of us lack and probably never had in the first place. Other qualities of imagery probably are much more widespread and differ from person to person in subtle degrees, not evidencing sharp discontinuities.

References

Ahsen, A. (1977). Eidetics: An overview, *Journal of Mental Imagery, 1*, 5–38.

Ahsen, A. (1979). Eidetics: Redefinition of the ghost and its clinical application. *The Behavioral and Brain Sciences, 2*, 594–596.

Allport, D. A., Antonitis, B., & Reynolds, P. (1972). On the division of attention: A disproof of the single channel hypothesis. *Quarterly Journal of Experimental Psychology, 24*, 225–235.

Braunstein, M. (1976). *Depth perception through motion.* New York: Academic Press.

Brooks, L. R. (1967). The suppression of visualization by reading. *Quarterly Journal of Experimental Psychology, 19*, 289–299.

Doob, L. W. (1964). Eidetic images among the Ibo. *Ethnology, 3*, 357–363.

Freides, D., & Hayden, S. P. (1966). Monocular testing: A methodological note on eidetic imagery. *Perceptual and Motor Skills, 23*, 88.

Giray, E. F., Altkin, W. M., & Barclay, A. G. (1976). Frequency of eidetic imagery among hydrocephalic children. *Perceptual and Motor Skills, 43*, 187–194.

Giray, E. F., Alkin, W. M., Roodin, P. A., Yoon, G., & Flagg, P. (1978). *The incidence of eidetic imagery in adulthood and old age.* Paper presented at the meeting of the American Psychological Association, Toronto.

Giray, E. F., Altkin, W. M., Vaught, G. M., & Roodin, P. A. (1976). The incidence of eidetic imagery as a function of age. *Child Development, 47*, 207–210.

Giray, E. F., & Barclay, A. G. (1977). Eidetic imagery: Longitudinal results in brain-damaged children. *American Journal of Mental Deficiency, 82*, 311–314.

Gray, C. R., & Gummerman, K. (1975). The enigmatic eidetic image: A critical examination of methods and theories. *Psychological Review, 82*, 383–407.

Gummerman, K., Gray, C. R., & Wilson, J. M. (1972). An attempt to assess eidetic imagery objectively. *Psychonomic Science, 28*, 115–118.

Haber, R. N. (1978). Visual perception. *Annual Review of Psychology, 29*, 25–59.

Haber, R. N. (1979a). Twenty years of haunting eidetic imagery: Where's the ghost? *The Behavioral and Brain Sciences, 2*, 583–594.

Haber, R. N. (1979b). Eidetic imagery still lives, thanks to twenty-nine exorcists. *The Behavioral and Brain Sciences, 2,* 619–629.

Haber, R. N., & Haber, R. B. (1964). Eidetic imagery: 1. Frequency. *Perceptual and Motor Skills, 19,* 131–138.

Haber, R. N., & Hershenson, M. (1980). *The psychology of visual perception* (2nd ed.). New York: Holt, Rinehart & Winston.

Kinsbourne, M. (1978). *Asymmetrical function of the brain.* Cambridge, England: Cambridge University Press.

Klatzky, R. (1984). *Memory* (2nd ed.). San Francisco: Freeman.

Kosslyn, S. M. (1980). *Mental imagery.* Cambridge, MA: Harvard University Press.

Leask, J., Haber, R. N., & Haber, R. B. (1969). Eidetic imagery in children: 2. Longitudinal and experimental results. *Psychonomic Monograph Supplements, 3,* 25–48.

Paivio, A. (1971). *Visual imagery and memory.* New York: Holt, Rinehart & Winston.

Paivio, A., & Cohen, M. W. (1977). *Eidetic imagery and figural abilities in children.* Paper presented at the Symposium on Current Directions in Imagery, Eidetic and Otherwise, conducted at the annual meeting of the American Psychological Association, San Francisco.

Perky, C. W. (1910). An experimental study of imagination. *American Journal of Psychology, 21,* 422–452.

Richardson, A., & Cant, R. (1970). Eidetic imagery and brain damage. *Australian Journal of Psychology, 22,* 47–54.

Roberts-Gray, C. (1979). The visualization continuum. *The Behavioral and Brain Sciences, 2,* 614.

Sheehan, P. W. (1966). Accuracy and vividness of visual images. *Perceptual and Motor Skills, 23,* 391–418.

Shepard, R. N. (1978). The mental image. *American Psychologist, 33,* 125–137.

Siipola, E. M., & Hayden, S. D. (1965). Exploring eidetic imagery among the retarded. *Perceptual and Motor Skills, 21,* 275–286.

Symmes, J. S. (1971). Visual imagery in brain-injured children. *Perceptual and Motor Skills, 33,* 507–514.

11

Where Is Eidetic Imagery? Speculations on Its Psychophysical and Neurophysiological Locus

JEREMY M. WOLFE

Thirty years of neurophysiological and psychophysiological research have yielded a fairly consistent picture of the sequence of processing steps in the human visual system. From the neuroanatomical evidence, we get a picture of visual information flowing from the retina to the lateral geniculate nucleus of the thalamus and from there to the primary visual cortex. Beyond the primary visual cortex, the path splits into several streams feeding a small multitude of "extrastriate" visual areas. An excellent introduction to the visual pathways can be found in Van Essen and Maunsell (1983).

Certain visual functions can be mapped onto the known anatomy. We know, for example, that the orientation of a line is not determined by the visual system until information reaches the visual cortex. Neurophysiology tells us that neurons in the retina and thalamus are insensitive to changes in orientation. We also know that, prior to the visual cortex, neurons are monocular. They respond only to the stimulation of one eye. Psychophysics tells us that visual effects that require orientation information can make use of information from either eye, suggesting again that orientation information is not available to the precortical visual system.

Where in the system does eidetic imagery happen? Given our knowledge about the sequence of visual processing, and the wealth of observations about eidetic imagery that can be found in the Habers' chapter (Chapter 10) in this volume, we can make some educated guesses. All of the assertions in this chapter about eidetic images come from material that can be found in Chapter 10.

Eidetic Images Are Not Retinal

The locus of the image is almost certainly not in the retina. "Photographic" images can occur at the retinal level. If one looks at a blank screen after looking at a visual

Jeremy M. Wolfe. Department of Psychology, Massachusetts Institute of Technology, Cambridge, Massachusetts.

stimulus, one can see a "negative afterimage." It is faithful representation of the stimulus, but all the colors are replaced by their complements. What was red appears green. What was bright appears dark. Eidetic images, by contrast, are positive, not negative. Positive afterimages exist, too, though they are generally seen only following very bright stimuli and then only in the dark.

All afterimages have certain properties. Most notably, they move when the eye moves. Eidetic images do not. Eidetikers can look around the eidetic image. If you try to look at the left-hand corner of an afterimage, you will find that the act of moving your eyes to the left causes the whole image to jump to the left and that the left-hand corner remains to the left of your center of gaze. Afterimages require fixation on a single point during their production. Eidetic images seem to require a series of fixations at different points around the stimulus. With a movement of the eyes, an afterimage can be moved so that it appears projected on another surface. Eidetic images resist such movement. Eidetic images can be wiped out by blinking. Visibility of afterimages is, if anything, enhanced by blinking.

Most of the objections to an aftereffect explanation would apply to any retinal explanation of eidetic images. Retinal effects are retinotopically localized. They are confined to the portion of the retina that was stimulated. Thus they move with the eyes, and so forth. Eidetic images, to the contrary, seem to be spatiotopically localized, albeit imperfectly. Spatiotopically localized objects exist in a perceived spot that is defined relative to other objects in the world and not relative to the position of the eyes. The spatiotopic localization of an eidetic image seems to be imperfect in that the Habers report that subjects can "slide" the image from one flat surface to another. A retinotopically localized image could be moved to any arbitrary location. A spatiotopically localized image could not be moved at all. The book you are holding and the print you are reading are spatiotopically localized. You cannot slide the print off the page. Apparently, if the print were an eidetic image, this would be possible.

From Retina To Visual Cortex

The nonretinotopic nature of eidetic images eliminates several loci beyond the retina. Processing of visual information into the first levels of the visual cortex is retinotopic. One line of evidence supporting this contention comes from the psychophysical study of aftereffects. Look at Figure 11-1b. The two regions contain bars of the same width and orientation. If you look at Figure 11-1a, you can see two regions with bars of different width. If you stare in between the two parts of 1a for 60 seconds and then switch your gaze back to a point in between the two parts of 1b, you will see that the two equivalent sets of bars now appear to be of different widths (Blackmore & Sutton, 1969). If, instead, you look in between the two fields in Figure 11-1c, you will note that the two fields are of different orientations. When you look back to a point in between the halves of 1b, you will see a "tilt aftereffect" (Campbell and Maffei, 1971; Gibson, 1937) in which the top and bottom appear to have different orientations.

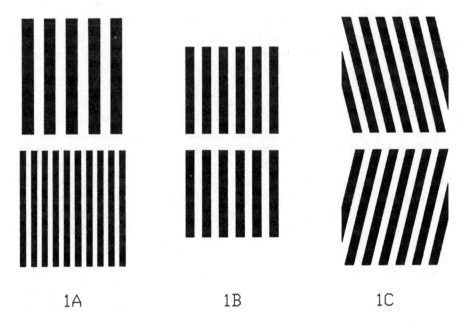

1A   1B   1C

FIGURE 11-1. Demonstration of two visual aftereffects. The top and the bottom halves of 1b are physically identical. Fixating between the two halves of 1a will change the apparent size of the bars in 1b while fixating between the two halves of 1c will change the apparent orientation of 1b.

In addition to these aftereffects of size and orientation, there are aftereffects of motion, depth, and color. Aftereffects are similar to, but distinct from, simple negative afterimages. For example, a body of work (reviewed briefly in Wolfe & Blake, 1985) indicates that the locus of these effects is the visual cortex, whereas negative afterimages are largely confined to the retina. One piece of this evidence is interocular transfer. If you look at Figure 11-1a or 1c with your left eye, you can still see an aftereffect when you look at 1b with your right eye (Blake, Overton, & Lema-Stern, 1981, Campbell & Maffei, 1971). (The transferred effect is weaker. You may need to look at the adapting stimuli for some time.) Clearly, an effect that can transfer from one eye to the other is not in the retina.

Though the effects are not retinal, they are retinotopic. Consider Figure 11-1c. If the spatiotopic layout were important, it should be possible to move your eyes all around the page and still produce the aftereffect. Eye movements would not alter spatiotopic relationships. However, with the tilt aftereffect, if you do look all around the page, there will be no effect.

Physiology concurs with psychophysics. The cells in the retina project in an orderly fashion to the cortex (via the thalamus), producing retinotopic maps in the primary visual cortex and in a number of subsequent, extrastriate visual areas. We would suspect, therefore, that eidetic images are not generated at or prior to the first processing stages in the visual cortex.

Two observations complicate this account. First, the Habers report that images are seen only with the eye that looked at the original stimulus. As noted in the discussion of interocular transfer, by the time we reach visual cortex, stimulation of one eye can affect what is seen in the other eye. In the normal case we would expect a phenomenon that occurs after the first levels in cortex to be binocular. However, there are some effects that are known to be cortical but that are, nevertheless, monocular. Aftereffects of color (e.g., the McCollough effect—McCollough, 1965; White, Petry, Riggs, & Miller, 1978) do not show normal interocular transfer. Further, neurons in the primary visual cortex that seem to be involved in the processing of color seem to be largely monocular (Livingston & Hubel, 1984). It is not impossible, therefore, for a visual phenomenon to be both cortical and monocular. The materials used in eidetic imagery experiments tend to be colorful, providing one possible explanation of the monocularity. Another possible source of monocularity is "utrocular" discrimination, the ability to name the stimulated eye when only one eye is stimulated (Blake & Cormack, 1979; Enoch, Goldman, & Sunga, 1969; Smith, 1945; though see Barbeito & Ono, 1984). Utrocular discrimination is quirky and is based on a strange, visceral "feeling" in the eye. Nevertheless, it is evidence for the preservation of some monocular information into and beyond the primary visual cortex.

The second complication is the report that the two slightly different images, each formed in one eye, can be fused to produce an impression of stereoscopic depth (Julesz, 1971; Stromeyer, 1970). Stereopsis is thought to occur in a specific location at or before the neural locus of aftereffects (Wolfe, 1986; Wolfe & Held, 1982). If eidetic images are formed after this level in visual processing, those images should not be available as input to a stereopsis mechanism. The eidetic stereopsis report is unusual for two reasons. First, the subject was an adult, while most other evidence about eidetic imagery is obtained from children. Second, the report is unique. No replication has been published. On the other hand, the Habers cite evidence that eidetic images can be superimposed, though these studies did not involve stereograms. For the purpose of a search for the locus of eidetic imagery, stereopsis is the important aspect of the Stromeyer observation. The issues raised by Stromeyer's experiment can be settled only by further research. Until such research is done, it would seem unwise to place too much weight on this finding.

Experimental Tests

Our rejection of several loci for eidetic imagery is based on *post hoc* comparisons between reports on such imagery and the psychophysical and physiological data on the order of visual processing. These hypotheses could be tested directly. For example, if, contrary to our expectations, eidetic images are formed at or prior to the neural locus of aftereffects, then it should be possible to use such images as stimuli to produce aftereffects. Suppose a child was asked to form an image of Figure 11-1c. According to reports, such an image would take just a few seconds to develop and could last for several minutes. The magnitude and the duration of aftereffects are functions of the length of time that the inducing stimulus is viewed (e.g., Blake et al., 1981; Wolfe & O'Connell, 1986). An aftereffect would be produced by viewing the physical stimulus for the few seconds needed to establish the eidetic image. However, after a few minutes of viewing the image, that aftereffect would be gone. Any aftereffect that was measured after viewing the image would have to be attributed to adaptation to the eidetic image. Results of this sort would be evidence against the model that we are proposing here. A possible variant might be to attempt to produce an eidetic motion aftereffect. This would not only help us to test hypotheses about the locus of eidetic images but also enable us to know if moving eidetic images exist at all.

A second experiment could cast more light on the monocular nature of eidetic images and on their neural locus. Suppose that a child looks with his or her right eye at a pattern of vertical lines and builds up an eidetic image. Those lines are removed, and a pattern of horizontal lines is presented to the left eye. Again, the child builds up an image. What is seen when both images are viewed in the same time and place? If real stimuli are used, the answer is "binocular rivalry." The vertical and horizontal lines compete with each other, and at any one spot in space and time only one orientation is seen. The other grating is perceptually suppressed (Walker, 1978). The neural locus of binocular rivalry is known to be beyond that of aftereffects (Blake & Overton, 1979; O'Shea & Crassini, 1981; Wolfe & Blake, 1985) but still in the retinotopic portion of the visual system. Since eidetic images are not retinotopic, we would predict that orthogonal images formed in each eye would not produce rivalry. The Habers report that two images can be combined to form composites. It seems likely that composites would be seen even if the two images were in different eyes.

Fading of Eidetic Images

Eidetic images are reported to fade in "meaningful" pieces. This would seem to be a useful bit of information in the search for the locus of these images. It could be proposed that images that fade object by object or feature by feature are probably located at a fairly late stage in visual processing. Unfortunately, fading data are suspect. The situation seems very similar to the fading of another type of image, the stabilized image. If a physical image is stabilized on the retina, that is, if it is not allowed to slide across the retinal surface when the eyes move, it will fade and vanish within a few seconds. Initial reports held that the fading was structured (Pritchard, Heron, & Hebb, 1960) and that the locus of this effect must be central and not retinal. However, subsequent work (e.g., Schuck, 1973) has demonstrated that the "structure" is in the verbal reports of fading and not in the fading itself. The problem is that it is very difficult to describe fading if bits and pieces are disappearing at random. The tendency is to report the disappearance of nameable chunks. Since this is all the more likely to be the case with children, the main subjects in eidetic imagery experiments, the reports of meaningful fragmentation of eidetic images should be treated very cautiously.

Eidetic Imagery and Mental Imagery

The psychophysical mapping of visual processing becomes less detailed and less assured beyond the level of binocular rivalry. Physiology has not yet found a locus for rivalry, and its understanding of subsequent processing is limited. Nevertheless, we can identify a few more landmarks in visual processing that are relevant to the search for a neural locus of eidetic imagery. One of those landmarks is mental imagery. Unlike eidetic imagery, mental imagery is a common, even universal, phenomenon. Consider the following question: How would you get your bed out of your bedroom and into another room? Most people, in answering such a question, conjure up an image of the bed and manipulate that image in order to determine if it will fit through an image of the door. Research has shown that these images are rotated and displaced in a very lawful manner. For example, images seem to rotate at a constant rate (e.g., Cooper & Shephard, 1984).

A little is known about the neural locus of imagery. First, psychophysically, it is known that images exist in some sort of spatial array. If a subject is asked to imagine a letter to the left of a fixation spot, his or her ability to detect that letter in that location is enhanced. The detectability of that letter in different locations and the detectability of different letters in the same location are not enhanced (Farah, 1985). It is not known if this spatial representation for mental imagery is retinotopic or spatiotopic.

Farah (1984) has reviewed the neuropsychological literature and concludes that patients with lesions of the posterior part of the cortex of the left hemisphere are most likely to report an inability to generate images. Experimental studies using both linguistic and nonlinguistic stimuli seem to support this conclusion. Much more work needs to be done. For example, knowing where mental images are generated is not the same as knowing the spatial array that they inhabit once generated.

Eidetic images seem to resist mental manipulations. This is not complete. The Habers report that children can "slide" images around on a blank sheet of paper and that they can push one imaged letter aside to make room for another, but there do not seem to be reports of children rotating eidetic images or moving one part of an image relative to others. It is possible that no one has ever asked the correct questions, and it would be instructive to know what would happen if eidetic images were tested with the paradigms that have been applied to mental images. Eidetic images fade with time and are interfered with by verbal rehearsal. Neither of these perils seem to afflict mental images. Print makes for bad eidetic images. To the contrary, letters are standard stimuli in mental imagery experiments.

Our knowledge is too sketchy to say with assurance that eidetic images occur "before" or "after" mental images in the visual system. There are at least two obstacles to making such a statement. First, the psychophysical locus of mental imagery is not clearly established. Obviously, it does not require a physical stimulus on the retina. However, some workers (e.g., Farah, 1985) think that images, wherever they are generated, are inserted into the visual pathway at a fairly early locus. Second, once beyond the level of binocular rivalry, "before" and "after" become somewhat problematical terms since it is clear that higher visual processing is characterized by a great deal of top-down as well as bottom-up processing. Nevertheless, we may conclude, on what information we have, that the locus of eidetic imagery is not the *same* as that of mental imagery.

Eidetic Imagery and Perception

Let us now leap to what could be considered one "end" of visual processing, the spatiotopically organized representation of the world that we loosely call "visual perception." Though eidetic images seem to be spatiotopic, they do not seem to be the same as the final working representation of the world.

First, eidetic images are imperfectly spatiotopic. As noted previously, they can be moved a little. We cannot move objects in our normal representation. Second, the Habers report that verbal rehearsal seems to interfere with eidetic images. There does not appear to be a parallel in the normal representation of the world. Finally, the Habers report that children never mistake eidetic images for the real thing. Two events occurring in the same neural locus should be confused with one another. Thus, for example, electrical stimulation of the visual cortex produces the perception of a flash of light. This is indistinguishable from a "real" flash. If eidetic images occupied the same neural locus as normal perceptions, we would expect confusions between the two experiences.

What and Where Are Eidetic Images?

Eidetic images are not by-products of early visual processing, nor are they isomorphic with the final representation of the world. They seem to lie in between. One of the difficult problems in visual perception is to understand how the system transforms retinotopic input into a spatiotopic representation (see Pinker, 1984, for a discussion). Perhaps eidetic images arise out of that process of transformation. The Habers note that eidetic images are not generated in a single glance but require a series of fixations on different parts of the stimulus over a few seconds. Each successive fixation must be analyzed for its content and then fitted into a spatial framework. This process of integration over multiple fixations is vital to the construction of normal spatiotopic vision. In normal vision, we go on to fit the current scene into our understanding of the larger world around us. Thus you know about the layout of the room you are in, and that knowledge includes parts of the room that are currently hidden from sight.

Eidetic images seem to be more restricted. They may represent the integration of a small amount of information into a reasonably spatiotopic representation of a region of the visual world. Further integration seems to be needed to create a coherent representation of visual space. An eidetic image may be one of the pieces that builds this larger representation. In standard adult vision, these intermediate steps occur fast and outside of conscious awareness (see Wolfe, 1983). Perhaps eidetic imagery is an abnormal state in which a normally automatic process becomes accessible to introspection. If this could be proven, eidetic imagery would acquire an important role as a tool in the study of standard visual perception. It will always remain a fascinating phenomenon in its own right.

Acknowledgments

This paper was prepared with the support of grants from National Eye Institute–National Institutes of Health and the Whitaker Health Sciences Fund. I thank Richard Held,

Deborah Fein, and Martha Farah for useful discussions and Ralph and Lyn Haber for the material on which these speculations are based.

References

Barbeito, R., & Ono, H. (1984). Stereodeficient observers cannot make utrocular identifications. *Investigative Ophthalmology & Visual Science*, (Suppl 25), 295.

Blake, R., & Cormack, R. H. (1979). On utrocular discrimination. *Perception and Psychophysics, 26*, 53–68.

Blake, R., & Overton, R. (1979). The site of binocular rivalry suppression. *Perception, 8*, 143–152.

Blake, R., Overton, R., & Lema-Stern, S. (1981). Interocular transfer of visual aftereffects. *Journal of Experimental Psychology: Human Perception and Performance, 88*, 327–332.

Blakemore, C., & Sutton, P. (1969). Size adaptation: A new aftereffect. *Science, 166*, 245–247.

Campbell, F. W., & Maffei, L. (1971). The tilt aftereffect: A fresh look. *Vision Research, 11*, 833–840.

Cooper, L. A., & Shephard, R. N. (1984). Turning something over in the mind. *Scientific American, 253*, 106–114.

Enoch J., Goldman H., & Sunga, R. (1969). The ability to distinguish which eye was stimulated by light. *Investigative Ophthalmology & Visual Science, 8*, 317–331.

Farah, M. J. (1984). The neurological basis of mental imagery: A componential anlaysis. *Cognition, 18*, 245–272.

Farah, M. J. (1985). Psychophysical evidence for a shared representational medium for mental images and percepts. *Journal of Experimental Psychology: General, 144*, 91–104.

Gibson, J. J. (1937). Adaptation with negative aftereffect. *Psychological Review, 44*, 222–244.

Julesz, B. (1971). *Foundations of cyclopean perception.* Chicago: University of Chicago Press.

Livingston, M. S., & Hubel, D. H. (1984). Anatomy and physiology of a color system in the primate visual cortex. *Journal of Neuroscience, 4*, 309–356.

McCollough, C. (1965). Color adaptation of edge detectors in the human visual system. *Science, 149*, 1115–1116.

O'Shea, R. P., & Crassini, B. (1981). Interocular transfer of the motion aftereffect is not reduced by binocular rivalry. *Vision Research, 21*, 801–804.

Pinker, S. (1984). Visual cognition: An introduction. *Cognition, 18*, 1–63.

Pritchard, R. M., Heron, W. & Hebb, D. O. (1960). Visual perception approached by the method of stabilized retinal images. *Canadian Journal of Psychology, 50*, 642–644.

Shuck, J. R., (1973). Factors affecting reports of fragmenting visual images. *Perception and Psychophysics, 113*, 382–390.

Smith, S. (1945). Utrocular or 'which eye' discrimination. *Journal of Experimental Psychology, 35*, 1–14.

Stromeyer, C. F. (1970). Eidetikers. *Psychology Today, 4*, 76–80.

Van Essen, D. C., & Maunsell, J. H. R. (1983). Hierarchical organization and functional streams in the visual cortex. *Trends in Neuroscience, 6*, 370–375.

Walker, P. (1978). Binocular rivalry. Central or peripheral selective processes? *Psychological Bulletin, 85*, 376–389.

White, K. D., Petry, H. M., Riggs, L. A., & Miller, J. (1978). Binocular interactions during establishment of McCollough effects. *Vision Research, 18*, 1201–1215.

Wolfe, J. M. (1983). Hidden visual processes. *Scientific American, 248,* 94–103.

Wolfe, J. M. (1986). Stereopsis and binocular rivalry. *Psychological Review, 93,* 269–282.

Wolfe, J. M., & Blake, R. (1985). Monocular and binocular processes in human vision. In D. Rose & V. G. Dobson (Eds.), *Models of the visual cortex,* (pp. 192–199). Chichester, UK: Wiley.

Wolfe, J. M., & Held, R. (1982). Binocular adaptation that cannot be measured monocularly. *Perception, 11,* 287–295.

Wolfe, J. M., & Held, R. (1983). Shared characteristics of stereopsis and the purely binocular process. *Vision Research, 23,* 217–227.

Wolfe, J. M., & O'Connell, K. (1986). Fatigue and structural change: Two consequences of visual pattern adaptation. *Investigative Ophthalmology & Visual Science, 27,* 538–543.

III

CASE REPORTS
AND CASE STUDIES

12

Trilingual Hyperlexia

YVAN LEBRUN
CLAUDIE VAN ENDERT
HENRI SZLIWOWSKI

> *The importance of the Idiot-Savant lies in our inability to explain him, he stands as a landmark of our own ignorance and the phenomenon of the Idiot-Savant exists as a challenge to our capabilities* (A. HOLSTEIN in *Horwitz, Kestenbaum, Person, & Jarvik, 1965* p. 1078.)

The word "hyperlexia" has been given various meanings since it was first introduced by the Silberbergs in 1967. However, there is now a fairly general consensus that the word should be used to refer to an abnormal condition characterized by an ability to read out written words that far exceeds the other verbal skills of the individual and that would not have been predicted on the basis of his or her relatively low level of general intellectual attainment. In other words, "hyperlexia" denotes the surprising expertise that a number of individuals with mental deficiency and restricted language functions have in calling words by sight. In addition to their limited cognitive development and language delay, hyperlexics more often than not exhibit behavioral disorders. These may range from restlessness and low level of frustration tolerance to severe autistic withdrawal. (For an extended discussion, see Aram and Healy, Chapter 4, this volume.)

Hyperlexia was noted long before it was identified as a nosological entity and was given a specific name. Early observers tended to regard it as just one of those strange gifts that some mentally retarded persons exhibit, such as calendar calculation skills or the ability, not infrequently found in autistic children, to reproduce verbatim parts of conversations or TV commercials heard weeks and sometimes months before.

In recent years hyperlexia has been given more systematic attention. Hyperlexics have been studied both clinically and experimentally. A sizable body of reliable information on hyperlexics shows that hyperlexia is not a strictly uniform syndrome. There may be important interindividual differences; moreover, despite

Yvan Lebrun and Claudie Van Endert. Neurolinguistics Department, School of Medicine, V.U.B., Brussels, Belgium.
Henri Szliwowski. Neurology Unit, University Hospital, U.L.B. Brussels, Belgium.

the available information, the pathophysiology of the condition is still poorly understood. Therefore every new detailed study of hyperlexic subjects is likely to help us gain a better insight into the nature and origin of hyperlexia.

In the section that follows we describe a hyperlexic child who, among other peculiarities, could read out words and short sentences in three different languages.

The History and Abilities of Isabelle

The patient, Isabelle, was a right-handed white girl, born on July 10, 1974. At the time of birth, her father was 33 and her mother 27 years old. Both were in good health. Nine years before, the father had undergone cobalt therapy for Hodgkin's disease limited to the cervical level.

Pregnancy had been uneventful, except that during the 2nd or 3rd month the mother had been in contact with rubella. A blood investigation done at the time is said to have been negative.

At birth, Isabelle's weight was 3.2 kg. The girl was 50 cm tall, and her head circumference was 31 cm, more than two standard deviations below the mean, indicative of microcephaly. Neither the parents nor their relatives ever presented with developmental disorders of the central nervous system, except for one of the mother's sisters, who had petit mal epilepsy between ages 4 and 11. The mother's brother was operated on at age 19 because of a brain tumor. Isabelle's motor development was a little slow, though not abnormal: head control at 3 months, sitting position at 10 months, standing at 13 months, and walking at 18 months. At 10 years of age, when we examined her, she had an abnormal gait and ran awkwardly.

At age 18 months Isabelle had convulsions affecting the left side of her body and lasting for 3 hours (status epilepticus). The convulsions could not be controlled even with high doses of diazepam and phenobarbital. There was no fever.

During the ensuing 8 years, antiepileptic drugs were administered, and the little girl showed only occasional fits or absences. At regular intervals EEGs were obtained. Some of them revealed paroxysmal activity, while others were normal. A brain scan did not show any malformation; in particular, the ventricular system did not appear enlarged. Cranial circumference remained below normal (see Figure 12-1).

Repeated chromosomal investigations proved normal, and the existence of a prenatal infection, such as toxoplasmosis, cytomegalovirus, or rubella, could be ruled out. The cause of Isabelle's microcephaly could not be discovered.

The girl's psychomotor and intellectual development was delayed, as was language acquisition. At age 4 years 9 months, Isabelle's I.Q. on the Terman-Merrill was 55; her mental age was considered to be 2 years 8 months. At 7 years 9 months, her scores on a variety of tests, including Leiter's International Performance Scale, the Minnesota Preschool Scale, and the Standard-Binet Intelligence Scale pointed to a mental age between 4 and 5 years.

Isabelle was an affectionate and outgoing girl. However she was hyperactive and tended to be difficult to control; she would often have tantrums when her

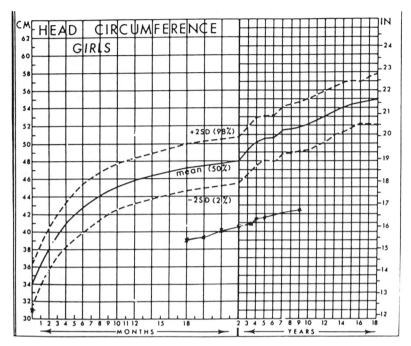

FIGURE 12-1. Isabelle's head circumference at various ages (18 months through 9 years) compared with the values provided by Nellhaus (1968) *Pediatrics, 41,* 106–114.

wishes and whims were not complied with. Her mother was inclined to overprotect her. Isabelle spoke her first words when she was 15 months old. From then on, language development was abnormally slow despite speech therapy. At home and in the remedial school she attended, Isabelle spoke Dutch. However, her father's mother tongue was French, and some of her relatives spoke French. She therefore knew some French in addition to Dutch.

Her oral comprehension was difficult to assess, since she was not always willing to follow instructions. When she failed to carry out a verbal command, or when she carried it out incorrectly, it was not always clear whether this was because she had not understood the direction or because she did not want to obey it. Similarly, when questions put to her were not answered, it was often difficult to ascertain whether she had not understood them, had not paid any attention, or had not cared to answer. Moreover, in formal testing it was repeatedly observed that Isabelle tended to give more inappropriate responses in the second part of the test; it looked as if the test was beginning to bore her and as if she no longer wanted to concentrate on what she was doing. Her test results, therefore, were not fully reliable. However, there can be no doubt that Isabelle's oral comprehension was noticeably below normal. For instance, at nearly 9 years of age she was given a standardized Dutch vocabulary test requiring her to point to one of the four pictures corresponding to the verbal item pronounced by the examiner. Her score on this task revealed a psycholinguistic age of 4 to $4\frac{1}{2}$ years. This result was confirmed by a repeat test a few months later.

Isabelle's speech production in everyday situations was usually copious but difficult to understand because of her defective pronunciation and limited command of vocabulary and syntax. In addition, she appeared ignorant of sociolinguistic rules: She would change the topics of conversation without any warning, would often interrupt her speech partner, and did not always react to questions. When she did answer a question, her reply could be completely inappropriate. Moreover, she sometimes seemed to engage in a conversation with someone who was not present and to ignore her actual speech partner. However, she switched between languages appropriately.

Isabelle's underdeveloped speech was replete with word and phrase repetitions and with embololalias, especially *maar* ("but") and *ja maar* ("yes but"). Stereotyped phrases kept cropping up, for example, *Die doet het toch* ("he does it all the same"). She would frequently add [ə] to final consonants or else repeat this final consonant a few times, for example, [wa: r: r: r: r:] (*waar*, i.e., "true").

During the summer of 1979 (the girl was then 5 years old and her active command of oral language was still very limited), Isabelle's mother was surprised to discover that her daughter could identify the titles of her parents' two daily papers, *Le Soir* and *De Standaard*. For instance, one day the girl spontaneously pointed to a van on which *Le Soir* was written, and she made it clear that she recognized the name. The mother decided to try to teach her daughter some written language. She wrote three Dutch substantives in block letters on separate cards. Isabelle soon learned to identify these three words: She would correctly point to the card corresponding to the item pronounced by her mother. In about two months the child's reading vocabulary could be extended to 15 words. Then Isabelle learned to pronounce these words. Thereafter, whenever the mother added a new item, her daughter was taught to read it aloud.

In April 1982, after about 20 months of exercises with Dutch words, the mother introduced French words, which Isabelle learned to recognize with the same facility. Indeed, her pronunciation when reading words aloud was noticeably better than in spontaneous speech, both in Dutch and in French. When the child's reading vocabulary numbered about 300 words in either language, she was taught to read aloud short sentences. Isabelle was given illustrated books that could be looked at while a cassette was being played, the words and sentences in the book corresponding to those in the recording. Isabelle easily learned to relate the written to the spoken items and spontaneously repeated the spoken items while pointing to the written ones.

In July 1983, some 15 months after French words were first introduced, the mother started to teach her daughter English words and short sentences. Initially she used separate cards but later on bought her daughter illustrated books and cassettes. The child's English pronunciation while reading aloud was quite intelligible and stood in sharp contrast to her defective pronunciation of her mother tongue in spontaneous speech.

The little girl could also be taught some limited writing skills. Using letters written on separate cards, she learned to supplement a missing letter to a word she was familiar with. For instance, if shown the letters *ON* she would promptly put a *Z* in front of them so as to form the Dutch word *ZON* ("sun"). However, she could not be taught to form a whole word by herself, even if she was given all the letters she needed and was told which word she was to form. Isabelle could not remember the alphabet. Although she loved to color and to scrawl, she was very awkward at copying letters and figures. She was unable to write words from memory.

At the same time at which she was teaching her daughter words, her mother also made her acquainted with figures. Once she could recognize the numbers from 1 to 20, Isabelle started to take an interest in calendars and thus learned to identify the names of the days. However, the little girl never used these names in spontaneous speech. Indeed, even at 10 years of age, she hardly ever used any word referring to a time division.

Isabelle obviously enjoyed calling words by sight and would spontaneously read aloud words appearing in advertisements, TV commercials, newspaper headlines, and so forth. Moreover, from 7 years of age on she was able to apply phoneme–grapheme correspondence rules, which she had never formally been taught, as she managed to read aloud a number of words her mother had not herself introduced. At 10 years of age, the child proved able to read Dutch nonsense monosyllables and to some extent Dutch nonsense disyllables. It should be pointed out, however, that in Dutch, so-called phonemic reading is relatively easy because of the fairly great regularity of spelling. On the other hand, in calling words by sight, our little patient clearly paid due attention to the order in which the letters stood, since she correctly distinguished between palindromes such as *"pot"* versus *"top"*, *kip* versus *pik*, ("chicken" versus "pick"), *tien* versus *niet*, ("ten" versus "not"), and *geel* versus *leeg*, ("yellow" versus "empty").

When her parents had visitors, or when she accompanied her parents on a visit to friends or relatives, Isabelle was often eager to show her reading skills. Whatever the circumstances, she would immediately take one of her reading books and start to read aloud, imperatively demanding the adult's attention.

In Dutch, Isabelle understood to a large extent what she read aloud, provided that sentences were kept simple. Indeed, she was able to match a written sentence with one of four pictures, even when the sentence was *De jongen staat in de zon* ("The boy is standing in the sunshine"), and there were foils such as a picture representing a *man* standing in the sunshine. She could also match a given picture with one of two written sentences. However, she could not deal with semicomplex and complex sentences. Her comprehension then was by no means age-appropriate. (She was ten years old at the time of examination.)

Interestingly enough, Isabelle hardly ever followed an instruction given in writing, even if she had read it aloud correctly. Since one could not be sure that this was not due, at least in part, to her waywardness, we had her read aloud simple sentences containing a piece of information in which she might legitimately have been expected to take an interest, such as *In de jas van Klodie zit snoep* ("there are sweets in the coat of Klodie[1]) or *In de tas van Klodie zit krijt voor Isabelle* ("there is chalk for Isabelle in Klodie's handbag). Such written sentences usually failed to elicit any reaction. However, if the sentence that the child had just read aloud was

---

1. "Klodie" stands for Claudie Van Endert, the one of us who saw Isabelle the most frequently and who did the testing reported here.

repeated orally by the examiner, *then* Isabelle most of the time showed the expected reaction, for example, she would go and fetch the sweets or the chalk. Similarly, when a written instruction failed to be followed although the child had read it aloud correctly, it often sufficed to repeat the order orally for it to be carried out. Again, if the very same sentence was used first in a multiple-choice test and on another occasion to refer to something the child should normally have been interested in, it would usually be dealt with adequately in the first, but not in the second, situation. All this strongly suggests that Isabelle was hardly able to derive useful information from what she read. Although to a large extent she understood what she deciphered, she failed to adjust to the written message in any practical sense. She seemed largely unable to incorporate written information into her spontaneous behavior. It looked as if our patient was reading for literal meaning but not for pragmatic meaning. Reading aloud was a game or a beloved exercise but was not put to practical use.

Discussion of the Case

At the time of examination, Isabelle had for several years shown reading skills that were not commensurate with her other verbal abilities, all of which were noticeably limited. This child therefore presented with the syndrome of hyperlexia. However, a number of features distinguished her from similar cases reported earlier.

Reading Aloud

To begin with, Isabelle could read aloud in three languages: Dutch, French, and English. Dutch was her mother tongue, and it was in this language that her reading capabilities were the best developed. It was also the language that she knew the best. She could read a number of French words and sentences, and used this language on occasion with her father and her father's relatives. Her command of French was even more limited than her command of Dutch. Finally, she could read approximately as many words and sentences in English as in French, but she never spoke English. English was used exclusively for reading purposes. No such case of trilingual hyperlexia seems to have been reported before.

In contradistinction to a number of hyperlexics, Isabelle did not show any precocious reading skills. Not until she was 5 years old was it discovered that she could recognize the titles of her parents' daily newspapers. Never before had her mother noticed any reading abilities.

Again, Isabelle's capacity for reading never exceeded that of her age-mates. To be sure, at 10 years of age our patient could read in three different languages, but 10-year-old children who are given a balanced trilingual education read in their three languages at least as fluently as Isabelle did in hers. In other words, the girl's reading skills did not surpass those of children of the same age; they were striking only in comparison with her other verbal abilities. Using the phrases coined by Philipps (1930), one might say that Isabelle's hyperlexia was a "personal talent," not a "social talent," that is, her ability to read aloud written words was considerably greater than might have been expected on the basis of her overall intellectual and linguistic development; on the other hand, it did not distinguish her from her age-mates.

Hyperlexic children are often reported to have developed reading skills spontaneously. Their parents are said never to have encouraged their interest in written material, let alone to have taught them to read. In the present case it is plain that the mother was instrumental in Isabelle's acquisition of reading. Indeed, without her mother's constant coaching, it is doubtful whether Isabelle would ever have become hyperlexic.

In some hyperlexic children reading aloud appears to be a compulsive behavior. For instance, most of the patients observed by Mehegan and Dreifuss (1972) would instantly and indiscriminately begin reading any available material, and attempts to divert them met with resistance. Although Isabelle was keen on reading aloud and liked to show people how well she could read words, she was certainly not an obsessive reader; it was possible to divert her from reading. However, like most hyperlexic children, she took an unusual interest in written material. If given a book with many color illustrations, she would direct her attention to the printed words rather than to the pictures. She preferred coloring over words to coloring outline drawings, and cutting out words to cutting out images. She spent much more time reading aloud, coloring, and scrawling than playing with toys.

Reading Comprehension

The view is often expressed that hyperlexics do not understand much of what they read aloud. For instance, Elliott and Needleman (1976) speak of hyperlexic children as mental retardates showing "an extraordinary advanced ability to recognize words, frequently without comprehension of their meaning," and they insist that "hyperlexics read without comprehension" (p. 344). As we reported previously, Isabelle, in a multiple-choice test using Dutch, was able to match a picture and a simple sentence, even when the picture to be selected and one of the foils were semantically related. A similar observation was made by Healy, Aram, and Horwitz (1982), who found that those of their 12 hyperlexic patients who "could attend to connected prose evidenced comprehension of short literal sentences associated with a pictorial stimulus" (p. 20). A number of hyperlexics, then, are able to derive semantic information from the sentences they read aloud. Indeed Isabelle understood short sentences well enough to match them with the appropriate pictures even if the foils were semantically close to the pictures to be selected. On the other hand, she seemed to have difficulty in organizing a motor behavior on the basis of written information: She hardly ever carried out written instructions, even though she read them aloud correctly, and she rarely responded to written messages that might legitimately have been expected to arouse her interest, even when the syntactic structures and the vocabulary of these messages were similar to those used in the tests requiring a picture choice in response to a single sentence.

Her main problem, then, does not seem to have been that she could not understand what she read aloud, but rather that she could not plan a behavior of some complexity in accordance with information given in writing. Such absence of reading pragmatism in a hyperlexic child seems not to have been reported before. However, it may conceivably have existed in some of the subjects of published cases of hyperlexia but may have passed unnoticed because the testing or observation procedure did not aim at distinguishing between reading for literal meaning and reading for pragmatic meaning. For instance, Mehegan and Dreifuss (1972) note that only 2 of their 12 hyperlexic patients followed instructions written on the blackboard. It is not known whether the 10 children who failed to follow written directions could not understand them or could not act them out.

Because a dissociation between understanding written instructions and acting them out has not formally been noted in previous cases of hyperlexia, one might doubt that it really existed in Isabelle's case. To this we can reply that such a dissociation is not unknown in brain pathology. A left-hemisphere lesion may render a patient incapable of following written directions, although he or she has decoded them and does not otherwise show apraxic symptoms. Albert, Yamadori, Gardner, and Howes (1973) have described a right-hander who, after having had neurosurgery for a glioma in the left temporo-occipital region, generally would not react to such written commands as "Cough" or "Close your eyes" However, specially devised tests showed that he could identify written words. Accordingly, his failure to carry out even one-word commands cannot be ascribed to a simple reading impairment. Most probably the patient could not turn a written message into a motor course of action. Again, a number of clinical observations strongly suggest that right-brain-damaged dextrals with so-called unilateral left neglect in fact can perceive verbal and nonverbal stimuli coming from the left but are unable to incorporate them into an appropriate motor reaction (Lebrun, 1985).

It appears, then, that cerebral pathology may prevent an individual from translating a verbal message into a corresponding motor behavior. Perhaps such an impairment is to be found in some hyperlexic children. These children, it would seem, find it difficult to adopt a course of action that would be directly consequent upon the written information they have decoded. The core of this disability may be a defective visuo-motor association. As a matter of fact, Cobrinik (1974), in examining six psychotic children showing what seems to have been hyperlexia, found that all of them had abnormally low scores on the Bender-Gestalt Visual Motor Test and on the Digit Substitution subtest of the WISC. Cobrinik concluded that his patients found it difficult to translate a visual percept into its motor counterpart. Perhaps our patient's lack of reading pragmatism should be viewed as a particular form of the inability to incorporate visual information into an appropriate motor response.

That Isabelle understood considerably more than she was able to turn into action should not be taken to mean that hyperlexics understand everything they read aloud or, conversely, that they read only the words they can understand. Comprehension of written material is not always on a par with technical reading. For instance, although he read aloud correctly 37 of the second 50 words of the Peabody Picture Vocabulary Test, the hyperlexic patient of Aram, Rose, and Horwitz (1983) could match only 19 of them with the corresponding pictures. There was, then, an obvious discrepancy between oral reading and semantic comprehension of words in this patient. However, it is doubtful whether such a discrepancy is characteristic of hyperlexia. Normal school children also are able to read aloud more words than they can understand. Niensted (1968), for instance, found that in 26 of the 45 normal public school pupils whom she tested, word-list reading was at least 1 year ahead of silent comprehension.

On the other hand, it may be observed that the tests that were used to assess reading comprehension in hyperlexics were sometimes ambiguous. For instance, Aram *et al.* (1983) report that their hyperlexic patient had great difficulty in completing such frames as "boy-girl," "man– . . . ." The authors interpret this difficulty as an indication of the patient's "very limited (reading) comprehension" (p. 519). It could be, however, that the patient's failure to complete such frames was due to a defect in logical reasoning rather than to a comprehension deficit. Perhaps the patient did understand the three terms of the frame but could not see that they formed a kind of geometric proportion that was to be completed. Obviously, the task calls for more than just word comprehension, and since the patient had a psychometrically measured IQ in the 60 range, he may have been unable to grasp the meaning of the task. His test results, therefore, do not unequivocally point to an impairment of reading comprehension *per se*. Clearly then, the problem of how much semantic information hyperlexic children can derive from what they read aloud needs to be investigated further. At all events, it is plain that hyperlexia cannot simply be equated with the behavior of some adults with severe sensory aphasia who read aloud correctly, even though they do not evidence any comprehension of the words and sentences they call by sight (Lebrun & Devreux, 1983).

Spontaneous Speech

A number of hyperlexic children have little spontaneous speech. For instance, one of the patients described by Mehegan and Dreifuss (1972) used only "grunts, high-pitched squeals, and a rumbling vocalization resembling an animal's roar" (p. 1107). At age $4\frac{1}{2}$ the patient described by Aram *et al.* (1983) produced only [a-a] for mama and [a-i] for daddy. As a man in his 40s, he still used "very little spontaneous speech" (p. 519). In our case, onset of verbal production was delayed (the exact date of this onset is not known). For several years Isabelle's speech, though not sparse, seemed to have little communicative value, since it was highly echolalic and repetitive. At 10 years of age, speech production was copious and most of the time appeared to have communicative intent. However, it remained highly defective. It contained many stereotyped phrases, some of which seemed to have been originally delayed echolalias from school, such as *En mooi tekenen eh* ("You should draw neatly"). A number of these phrases were ritualized; they were invariably produced when a particular situation occurred. Aram *et al.* (1983) also noted "a considerable amount of stereotyped connected phrases, such as "keep these in order", "You must think first", "Cover your mouth when you yawn" (p. 519), in their patient's spontaneous speech.

Pronunciation

We note further that, as in a number of previously reported cases, Isabelle's pronunciation was markedly better in reading aloud than in conversation. Indeed, her

English pronunciation was not bad at all, and someone hearing her read English words and sentences would never have suspected that her Dutch pronunciation in communicative situations was so defective. How is it possible that someone who is able to learn to articulate foreign words so well should pronounce the words in her own mother tongue so poorly? Could it be that hyperlexic children like Isabelle, who pronounce words considerably better when reading aloud than when speaking spontaneously or in response to questions, have formed at the cerebral level not one but two sets of articulatory habits—one that has developed in the context of verbal interaction with the environment and has remained crude and labile, and another that has developed in the context of calling written words by sight and is much better shaped?

The notion that Isabelle may have developed two sets of articulatory engrams (verbo-motor engrams) instead of one seems to receive some support from an observation made by Alajouanine, Pichot, and Durand (1949). These authors reported on a bilingual adult (French and English) in whom speech apraxia resulting from a stroke affected articulation consistently more in one language than in the other. This suggests that in the patient the neural substrate of speech production in one language was, at least in part, distinct from that in the other language. As a matter of fact, it is often assumed that in so-called coordinate bilinguals the two language systems are kept separate because they are subserved by neuronal networks that are, to some extent, specific to each language (Paradis & Lebrun, 1983). Therefore it is not inconceivable that Isabelle may have behaved somewhat like a coordinate bilingual, developing two sets of verbo-motor engrams, one of which was used for communicative purposes and the other for reading aloud. That articulatory skills were acquired in two different settings, one communicative (interactive speech) and the other metalinguistic (reading aloud), may have been instrumental in bringing about two different sets of articulatory engrams. As a matter of fact, there are indications that when two languages are acquired in vastly different contexts, or by using different teaching methods, they may have different cerebral organizations, so that in case of cerebral damage, one may be more affected than the other (Lebrun, 1976). Isabelle, then, may have been bilingual in her own mother tongue, having developed two sets of articulatory skills that were somewhat independent of one another.

Other Special Talents

Some hyperlexic children have more than one talent; that is, in addition to their reading skills, they possess another aptitude that stands in sharp contrast to their overall retardation. The patient of Aram *et al.* (1983), for instance, was a date calculator: Given a specific date he was able to say the day of the week on which this date fell. In contrast, Isabelle had no remarkable ability other than her hyperlexia. To be sure, she was very fond of calendars, but she was no date calculator. She could neither draw nor write. She could not calculate and had no musical talent. And she never gave evidence of special mnemonic power. Except for her hyperlexia, she was a very ordinary microcephalic child with a moderate mental handicap.

Language Deficits in Parents

In their chapter on hyperlexia Aram and Healy (Chapter 4, this volume) stress the frequent existence of language-learning deficits among the paternal relatives of hyperlexic children. They suspect that there may be a relationship between dyslexia and hyperlexia and that hyperlexia may be genetically transmitted. Our case does not really confirm this surmise. Isabelle's parents never had reading problems, and both of them enjoyed reading. And only one relative, a nephew on the paternal side, could be found who had had dyslexia. Moreover, there are some discrepancies in the opinion expressed by Healy *et al.* (1982) that "hyperlexia may actually represent a subgroup of dyslexia" (p. 19). Unlike hyperlexics, dyslexics do not enjoy reading, are not precocious readers, and do not read as well as their age-mates. Dyslexia and hyperlexia, then, are phenomenologically different. Moreover, it is uncertain whether they are genetically related. Accordingly, it is probably better to view them as two separate entities, even though in the long run each represents an underachievement in the acquisition of reading skills.

Conclusion

Isabelle, a microcephalic girl, showed one mental capacity—reading aloud in three languages—that was far beyond her overall retarded functional level, although not higher than her age-mates' ability. Her reading skills could never have been predicted on the basis of her limited linguistic and mental development. In contradistinction to other idiot savants, whose brilliance in some particular field, for example, date calculation or mental arithmetic, remains unsurpassed, Isabelle was remarkable only in comparison with herself.

In order to somewhat improve the little girl's condition we recommended that the mother should change her approach to the development of reading skills in her daughter. We explained how crucial it was that Isabelle should acquire some pragmatic reading skills. We suggested a number of exercises that were likely to help the girl discover how useful reading could be and to teach her to react adequately to the written messages she would decode. But the mother did not appear willing to take our advice. Indeed, she seemed to resent the approach we were suggesting and indicated that she might try to teach her daughter to "read" in a fourth language! We do not know whether she eventually achieved her end and turned her child into a quadrilingual hyperlexic.

References

Alajouanine, R., Pichot, P., & Durand, M. (1949). Dissociation des altérations phonétiques avec conservation relative de la langue la plus ancienne dans un cas d'anarthrie pure chez un sujet français bilingue. *L'Encéphale, 28,* 245–265.

Albert, M., Yamadori, A., Gardner, H., & Howes, D. (1973). Comprehension in alexia. *Brain, 96,* 317–328.

Aram, D., Rose, D., Horwitz, S. (1983). Hyperlexia: Developmental reading without meaning. In R. Malatesha & H. Whitaker (Eds.), *Dyslexia: A global issue* (pp. 517–531.) The Hague: Nijhoff.

Cobrinik, L. (1974). Unusual reading ability in severely disturbed children. *Journal of Autism and Childhood Schizophrenia, 4,* 163–175.

Elliott, D., & Needleman, R. (1976). The syndrome of hyperlexia. *Brain and Language, 3,* 339–349.

Healy, J., Aram, D., & Horwitz, S. (1982). A study of hyperlexia. *Brain and Language, 17,* 1–23.

Horwitz, E., Kestenbaum, C., Person, E., & Jarvik, L. (1965). Identical twin—"idiot savants"—calendar calculators. *American Journal of Psychiatry, 121,* 1075–1079.

Lebrun, Y. (1976). Recovery in polyglot aphasics. In Y. Lebrun & R. Hoops (Eds.). *Recovery in aphasics* (pp. 96–108). Lisse: Swets & Zeitlinger.

Lebrun, Y. (1985). Disturbances of written language and associated abilities following damage to the right hemisphere. *Applied Psycholinguistics, 6,* 231–260.

Lebrun, Y., & Devreux, F. (1983). Alexia in relation to aphasia and agnosia. In R. Malatesha & H. Whitaker (Eds.), *Dyslexia: A global issue* (pp. 191–209). The Hague: Nijhoff.

Mehegan, C., & Dreifuss, M. (1972). Hyperlexia. Exceptional reading ability in brain-damaged children. *Neurology, 22,* 1105–1111.

Nellhaus, G. (1968). Head circumference from birth to 18 years: Practical composite of international and interracial graphs. *Pediatrics, 41,* 106–114.

Niensted, S. (1968). Hyperlexia: An educational disease? *Exceptional Children, 35,* 162–163.

Paradis, M., & Lebrun, Y. (1983). La neurolinguistique du bilinguisme: Représentation de deux langues dans un même cerveau. In M. Paradis & Y. Lebrun (Eds.), *La neurolinguistique du bilinguisme* (pp. 7–13). *Langages, 72,* (18). Paris: Larousse.

Philipps, A. (1930). Talented imbeciles. *The Psychological Review, 18,* 246–255.

Silberberg, N., & Silberberg, M. (1967). Hyperlexia: Specific word recognition skills in young children. *Exceptional Children, 34,* 41–42.

13

Elly: A Study in Contrasts

LOLA BOGYO
RONALD ELLIS

> *Elly knew the whereabouts of every cookie shelf in every supermarket in the Northern Berkshire area of Massachusetts. There was not a location, not an orientation in her world that she did not have memorized.* (PARK, *1967*)
>
> *When she was given a box of 48 crayons to add to her set of 64, she knew by some process of her own that she had 112, although she had not yet learned to perform addition that involves carrying.* (PARK, *1967*).
>
> *At 13, she knew the prime factors of all the numbers from 1 to 1000 and beyond, and would write them on request—write them because she could not pronounce them* (PARK & YOUDERIAN, *1979*).

"She looked through human beings as if they were glass. She created solitude in the midst of company, silence in the midst of chatter" (p. 5). Thus Clara Claiborne Park (1967) described her daughter, Elly—a child who came to be labeled "autistic." Brilliantly chronicled in her mother's book, *The Siege: The First Eight Years of an Autistic Child*, Elly's early functioning was, in many respects, gravely impaired. She was delayed in sitting, standing, and walking; developed no active exploratory play; spoke only a few words before age 5; and seemed to exist in a world of her own, oblivious to the people around her. While other children played and laughed together, Elly sat alone, preferring to rock back and forth or engage in repetitive isolated play. She did not seek comfort in the laps of her parents, did not call "Mama" or "Dada," and seemed blind and deaf to the presence of other human beings. In many realms, her functioning was—and is—retarded, relative to others her age.

And yet, even as her parents first began to suspect that something might be wrong, Elly demonstrated exceptional abilities—some that were exceptional only relative to her many areas of impairment, some that seemed extraordinary by any standard. Some of these exceptional abilities appeared to disappear as she grew older, while others have persisted and continue to astonish.

It is these exceptional abilities—both the relative and absolute—that are our focus in this chapter. In the sections that follow, we describe some of these abilities

Lola Bogyo. North Shore Children's Hospital, Salem, Massachusetts.
Ronald Ellis. Boston University School of Medicine, Boston, Massachusetts.

in detail while attempting to sketch the backdrop of impairments against which they shone. We also raise the question that was in the back of our minds as we worked with Elly: What can we learn by studying these exceptional abilities; what can they tell us both about autism and about cognition in general?

Memory

> A mother with an abnormal baby is always testing. On our walks I would deliberately lag behind and let her lead me home. She never hesitated, never took a wrong turn. A single visit and her knowledge was infallible. (Park, 1967, p. 152)

By age 2, Elly was suspected of being developmentally delayed. She was just beginning to walk, had spoken only a handful of words—each generally only once or twice before they seemed to disappear—and seemed locked inside her own self-contained world. Hospital tests found no evidence of any physical deficiency. Doctors told her parents to wait—and watch. Her mother recalls that "We watched, with ever sharper and more experienced eyes. . . . Speechless, uncomprehending, unable to care for her physical needs, Elly was retarded in every functional way" (Park, 1967, p. 30).

But even as Elly fell further and further behind her peers, signs of a remarkable memory began to appear. In *The Siege* her mother recounts an early episode—astounding then, but later to be seen as characteristic of this paradoxical child. Elly was 2 years old and had been walking for only 3 months when one day she disappeared. After a frantic search she was finally found, crawling on the painted cross-stripes and arrows of a parking lot several blocks away. Elly had never walked to this place before and had traveled the route only once, pushed in a stroller by her mother. She had been fascinated then by the bold markings on the ground—enough, it seemed, to undertake an expedition of her own. One trip and the route had been firmly fixed in her memory—well enough for successful navigation on her own wobbly legs.

And so it was in general. One trip, one exposure to something new, and the information seemed stamped in the mind of this child who seemed oblivious to much of the world around her. Elly's communication skills were very limited, but her tantrums—her shrieks and wails—belied her remarkable memory. Like most other autistic children, she had difficulty tolerating change and responded to alterations in routine with cries of despair. Elly noticed minuscule changes, demonstrating that she remembered exactly how things had been. A slight variation in the pattern of lights in the building across the street or a glass positioned in other than its usual place in the dishwasher was enough to produce cries of despair. No change seemed too small to escape Elly's notice—she appeared to have the tiniest physical details of her environment imprinted indelibly on her mind.

Elly's impressive memory was not limited to locations and routes. She seemed to retain detailed information about her experiences even before she had words with which to label them. That this was so became evident only later, at the age of 5 or 6, as Elly began to use language to comment on her world and thus to reveal to others the information that she had previously stored. Her mother relates, for example, how Elly, at age 6, one day exclaimed "*Curved* stairs!" as she walked past a neighbor's house. She had just acquired the word "curved" and had not visited that house in over a year. Mrs. Park remembers, "I rang the bell in some excitement. I myself had never noticed the staircase, though I had been there more often than Elly. I might have known I could rely on her. As we entered the hall, I saw that it swept up and around in a splendid curve" (Park, 1967, p. 204).

As Elly's language skills developed, it became possible to see more accurately what she retained. Her progress in acquiring basic language skills was very slow. At age 9 her speech was still largely unintelligible to strangers, and at age 12, although she could generate sentences, her grammar remained that of someone laboriously acquiring a foreign language: "Get cookie for some people where is hungry." Nonetheless, by about this age it became possible to ask Elly what she remembered and to understand her spontaneous comments about the past.

Her recall of specific details was astonishing. She could easily remember minutiae of a visit years ago, such as what day of the week the visitor came, what she said, where they walked, and who bought what kinds of candy at the village newsstand. In her own broken syntax Elly repeated conversations of interest to her frequently and obsessively, recalling facts the disseminator had long since forgotten—the differences between hepatitis A and hepatitis B, the names and characteristics of various cloud types, the distances between planets.

Numbers have always held a particular fascination for Elly, and, especially during her adolescent years, her memory for number facts was extraordinary. At age 13 she knew all the prime numbers from 1 to 1,000 and, if presented with a nonprime, could immediately state its prime factors (see the next section for further discussion). At present, astronomy holds a special fascination for Elly, and she effortlessly remembers reams of number facts concerning interplanetary distance.

Since early childhood, Elly has been obsessed with ordering and categorizing information (see the discussion in the next section). She spontaneously compiles mental lists of information she encounters and retains. Current lists include, for example, "things bank tellers say" (e.g., "Please wait for your change," "Thank you very much," "There you are!," "Have a good day!") and contain *all* the instances that Elly has ever come across. Her lists multiply effortlessly in number and length—radio station call signs, symptoms of colds, ways to say "thank you"— without seeming to tax her memory.

How can we explain these feats of memory in someone who was—and is—so seriously impaired in many respects? It is one thing to assert that some functions have been "spared" and are normal in an otherwise impaired child; it is quite another to assert that they are "extraordinary." This general pattern of striking talent in the context of serious disability occurs too often to allow us to view Elly as a unique or isolated case. It prompts us to consider whether the talents might not be linked to the deficits—in some sense, a product of the impairments themselves. To examine this intriguing possibility more generally, let us first discuss another realm in which Elly's abilities seemed extraordinary and then explore the possible relationships between her strengths and weaknesses.

Calculation and Inferential Skills

> Elly has the kind of mind that given the series 2, 4, 6 . . . will spontaneously supply
> 8 and carry the series to 100. . . . It is simply apparent to her that that is what is there
> to be done—that the system itself demands it. (Park, 1967, p. 240–241)

We first met Elly when she was 23 years old. Although she knew it was "polite"
to talk with guests, her ability to carry on a simple conversation was severely
limited. She had learned rudimentary social conventions (e.g., to say "thank you"
when given a present, to return a greeting) but seemed to have little "social
sense." She appeared very awkward and ill at ease. We groped for something that
might interest and engage her and, knowing of her fascination with numbers,
decided to show her our new computer. We walked to the lab and decided to
demonstrate how quickly the machine could calculate. Before submitting a problem to the computer, we gave Elly paper and pencil so that she could perform the
calculation herself. We dictated the problem to her—a multiplication of two
three-digit numbers. Elly paused briefly and, without touching the pencil or paper, responded with a series of six numbers. Somewhat taken aback, we typed the
problem into the computer; it produced the same solution, at a speed not much
faster than Elly's. Unsure if we were to believe what we had seen, we gave Elly a
few more calculations, and in each successive case, she responded more quickly,
her answers unfailingly correct.

    This surprising display of facility in calculation, which stood in marked con-
trast to Elly's halting speech and fragmentary comprehension, was, for us, only
the most preliminary glimpse of Elly's exceptional capabilities. Before long, we
had witnessed many examples of her skill with numbers and rules and had learned
of her fascination for the creation and elaboration of systems involving number
and order. It became clear that at the root of these systems lay a remarkable
ability to induce the rules and regularities that characterized any set of items—
numbers, words, objects, or events. Elly not only induced these rules, she systematically and obsessively explored all of their possible applications. From numbers,
colors, and common objects she created complex, intricately ordered systems,
some of which she used, it seemed, to structure her world, and some of which she
merely played with, endlessly delighted by their order.

    Before we describe some of these systems, let us look back and see how these
abilities first emerged. As soon as she could manipulate objects and well before
she talked or counted, Elly was clearly fascinated by order and patterns.

> At two and three it had been blocks in parallel rows or a deck of cards made to stand
> vertical in the cracks between the floorboards, each card a neat half inch from the next.
> At age 4, it had been configurations of washcloths and cookies unerringly kept track of
> by a baby who had no words for number but who knew at once if any were missing,
> and how many. Elly could grasp an ordering principle with astonishing rapidity. She
> needed only to be presented with the opportunity to arrange objects by shape, color,
> and size, and later, by kind and function, and she would do so. (Park, 1967,
> p. 231–232)

At age 5, when Elly was using only a handful of words, she incorporated into her tiny vocabulary the terms "square," "triangle," and "hexagon." More interesting to her than birthday parties or friends was the fact of an ordered system of shapes—different labels corresponding to different numbers of sides. Elly knew "pentagon," "hexagon," "heptagon," and "octagon" well before she knew "sister" or "cousin" or could produce a simple sentence. She delighted in ordered systems wherever she found them and extrapolated rules as soon as she discovered them. Her mother describes teaching Elly, at age 8, that the plural of "man" is "men"; she had drawn pictures of one man and many to illustrate the concepts. She relates that "the next day, Elly, totally absorbed, produced five pictures of her own. One was a reproduction of my man–men original. Next came MAMA–MEME, illustrated, of course, by one mama and several, followed by DADDY–DEDDY, SARA–SERE, and MATT–METT, each illustrated with a single figure and a group" (Park, 1967, p. 243). From a single instance, Elly induced a pattern— "a" means one, "e" means many—and extended it to the world around her.

Elly's father, David Park, and Phillip Youderian have described the development of her mathematical ability and its application to the creation of elaborate ordered systems (Park & Youderian, 1974). We draw from their account for our description here of a few of Elly's remarkable abilities.

Elly first began to demonstrate an interest in numbers and arithmetic when she was 11 years old. Prior to that, her mother had worked with her at home, teaching her arithmetic up through fractions, knowledge that Elly acquired "unenthusiastically, but easily" (Park & Youderian, 1974, p. 314). At 11, however, she began calculating, especially factoring, endlessly and obsessively, apparently for her own pleasure. Numbers were, it seemed, more interesting than people, and relationships between numbers were rule-bound and predictable. It should be stressed that Elly's fascination with numbers was not simply the abstracted, distanced interest of a budding mathematician. Numbers were emotionally charged for her—potent embodiments of good and bad. As Park and Youderian (1974) recount, "Some she liked, some she hated. Cars whose license plates bore the number 75 were kicked ritually but with passion. Numbers changed without warning, amid the tears of real pain, from 'good,' as she put it, to 'hate' (p. 314). Some numbers were "too good" to utter and produced intense shivers of excitement."

Prime numbers were of particular interest to Elly; she spent days calculating all the ways of factoring a particular number. By age 13 she could list, on request, all the prime numbers from 1 to 1,000 and beyond. The primes as a class were invested with strong affective valence, but two prime integers, in particular, stood out among the rest: 7, a good number, and 3, a very bad one. Elly endlessly explored the composites and combinations of these numbers, working for hours on end, content in her abstract isolated world. She discovered, among many other things, that the delightful formal symmetry of the integer 10,001 could be generated unexpectedly by multiplying 73×137. This formal symmetry was used to produce integers possessing a duplicating structure, as in the following examples:

$$10,001 \times 137 \quad = 1,370,137$$
$$10,001 \times 7,003 = 70,037,003$$
$$10,001 \times 7,337 = 73,377,337$$

Elly correctly inferred that she could generate formal duplication without directly using the integer 10,001 but by embedding its factors in her calculations:

$$37 \times 37 \quad = 1,369$$
$$1,369 \times 73 \quad = 99,937$$
$$99,937 \times 137 = 13,691,369 \text{ (formal duplication)}$$

Elly also found that she could encrypt selected integers within her duplicating structures by the formation of composites and then retrieve the original digits in a delightfully altered form by further manipulations:

$$13,691,369 \times 53 = 725,642,557 \text{ (53 is encrypted)}$$
$$725,642,557 \div 37 = 19,611,961 \text{ (a formal duplication)}$$
$$19,611,961 \div 37 = 530,053 \text{ (53 appears in duplicate!)}$$

These were the sorts of calculations that Elly performed for days and weeks and months on end. Wherever there were patterns, however complex or subtle, Elly discovered them; wherever instances adhered to some underlying rule, that rule was induced. On her own she discovered a means of telling at a glance how many ways a number could be factored. She explored her world of numbers until it had become for her predictable and ordered.

Intrigued by these anecdotal accounts of Elly's calculation and inferential abilities, we sought to explore her skills more systematically. We wanted to know whether her uncanny ability to detect regularities and rules was limited to the domain of numbers or whether it extended further. We chose some tasks that were language based and others that used visual patterns.

Because Elly's language skills were still limited—her speech agrammatical, her comprehension impaired for complex messages—we began with a "nonverbal" test, Raven's Progressive Matrices. This test, which contains a series of problems graded in difficulty, is designed to measure an individual's aptitude for abstraction and rule induction. The problems are presented visually and require little instruction. Each problem consists of a pattern or matrix from which a piece is missing; the subject is given a set of alternatives and must choose the piece that completes the whole. Simple problems consist of a homogeneous pattern (e.g., a grid of dots) from which a piece has been "cut out." More difficult problems present patterns consisting of disparate elements related by subtle and complex rules; simultaneous variations on several different dimensions (e.g., shape, size, orientation) must be attended to in order to deduce the underlying regularities. Normal adult subjects find the solutions to initial problems quickly and easily; they falter and slow down for painstaking analysis as the problems become more complex.

Watching Elly perform this task, one might have thought that she had designed it in a moment of absorption. She needed no instruction and quickly began to turn the pages, pausing only to glance briefly at the patterns and to point immediately at the missing piece. We waited for her to slow down and falter. We waited in vain. Her response latencies to all but the few most difficult problems were under 5 seconds. She made errors on 3 of 60 problems, scoring well above the 95th percentile for "normal" adult subjects; all of her errors she quickly corrected when she was asked to try again and work more slowly. Her parents were not surprised; apparently she had performed similarly at age 11, when evaluated by a psychologist.

Given her level of performance, it was clear that the limits of Elly's abilities had not been tested. We ordered the Advanced Progressive Matrices, a set constructed specifically to assess the skills of gifted individuals. Again we watched with amazement as Elly turned the pages more quickly than we could consider the choices. Once again, she scored above the 95th percentile, this time being compared to graduate technical and medical students.

Given Elly's limited language skills, we wondered whether she actually knew and could articulate the rules governing patterns or whether she had somehow been able to guess which pieces would make the wholes "look right." We went back over the problems, asking Elly to explain her choices. Despite her stilted broken sentences, she was unfailingly able to name the relevant dimensions and features, to articulate the rules governing their progressive alterations, and to describe how an extrapolation of those rules generated the correct pattern. It was clear that to Elly these rules and regularities were obvious, self-evident in the designs themselves. She seemed puzzled that the solutions needed any explanations at all—as if we had asked her what shaped peg would best fit in a round hole.

Later we began, with low expectations, to explore Elly's verbal reasoning skills. We knew that she had not mastered the rules of the grammar sufficiently to consistently produce well-formed sentences. A test designed to delineate the nature of language deficits in language-impaired patients documented articulation difficulties, naming errors, comprehension problems, deficient prosody and fluency, and frank errors of grammar. More important, perhaps, we were well aware that Elly had great difficulty inferring the meaning of colloquial expressions, turns of phrase, aphorisms, and proverbs. Her interpretations were generally completely literal. "Strike while the iron is hot!" was interpreted as "Iron the clothes," and "Shallow brooks are noisy" as "Shallow brooks can splash a lot than deep brook." Even familiar turns of phrase were incomprehensible, unless their meaning had been explicitly taught. "What's new?" elicited responses such as "We have a new car," and "I feel blue" produced only stares of confusion.

It was clear to us, however, that much of our colloquial speech is not, in fact, rule bound but is determined by social convention. We knew also that Elly's failure to apply the "rules" of the language consistently might speak more to their lack of absolute regularity than to her inferential skills. We gave Elly one task that required her to formulate the similarities between different things (e.g., a dog and a lion, north and west, praise and punishment). Despite her language impairments, she scored above average for adults and could easily detect similar features, whether physical or functional.

Impressed by her success, we gave her a verbal analogies task: "Red is to color as circle is to _____,"; Then is to now as past is to _____,"; "Slow is to quickly as good is to _____." Elly produced the answers to such problems quickly and easily. She succeeded even with the items based on syntactic relations, for example, "Your is to my as yours is to _____." As long as the relations were rule-bound, she had no trouble inducing the relationships and applying the rules.

On her own, however, the regularities that Elly notes about language are different from ours. She is not likely to note that a particular person always exaggerates or puts on airs; rather, she is keenly attuned to structural similarities in words, enough so to create labeled categories. Words that are "fluffy in the middle," for example, are words like "motor," "water," and "robin," which contain a tall middle consonant surrounded by a symmetrical arrangement of vowels and short consonants. She has made lists of them. Other lists contain words with common roots or affixes, for example, "production," "reduction" "seduction," "conduction." Even before she could read, Elly spent hours poring over the dictionary finding regularities: shelf/shelves, elf/elves, and so forth.

Elly's bent to induce rules and extend their applications has even made her an inventor of terms. She speaks of "painto's," "spello's," "speako's," and "reado's." Of course. What could be more natural—or more characteristic of Elly? Type is to typo as paint is to _____. The blank must be filled. Elly could no more fail to apply a rule than a fish could fail to swim.

Exceptional Abilities and Deficits—Two Sides of the Same Coin?

In the end Elly presents us with a challenge. How can we explain these exceptional abilities, particularly against their background of severe and continuing impairments? As we have noted, too many autistic-like children demonstrate similar exceptional abilities to allow us to view Elly as a unique or isolated case. This repeated co-occurrence of deficits and special talents prompts us to consider the possibility that the two are tightly linked—that the exceptional abilities are, in a sense, the "flip side" of the characteristic autistic impairments. This possibility carries with it the intriguing corollary that "average," nonexceptional abilities are the price that most of us pay for overall "normal" cognitive and emotional functioning, that normal functioning places limits on the development and/or exercise of isolated exceptional abilities.

Review of Elly's Deficits

To consider this idea, let us look more closely at Elly's deficits—the realms in which her functioning is impaired—and sketch out the possible consequences of such impairments. Two major realms of deficiency were—and are—most striking. First is the sphere of social functioning. Even today, Elly has enormous difficulty reading and interpreting social cues. She, whose inferential skills are so impressive, cannot intuit whether particular actions or comments would be socially inappropriate. She does not discern that a listener might be bored, uninterested, or confused.

Elly has learned to behave in socially acceptable ways as she learns most things, that is, by memorizing rules or instances: It is not nice to scratch oneself in public, to draw attention to someone's handicaps, to interrupt a conversation. These rules must be learned one by one. They are not obvious to Elly. Social concepts such as embarrassment and envy are completely foreign and incomprehensible to her. They cannot easily be explained to one who does not feel them. Elly misses the social cues that normal 6-year-olds pick up with ease.

The second realm in which Elly was—and is—severely impaired is that of language. As a young child, she was essentially mute and uncomprehending. She began to acquire and retain words at about age 5, but the process of language development was slow and arduous. She learned with none of the ease and automaticity that characterize language acquisition in most children. For years the words and phrases were indistinct mumbled sounds, which were incomprehensible to strangers, and often to friends and family.

Even today, after many years of painstaking drill and study, Elly's speech resembles that of a foreigner struggling to gain control over an alien grammar. Discussing the relationship between a bat and a ball, she says, "They are both go with the baseball game"; explaining kitchen rules, she writes, "Never to put iron knives in the dishwasher." When the messages she seeks to convey are more complex, her grammar becomes more distorted and difficult to understand.

And what of Elly's comprehension? It is difficult to assess what Elly understood as a young child, since she did not respond to language in any way. Had she not reacted to the click of the dishwasher or the drop of a pin, her parents would have thought she was deaf. Elly's responsiveness to language, like her expressive abilities, has developed slowly. Her ability to comprehend is still impaired today, although she generally functions reasonably well by understanding individual words and their probable meaning in combination. Her ability to understand verbal messages is compromised by two separate deficits—one involving syntax and the other, pragmatics.

Elly's difficulties in decoding syntax are subtle; they become clear only when the meaning of a sentence depends critically on grammatical elements—functors such as "from," "by," and "for," or markers of tense or number. She confuses, for example, the meanings of sentences such as "Food is bought by the man" and "Food is bought from the man." She has difficulty when sentences become long and contain complex grammatical clauses, for example, "The dog whom the cat chased won the race with the squirrel."

At present, however, Elly's ability to comprehend verbal messages seems more compromised by her difficulties in grasping pragmatic constraints than by her syntactic deficits. Clearly, the meaning of a sentence often depends on much more than the meaning of the words and the grammatical rules that connect them. Linguistic and social conventions, social context, tone of voice, and facial expression are some of the factors that must be considered in interpreting a message. "You're some friend!", for example, has two diametrically opposed meanings, depending on the tone of voice. "I'm starting to feel cold" often means "Would you please close that window?" "How are you?" calls for different responses, depending both on the speaker (friend vs. stranger) and on the sentence prosody.

Elly, not surprisingly, is lost in this domain of pragmatics. She interprets statements literally, unable to decode the social cues or to understand the speaker's motivations. She has learned through explicit instruction the proper responses to some conventional phrases (e.g., "How are you?" "Fine!") but cannot master all the subtle context-dependent cues. Elly has also learned the meanings of some common sayings and turns of phrase and uses these gleefully as useful shorthands; she explains, " 'You're treading on thin ice!' means 'Watch out! Might get in trouble.' Ice might break." The meaning of each of these sayings has been explicitly taught; Elly is unable to infer their meanings from the contexts in which they are used.

Elly's most striking deficits, then, relate to language and social functioning. She cannot easily read social cues, has not mastered social conventions, and does not understand complex social motivations or effects. She has difficulty decoding syntax and fails to grasp the pragmatic aspects of language use. These impairments have clearly been central to Elly's "disability" since early childhood.

Deficits and Their Likely Consequences

In trying to understand the basis for Elly's exceptional abilities, it seems useful to consider the likely consequences of her impairments—both their immediate effects and the indirect effects of Elly's struggle to cope.

We think that many, if not all, of her talents can best be understood as "by-products" of her impairments. While clearly speculative, the relationships we posit seem to make sense of this paradoxical pattern of great strengths and weaknesses.[1]

For a child unable to read social cues or understand verbal messages, the world can only be an overwhelming, frighteningly unpredictable place. The child is bombarded by a constant barrage of sounds and sights that cannot be made manageable by the imposition of meaning. Events and interchanges cannot be consolidated and coded in terms of intents or effects; it is not possible to condense the welter of information by "getting the point." Things that people do or say make no sense; there is constant confusion.

---

1. It is fascinating to ponder possible causes of these impairments and to ask whether they might be related in some way. The rules of social interchange are clearly subtle and context-dependent; what is acceptable in one situation is totally unacceptable in another. Pragmatic aspects of language are similarly context-dependent and require the interpretation of subtle social cues. We might ask, How do we—most of us—acquire a sense of social appropriateness, master the rules of social intercourse, and learn to read social cues? The process is surely complex and poorly understood, but one point is obvious—we learn by participating in and observing social interactions. We watch what people do and gauge the reactions of others. We try our hand in the social arena—and learn quickly through our failures. Elly, of course, did none of this. She did not socialize with others. She did not seek the affection or approval of her parents or peers. Elly was a nonsocial being from early childhood on, alone in the midst of a bustling household. We learn early, through experience, the basic rules of social interchange and the keys to decoding expressions, shrugs, and sighs, but Elly did not. Locked in her own world, Elly also did not attend to the linguistic communications of others. Her difficulties with syntax are strikingly similar to those of a child who was literally locked away from others during early childhood (see *Genie* by Susan Curtiss, 1977). This similarity raises the possibility that childhood exposure and attention to language may be necessary for the "automatic" acquisition of syntax characteristic of normal development.

How might such a child cope? Useful strategies seem clear: (1) Focus on nonsocial, physical attributes of the world, which can be understood and predicted; (2) attempt to order the confusion around you by noting regularities and patterns; (3) cling to routine, to sameness, wherever and whenever possible, to ensure predictability; (4) explore rule-governed systems, like the realm of mathematics, fully and obsessively, to produce a sense of predictability and control; (5) create your own completely rule-governed systems and use them to order your world.

Such strategies might explain many of Elly's behaviors, but can they explain her exceptional skills? We think that they can, when viewed in conjunction with the impairments themselves. For a child who cannot appreciate "the point" of an event or conversation, there is no way to consolidate and interpret information. The "raw data"—the physical details and actual words—are retained because they are not "processed" en route to meaning, to be discarded later as unnecessary, once the point has been derived. Many small physical details are remembered because it is they, rather than the social interchanges, that are the primary focus of attention. Some bits of information are particularly attended to or rehearsed because they relate to things the individual greatly cares about—order, patterns, predictability.

Consider Elly's mathematical feats, for example. Were they really so extraordinary? If a "normal" child has spent years of her life focusing on numbers and performing calculations day in and day out, would she not have begun to note certain regularities and induce general rules? And what of Elly's remarkable ease in discerning the patterns and rules inherent in complex visual arrays? Is it too farfetched to imagine that this is the result of practicing a general skill infinitely more intensely and persistently than others? Elly is, after all, the child of two extremely bright professors; surely her "native endowment" includes a general quickness to learn and retain information in realms not compromised by her disabilities.

If these possibilities seem plausible, then it is not Elly's abilities themselves that are extraordinary but the ends toward which they are put. It is not her calculation skills that are most striking but her obsession with calculation. It is not her memory for prime numbers that is astounding but her single-minded dedication to exploring them. It is not her recall of tiny details that is remarkable but the fact that she should focus on them.

It seems noteworthy that as Elly has progressed and become more "normal," her exceptional abilities are much less in evidence. When she is asked about details of past events, Elly often reports that she "can't remember." When queried about prime numbers, she cannot always recall the pertinent facts. She can, when she concentrates, still attend intensely to her physical environment. But her mind is on other things.

Rules of order no longer completely dominate Elly's life. She still cares deeply about systems and what *should* happen according to some rule, but she can practice "being flexible." She spends little time alone devising complex rule-governed universes, preferring to spend time with family and friends. She still notes regularities and catalogs patterns wherever they exist but more as a hobby than as a passion.

Thus it seems that as Elly has become more like the rest of us, both her weaknesses and her strengths have been moderated. She is no longer a child locked in a world of her own and no longer a nonsocial being. She is a young woman with friends and social interests—and less need or time for creating and cataloging order.

References

Curtiss, S. (1977). *Genie: A psycholinguistic study of a modern-day "wild child."* New York: Academic Press.

Park, C. C. (1967). *The Siege: The first eight years of an autistic child.* New York: Harcourt, Brace, and World.

Park, D. & Youderian, P. (1974). Light and number: Ordering principles in the world of an autistic child. *Journal of Autism and Childhood Schizophrenia, 4,* 313–323.

14

Case Study of a Musical "Mono-savant": A Cognitive–Psychological Focus

NEIL CHARNESS
JANE CLIFTON
LYLE MacDONALD

The Mono-savant and Intelligence

The phenomenon of the "idiot savant" has attracted the interest of psychologists for many years but particularly following the rise of the concept of intelligence and the successful marketing of intelligence tests. An "idiot savant" is usually defined as someone with very low intelligence who is highly skilled at a single activity. The term has also been extended to cover autistic children with unusual ability (e.g., Rimland, 1978). Usually, "highly skilled" means that the skill is exercised at a level markedly greater than that of a normally intelligent adult in the culture. Because of the perjorative aspect of the term "idiot" in "idiot savant," we have decided to coin the term "mono-savant," meaning a mentally retarded person with highly developed skills in (and knowledge of) one domain.

"Intelligence" is a term that few people can agree upon, as evidenced by the diversity of approaches to studying it, for example, Resnick (1976), and the attempts to redefine and restructure the concept by Sternberg (1977) and Gardner (1983). We are going to take "intelligence" to mean learning ability, because this feature seems to be what motivates the investigation of mono-savants. The mono-savant is a paradoxical individual, since low intelligence-test scores and the relative lack of ability to acquire the life skills that are valued in society stand in sharp contrast to the finely honed single skill that the individual has acquired. We intend to address two central questions with our case study: (1) Does the mono-savant represent information about his or her skill in the same way as an intellectually normal person? (2) How can a mentally retarded person acquire a highly developed skill?

The mono-savant is of interest to neuropsychologists because usually there is evidence of brain damage in the mono-savant's case history, though the evidence is

Neil Charness and Jane Clifton. Department of Psychology, University of Waterloo, Waterloo, Ontario, Canada.
Lyle MacDonald. Algoma District Mental Retardation Service, Sault Ste. Marie, Ontario, Canada.

often circumstantial, for example, retrospective reports of birth trauma or of epilepsy. We are reporting the case of a musical mono-savant, J. L., who has definite clinical evidence of damage to the left cerebral hemisphere. Since the talents exhibited by mono-savants involve functions usually associated with the right cerebral hemisphere (e.g., music, art, mechanical ability), it is of interest to examine their performance in detail. The attempt to localize musical function in the cortex via these cases is risky at best. In many cases the time of the apparent injury is unclear, and if the damage occurred early enough, there is the question of possible reorganization of function.

One case history in the popular press (Blank, 1982; Monty, 1981) portrays the musical mono-savant as someone who sat around listlessly, exhibiting no apparent talent, until suddenly, in the middle of the night, he sat down in front of a piano and started to play whole concertos flawlessly. That is, the mono-savant is seen as someone with mysterious powers, who acquires skill in ways quite different from those of normally intelligent people. This sudden appearance of a high degree of skill or of a rapid-acquisition function is counter to the rule of thumb in cognitive psychology that a complex skill can be acquired only after many hundreds or thousands of hours of practice (Bryan & Harter, 1899; Ericsson & Faivre, Chapter 24, this volume; Lindsay & Norman, 1977; Simon & Chase, 1973). The contrast between poor general learning ability and the alleged rapid skill learning leads some theorists to question whether intelligence is a unitary construct (as in the case of the g factor of Spearman) or whether there are multiple intelligences (Gardner, 1983), each calling on specialized neural circuitry.

The Case of J. L.

The musical mono-savant whom we have studied, J. L., is a 36-year-old severely mentally retarded man, institutionalized from age 15 on. Testing shows no known chromosomal abnormalities. He was born about $2\frac{1}{2}$ months premature. (During a recent interview, his parents reported that he was more premature than is indicated in the medical case history, namely, that he was born at 6 months). His mother is reported to have had three miscarriages before him and one subsequently.

J. L. suffered from retrolental fibroplasia (probably induced by excessive oxygen given to him following his premature birth), which rendered him blind since infancy. His right eye was enucleated when he was 28. In addition to blindness, J. L. has suffered from severe epilepsy since age 6. (His parents now report he suffered his first episode at age 4). At the time of testing, he was experiencing an average of one grand mal seizure per month, usually going into status epilepticus, requiring intravenous administration of anticonvulsant medication. He also received daily administrations of Tegretol and Mysoline. J. L. is also moderate right spastic hemiplegic (onset reported at age $2\frac{1}{2}$ years, though his parents now report that he was always spastic). A series of EEG examinations reveal excessive slow-wave and spiking activity in the left hemisphere.

J. L.'s verbal communication skills are relatively poor, with frequent echolalia (automatic repetition of other speakers' words) and perseveration. To the extent that it is possible to test someone as severely retarded as J. L., his hearing (both ears) appears to be normal. He has no concept of money or time telling and does not know when he needs assistance. He is unable to brush his teeth, shave, or comb his hair, but he can dress himself, wash his face and hands unsupervised (the result of about a 1-year behavior modification program), and self-initiate his toileting. Although able to feed himself with a spoon with prompting, J. L. cannot tell when his bowl or plate is empty and will continue to go through the motions of feeding himself.

With respect to cognitive skills, J. L. is unable to discriminate correctly, through touch, a circle, square, and triangle, nor does he understand the concept of big and small. He does participate in a prevocational training program a few hours per day, and at the time of testing he was able to sort two objects, thread a nut on a large bolt with the help of a jig, and assemble a three-piece ball-point pen. He is virtually untestable with standard instruments such as the WAIS, though he was able to repeat five digits forward (none backwards). He did repeat a six-digit string but had some of the digits out of order. His relatively intact forward digit span is consistent with the finding by Spitz and LaFontaine (1973) that mono-savants have digit spans larger than those of the mentally retarded population as a whole. Although J. L. is virtually untestable on most standardized instruments, a rough estimate in terms of the types of activities given in the Vineland Social Maturity Scale is that he is at the development level of a 2-year-old.

Early Development

A recent interview with his parents revealed that J. L. never crawled and had trouble learning to walk, doing so at $2\frac{1}{2}$ to 3 years. He started playing with the piano in his home at around age 3. He never had any formal instruction in music, although his family was musically oriented. The family used to hold sing–songs; his mother's sisters were in a band, and his uncle played trumpet. His grandmother played piano skillfully enough to give concerts. J. L. started to talk at about age 3 and exhibited what his parents termed "parrot" speech, repeating words. Though blind, J. L. was good at recognizing people by their voices.

J. L.'s grandmother played piano with him and encouraged him to practice, though evidently did not instruct him formally. His parents report that initially he was not very good at the piano, but he practiced for many hours, even getting up in the middle of the night to play. He is reported to have spent practically all day at the piano. He listened to records of all types, big bands, semiclassics, Irish folk tunes. He also listened to the radio a great deal. He improved tremendously over the years.

Although J. L. appears to be emotionally flat in normal interaction, he does seem to enjoy playing music and is quite reluctant to leave the music room following our studies, even after hours of playing. He does exhibit a sense of humor over the keyboard. His parents relate a story of him listening to someone play a familiar tune badly on the piano. J. L. went over to the keyboard and played the same wrong notes, laughing, and then played the melody the correct way. It is difficult to assess how much encouragement J. L. received for playing music. If a recent statement by his parents is any guide ("J. L.'s music ability gives him a reason for living"), he probably had considerable external as well as internal motivation for practicing.

Music Skills

J. L. is highly skilled at playing keyboard instruments with his good left hand, and he uses his left foot to play both piano and organ pedals. (When we have played a tape of his performance informally to naive listeners, they are always surprised to find out that he plays with one hand.) He can play the piano, organ (learned 5 or 6 years ago), melodica, and harmonica, and strum a guitar. He exibits absolute pitch in that when a tune or chord is played, he can reproduce the same notes on the piano or organ with little hesitation. He very occasionally transposes the notes or chord to a different octave. He has developed rather ingenious fingering techniques for the piano and organ such that he can produce the melody and harmony lines for pieces, although he has to engage in some digital gymnastics to do so. His playing features fine attention to rhythmic nuances, inclusion of embellishments, and attention to the dynamics of a vast array of different musical genres, including Broadway musicals, jazz, classical music, opera, and popular music.

His repertoire of known pieces seems to be quite large. He seems to have some of them indexed by name as well as by sound. Thus, if you ask him to play the *William Tell* Overture, "The Moonlight Sonata," or Carol King's "Tapestry," he can usually do so. If you hum or whistle the tune from a piece, he can then play the piece. It is difficult to judge how well he knows a piece, that is, how faithfully he reproduces the notes of a score, because of the modifications he makes to accommodate to one-handed playing.

When he plays spontaneously, J. L. often cannot report the name of the piece he is playing or has an idiosyncratic name for it. He is quite good at shadowing or playing with another pianist on the same keyboard. He is also able to join in jazz improvisation. He will also hum or sing some of the words to the songs that he plays and seems more fluent at this than at normal speech. He occasionally imitates other instruments (e.g., trumpet) or vocalists (e.g., Louis Armstrong) with his singing. He usually sings in a very high pitched voice that is markedly different from his normal speaking voice, perhaps to maintain the same absolute pitch as the original recording, since in many cases he is imitating female vocalists.

J. L. is quite capable of transposing a piece to a different key in order to accommodate another pianist sitting with him at the same keyboard or to avoid a nonfunctioning key on the piano in his ward. He can also improvise imitations of styles of playing, such as playing a piece in "boogie-woogie" style, or insert elaborations, such as trills, into a classical piece. In short, his virtuosity at the keyboard is quite out of line with his everyday level of functioning in the institution.

How does J. L. manage to deal so effectively with the vocabulary of music when functioning so poorly with his native language of English? The discrepancy must be due, at least in part, to the localization of language functions in the left hemisphere and to J. L.'s documented left-hemisphere damage. Marin (1982), in a thoughtful review of the neurological aspects of music, points out that there are many cases indicating that language functioning could be impaired by brain damage with virtually complete sparing of musical functioning, so-called aphasia without amusia. There are also many cases of the reverse: amusia without aphasia. However, there are also cases of aphasia with accompanying amusia, and there is some conflicting literature on the lateralization of musical processes (see also Judd, Chapter 6, this volume), suggesting that for skilled musicians the left hemisphere is more deeply involved in music processing, whereas for less skilled people music is processed more effectively in the right hemisphere.

In the literature on mono-savants, the suggestion has been made that the mono-savant represents the case of a "tape-recorder" type of performance. That is, the mono-savant is unable to abstract information but rather deals with it literally, implying a sensory or perceptual encoding of domain-related information. That musical mono-savants are frequently found to possess absolute pitch tends to support this tape-recorder notion. Skilled people, on the other hand, generally are more likely to represent domain-related information in a hierarchical structure, nesting low-level information under general abstract principles that represent elaborate recodings of the stimulus material (see Charness, Chapter 22, and Ericsson & Faivre, Chapter 24, this volume). As outlined in the Charness chapter on expertise, skilled musicians are not better than their less skilled counterparts on all music tasks but only on those that allow them to tap their knowledge of chord and melody conventions. We attempted to discover whether J. L. represents information about music literally or, as do normal musicians, in a structure that reflects the conventions of Western tonal music.

To determine whether J. L. represents musical knowledge in a manner similar to that of other skilled individuals, two types of musical recall tasks were administered. In one set of tasks (Experiment 1), J. L.'s recall of melodies and his sensitivity to melodic structure were assessed. In the second set (Experiments 2a and 2b), J. L.'s chord recall was examined to determine whether he was sensitive to common harmonic structures or simply recalled chords as collections of unrelated notes. All experiments were carried out in the music room at J. L.'s institution.

Experiment 1: Assessing J. L.'s Recall of Melodies

Deutsch (1980) found that skilled musicians could recall and transcribe 12-note melodies more accurately when the sequences followed certain structural rules and were temporally grouped in accordance with that structure than when they were not structured or not appropriately temporally grouped. Deutsch's structured sequences can be economically described as a hierarchical set of patterns. A lower level pattern of 3 or 4 notes is repeated on each element of a higher order sequence. The elements of a sequence are chosen from an alphabet such as a major scale or the elements of a triad. Examples of structured and unstructured sequences are shown in Figure 14-1.

Preliminary work showed that J. L.'s reproduction of brief melodies was perfect for melodies of up to 5 notes and that he could recall some melodies of as many as 8 notes perfectly. Thus his note span is between 5 and 8 notes. All studies

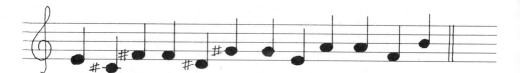

Sequence structured in groups of three

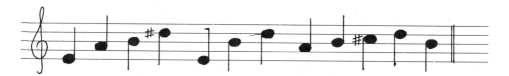

Unstructured sequence

FIGURE 14-1. Examples of structured and unstructured melodic sequences.

of J. L.'s musical ability have used reproduction, or playing what he has heard, as the index of recall, since J. L. did not seem capable of understanding other recall or recognition tasks. We predicted that if J. L. were sensitive to musical structure of the type described by Deutsch, he would be able to reproduce longer sequences of notes if they are structured. We also predicted that J. L.'s recall performance on structured and unstructured sequences would be influenced by temporal grouping in a manner similar to the recall of the skilled musicians in Deutsch (1980). In addition, the effects of familiar and unfamiliar musical alphabets on recall were compared in this study.

Method

STIMULI

Eighty-eight sequences from 3 to 24 notes in length were generated. Half of the sequences of each length were based on a conventional E-major scale, and half were based on a less common E whole-tone scale. These alphabets were chosen because the proportion of black notes in each (4 out of 7 and 3 out of 6, respectively) were similar. Half of the sequences longer than 4 notes were structured, and half were unstructured. Structured sequences were constructed similarly to those used by Deutsch. Temporal grouping was effected by introducing a pause between otherwise equally spaced notes. The duration of such pauses was about equal to the duration of a note in the sequence. Sequences of 12 or 24 notes could be unstructured or structured in groups of three or four. They could be temporally grouped in threes or fours or not at all. Thus some sequences were temporally grouped in accordance with structure, and some were temporally grouped in conflict with structure. A detailed breakdown of the types of sequences is shown in Table 4-1.

TABLE 14-1. Types of Sequences Used in the Melody Span Task

Length:	3	4	6	8	12	16	18	24
Number:	4	4	8	8	24	8	8	24

Lengths	Sequences types			
3,4	W;W;M;M			
6,18	W;US,NTG;	M,US,NTG		
	W,US,TG3;	M,US,TG3		
	W,S3,NTG;	M,S3,NTG		
	W,S3,TG3;	M,S3,TG3		
8,16	W,US,NTG;	M,US,NTG		
	W,US,TG4;	M,US,TG4		
	W,S4,NTG;	M,S4,NTG		
	W,S4,TG4;	M,S4,TG4		
12,24	W,US,NTG;	M,US,NTG;	W,S3,TG3;	M,S3,TG3
	W,US,NTG;	M,US,NTG;	W,S3,TG4;	M,S3,TG4
	W,US,TG3;	M,US,TG3;	W,SE,NTG;	M,S3,NTG
	W,US,TG3;	M,US,TG3;	W,S4,TG4;	M,S4,TG4
	W,US,TG4;	M,US,TG4;	W,S4,TG3;	M,S4,TG3
	W,US,TG4;	M,US,TG4;	W,S4,NTG;	M,S4,NTG

Note. Symbols: W, whole-tone-scale alphabet; M, major-scale Alphabet; US, unstructured; NTG, not temporally grouped; S4, structured in groups of four; S3, structured in groups of three; TG3, temporally grouped in threes; TG4, temporally grouped in fours.

PROCEDURE

Stimuli were played on a Yamaha organ in the music room and recorded on tape. Notes within a sequence were played at a rate of 2 per second, except when pauses were introduced for temporal grouping. J. L. later heard each taped sequence once and attempted to reproduce it on the same instrument. His hand on the keys was videotaped, so that his responses could be scored later. Sequences were presented in ascending order of length, and order of presentation was randomized within lengths. J. L. was permitted to warm up by first playing ad lib for a few minutes.

Results

J. L.'s responses on sequences up to and including a length of 6 notes were perfect. On sequences of 8 notes he recalled 2 of 8 sequences completely correctly, and on the remaining 6 he made one or two errors, for example, omitting or repeating a note. On sequences of 12 notes he was completely correct on 3 of 24 sequences. These 3 were structured sequences in which the temporal grouping agreed with the structure. J. L. was not correct on any sequences longer than 12 notes, and testing was discontinuted during the 24-note sequences. His performance on sequences longer than 12 notes was not analyzed. (As a control, we also had another ear-trained musician on staff attempt the same tasks as J. L., telling him the starting note for the sequences in order to control for his lack of absolute pitch. He had great difficulty doing this as well as the chord task that followed, replaying many notes, with a span of around 4 notes if corrections were allowed.)

Two scoring systems were used to assess J. L.'s performance on 12-note sequences. The first system was similar to the procedure used by Deutsch (1980): Pitches correctly recalled in their correct serial positions yielded a percentage correct for each sequence. The percentage recall for each condition is shown in Table 14-2. The results from the analogous conditions in Deutsch's study are shown for comparison.

A single-factor, unweighted means analysis of variance (ANOVA) was performed on J. L.'s recall of four types of sequences. The first type was temporally grouped congruent sequences with structure (e.g., structured in 3's and temporally grouped in 3's). The second type consisted of sequences with temporal grouping incongruent with structure (e.g., structured in 4's but temporally grouped in 3's). The third type consisted of structured sequences that were not temporally grouped. The fourth type consisted of all of the unstructured sequences combined across temporal grouping.

The effect of sequence was reliable, $F(3, 20) = 5.11$, $p < .01$. Tukey tests on the means showed that J. L.'s performance on structured sequences with congruent temporal grouping was significantly better ($p < .05$) than his performance on unstructured sequences and structured sequences with incongruent temporal grouping. Structured sequences with no temporal grouping were intermediate in performance and did not differ reliably from any of the other groups.

J. L.'s percentages correct on major-scale and whole-tone sequences were 51% and 35%, respectively. Although this difference is not reliable, J. L. was not insensitive to alphabet. His responses rarely included notes outside the appropriate alphabet, even for sequences he could not recall. There were only 3 notes played in the entire session that were extraneous to the alphabet of the sequence being tested. J. L. appeared to be familiar with both alphabets.

J. L.'s performance on a reproduction task was in many ways analogous to the performance of skilled musicians on a transcription recall task. Unlike Deutsch's

TABLE 14-2. J. L.'s Performance on 12-Note Sequences

Sequence type	Number of items	Percentage of correct notes	Chunk score percent correct	Percentage of correct notes (Deutsch, 1980)
Structured, congruent temporal grouping	4	85.4[a]	77.5[a]	90.7
Structured, no temporal grouping	4	47.9[ab]	47.5[ab]	93.5
Structured, incongruent temporal grouping	4	31.2[b]	40.0[ab]	56.4
Unstructured	12	31.2[b]	14.2[b]	59.2

Note. Means within a column that share a common superscript letter do not differ at the .05 level (Tukey test). The Deutsch (1980) column represents averaged results from analogous conditions for her Experiments 1 and 2.

subjects, however, J. L. could not be expected to know that each sequence contained 12 tones, and his responses sometimes contained more or less than this number. The first scoring system used was insensitive to instances in which J. L. omitted or added a note in a sequence but recalled a large chunk of the original sequence displaced from the appropriate serial position. An alternative scoring system was used, in which J. L. was allotted a point for a group of 3 adjacent notes correctly recalled from the sequence, regardless of the serial position of the group of notes. Each note of the group or chunk above 3 was given a point. Thus a perfectly recalled sequence would yield ten points.

An ANOVA on the chunk scores obtained using the second scoring system yielded a reliable effect of sequence type, $F(3, 20) = 4.17$, $p < .025$. The means are shown in Table 14-2. Tukey tests showed a reliable difference between the sequences temporally grouped congruent with their structure and the unstructured sequences. Performance on structured sequences with no temporal grouping and on structured sequences with incongruent temporal grouping was intermediate, and these groups did not differ reliably from any others. Using the chunk scoring system had little effect, except possibly to indicate that J. L. recalled more of the structured sequences with incongruent temporal grouping than is indicated by the percentage of notes recalled in correct serial position.

Discussion

J. L. is clearly sensitive to musical structure and can reproduce structured patterns better than random arrangements of notes. His recall of structured sequences is strongly enhanced by appropriate temporal grouping. This effect may be more marked than that found by Deutsch for three reasons. First, in Deutsch's study only 12-note sequences were presented, whereas in our study shorter sequences had been presented earlier in the testing session. Thus, without temporal grouping, with a weak expectation of sequence length, it might be more difficult for anyone to recall exactly 12 notes and to pin down the serial positions of the chunks recalled.

Second, reproduction, in contrast to transcription, leaves no permanent record of how many notes have been recalled. Both of the explanations of J. L.'s sensitivity to temporal grouping of structured sequences can be examined by testing skilled musicians. We would predict that randomization of sequence lengths would be detrimental to the recall of structured sequences without appropriate temporal grouping to clearly mark the number of notes. In addition, requesting reproduction rather than transcription, while detrimental to performance levels in general, should be particulary damaging to performance on structured sequences with inappropriate or no temporal grouping.

A third explanation of J. L.'s sensitivity to temporal grouping is not concerned with how the methodology used reduces the probability of recalling the correct number of notes and placing the recalled chunks correctly. It seems probable that J. L. relies on small temporal groups to produce recalls of the appropriate length and uses no other cues or strategies for generating enough notes. Thus J. L. would be particularly hurt by the absence of temporal groups.

It is not clear how J. L responds to the musical alphabet. He seems to be quite capable even with an unfamiliar alphabet. It is possible, however, that he recalls a note set rather than a whole-tone scale. This could be further tested by using a larger number of alphabets in a session, thus preventing him from learning an unfamiliar alphabet in the course of a session.

Experiment 2a: Assessing J. L.'s Recall of Chords

In most studies of skill it has been found that skilled individuals recall meaningful or conventional domain-specific materials better than meaningless or unconventional material (e.g., see Charness, Chapter 22, this volume). This is in contrast to the belief that mono-savants have little or no abstraction capability and tend to recall everything within their skill domain exactly and concretely. In the first of two experiments on chord recall, J. L.'s memory for conventional and unconventional chords was compared.

Method

STIMULI AND PROCEDURE

We prepared 30 conventional and 30 unconventional 4-note chords. There were several types of conventional chords. Major and minor chords, with the bottom note repeated an octave higher, were included. In addition, dominant seventh and supertonic seventh chords were included. These contain the same notes as major and minor triads, respectively, but instead of repeating one of the chord notes in a different octave, a note is added a minor seventh above the root of the triad. Unconventional chords were created by altering any nonduplicated note of a chord by a semitone, with the restriction that the alteration not yield a conventional chord. The unconventional chords sound dissonant to a Western listener. Chords could be presented in any inversion, and several keys were used. The order of chord presentation was randomized, with the constraint that no more than 3 conventional or unconventional chords appeared successively.

Chords were recorded on the same instrument used in Experiment 1. J. L. heard each chord and attempted to reproduce it on the organ. His responses were videotaped.

Results and Discussion

J. L. was completely correct on 21 of the 59 scorable chord trials. On 31 of the 42 chords that spanned an octave, however, he omitted the top note, which is the same as the bottom note but an octave higher. This type of error does not change many of the characteristics of the chord, in that every note chroma or note name present in the original is present in the response. When responses that included all the appropriate chroma and no others were scored as correct, J. L. was correct on 55 of the 59 chords, responding in a parsimonious manner suitable for one-handed adaptations. J. L.'s performance on conventional and unconventional chords did not differ. There were no differences between the mean times to reproduce conventional and unconventional chords: The means were 2.00 and 1.99 seconds, respectively. Since J. L.'s span for unrelated notes is about 6, differences between conventional and unconventional chords might not be expected to emerge since each chord contained only 4 notes.

Experiment 2b: A Supplementary Test of J. L.'s Recall of Chords

In this experiment we examined J. L.'s performance on sets of 2, 3, and 4 sequentially presented 4-note chords (containing 8, 12, and 16 notes).

Method

STIMULI AND PROCEDURE

We generated 108 chord sets varying on two factors of three levels each. The first factor was chord-set size. Of the 108 chord sets, 36 contained 2 chords, 36 contained 3 chords, and 36 contained 4 chords. The second factor was chord-set type. The first 36 of the chord sets contained conventional chords with a common tonal center, referred to as "conventional related sets." The second 36 sets contained conventional chords with no common tonal center, referred to as "conventional unrelated sets." The final 36 sets consisted of unconventional chords that did not, being unconventional, have a common tonal center. These are referred to as "unconventional sets." The types of chords used in the conventional sets differed slightly from those used in Experiment 2a. Major, minor, and dominant seventh chords were used, but diminished seventh chords were used rather than the supertonic seventh chords. As in Experiment 2a, unconventional chords were generated by altering a nonduplicated note of a conventional chord by a semitone.

The procedure followed that of Experiment 2a, with the constraint that within a chord set, a chord was played every 1.5 seconds.

Results

A sequence was scored correct if all the chords within it were correct according to the scoring system adopted in Experiment 2a. Thus, if all note chroma present in the original chord were present in the response, and if there were no extra chroma, a chord was considered correct. Because of difficulties in determining J. L.'s reponse from the videotape, 4 of the 108 chord sets were dropped from the analyses.

A 3×3 unweighted means ANOVA was performed. Chord-set size varied from 2 to 4 chords. The types of chord sets were related unconventional chords, unrelated conventional chords, and unconventional chords. There was a highly significant effect of set size, $F(2, 95) = 16.41$, $p < .001$. Recall decreased with increasing set size. The effect of set type was reliable, $F(2, 95) = 4.08$, $p < .025$; sets of unconventional chords were recalled more poorly than sets containing related or unrelated conventional chords. The results of the analysis are shown in Table 4-3.

TABLE 14-3. J. L.'s Performance on Chord Sets

Number of chords in a chord set	Chord-set type—percent correct		
	Related conventional	Unrelated conventional	Unconventional
2	75.7 (9/12)	83.3 (10/12)	45.4 (5/11)
3	54.6 (6/11)	33.3 (4/12)	10.0 (1/10)
4	16.7 (2/12)	8.3 (1/12)	8.3 (1/12)

Note. Parentheses contain the proportions for scorable trials.

A separate analysis showed no reliable differences between conventional related chord sets and conventional unrelated chord sets.

A 2×4 unweighted means ANOVA was performed in which J. L.'s responses to single chords were included in addition to his responses to larger chord sets. The first factor was set type, which had two levels. Single conventional chords, related conventional chord sets, and unrelated conventional chord sets were combined and considered to be conventional chord sets. The second factor was set size, which varied from 1 to 4 chords.

Trend analysis was performed on the set-size main effect and on the interaction of set size and set type. J. L.'s recall performance on single chords, regardless of type, was high. Enlarging the chord sets decreased J. L.'s performance and eventually would be expected to decrease performance to similar floor levels on both conventional and unconventional chord sets. If J. L's performance on unconventional sets falls at smaller set sizes than his performance on conventional sets, the quadratic component of the Set Size × Set Type interaction would be significant. This quadratic component reflects the difference in degree and direction of curvature in the set-size effect for the conventional and unconventional chord sets.

There was a significant effect of set type, $F(1, 155) = 9.84$, $p < .01$. Conventional chord sets were better recalled than unconventional chord sets. The linear component of the set-size effect was reliable, $F(1, 155) = 104.55$, $p < .01$, and accounted for 98% of the variability due to set size. No other components of the set-size effect

TABLE 14-4. J. L.'s Recall of Conventional and Unconventional Chord Sets

Set size	Chord-set type—percent correct	
	Conventional	Unconventional
1 chord	96.6[a] (28/29)	90.0[a] (27/30)
2 chords	79.2[a] (19/24)	45.5[ab] (5/11)
3 chords	43.5[ab] (10/23)	10.0[b] (1/10)
4 chords	12.5[b] (3/24)	8.3[b] (1/12)

Note. Means sharing a common superscript do not differ at the .01 level (Tukey test). Parentheses indicate proportions for scorable trials.

were significant. J. L.'s performance decreased as set size increased from 1 to 4 chords.

The trend analysis of the Set Type × Set Size interaction yielded a reliable quadratic component, $F(1, 155) = 5.14$, $p < .05$, which accounted for 99% of the interaction variability. A set of pairwise Tukey comparisons also supported the claim that J. L.'s performance on unconventional chord sets dropped more rapidly than his performance on conventional chord sets as set size increased. On both conventional and unconventional sets, J. L.'s performance on single chords was reliably better than his performance on 4-chord sets. When sets of 2 chords are considered, however, J. L.'s performance is only reliably above his performance on 4-chord sets when they consist of conventional chords. The results of this analysis are presented in Table 14-4.

Discussion

J. L. seemed to have no difficulty in analyzing single chords into their component chroma very quickly, regardless of the conventionality of the chords. This contrasts with other results suggesting that skilled musicians are poor at analyzing unconventional chords (Beal, 1980, 1985; Clifton, Inch, & Charness, 1985).

The amount J. L. could recall seemed to be the primary limitation on his performance on larger chord sets. He did not seem to rely heavily on tonal center in the chord task; perhaps more subtle measures of his recall performance would show a reliable difference between related conventional and unrelated conventional chords.

J. L.'s recall advantage for conventional chord sets indicates that he represents such sets more efficiently than unconventional chord sets. This advantage may occur in at least two ways: he may simply be faster at processing conventional material, thus demanding less working memory, or he may have more abstract representations of conventional chords but be forced to remember unconventional chords as sets of unrelated notes. The first explanation is less probable, because latency data on single-chord recall showed no differences between conventional and unconventional chords.

J. L.'s performance on both the melody and the chord recall tasks indicates that he is sensitive to many of the same musical factors (e.g., scale structure, temporal grouping) that musicians are sensitive to.

Learning Tunes

We attempted another experimental procedure with J. L. following the chord-set task. It was obvious that J. L. had built up an extensive repertoire of music. Anecdotal accounts suggested that he could learn a new piece very quickly, perhaps after one hearing. In fact, following Experiment 1, we noticed that when playing ad lib, J. L. was attempting to repeat several of the artificial melodies that we had presented to him. This supposed rapid learning of new melodies stands in marked contrast to J. L.'s inability to learn other sequential tasks, such as washing his hands. We attempted to use a trials-to-criterion learning procedure with a new set of melodies that were above his span, namely, 16-note sequences. Again, we used structured and unstructured sequences that also varied in both temporal grouping (grouped in 4's or ungrouped) and scale type (E major v. E whole tone).

In this procedure we played a tune, waited for J. L.'s recall attempt, and then replayed it if he was incorrect on any note. As a control, we tried a digit-span task on alternate trials that was isomorphic in that single digits were substituted for the note values. The task failed miserably. J. L. perseverated with his first recall attempt no matter how many times we replayed the melody, or digit string. We gave up after a few trials.

Either J. L. misunderstood the task demands or he was simply incapable of learning with this somewhat artificial procedure. One potential problem is that the melodies were constrained to equal-duration notes and that rhythm, apart from simple grouping, may provide an important cue for segmenting long melodic sequences. At any rate, we have not yet devised a procedure for properly investigating how J. L. acquires new melodies. It is also possible that, as he continues to suffer from additional epileptic seizures, his learning ability is diminishing. In summary, there is no evidence that J. L. learns new musical information extraordinarily quickly. These results contrast with those obtained by Sloboda, Hermelin, & O'Connor (1985). The autistic savant that they studied was quite successful memorizing a conventional piece and had considerable difficulty with a modern tonally unconventional piece.

Skill and the Mono-savant

J. L. is probably one of the lowest functioning musical mono-savants reported in the literature. Most of the others had verbal IQs in the low-normal to moderately retarded range and could carry on conversations and even say something about how they practiced or represented musical information. The case of J. L. clearly rules out, for instance Hoffman's (1971) speculation that for the development of a mono-savant "it would seem reasonable to assume that a minimum level of cognitive functioning is necessary for the achievement of these mental abilities (possibly, IQ greater than 50–60). Below that minimum level, it is highly unlikely that any amount of motivation or environmental favorability would enable the individual to develop the abilities" (p. 20).

J. L. clearly has a damaged left cerebral hemisphere and is further handicapped by his blindness, epilepsy, and hemiplegia. Nonetheless, he has managed to build up an extensive repertoire of musical knowledge and has found clever ways to use his one good hand to play music on keyboard instruments.

In answer to the first question raised in the introduction—whether the mono-savant represents information about a skill domain in the same way as a normal person—it is clear that J. L. is sensitive to dimensions of music to which normal musicians are also sensitive, namely, tonal features such as scale, and temporal features such as rhythmic grouping. His melody and chord spans are large, at least compared to his digit span of 5, though probably not out of the range of span for normally intelligent musicians. Although he has absolute pitch, a rare ability even for musicians, it is known that absolute pitch is trainable (see the discussions by Charness, Chapter 22, and by Ericsson & Faivre, Chapter 24, this volume). In short, J. L.'s representation of musical structure is similar to that of normally skilled musicians. He is not necessarily endowed with a specialized "module" for encoding and reproducing any and all musical sequences.

Nonetheless, J. L. is better at dealing with unstructured materials than would be predicted by the research with normally skilled musicians. This may be due to his rather specialized personal history of finding his own way to achieve musical fluency, without the "benefit" of normal training in musical theory. It may also be due to inadequate controls in the literature on normal musicians, who often, at least for chord memory tasks, are music students rather than professionals.

J. L.'s history is replete with accounts of how much time he spent at the piano when he was young. He did *not* start off playing music like a concert pianist when he first sat down to play at the age of 3. It is not too surprising that a blind, hemiplegic child would find the production of musical sounds a highly reinforcing activity. There was very little else in his environment over which he could exhibit much control. The many thousands of hours of practice that he engaged in provided him with experience similar to that of normally intelligent sighted musicians. Although his repertoire of musical pieces is large, it is probably not out of the range of that of many skilled professional pianists. That he seemed familiar with a whole-tone scale (Experiment 1) may not be that surprising for someone who has experimented a great deal on the keyboard. Unfortunately, we have no way of knowing how much "modern" music he has listened to or has attempted to play.

Apparently his learning rate is not out of the ordinary, at least for the artificially constrained set of tunes that we generated. In music, unlike the case in other domains such as chess, there are no truly random configurations of elements. Even random assemblages of notes do not violate any official rules for composition, though they do violate certain conventions for euphonious music. Thus the artificial melodies used here are less artificial than are the random board configurations used to look at skill in chess (see Charness, Chapter 22, this volume). If J. L. were extraordinarily sensitive to musical structure, it should have been apparent with these melodies. The tape-recorder model of the mono-savant is obviously an inadequate explanation of J. L.'s performance. Similarly, the notion that the mono-savant cannot abstract information is contradictory to J. L.'s sensitivity to musical scale and temporal congruity.

Thus we have to conclude that the skill that J. L. exhibits in music is comparable to the skill that normally intelligent musicians develop in the sense that J. L. and normal musicians both acquire cognitive structures that code (and enable reproduction of) selective aspects of musical information as opposed to nonabstractive, sensory representations. Miller (1987) arrived at similar conclusions in a study of a developmentally delayed 5 yr old musical savant. It seems that intense practice, together with an intact neurological substrate for coding a musical symbol system (e.g., Deutsch & Feroe, 1981), are sufficient to explain J. L.'s performance. Aligning with Ericsson and Faivre's (Chapter 24, volume) view, we can speculate that the need to master some aspect of his impoverished perceptual and motor environment was the motivating force that kept J. L. working at the piano for the many hours necessary to acquire a high level of skill.

From the perspective of neuropsychology, the conjunction of J. L.'s obvious left-hemisphere damage, his impaired language functioning, and his high level of musical skill raises questions about whether the right hemisphere is specialized to encode musical information. Two of the other musical mono-savants discussed in the literature, X. (Minogue, 1923) and Harriet G. (Viscott, 1970), also showed abnormalities in functioning consistent with left-hemisphere damage. Judging by other cases, however, such as S. (Anastasi & Levee, 1960), who apparently had damage to the right hemisphere, it is clear that there are no hard-and-fast rules that music must develop in the right hemisphere. The only case with autopsy data for an individual with skill in mathematics, music, and calendar calculation showed diffuse neuronal loss throughout the brain but most particularly in the temporal lobes and in the Broca area (Steinkopf, cited in Hill, 1978). J. L.'s reported skill at being able to recognize people's voices, even after a brief interaction and a long temporal interval, also suggests that some aspects of speech perception can be carried out successfully by the right hemisphere, a finding that fits with some of the literature.

It is perhaps not surprising that many mono-savant skills have been characterized as "right-hemisphere" tasks. Mental retardation is almost always characterized by poor language performance. It is often the slow development of language functioning that triggers the diagnosis of mental retardation. Perhaps it is to be expected that those individuals who have so little success with language functioning find alternate symbol systems (e.g., music, art), and possibly an alternate hemisphere, for self-expression.

Nonetheless, there are many mentally retarded and physically handicapped members of our society who have *not* acquired a high level of skill at any task. There is a very low incidence of mono-savants in institutions for the mentally retarded: Hill (1978) puts the rate at 1 in 2,000 residents of institutions and also notes that for published cases males outnumber females by about 6 to 1. Then if the drive theory of skill acquisition is correct, these findings suggest that the personality characteristics (and their underlying neural substrate) necessary to engender high levels of motivation are not found in many people. It also becomes important to ask how to motivate people to put in the many hours necessary to become skilled. In particular, a better understanding of why some mentally retarded individuals develop a high degree of skill, even in a narrow area such as musical performance, may hold out the promise of helping their peers to acquire the everyday skills that develop so readily in normally intelligent people.

Acknowledgments

This project was supported by a grant from the Natural Sciences and Engineering Research Council of Canada (NSERC—A0790) and by a Sabbatical Leave Fellowship from the Social Sciences and Humanities Research Council of Canada (SSHRC—451-84-4284) to the first author during his stay at the Mental Performance and Aging Lab, Veterans Administration

Outpatient Clinic, Boston. We gratefully acknowledge cooperation from the Ontario Ministry of Community and Social Services. We are also grateful to Barry Wills, Systems Design Department, and Christine MacKenzie, Kinesiology Department, University of Waterloo, for guidance in this project, and to William Milberg, Deborah Fein, and Loraine Obler for critical comments on earlier drafts. Finally, we would like to thank J. L., a very special person, and his parents.

References

Anastasi, A., & Levee, R. F. (1960). Intellectual defect and musical talent: A case report. *American Journal of Mental Deficiency, 64*, 695–703.

Beal, A. L. (1980). *Musical judgements and musical skill: Overtones in auditory memory.* Unpublished doctoral dissertation, University of Waterloo, Waterloo, Ontario.

Beal, A. L. (1985). The skill of recognizing musical structure. *Memory and Cognition, 5*, 405–412.

Blank, J. P. (1982, December). The miracle of May Lemke's love. *Reader's Digest*, pp. 49–54.

Bryan, W. L., & Harter, N. (1899). Studies in the telegraphic language. The acquisition of a hierarchy of habits. *Psychological Review, 6*, 345–375.

Clifton, J. V., Inch, R. L., & Charness, N. (1985, June). *Effect of tonality and chord quality on chord judgments by musically skilled and unskilled people.* Paper presented at the meeting of the Canadian Psychological Association, Halifax, Nova Scotia.

Deutsch, D. (1980). The processing of structured and unstructured tonal sequences. *Perception and Psychophysics, 28*, 381–389.

Deutsch, D., & Feroe, J. (1981). The internal representation of pitch sequences in tonal music. *Psychological Review, 88*, 503–522.

Gardner, H. (1983). *Frames of mind: A theory of multiple intelligences.* New York: Basic Books.

Hill, A. L. (1978). Savants: Mentally retarded individuals with special skills. In N. R. Ellis (Ed.), *International review of research in mental retardation* (Vol. 9). New York: Academic Press.

Hoffman, E. (1971). The idiot savant: A case report and a review of explanations. *Mental Retardation, 9*, 18–21.

Lindsay, P. H., & Norman, D. A. (1977). *Human information processing* (2nd ed.). New York: Academic Press.

Marin, O. S. M. (1982). Neurological aspects of music perception and performance. In D. Deutsch (Ed.), *The psychology of music.* New York: Academic Press.

Miller, L. K. (1987). Developmentally delayed musical savant's sensitivity to tonal structure. *American Journal of Mental Deficiency, 91*, 467–471.

Minogue, B. M. (1923). A case of secondary mental deficiency with musical talent. *Journal of Applied Psychology, 7*, 349–352.

Monty, S. (1981). *May's boy.* Nashville: Thomas Nelson.

Resnick, L. B. (Ed.). (1976). *The nature of intelligence.* Hillsdale, N.J.: Erlbaum.

Rimland, B. (1978, August). Inside the mind of the autistic savant. *Psychology Today*, pp. 69–80.

Sloboda, J. A., Hermelin, B., & O'Connor, N. (1985). An exceptional musical memory. *Music Perception, 3*, 155–170.

Viscott, D. S. (1970). A musical idiot savant. A psychodynamic study, and some speculations on the creative process. *Psychiatry, 33*, 494–515.

15

Talent in Foreign Languages: A Case Study

LORIANA NOVOA
DEBORAH FEIN
LORAINE K. OBLER

Few adults ever attain native levels of proficiency in a second language. Selinker (1972), for example, posits that a mere 5% of the adult population is capable of attaining nativelike competence in languages after puberty. There are a number of explanations in the psychological and psycholinguistic literature for this small percentage (see Schneiderman & Desmarais, Chapter 5, this volume). They include psychological variables such as motivation, empathy, and tolerance for ambiguity (Gardner & Lambert, 1972) and pragmatic variables such as time and energy available to devote to second-language learning (Snow & Hoefnegel-Hohle, 1978). As to neurological or neuropsychological variables related to second-language acquisition, the only work to date suggests unusual hemispheric lateralization and, in particular, right-hemisphere involvement in at least the early stages of second-language acquisition (Albert & Obler, 1978). To explore whether identifiable neuropsychological factors (such as exceptional verbal memory or visuospatial deficits) would be associated with second-language facility, we conducted an extended exploratory case study of a talented second-language learner.

Portrait of C. J.

C. J., our subject, was selected as a result of advertising for subjects in language departments of local universities and consulting with numerous colleagues. We required a subject who had learned several languages postpubertally (and only one

Loriana Novoa. Department of Curriculum and Instruction, College of Education, Florida International University, Miami, Florida; and Department of Pediatrics, Genetics Division, University of Miami Medical School, Miami, Florida.
Deborah Fein. Laboratory of Neuropsychology, Boston University School of Medicine, Boston, Massachusetts; and Department of Psychology, University of Connecticut, Storrs, Connecticut.
Loraine K. Obler. Program in Speech and Hearing Sciences, Graduate School and University Center of the City University of New York, New York, New York; and Aphasia Research Center of the Boston University School of Medicine, Boston, Massachusetts.

prepubertally), quickly, and to nativelike proficiency. Very few names were suggested; C. J. was selected from among this group because he would be available for testing over the course of a semester. We interviewed native speakers of the different languages C. J. speaks and asked them to evaluate C. J.'s abilities, accent, and fluency.

We first interviewed C. J. about his language-learning history and general background. The interview included questions regarding his developmental milestones and growth, family history, school and academic performance, parental expectations and interactions, and the Geschwind cluster of neuro-immuno-endocrinological factors linked to left-handedness and exceptional abilities (Geschwind & Galaburda, 1985a, 1985b, 1985c). We also asked our subject whether there was any other information related to his exceptional abilities in language that might help us to better understand his talent.

C. J. is a 29-year-old left-handed single Caucasian male who, at the time of testing, was a graduate student in international education, specializing in curriculum development. C. J. was a native speaker of English who grew up in a monolingual home. He does recall hearing some French spoken in one of the communities in which he lived while growing up, and Latin was used in the church services he attended regularly in childhood. However, C. J.'s first true experience with a second language came at age 15, with formal instruction in French in high school. Because he excelled in French classes, C. J. decided also to study German while in high school. In addition to 2 years of formal and traditional instruction in German, C. J. studied Spanish and Latin for one semester each during his early high school years.

In college C. J. majored in French language and literature and spent his junior year, at age 20, in France. A brief visit to Germany while studying in France evidently "restored" the German he had studied during high school. C. J. reports that just hearing the language spoken for a short time was enough for him to recover his lost fluency.

Upon graduation from college, C. J. accepted a government position in Morocco, where he reports having learned Moroccan Arabic through both formal and informal instruction and immersion. Although Moroccan Arabic was evidently more difficult for him than the Romance or Germanic languages because of the greater linguistic distance from English, C. J. reports having learned it with unusual ease relative to his peers. Subsequently, C. J. also spent some time in Spain and Italy, where he apparently "picked up" both Spanish and Italian in a "matter of weeks." He reports that contact with the media and informal gatherings with native speakers were particularly useful and effective means for him to acquire these languages rapidly. Native speakers of all his languages confirm C. J.'s reports of his nativelike abilities, including lack of foreign accent and the ease and speed of his language acquisition.

C. J. and his identical twin brother are the eldest of four siblings. The twins are the only family members who are not right-handed. C. J. shows mixed handedness: Fine motor abilities, such as writing and drawing, are executed with his left hand; gross motor abilities and tasks requiring strength, such as batting and bowling, are usually carried out with his right hand. When C. J. first attempts a new motor task, he always uses what he considers his dominant hand, that is, the left one. If he cannot execute the task with the left hand, he will then try the right.

Although C. J. and his twin brother were born 1 month prematurely and put into an incubator, evidently all developmental milestones were achieved normally. He reports no knowledge of possible prenatal and/or perinatal difficulties. He recalls having had the usual childhood diseases and scarlet fever all before the age of 6. Recovery from all was uneventful.

C. J. reports that, in general, his academic performance throughout childhood and adolescence was quite good, despite his family's frequent moves and his frequent changing of schools. He suggested that perhaps because he and his twin brother were extremely close, the disruptions of moving were not particularly problematic.

Evidently, C. J. was somewhat slow in learning to read, although his first-language acquisition was apparently normal. Once the basic reading skills were mastered, however, he had no difficulty maintaining an adequate level of performance. To this day, he reports that reading is slow and somewhat laborious, regardless of the language and/or material involved. Otherwise, C. J. believes that he was essentially a good student throughout his school years and was generally quite good in mathematics, sciences, graphic arts, and music. On the other hand, he reports poor performance in athletics and believes that he has extremely inadequate skills relating to directionality and spatial orientation, such as in reading maps or finding his way.

Of the information available to C. J. and his mother, C. J. reports a number of positive items in relation to the Geschwind cluster. In addition to his left-handedness and his being a twin, C. J. reports having allergies and hives. C. J. also reports that it is possible that a maternal grandfather was diagnosed as schizophrenic. In addition, C. J. recognized prepubertally that he is homosexual and believes this to be particularly significant in regard to understanding his language-acquisition talent. C. J. explains that he realized from a very young age that he was "different" and therefore chose to be distinctive in particular ways. Doing well in language learning as opposed to athletics, by his analysis, distinguished him markedly from other high school males. C. J.'s twin is also left-handed; he is not reported to have done either notably poor or notably well in learning language, although C. J. suggests that this may be due partly to a lack of opportunity.

Neuropsychological Test Results

C. J. was given a series of neuropsychological tests to assess his general intellectual functioning and examine some specific cognitive functions that might be expected to be associated with exceptional second-language aptitude. Although we focused primarily on tests measuring memory and language abilities that might be particularly pertinent to second-language acquisition, we also assessed abstract reasoning, visuo-spatial functioning, mental control and response set, and sensorimotor abilities.

General Cognitive Functioning

In many respects C. J.'s functioning was in the range of average to high average. On the WAIS-R, C. J. scored a Verbal IQ of 105 and a Performance IQ of 110, for a

Full-scale IQ of 107. Thus there was no marked verbal–performance discrepancy, and his performance was not out of the ordinary. There is some scatter across the WAIS-R subtests, with low scores (25th percentile) on sequencing cartoon pictures and on abstracting similarities between a pair of words, and with highest scores (91 percentile) on vocabulary and pairing digits with symbols. It is interesting that C. J. did not do particularly well on abstracting the common properties of two words. His answers tended to be either concrete (a table and a chair both "have legs") or somewhat idiosyncratic or attentive to form rather than meaning (a poem and a statute both "have lines," and work and play both "have four letters"). Similarly, on a multiple-choice proverb interpretation test (Gorham Proverbs), C. J.'s performance was average. He missed the point of some proverbs, and on others he chose a rather concrete interpretation of the proverb rather than an abstract restatement. On the arithmetic subtest, C. J.'s performance was average; he did not know the correct procedures for doing the more difficult problems and was slightly impulsive and sloppy in his calculations on some of the easier items.

It is interesting that C. J.'s two best performances on the WAIS-R were on tests plausibly closely tied to language acquisition. One high score was on Vocabulary, in which he was asked to define words of increasing difficulty. Not only did he know most of the difficult words, but he was easily able to give accurate one-word synonyms for many of the harder words, such as "burden" for "encumber," "foreboding" for "ominous", and "palpable" for "tangible." He scored at about the same level on the Vocabulary subtest of the Shipley-Hartford Institute for Living Scale, which uses a multiple-choice vocabulary format.

The other WAIS-R subtest on which C. J. did very well was Digit Symbol. On this subtest the subject is asked to place symbols in blank spaces below a series of digits, using a code at the top of the page as a guide. Individuals tend to score better if they are, in fact, learning the code rather than merely continually referring to it. That C. J. did learn the code was demonstrated by using Edith Kaplan's modification of the test, in which the subject is asked to recall the digit-symbol pairings from memory immediately after the test is given. C. J. recalled all nine pairs without error, a superior performance, and retained all nine perfectly after a 20-minute delay. This subtest, which requires acquisition or at least use of a code transforming a known series of symbols to a previously unknown series, bears an obvious relationship to new-language acquisition.

C. J. also did very well on two other tests of higher cognitive functioning. On Raven's Progressive Matrices, which requires the subject to decide which of six choices correctly completes a pattern with a piece missing, C. J. scored at the 95th percentile. On the Shipley-Hartford Abstraction subtest, the subject must figure out what relations obtain among a series of letters, numbers, or words, and then complete the pattern (e.g., surgeon 1234567_____snore 17635_____ rogue_____). On this subtest C. J. did almost as well as he did on the Shipley-Harford Vocabulary subtest; he scored at about the 93rd percentile on the two subtests combined. Again, his few errors on the Abstraction subtest seemed to be due as much to impulsivity as to inability to figure out the rule. Thus on these two tests (Raven's and Shipley-Hartford), in which a rather abstract pattern must be apprehended and completed by the subject, C. J. did very well.

In summary, C. J.'s overall intellectual functioning, as measured by traditional IQ tests, is not out of the ordinary. In particular, he does not use words or even proverbs in a very abstract or sophisticated way. However, there are some areas of outstanding ability or skill. These include vocabulary, acquisition of a new code, and the ability to perceive and complete formal patterns. This facility with patterns obtains in both verbal and visual realms, despite his otherwise relatively poor performance in visuo-spatial tasks.

Specific Language Aptitude

We administered the Modern Language Aptitude Test (MLAT) as a further measure of C. J.'s second-language abilities. The MLAT (Carroll, 1959) was designed to provide an indication of an individual's probable degree of success in learning to speak and understand a foreign language. It is also useful in predicting success in learning to read, write, and translate a foreign language. The subtests include Number Learning, Phonetic Script, Spelling Clues, Words in Sentences, and Paired Associates. They measure aspects of memory and phoneme appreciation, sound–symbol association ability, and sensitivity to grammatical structure.

Consistent with his performance on the WAIS-R Digit Symbol subtest, C. J. performed at or almost at ceiling on the three subtests requiring learning a new code system, whether it was English numbers to new words, English words to nonsense words, or a new phonetic transcription system. He also scored near ceiling on the test that required him to retrieve a word based on only the consonants of that word. However, he was only at the 50th percentile on the Words in Sentences subtest, which required him to judge which two words serve the same functions in two English sentences. Thus, what might be termed his "conscious appreciation of grammatical structure" was only average.

On a test of verbal fluency, where he was required to give as many words beginning with a given letter as he could think of in 1 minute, C. J. scored in the high-normal range. His word lists included such low-frequency words as "facetious," "frenzy," "anorexic," "asterisks," "sedentary," and "stevedore."

C. J. was asked to provide a written description of a standard picture stimulus. He provided an adequate description of the story, with nothing remarkable in it. However, he did make two minor grammatical errors (e.g., "oblivious of"). Thus, as on his general cognitive test, C. J.'s strengths appear to be in the acquisition of new codes rather than in the higher conceptual manipulation of verbal material.

Visuo-spatial Functions

It is suggested by Schneiderman and Desmarais (Chapter 5, this volume) that exceptional second-language aptitude may be associated with a compromised visuo-spatial system. They suggest that mild to moderate deficits in visuo-spatial functions may be a frequent concomitant to second-language aptitude. C. J.'s strengths certainly did not lie in visuo-spatial areas, but his skills on these tests were generally within the average range. He actually scored quite well (84th percentile) on assembling puzzles on the WAIS-R, even when those puzzles relied completely on the appreciation of outer configuration, a heavily "right-hemisphere" visual strategy. His score on Block Design on the WAIS-R was at an average level. He was unable to solve one puzzle, the one requiring perhaps the most appreciation of visual form (# 7). His copy of the Rey-Osterreith complex figure was normal, well organized (starting with the base rectangle and then adding details), and quite accurate. He had no difficulty making right–left discriminations on pictured body parts and articles of clothing. He did score at the low end of the average range on the Hooper Test of Visual Organization, which requires the subject to assemble mentally and name a cut-up drawing representing an object. He had difficulty with the mental rotations involved and was frequently observed to rotate the book. He did tend to fail items on this test that require the most appreciation of configuration information; if a small part of the picture looked like a thing in itself, he was sometimes inclined to give this as a response.

C. J. was also asked to visualize the alphabet, and name every capital letter that had a curve in it, and then to think through the alphabet and name every letter that rhymes with "tree." For normal right-handed males, the second of these tasks is generally considered to be more dependent on left-hemisphere functioning, whereas naming curved letters is more dependent on right-hemisphere functioning. (Edith Kaplan, personal communication, 1985, March). C. J. did not show any dissociation between these two tasks. His quick time and few errors on both were normal and did not differ from each other, suggesting no strong bias toward either left- or right-hemisphere processing styles.

Musical Ability

In the popular lore it has sometimes been suggested that a "good ear" for language is also a "good ear" for music. C. J. was given the Seashore Test of Musical Ability. The three subtests given were immediate memory for tonal sequences, rhythmic sequences, and pitch discrimination. C. J. did somewhat better on the Tonal Memory (61st percentile) than he did on rhythm (28th percentile) and Pitch (40th percentile), but all scores were in the average range.

Memory

It has also been suggested that second-language acquisition may reflect underlying strengths in verbal memory or a strong general memory. Indeed, C. J.'s verbal memory was clearly outstanding. As mentioned before, he incidentally learned the entire digit–symbol code on the WAIS-R and retained it perfectly after 20 minutes. On the Rey Auditory Verbal Learning Test, C. J. showed an average learning curve for his age but retained this unrelated list of words virtually perfectly after 20 minutes. He showed a high-average (84th percentile) performance on Paired Associates on the Weschler Memory Scale and retained most of this list even after a 2-week interval. His outstanding performance, however, was on retention of prose passages, both immediately and on delay. His performance was above the 99th percentile on this task. On the other hand, his score on Digit Span was not out of the ordinary (6 forward and 7 backward), with a slightly lower score on Digits Forwards probably being due simply to fatigue or impulsivity. In contrast, on visual recall of the Rey-Osterreith figure and on recall of the visual figures from the Weschler Memory Scale, his performance was average.

Personality

It has been suggested that personality or cultural factors may play a role in second-language acquisition. Schneiderman and Desmarais (Chapter 5, this volume) discuss in some detail the notion that a willingness to adopt the identity of, or to be taken for, someone in another culture may significantly influence the readiness with which foreign accent and grammar are picked up. With regard to accent, in particular, for which C. J. is also outstanding, they suggest that one must be willing not only to sound like someone from another culture but also to give up the protection that foreign accent confers. In other words, native speakers may make allowances for grammatical errors when the speaker is obviously not a native speaker, and thus the person may be protected from sounding foolish. The "risk taking" of a certain sort, or the failure to be strongly identified in a conservative fashion with a "mainstream" member of one's own culture, may indeed apply to C. J. As mentioned several times previously, C. J.'s responses were very quick, costing him somewhat in accuracy, since he made occasional impulsive errors. Furthermore, he sees himself as something of a maverick and has not settled down with any steady occupation. His sexual orientation may also relate to this way in which he sees himself, as cause, as effect, or as some combination of the two.

Personality testing with the Thematic Apperception Test (TAT) and the Rorschach test revealed little of significance. C. J. tended to give many popular responses and was somewhat guarded in being willing to predict the future in his TAT stories. He did try to give some intellectualized abstract symbolic responses on the Rorschach, and these were generally less successful than his popular responses. The record showed many animal reponses and little in the way of human content or human movement, perhaps contradicting the theory of Guiora, Brannon, and Dull (1972) that individuals who are more empathic are those who have better accents in foreign-language learning.

Neuropsychology and Second-Language Facility

Clearly, generally superior cognitive functioning is not necessary for exceptional second-language acquisition. C. J.'s IQ scores, plus his ability to manipulate abstract verbal concepts and his general fund of information, were at average levels. His musical ability was also average, as was his ability to solve visual problems such as reproducing block patterns. He also complained of a lack of ability to read maps and learn new routes, and he had some difficulty in performing mental rotation problems.

Furthermore, no marked discrepancy was seen in his overall problem-solving style—his cognitive approach was not in any obvious way favoring a "left-hemisphere" versus a "right-hemisphere" style.

C. J.'s memory was not exceptional for all material–visual memory for figures was merely average. However, his verbal memory was exceptional, both for English passages and for acquiring new verbal codes. Furthermore, his performance was quite good on tasks requiring the perception and completion of formal patterns whether the stimulus was abstract visual symbols or the relations between series of words (as long as the relation was formal and not semantic).

To the extent that one can argue from a single case, C. J.'s pattern of strengths and weaknessess is consistent with some theories of second-language acquisition and contradicts others.

C. J. provides a counterexample to the lay belief that good second-language abilities are related somehow to a "musical ear." Contrary to what some may expect, exceptional IQ is not a *sine qua non* for good second-language acquisition, nor does Guiora *et al.'s* (1972) notion that superior capacity for empathy is required for nativelike accent in a second language receive support from C. J.'s case. C. J.'s personality characteristics, however, might be taken to support the idea discussed by Schneiderman and Desmarais (Chapter 5, this volume) that high motivation, a nonconformist self-concept, and a willingness to take risks may be associated with second-language facility, especially in accent.

It is not immediately obvious that ability for prose recall in a first language would necessarily be linked with second-language talent. C. J.'s exceptional verbal memory, in contrast to his visual memory and his overall intellectual ability, would at least raise the possibility that exceptional verbal memory would be strongly linked to second-language talent in other individuals as well. Clearly, exceptional memory for other types of material is *not* necessary, since C. J.'s memory for digits and for visuo-spatial and musical material was not remarkable.

It is a provocative, but not an unexpected, finding that C. J. performed particularly well on the Shipley-Hartford test and on Raven's Progressive Matrices, both requiring appreciation and completion of formal patterns. Perhaps the ability to extract patterns from complex input contributes to appreciating patterns in foreign-language input.

Although C. J. does not show any frank visuo-spatial deficits on neuropsychological testing, his visuo-spatial skills are clearly inferior to his verbal abilities, and he reports subjective difficulty with various visuo-spatial skills, such as map reading and finding his way around. This may be taken as weak support for the Schneiderman and Desmarais hypothesis that second-language talent is associated with visuo-spatial deficits. One theoretical possibility is that C. J.'s exceptional ability rests on a more bilateral organization for language than right-handed males as a group show. As with females who may generally show such a pattern (Obler & Novoa, in press), verbal skills appear to benefit from bilateral organization, whereas for the same individuals visuo-spatial abilities seem to suffer.

As mentioned before, there are several items in the Geschwind-Galaburda cluster in C. J.'s history (mixed handedness, homosexuality, allergies, twinning, and the possibility of schizophrenia in a grandfather). As discussed in the introductory chapter to this volume, Geschwind and Galaburda (1985a, 1985b, 1985) postulate a high coincidence of non-right-handedness, autoimmune disorders, learning disorders, and talents. They suggest that the talents as well as the disabilities can be explained by a hormonal factor present in the third or fourth month of fetal life, when the right hemisphere is developing faster than the left. This hormonal factor delays cell migrations for certain zones of the left hemisphere, resulting in effective "lesions" and leading to hypertrophy in corresponding areas of the right hemisphere or in areas surrounding the "lesion" in the left hemisphere. The talents discussed by Geschwind and Galaburda (mathematical, artistic, architectural, engineering, musical, and athletic) all can be considered to rest more heavily on right-hemisphere processing. Geschwind and Galaburda (1985a) do allude to the possibility that such individuals "may have elevated skills related to unaffected regions on the left" (p. 432), but they do not specify what such left-hemisphere talents might be. We suggest that C. J., with his slowed development and persistent mild difficulty in reading contrasting with his exceptional ability in second-language acquisition, may constitute an example of such a case.

References

Albert, M., & Obler, L. (1978). *The bilingual brain—Neurospychological and neurolinguistic aspects of bilingualism.* New York: Academic Press.

Carroll, J. (1959). *Modern Language Aptitude Test.* New York: Psychological Corporation.

Gardner, R., & Lambert, W. (1972). *Attitudes and motivation in second language learning.* Rowley, MA: Newbury House.

Geschwind, N., & Galaburda, A. (1985a). Cerebral lateralization: Biological mechanisms, associations, and pathology: 1. A hypothesis and a program for research. *Archives of Neurology, 42,* 428–459.

Geschwind, N., & Galaburda, A. (1985b). Cerebral lateralization: Biological mechanisms, associations, and pathology: 2. A hypothesis and a program for research. *Archives of Neurology, 42,* 521–552.

Geschwind, N., & Galaburda, A. (1985c). Cerebral lateralization: Biological mechanisms, associations, and pathology: 3. A hypothesis and a program for research. *Archives of Neurology, 42,* 634–654.

Guiora, A., Brannon, R., & Dull, C. (1972). Empathy and second language learning. *Language and Learning, 22,* 111–130.

Obler, L., & Novoa, L. (in press) Gender similarities and differences in brain lateralization. *Genes and Gender, V.*

Selinker, L. (1972). Interlanguage. *International Review of Applied Linguistics, 10,* 209–231.

Snow, C., & Hoefnegel-Hohle, M. (1978). The critical period for language acquisition: Evidence from second language learning. *Child Development, 48,* 1114–1128.

16

A Portrait of the Artist
as a Brain-Damaged Patient

AVRAHAM SCHWEIGER

Artistic Talent and the Brain

Are the brains of artistically talented individuals structurally different from the brains of normal individuals who are not endowed with artistic ability? To discuss this question, we need definitions of art and artistic talent. For the purpose of this chapter, I define "art" as an aesthetic, nonverbal medium the artist uses for communicating symbolized emotions to some receptive audience. Art resembles language in that it communicates meaning, but art is based on intuitive, affective referents, whereas language as a rule conveys more precise referents. "Artistic talent" is taken here as the relatively superior ability to transform affective experiences into visible forms conveying emotional meaning to at least a segment of the creator's community.

Since there is evidence linking emotional expression and perception to the right hemisphere, it has been speculated (see, e.g., Levy, 1983) that artistic performance is especially associated with the right hemisphere (see discussion in Gardner 1974; 1982b). For example, impaired art in right-brain-damaged artists was described by Jung (1974). Furthermore, cases of artists who continued their creative output after damage to the left brain have been reported (e.g., Alajouanine, 1948; Bonvicini, 1926). Cases have also been reported, however, of artists with impoverished artistic production following left-hemisphere strokes (e.g., Zaimov, Kitov, & Kolev, 1969) and of other artists with spared artistic creativity following right-brain lesions (e.g., Ball, 1982). Such a distribution of cases is clearly sufficient to undermine a simplistic attribution of artistic creativity to either side of the brain alone.

Perhaps a better distinction to draw is that between competence and performance. As with perception and production of linguistic material, we suspect that production of art objects may be impaired while artistic appreciation is spared. Moreover, with the right-brain-damaged artist, as in the case study that follows, we may demonstrate that the artist's competence—that is, his or her ability to conceive of an artistic work—is intact, while the performance, or productive realization, of the work is impaired.

Avraham Schweiger. Psychology Department, University of California at Los Angeles, Los Angeles, California.

A necessary but not sufficient component of being a talented artist is the ability to execute art objects. Indeed, we might draw a distinction between individuals who have this skill alone, for example, those who limit themselves to drawing portraits of passersby on the sidewalk, and those artists whose work is appreciated by a given culture because it perceives a greater investment of meaning in the work. As we shall see in the case study that follows, it is possible for these two levels of artistic talent to be differentially affected by brain damage: The creative may remain in the face of severely impaired artistic skills.

In this book we focus on the possibility that unusual brain structures underlie the exceptional abilities of individual artists. Naturally, environmental factors such as education, exposure, criticism, and encouragement are crucial factors to becoming an artist (see Gardner, 1973, 1982a, and Winner, 1982, for a more extensive discussion). To focus on the neuroanatomical component of artistry for this chapter, I have chosen to report on a brain-damaged artist because his artistic and linguistic functioning has been rendered more "transparent" to investigation by the systematic impairment resulting from the brain damage (Gardner, 1982b).

The Case of L. D

L. D. is a self-taught fashion designer who never attended college. He has been involved in drawing, by his own report, since approximately the age of 5. His father was in the clothing business and a designer as well. L. D. has designed fashion clothes for men and women, and accessories for manufacturers, including leather items, buckles, coins, and emblems. In addition, he has designed window displays for specialty shops.

L. D.'s 59 years have, by his report, never been boring. Prior to and during his 38-year career as a designer, his jobs included undercover work for the Defense Department and attempts at comedy writing. A true *bon vivant*, L. D. was married to and divorced from two models. Our patient made a good deal of money and squandered it as rapidly as he made it, living extravagantly and enjoying travel, alcohol, cigarettes, and rich food at the best restaurants in town.

In October 1982 L. D. suffered a stroke that resulted in an infarct in the posterior distribution of the right middle cerebral artery. The CT scan showed a low-density area in the parietal lobe, extending into the occipital lobe (see Figure 16-1). A resting PET scan indicated an area of hypometabolism in the same area shown by the CT scan to have structural damage; this area of hypometabolism was slightly larger than that shown on the CT scan. Initially, there was a mild left homonymous hemianopsia, which cleared within 2 months following the stroke. Other sensory and motor systems remained essentially intact, so that 2 years after the stroke, the patient ambulated normally and even drove his car.

Poststroke Test of L. D.'s Abilities

During initial testing L. D. presented with mild, fluent aphasia, with occasional literal and verbal paraphasias and moderate word-finding difficulties. His writing

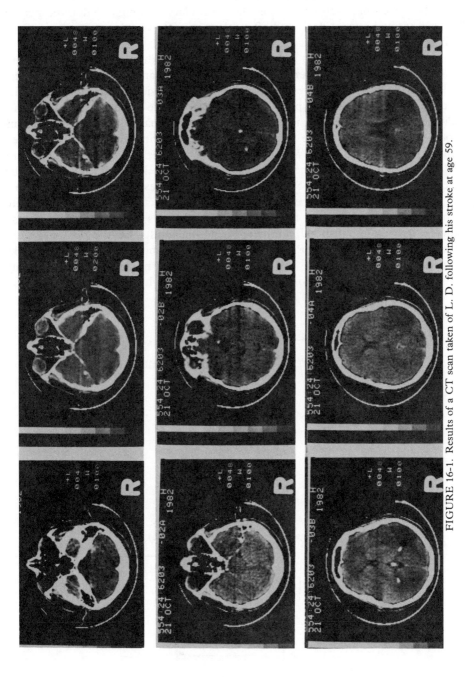

FIGURE 16-1. Results of a CT scan taken of L. D. following his stroke at age 59.

was moderately impaired. One striking aspect of L. D.'s language is that despite his paraphasias and anomia, and considering that his formal education ended at his graduation from high school, he uses the vocabulary of a highly educated person (he used to read a great deal) and often uses correctly very low-frequency words such as "ubiquitous," "myriad," and "propitious."

L. D. has always been a right-hander. Moreover, there is no left-handedness in his family. Therefore he was diagnosed as a crossed aphasic, since it is unusual for language disturbance to result from a right-sided lesion in a right-hander. His concomitant selective visuo-spatial deficits, however, are more consistent with his right-hemisphere lesion. For instance, he was (and remained for 2 years after his stroke) unable to render the third dimension in drawing an object, even when copying it (see Figure 16-2). When seen initially at 2 weeks poststroke, our patient could not complete even the simplest of Koh's Block Design figures of the Wechsler Adult Intelligence Scale. Subsequently, he has been able to complete a few of the simplest ones, albeit with considerable difficulty, exceeding 1 minute each time, whereas the limit for normal performance is 1 minute, with the easy figures requiring less than half a minute for normal adults. On the Benton Three-Dimensional Constructional Praxis Test (where three models of blocks and sticks are presented to the patient, who must build identical models from the separate parts), L. D. received a score of 25 out of a possible 29, which represents a defective

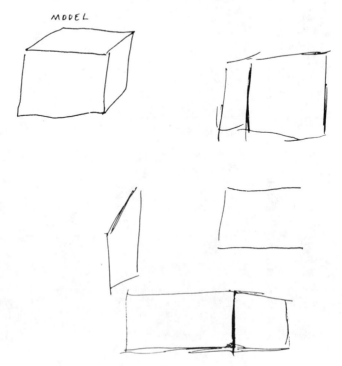

FIGURE 16-2. L. D.'s attempts, shortly after his stroke, to render the third dimension in copying the model of a cube.

performance both from a normative standpoint (98% of normal persons scored above 26) and when considering our subject's profession.

L. D. showed great difficulty in performing a test that requires a coordination of perspectives. In this test, fashioned after Piaget's theories and testing schemes, the patient is shown a board with three cones of different sizes that represent mountains. The patient is asked to choose, on a multiple-choice card, the correct depiction of the three "mountains" seen from different locations around the board. To perform correctly, the patient needs the ability to transform perspectives in his or her mind and match the correct one to the response case. L. D.'s performance was at chance level, whereas most normal persons perform at 100%. These results suggest a visuo-constructive impairment consonant with his difficulty in organizing visual objects in three dimensions. It should be emphasized that L. D. was keenly aware of his shortcomings on all the tests on which he performed poorly; he expressed great frustration at his inability to draw three-dimensional cubes and other objects he previously had designed.

In contrast with these impairments, L. D.'s rendering of two-dimensional

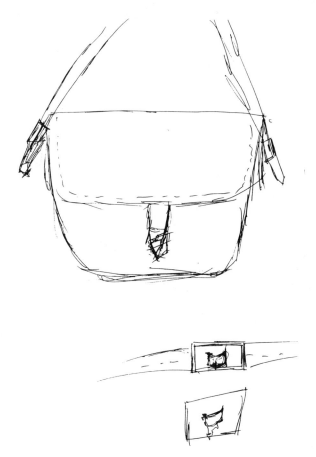

FIGURE 16-3. L. D.'s rendering, shortly after his stroke, of objects he had designed prior to his stroke.

objects that he designed premorbidly was almost intact (see Figure 16-3). In addition, on other visual tests requiring two-dimensional processing (e.g., the Hooper Visual Organization Test, the Judgment of Line Orientation Test, the Goldstein-Scheerer Stick Test), he showed no impairment. It seems, therefore, that L. D.'s lesion caused a regression, at least on the productive side, to an earlier, simpler stage of rendering objects in two dimensions, much like young children.

These facts suggest a specific dissociation demonstrated by the case of L. D.—that between two-dimensional and three-dimensional representation. Let us consider Figures 16-2 and 16-3. Rendering a two-dimensional object presented no difficulty for L. D. in terms of the relations among the lines making up the various aspects of the design. Attempting to draw a three-dimensional "simple" cube, by contrast, even copying from a model, proved to be too complex a task. To do that, L. D. needed to perform some abstract mental transformation of visual images (to decide, for instance, at what angles certain lines should be in order to denote the third dimension) that he could no longer carry out. Accordingly, he performed poorly on tests that require such manipulations of visual forms (e.g., the Benton Three-Dimensional Constructional Praxis Test, the test requiring coordination of perspectives, and Koh's blocks). Here we can see a dissociation between the ability to conceive of an object and the rendering of it in three dimensions so as to make it look real. It is as if L. D. regressed here to the level of a young child who has not yet learned to render perspective on paper. Yet, L. D. clearly retained his ability to perceive and to conceive old and new designs. It seems also that to copy an object is more than just to see it "as it is"; there is a process of "breaking down" the visual stimulus into its (more or less) retinal image, followed by a reorganization on the paper. That is, lines must be treated abstractly, apart from the object they form, so that their individual contribution to the illusion of a three-dimensional object can be manipulated. It is the latter ability that L. D. seems to have lost.

The remarkable fact about L. D. is that despite his impairment in drawing three-dimensional objects, he can still appreciate the subtleties of fashion clothes, of visual displays in shops, and of art objects. In fact, 2 years following the stroke, he returned to work in his profession, albeit part-time and at a reduced capacity, mostly managing projects but not designing, since he can no longer realize his ideas well on paper. More recently, L. D. has undertaken a project involving a new line of fashion attire, in which he is responsible for setting a display within a department store as well as for designing the items. To circumvent his deficits in rendering, L. D. hired someone to execute his ideas on paper. His aphasia has improved to the extent that despite his word-finding difficulties, he can describe his ideas verbally in sufficient details that another artist can render them. Once this initial rendering is on paper, L. D. can use his intact perceptual skills to supervise corrections or additions.

Conclusion

Thus the case of L. D. demonstrates a dissociation between conceiving an art object and realizing it. L. D. claimed that he could see in his mind exactly what he was trying to render on the paper, yet he failed to do so. An artist, then, may be capable of conceiving aesthetic ideas in the abstract, perhaps in terms of imaginary relations but yet quite specific in details, without being able to execute them. The materialization of a piece of art can be separated from its conception, provided that there are ways of transmitting it so that someone other than the artist can execute it.

Finally, we turn to the combination of language and artistic impairment in L. D. It is not uncommon to find in the literature on cases of brain-damaged artists a dissociation between language and artistic production (e.g., Gardner, 1982a, 1982b; for a review of the same dissociation in musicians, see Judd, Chapter 6, this volume). That is, there are reported cases of artists with impaired language but with intact artistic production (Alajouanine, 1948) and cases of artists with impaired artistic production but with no aphasia (Jung, 1974, and an unpublished case of an architect I had the opportunity to examine, who sustained bilateral posterior lesions and could no longer design anything but who showed no aphasic symptoms). Such reports are taken as a demonstration of the functional independence of art and language. The inference drawn in such cases is that such independence of art from language indicates separate underlying anatomical substrates serving these two abilities. As discussed previously, L. D. suffered damage to both systems from a single lesion. Unfortunately, only speculations can be offered at this point. Perhaps, L. D. somehow acquired language in a visuo-spatial fashion, so that the two systems evolved together functionally as well as anatomically. Alternatively, L. D.'s brain could be one of the few (perhaps about 1% in the population) with linguistic functions specialized in the right hemisphere, while visuo-spatial skills also involve that hemisphere, so that it is their contiguity that is responsible for L. D.'s symptoms.

References

Alajouanine, T. (1948). Aphasia and artistic realization. *Brain*, *71*, 229–241.
Ball, M. (1982, August 14). Lyrical abstract expressionism. *Artweek*, pp. 5–7.
Bonvicini, G. (1962). Die aphasie der Malers Vierge. *Wiener Medizinische Wochenschrift*, *76*, 88–91.
Gardner, H. (1973). *The arts and human development*. New York: Wiley.
Gardner, H. (1974). *The shattered mind*. New York: Vintage Books.
Gardner, H. (1982a). *Art, mind and brain*. New York: Basic Books.
Gardner, H. (1982b). Artistry following damage to the human brain. In A. W. Ellis (Ed.), *Normality and pathology in cognitive function*. New York: Academic Press.
Jung, R. (1974). Neuropsychologie und Neurophysiologie des kontur und Formsehens in Zeichnung und Malerei. In H. H. Wieck (Ed.), *Psychopathologie Musischer Gestaltungen*. Stuttgart–New York: F. K. Schattauer.
Levy, J. (1983). Individual differences in cerebral hemisphere asymmetry: Theoretical issues and experimental considerations. In J. B. Hellige (Ed.), *Cerebral hemisphere asymmetry*. New York: Praeger.
Winner, E. (1982). *Invented worlds*. Cambridge, MA: Harvard University Press.
Zaimov, K., Kitov, D., & Kolev, N. (1969). Aphasie chez un paintre. *Encephale*, *68*, 377–417.

17

Paul: A Musically Gifted Autistic Boy

DOROTHY LUCCI
DEBORAH FEIN
ADELE HOLEVAS
EDITH KAPLAN

In this chapter we describe the history and current functioning of a 13-year-old black, right-handed, musically talented autistic boy, whom we will call Paul. In the first section we present his general development, and in the second, a description of the music-related aspects of his development. In the third section we describe the results of music testing, and in the fourth, the results of neuropsychological assessment. We conclude with some speculations about musical talent and autism.

General Developmental History

Paul was the product of an unplanned pregnancy; his mother was a single 18-year-old woman living with her own mother and enrolled in a state college. The father has been in intermittent contact with Paul and his mother through the years but lives out of state and does not participate in planning Paul's life. Paul's mother currently works at management level in community service and continues to have a close and supportive relationship with her own mother.

Pregnancy was generally uneventful, except for an episode of bleeding in the 4th month and a falling down a flight of stairs in the 6th month. Paul's mother was overweight during pregnancy and had occasional, but not heavy, alcohol use. Paul was born prematurely at 36 weeks gestation and weighed 5 lb. 10 oz. A spinal anesthetic was used. Labor lasted $4\frac{1}{2}$ hours, and Apgar scores were 5 at 1 minute and 6 at 5 minutes, with color noted to be poor. Paul was in the "preemie" unit for 24 hours. At 2 weeks he was noted to have some problems in breathing, secondary to fluid not draining out of his lungs. He did not sleep through the night until approximately 10 years of age. Motor milestones were apparently normal, except that he did not crawl; reportedly, he walked at 8 to 9 months. Babbling, which

Dorothy Lucci. Laboratory of Neuropsychology, Boston University School of Medicine, Boston, Massachusetts.
Deborah Fein. Laboratory of Neuropsychology, Boston University School of Medicine, Boston, Massachusetts; and Department of Psychology, University of Connecticut, Storrs, Connecticut.
Adele Holevas. League School of Boston, Newton, Massachusetts.
Edith Kaplan. Boston University School of Medicine, Boston, Massachusetts.
310

began at 5 to 6 months, dropped out by 12 months. The exact development of language is unclear, but by age 3 spontaneous speech was not in evidence. Paul would point when he wanted something. His mother's impression, however, was that he could speak to some extent but did not want to. Paul was seen for regular medical checkups in early childhood. Despite a lack of feeding problems, a question of dehydration was raised by a physician when he was 15 months old; no other health problems were noted.

Paul's health generally has been good. He carries sickle-cell trait from his father. The only available EEG, taken when he was 6 years old, showed "right anterior temporal/right frontal sharp wave reversals, with one beta burst in the right anterior midtemporal region and some right sided slowing".

From the history Paul seems to be one of those autistic children who has a selective and fairly normal attachment to his mother. She reports that he had a good social smile, raised his arms to be picked up, loved being held, and generally seemed quite attached to her, including crying when she left him at his Headstart program at age 3. She knew that something was wrong, however, by age $2\frac{1}{2}$ or 3, since there was no speech and little interaction with others. He preferred to play alone and was quite compulsive and resistant to change. At that time his favorite playthings were trains and musical toys. His doctor suspected that he was deaf because he was so unresponsive, but his mother did not think so because he attended to the radio and to her voice.

Paul's mother also reports that he was hyperlexic. When he was between $2\frac{1}{2}$ and 3 years, he could read third- and fourth-grade books aloud, but with minimal comprehension.

He was also noted to be extremely good at remembering routes and directions. Even today, his memory is excellent; he seems to recall, in exquisite detail, events from when he was 2 and 3 years old.

Paul's mother identifies quite a few autistic behaviors as typical of Paul in the first 5 years; these include symptoms of autistic aloofness (being hard to reach or in a shell, ignoring people as if they did not exist, preferring to be alone, seeming to be able to do things but being unwilling to, leading others' hands to desired objects, and refusing to meet others' gazes), rigidity (being upset when things he was used to were changed, engaging in preferred activities for an unusually long time, becoming agitated by loud or unusual noises, and insisting that things be done the same way each time), and language abnormalities (echolalia, and knowing words but not using them for communication). His mother also notes three unusual skills: memory, music, and reading at age 3.

When Paul was 7 years old, his special education teacher described him as follows: Paul could speak up to seven-word sentences, but most of them were awkward or nonsensical. He showed significant comprehension and inferential problems for material that was lengthy or subtle. His reading comprehension and arithmetic were at first-grade level. He was unable to organize his substantial store of information. Paul needed help in controlling and modulating emotional outbursts. For instance, when another child threw a tantrum, Paul followed suit. Paul lacked the spontaneity and flexibility to interact socially. He paid attention to only two of the five other children in the classroom. He usually did not look at other children or call them by name. His primary means of interacting consisted of imitation, parallel play, and some outdoor chasing games. With guidance, he could play reciprocally but still preferred solitary play much of the time. His favorite free-time activities were drawing pictures of orchestras, listening to music and "conducting," or "playing drums" on anything he could find. Adults were easier for him to interact with, because they were more tolerant of his bizarre interactional style. When visitors entered the classroom, for example, Paul would stand up, say their name, and rapidly recite a social study lesson: "Hi ____, my name is Paul, in the summer, the temperature is between 70 and 100 and in the winter, the temperature is between 0 and 35 . . . ." He related best to his teacher, but still the impression was that the relationship served need fulfill-ment and that he was not genuinely attached to her. After Paul moved to another class, despite an apparent dependency during the year, he largely ignored this teacher.

Paul's current teacher describes 13-year-old Paul in similar terms, despite the progress Paul has made. Academically, Paul is 2 to 3 years below grade level in most areas. Socially, he continues to relate best to a few selected peers but is better able to initiate and sustain interactions; he is able sometimes to engage in limited turn-taking conversations on favorite topics and to ask appropriate rather than stereotyped questions. A true sign of empathic capacity was noted recently by his teacher: When a fellow student was leaving his school and going to a resi-dential school, Paul said "I feel sorry for____. He has to go to a live away school, I wouldn't want that." Paul has made significant progress in being aware of his own emotional states and the reasons for them, and can verbalize them quite well. He is still, however, described as anxious, withdrawn, and timid, often appearing confused by external events and his own feelings. Most of his free play is still solitary or parallel. His chosen leisure activities are drawing elaborate pictures of cartoons or buildings, listening to records, and playing with instruments.

Musical History

Paul's musical history is based on his mother's recollections. To begin, it should be noted that Paul had minimal formal instruction. He had eight weekly lessons on a full set of drums in the summer of 1982 but did not own a set of drums. There was a piano in the house for several months, but Paul did not receive any formal piano instruction. His mother is an amateur singer, and he did receive early exposure to classical records.

Paul's mother recalls that he would tap on his crib in definite and deliberate rhythms around the age of 7 months. She frequently placed a radio, tuned to a classical music station, in his crib or on the nightstand to help him with his sleep-ing problems. He showed a great fascination with all kinds of musical toys. As a toddler, he even lined up his toys and banged out "music" on them.

When Paul was 4 or 5 years old, he began to ask for specific recordings of his favorite pieces, usually symphonic. Now Paul purchases only classical records, even though he is familiar with all the popular artists.

When Paul was 7 years old, he attended rehearsals of his mother's jazz group, in which she was the lead singer. He started playing on the drums during breaks in the rehearsals and the musicians noticed he could reproduce long sequences after only one or two hearings. Eventually they invited him to play with them and incorporated his playing into their performance.

When Paul was 8 years old, a graduate music student spent 1 hour a week playing a conga drum with Paul. They would improvise together, playing a game in which each would imitate what the other had done and then add another improvisation. The student reported that Paul was better than he at the game and that the sequences got too long and complicated for the student to remember before they got too difficult for Paul.

When he was 9, Paul had 8 weeks of lessons on a full set of drums, which concluded with a small ensemble jazz recital. On the tape recording of the recital, Paul is a steady drummer, even when the piece becomes too difficult for the other children. In one selection he is featured as a soloist. Compared to the other players' solos, Paul's improvisation is much more sophisticated, confident, and competent—it is imaginative and elaborate, an impressive feat after only eight lessons and having no drums to practice on at home.

Paul's mother says that although he is most proficient at playing drums, when he was 10, he played a piano by ear "using all ten fingers." Paul was also exposed to gospel singing through his mother's group and, according to her, sometimes played piano accompaniment to her singing.

Paul's mother says that he has a beautiful singing voice and "perfect pitch" but that he will not allow anyone to hear him (she listens from another room). He now has his own synthesizer (acquired after the musical testing described in the next section) and a two-tape recorder on which he produces what his mother calls "operettas." He also will not allow anyone to listen to his taped compositions.

A friend of Paul's mother taught him the basics of conducting, and he is able to make correct conducting patterns for various meters. He often "conducts" while listening to music.

Paul is a great fan of the Boston Pops; Arthur Fiedler was an important figure in Paul's life. For a long period all his drawings and stories centered around Fiedler, and he would use Fiedler's name as a kind of incantation to help calm himself when he lost control. When Fiedler died, Paul had tantrums and was quite upset for several months. To the best of our knowledge, no one replaced the role Fiedler had in Paul's life.

Music Testing

Paul was seen by two of the authors—Paul's former teacher (D. L.) and a musician (A. H.)—in five 1-hour sessions to assess his musical ability. Paul came to his sessions willingly enough but was really not very happy to display his musical ability. This is consistent with what his mother reports, that is, that he will not allow anyone to listen to his taped compositions or to hear him sing. In fact, after the second session, Paul told his teacher that he could do better in the music sessions if he could play by himself. As a result, we decided to leave him alone in the room with two pianos and a synthesizer. He was told at the beginning of the third session that the two adults would wait outside until he wanted them to come in. When the session was almost over, he was told that it was getting close to the end in case he wanted the adults to join him, but he chose to have the room to himself the entire time. The two examiners were reduced to listening through the open door.

In addition to standardized testing, informal observations were made in three basic areas: (1) behaviors acquired primarily through training, such as pitch naming, music reading, and piano fingering; (2) the ability to imitate pitch, melody, rhythm, and chords, skills, it might be argued that would correlate with talent, at least in an untrained person; and (3) creativity in improvising on the piano, in exploring a new instrument (the synthesizer), and in elaborating on musical phrases.

Paul did not do well on musical behaviors that might be considered closely tied to formal training. He was unable to name pitches on the piano. When the examiner played the note F, Paul replied, "I think it's a G." When the examiner told him it was an F and then played a D, a minor third lower, he replied, "It's a minor." For the next several notes he was considerably off, and appeared to be guessing. Although he was not able to name any notes, he was aware of their relationships to one another, that is, generally how far apart they were and in what direction. Paul was also unable to read music. After he hesitated to read the first note of a melody, the examiner told him the starting note was a G. He then attempted to play the music by approximating intervals in the right direction. He played using only his index fingers, alternating fingers for each note in the melody.

In sharp contrast, Paul's ability to imitate various notes in combination was quite good. On eight of ten trials he was able to match the note the examiner played on her piano, sight unseen. In the remaining two trials, he played an adjacent white note and then quickly corrected himself. When the examiner played three-note melodies on her piano, Paul was able to imitate them quickly and accurately. If the three tones happened to make a triad, he would play them as a chord and in most cases identify them correctly, for example, "G minor," "F major." When the number of notes in the melody was increased to five, he was still able to play back the tones perfectly.

Paul's ability to imitate rhythmic sequences was equally impressive. Paul was able to copy all of the eight-beat rhythms, no matter how complex.

Paul could find and imitate triad chords but seemed to become distracted or bored by this and began experimenting by adding nonharmonic tones, often sevenths. In this context he mentioned Prokofiev as one of his favorite composers and indeed created some Prokofiev-like chords that were definitely not confined to the major–minor system.

To further assess these abilities, Paul was given the Seashore Measures of Musical Talents. The following brief descriptions of the Seashore subtests are taken from the manual:

PITCH. In the test of the sense of pitch, 50 pairs of tones are presented. In each pair the listener is to determine whether the second tone is higher or lower in pitch than the first. . . . LOUDNESS. Fifty pairs of tones are presented. The subject is to indicate for each pair whether the second tone is stronger or weaker than the first. . . . RHYTHM. Thirty pairs of rhythmic patterns comprise the sense of rhythm test. The subject is to indicate whether the two patterns in each pair are the same or different. . . . TIME. The test of the sense of time consists of 50 pairs of tones of different durations. The subject is to determine whether the second tone is longer or shorter than the first. . . . TIMBRE. The purpose of the timbre test is to measure ability to discriminate between complex sounds which differ only in harmonic structure. It consists of 50 pairs of tones; in each pair the subject is to judge whether the tones are the same or different in timbre or tone quality. . . . TONAL MEMORY. This test has 30 pairs of tonal sequences consisting of 10 items each of three-, four-, and five-tone spans. In each pair one note is different in the two sequences, and the subject is to identify which note it is by number. (Seashore, Lewis, & Saetveit, 1960, pp. 3–4)

Paul scored in the following percentiles for his mental age on each subtest: Pitch—92nd percentile; Loudness—89th percentile; Rhythm—96th percentile; Time—98th percentile; Timbre—98th percentile; Tonal Memory—99th percentile.

Paul was also examined on various improvisational and responsive tasks. In one session he was encouraged to play a phrase on the piano, and the examiner would "answer" it either sequentially, by adding a new musical idea, or by changing the harmony. In all cases Paul picked up the new material and incorporated it musically into his next phrase. At the end of the first session, Paul was encouraged simply to improvise on the piano. At times it was chaotic in that no apparent form or structure emerged; when allowed to play by himself for a few minutes, however, his composition had a definite development section and a conclusion, an E-major chord with rolled octaves in the left hand. The examiners felt that Paul was hampered by his lack of piano technique and was unable to implement his musical ideas.

In the second session the examiner brought along a small synthesizer. The first thing that Paul did was to try to pick out a familiar melody—a Prokofiev march—but he was unable to end the second phrase. Next he began to explore all the different timbres: violin, flute, and so forth. He started on a different pitch each time and successfully transposed the melody except for the last three notes. He also tried playing the timbres in different registers. The examiner then tested recognition of the synthesizer timbres, and he was completely accurate, with no hesitation. After he improvised a bit more, he asked if he could test the examiner in the same way with the timbres. When asked how he wanted to end the session, he played another improvisation on the piano with a very dramatically rolled final chord.

During the third session, when Paul was left by himself in a room with two pianos and a synthesizer, he started on the piano, playing with both hands, the left playing chords while the right played a melody. He would explore one musical idea for 2 or 3 minutes and then switch to something totally different. At one point he played a sequence moving down through five different keys. He spent a fair amount of time deliberately playing dissonant chords, which was "like one of my favorite composers." Next Paul turned to the synthesizer. Using the flute stop, he played a melody with his right hand while playing chords on the piano with his left hand. It was a surprisingly effective simulation of a flute-and-piano ensemble. His flute melody was idiomatic to the instrument, that is, containing trills and ornamentation. Then Paul began using rhythms on the synthesizer and played syncopated chords against it on the piano. He stayed with this longer than his usual attention span of 2 to 3 minutes. He changed the rhythm to a more complex one and played a synthesizer melody that was stylistically suited and rhythmically synchronized. He started changing the tempo of the rhythm and was able to adjust the melody instantly to the new speed.

Neuropsychological Testing

When Paul was 8 years 8 months, and again when he was 12 years 7 months, he was given a comprehensive neuropsychological evaluation. The pattern of results was essentially the same from one testing to the next, so we will discuss primarily the more recent findings. In addition to documenting Paul's musical ability on standardized tests, we were also concerned with investigating areas of cognitive function that might be expected to correlate with musical ability. In particular, we were concerned with exploring his motor skills, his auditory memory and memory in general, his ability to reproduce sequential material, and functions thought to be heavily dependent on the contribution of the right hemisphere, such as complex visuo-spatial abilities. We also present some background on general cognitive functioning and language.

General Cognitive Functioning and Language

At present Paul scores a Verbal IQ of 82 and a Performance IQ of 108 on the WISC-R, placing him within the average range of functioning. However, there is a great deal of variability among subtests. His functioning ranges from the 5th percentile for his age on tests of arithmetic, vocabulary, and coding (i.e., writing symbols paired to numbers according to a prearranged key), to the 84th percentile on assembling puzzles and recreating block patterns and to the 91st percentile on pointing out the missing pieces of pictures. Paul's teacher suggests that the reason for his low arithmetic score at present is that he has taken to using a calculator and has forgotten most of his multiplication tables. Digit span, acquisition of academic information, abstracting the similarities between pairs of words, and sequencing cartoon pictures are in the average range. On sequencing cartoon frames Paul did not appreciate the humor in any of the cartoon strips, but he did appreciate the basic social situations in which the people were involved.

Paul scored in the average range on Raven's Progressive Matrices, a test involving the apprehension of visual patterns and nonverbal analogous reasoning. He did very well in sorting a deck of cards by one of three variables (color, form, or number) and then shifting the basis on which the sorting is made depending on yes–no cues from the examiner. This test is generally considered to be a sensitive measure of frontal lobe function, in that it requires formation, maintenance, and appropriate shifting of response sets. Paul also showed good visual reasoning (normal for his age) in identifying the absurd aspects of pictures on the 1985 revision of the Stanford-Binet. He was able to notice, for example, that the bubbles produced by a skin diver were going down instead of up, and in another picture, that the wind was blowing the trees in the wrong direction compared to the way a girl was leaning.

Paul's language skills continue to be his most impaired area of functioning, as they have been throughout his development. However, this does not seem to be due to any specific linguistic deficit. His ability to repeat complex sentences is age-normal, as is his single-word expressive vocabulary. Verbal fluency (producing lists of words beginning with a given letter or in a particular semantic category) was also age-normal, except that, in typical autistic fashion, he took the instructions to produce a list of "fruits and vegetables" very literally, giving a list in which fruits and vegetables alternated.

Major linguistic deficits lie in his ability to express what he knows in complex syntactic utterances. His vocabulary score on the WISC-R, a test that requires oral definitions of words, was only at the 5th percentile, while he was at about the 50th percentile on simple one-word expressive naming. His reading comprehension has developed relatively well. Though not age-normal, it does not suggest severely impaired reading comprehension and seems to be more limited by his inability to understand connected passages than by single-word comprehension or decoding deficits.

There are two special aspects to Paul's language that are rather unusual. One is seen in his written language. He much prefers to print, especially in school, but can produce cursive writing on request. In either case, Paul tends to omit spaces between words. When asked to count the number of words in sentences he has written, he is generally correct, indicating that he does know the boundaries of words. When pressed to put in the appropriate spaces, he is able to do so, but there is still a tendency to slip back into running words together.

The second peculiarity in Paul's language is seen in his word choices: parts of sentences do not agree with each other; communicative intent changes in the middle of a sentence; and pronouns are misused (gender as well as singular vs. plural). Also, word choices indicate reduced sensitivity to the connotative meaning of words. For example: "Pound and yard both means something they weigh"; "Telephone and radio both have electricity"; "Candle and lamp both have light in them"; Join means "to come with . . . to come with the people"; What should you do if you cut your finger? "Tell a mother. . . . "; Why is it important for the government to hire people to inspect the meat in meat-packing plants? "So they won't spoil"; Why is cotton often used in making cloth? "So it can be warm, it's effective and more used."

Paul was given a set of experimental matching tasks of equal difficulty for normal children between 3 and 9 years of age. He performed at or near ceiling on matching different views of an object and on matching which two people showed the same facial affect, and which affect was appropriate to a situation, but he scored only 80% on matching pictures of individuals. His errors indicated that unless the discrimination was very easy, he tended to match on the basis of orientation in space and clothing similarities rather than facial configuration.

Thus Paul is generally functioning in the average range of intelligence, but he shows deficient performance on tasks requiring him to express complex ideas verbally and on face recognition, and superior performance on some visual constructional and visual remote memory tasks.

Motor Functioning

At age 8 years 8 months, Paul's arm coordination was somewhat low for his age, but his balance and gait were normal. Fine motor coordination was assessed by moving pegs (Annett, 1970), sequentially tapping fingers, and pronating and supinating each hand (Denckla, 1973). Performance was somewhat above average for Paul's age, with the right hand being especially good.

Visuo-Spatial Skills

This is clearly an area of relative strength for Paul. His visual scanning is rapid and efficient. His free drawings and copies are accurate and well planned but are not extraordinary for his age. The limits of his organizational ability are reached on the copy of the Rey-Osterrieth Complex Figure. Although he does start with the base rectangle, his approach is somewhat disorganized, and the final product is not totally accurate, but, again, this is within normal limits for his age. He draws cartoon characters, including people and animals, which might appear to demonstrate exceptional talent, except that they are stereotyped and have been often practiced. He does do very well relative to his age peers (84th percentile) on the block-reproduction and puzzle-assembly tasks of the WISC-R. All puzzles were assembled accurately and within time limits; on assembling the car, which is rich in internal detail, Paul got maximum-time bonus credits. He was also able to complete all the block designs, although he did not complete the last one within the time limit. On many of the items he got maximum-time bonuses, completing the design in less than 10 seconds. Paul always started his block reproductions on the left side, and the left side of the Rey-Osterrieth figure was somewhat expanded on immediate memory and was reproduced slightly better than the right side in the delayed condition.

When asked to visualize the capital letters of the alphabet and report which ones contain curves, Paul was able to do quite well and in reasonable time; however, he was almost twice as fast at reporting which letters of the alphabet rhyme with "tree." These tasks have been found to be sensitive to asymmetries in hemisphere functioning; Paul's asymmetry is suggestive of more efficient left-hemisphere processing. That Paul can use rhyming is demonstrated in the following birthday poem he wrote for a classmate ("Closkey" refers to Paul himself):

YOUKNOW
I KNOW JIMMYTHATS
MYGOO DFRIEND. I
KNOWLARRY, THEFUN
MUSTNOTEND, THERE'SANOTHER
PERSO N THAT'SINMYCLASS IS
KIMCHEE,WHWATCHOUTTOMMY,
HERECOMES CLOSKEY!THAT'S
ME!ANDWHEATHERYOULIKE
ALICEOR PETER OREVENKEVINTOO
I CAME TOS AYTHERE'S
NOONEELSELIKEYHOU
AND SO . . .
HAPPY
BIRTHDAY
TO YOU!
FROMPAUL TO TOMMY[1]

Memory

Finally, we come to an examination of Paul's memory capacity, which in many respects is the most unusual feature of his neuropsychologïcal profile. His overall memory quotient on the Denman Neuropsychological Memory Scale, 91, is quite consistent with his WISC-R IQ of 93. Furthermore, his verbal memory quotient was 83 (consistent with his Verbal IQ of 82), and his nonverbal memory quotient was 103 (consistent with his Performance IQ of 108). The same general difficulty with verbal material described previously is reflected in Paul's memory function. However, an examination of the Denman subtests reveals even more striking dissociations. Paul does well (84th percentile) on Paired Associate Learning, perhaps because it can be done as a rote memory task without the constraints of semantic processing. Furthermore, he maintains these memories, scoring at the 84th percentile (ceiling) on 20-minute recall of the pairs. However, his immediate recall of a prose story was quite poor (5th percentile). Delayed recall is at the same level as immediate recall. His lack of comprehension and active encoding of the story prevents efficient recall under either condition.

On remote verbal information (such as identifying Babe Ruth and Neil Armstrong, and listing the ingredients of gravy), Paul scores in the 25th percentile, not significantly different from his 50th-percentile score on remote nonverbal information, such as remembering what traffic, handicapped, and no-smoking signs look like. However, his 91st-percentile score on Picture Completion on the WISC-R suggests that his figural memory for more common objects is at a superior level; the lower score on the Denman Remotely Stored Non-Verbal Information subtest

---

1. To ensure anonymity, all names have been changed, but the meter, spacings, and punctuation have been preserved.

may be due to the verbal output requirements. Both immediate and delayed recall of the complex Rey-Osterrieth figure were average for his age.

Of particular interest was Paul's memory for musical tones and melodies and for human faces (subtests of the Denman). He performed at the 98th percentile on memory for musical tones and melodies, making only 2 errors out of 30 same–different judgments, both errors occurring on trials where he was distracted. In contrast, his memory for photographed human faces was quite poor (16th percentile).

Paul was also given the children's version of the California Verbal Learning Test, in which the subject gets five trials to learn a list of 12 words falling into three categories. Paul had an average learning curve for this list of words and, furthermore, was able to use the intrinsic semantic organization of the list to organize his recall. Interestingly, when he had mastered the list, by the fourth trial, he suddenly dropped his semantic clustering strategy and gave the list back in sequential order on the last trial. This is a varient of a normal strategy, described by Dellis, Kramer, Ober, and Kaplan (1987). Likewise, he did not show any sensitivity to proactive or retroactive interference; that is, recall of a second list after five presentations of the first list was quite good, and he was able to immediately recall the first list and to retain it after a 20-minute filled delay.

One quite remarkable aspect of Paul's memory was his incidental learning of the digit–symbol pairs on the Coding subtest of the WISC-R. Despite his slow performance and therefore his low score, and despite his having had only 90 seconds' exposure and only getting to do one line of the test, he was able to recall all nine of the digit–symbol pairs without any errors. This is a remarkably superior performance.

Sequential Memory Tasks

Because of the ordered nature of musical material, we were interested in whether Paul would show any outstanding ability on specifically sequential memory tasks. At age 8 years 8 months, his score was age-normal on Tapping Sequences and slightly below average on Digit Span (5 forward, 2 backward) from the McCarthy Scales of Children's Abilities. His Digit Span currently is within normal limits, although it is somewhat low for Digits Backwards (7 forward, 3 backward). On a test of nonverbal spatial pointing span, analogous to Digit Span (two-dimensional adaptation of Corsi blocks), Paul points accurately to six blocks preserving the sequence, and he can point to seven but loses the sequence. On testing his memory for objects on the 1985 revision of the Stanford-Binet, in which the subject is shown pictured objects one at a time and then is required to point to them sequentially on a large array, Paul did quite well (one standard deviation above the mean for his age). He recalled six objects in correct sequence, and eight objects by making some sequential reversals. Thus his sequential memory span for material of all types seems to be about equal and falls within the average range.

Discussion

Paul's scores on the Seashore Measures of Musical Talents provide objective confirmation of his musical talent. Factor analytic and other studies (reviewed by Judd, Chapter 6, this volume, and by Gardner, 1984) suggest several components to musical ability, including pitch discrimination, tonal memory, rhythm, and comprehension of complex patterns. Paul's test results and informal performances suggest that he excels in all of these components. His highest score (99th percentile) was achieved on Seashore's Tonal Memory, despite a history of very little actual music instruction. Judd (Chapter 6, this volume) reports that Tonal Memory is the only subtest in the Seashore battery on which professional musicians clearly show superior performance and that early excellent musical memory is probably the most reliable indicator of a prodigy or a musical savant.

Typically, the talent of autistic individuals involves fine-grained reproductions of stimuli but an unimpressive ability to generate unique patterns with them. (There are exceptions, however, such as the artists Richard Wawro and Elly, who are discussed by Bogyo & Ellis, Chapter 13, this volume.) We could not observe enough of Paul's musical productions to judge the extent of his capacity for creativity, but from his mother's reports and from what we were about to observe, we judge his ability to create and respond to musical ideas to be well above average. Often, individuals with extensive musical training are unable to improvise or compose with the fluency that Paul does. Paul's musical assertiveness and confidence are in marked contrast to his social and interpersonal style. It could be argued that the nonlinguistic dimension of music is for Paul a more satisfying means of expression than language. Whether or not this is the case, Paul's musical expression is well above average, and almost completely self-taught.

Consistent with the literature about other talented musicians, Paul demonstrated his interest in music at a very early age. He had no opportunity to play at that time, so his potential performance skills must remain in doubt, but by his mother's report, he was unusually interested in musical toys and in listening to classical music from very early childhood. This might be taken as support for those who suggest that some inclination or talent may be inborn and not explainable by practice effects.

Music is a solitary activity for Paul. It does not serve or promote social functions for him, except for a rudimentary reciprocal play that one can induce him to engage in. It fits very well into his self-absorbed world, and he guards his compositions and performances from the eyes of others. The potentially solitary character of music making may have been part of its original appeal for Paul.

The detailed neuropsychological examination affords an opportunity to examine skills and abilities that may be highly correlated with, or dissociated from, musical ability in Paul. The two significant areas of deficit in Paul's neuropsychological profile are language expressivity, and face matching and face memory, while areas of superior ability include some visuo-spatial functions, music discrimination, and some other aspects of memory. One cannot make a simple argument about hemisphere impairment to explain this pattern of ability. Language impairment combined with visuo-spatial superiority might lead one to posit left-hemisphere dysfunction and overreliance on right-hemisphere processing, but there are several reasons why a simple hemisphere argument will not adequately explain Paul's pattern. First, most of Paul's language functions, including repetition, verbal fluency, naming, and articulation, are intact—in fact, they are in the average range. Second, the alphabet-rhyming versus the curved-letters task dissociates in Paul in a direction suggesting left-hemisphere superiority. Finally, fine motor coordination is significantly better in Paul's right hand.

The two areas of dysfunction (expressive language and face recognition) compared to the areas in which Paul was average or superior suggest not left versus right hemisphere but another dichotomy. One could argue that language expressivity and face recognition are the most socially based of all the functions tested. If Paul (and other high-functioning autistic children) has a primary deficit in social motivation—that is, that he suffers from the lack of a strong innate interest in members of his own species and from a lack of desire to communicate with them—then one might expect impaired development in those cognitive functions most heavily dependent on social interaction. Another similarity between complex expressive language and face recognition is that there are areas of cortex devoted specifically to these functions. If social interest does not develop until quite late (or not at all), however, the child may not be motivated to take in the large amount of language and face data that these areas of cortex may need to develop into efficient systems (see Rimland & Fein, Chapter 25, this volume for a fuller discussion of this point.)

Music and visuo-spatial pursuits, in contrast, may be done asocially. They may be appealing to the autistic child for this reason and may show normal or superior development. Autistic children are drawn to pattern-generation activities of all sorts. The literature is replete with descriptions of autistic children who spend many hours arranging what are intended to be symbolic toys into abstract patterns based on their physical, and not their symbolic, properties. Within the higher functioning autistic population, for example, some of the paintings of Elly (described by Bogyo & Ellis, Chapter 13, this volume) are masterpieces of colored squares arranged in subtle and intricate patterns. The autistic boy described by Waterhouse (Chapter 18, this volume) has superior ability in the area of visual pattern recognition.

Music, too, can be seen as a patterned activity, which can be devoid of symbolic content if the listener likes and can be appreciated as abstract sequences of auditory patterns. Paul, therefore, can be seen in a sense as an auditory analogue to the visually talented boy described by Waterhouse. In the concluding chapter of this volume, Waterhouse presents a theory of special talent that posits a possible reorganization of undedicated cortex to an architecture that lends itself to pattern recognition. The findings of her case and of our own suggest further that this pattern-recognition cortex may be dedicated to one modality in particular, in that Paul was only average on the best single test of visual pattern analysis (Raven's) on which the Waterhouse boy excelled, whereas the Waterhouse boy was not especially talented at music.

In this volume Judd (Chapter 6) and Fein and Obler (Chapter 1) discuss the central role of memory in special abilities; Waterhouse (Chapter 26) suggests that reorganized cortex makes encoding of complex patterns easier and thus facilitates memory. Whether or not this notion of reorganized cortex proves correct, accounts of exceptional and domain-specific memory are very common in the lives of prodigies. Paul's case certainly supports the notion that outstanding domain-specific memory is associated with talent in that domain. His memory for musical and rhythmic patterns not only was exceptional in standardized tests but reportedly exceeded that of the graduate student in music with whom he played. His exceptional memory, however, was not limited to musical material. On paired-associate learning (in the verbal domain) and in incidental learning and recall of digit-symbol pairs, Paul was exceptional—and this despite limited verbal expressiveness and average verbal reasoning and vocabulary. In contrast, where one might expect that all aspects of sequential or auditory memory would be correspondingly good, they were not. Digit span, pointing span, and sequential memory for objects were merely average. This pattern of exceptional musical memory and verbal associative memory, with average memory for other sequential auditory and visual material, was unexpected. This raises the possibility that Paul has outstanding capacity for rote learning based on visual or acoustic properties but that semantically based learning is impaired and that one-trial immediate memory span is merely average.

The Waterhouse argument suggests that persons with special abilities are able to "see" or "hear," directly and immediately, higher order patterns in stimuli that others might have to analyze in a more laborious way. Paul's performance on the Seashore subtests also suggests that persons with special abilities not only "see" or "hear" higher order patterns but also can make more accurate and finer discriminations at the concrete sensory-perceptual level, perhaps consistent with Rimland's (1978) suggestion of focus on "high fidelity" physical characteristics. The ability to perceive the stimuli in a very fine grained way and the ability to see higher order patterns may be dissociated, and either or both may be necessary for the expression of a special ability.

Another possible basis for autistic special abilities is raised by Fein and Waterhouse (1985) and by Rimland and Fein (Chapter 25, this volume). They suggest that in some high-functioning autistic children, hyperfunction of the hippocampus, triggered by dysfunction of a complementary structure, the amygdala, or resulting from neurotransmitter imbalance, may result in abnormal *ease* in laying down new memories, particularly episodic, contextual, or associative memories. A similar notion is developed by Oscar-Berman (Chapter 9, this volume). David Bear and others have suggested that in some brain areas and with some psychological functions, epileptic discharge may result in hyperfunction rather than disrupted function of that area.

Thus there are several, albeit highly speculative, mechanisms by which the functional contributions of a particular brain region may be overrepresented in cognitive functioning. There is strong evidence, provided by Milner and others and reviewed by Judd (Chapter 6, this volume), that the right temporal region is necessary for tonal memory and timbre discrimination, at least in right-handed males. Paul's EEG abnormality involves his right midtemporal region. This raises the speculation that in Paul's case, hyperfunction of cortical and subcortical (hippocampal) tissue in this area contributes to his musical memory (and thus to his musical talent).

References

Annett, M. (1970). The growth of manual preference and speed. *British Journal of Psychology, 61*, 545–558.

Dellis, D., Kramer, J., Ober, B., & Kaplan, E. (1987). *The CVLT: Administration and interpretation.* San Antonio: Psychological Corporation.

Denckla, M. (1973). Development of speed in repetitive and successive finger movements in normal children. *Developmental Medicine and Child Neurology, 15*, 635–645.

Denman, S. B. (1984). *Denman Neuropsychology Memory Scale.* Charleston: Sidney B. Denman.

Fein, D., & Waterhouse, L. (1985, June). *Infantile autism: Delineating the key deficits.* Paper presented at the International Neuropsychological Symposium, Edinburgh, Scotland.

Gardner, H. (1984). *Frames of mind.* New York: Basic Books.

Grant, D. A. & Berg, E. A. (1948). A behavioral analysis of degree of reinforcement and ease of shifting to new responses in a Weigl-type card-sorting problem. *Journal of Experimental Psychology, 38*, 404–411.

McCarthy, D. (1972). *McCarthy Scales of Children's Abilities.* New York: Psychological Corporation.

Osterrieth, P. A. (1944). Le test de copie d'une figure complexe. *Archives de Psychologie, 30*, 206–356.

Raven, J. C. (1960). *Guide to the Standard Progressive Matrices.* London: H. K. Lewis; New York: Psychological Corporation.

Rimland, B. (1978). Savant capabilities of autistic children and their cognitive implications. In G. Serban (Ed.), *Cognitive defects in the development of mental illness.* New York: Brunner/Mazel.

Seashore, C., Lewis, D., & Saetveit, J. (1960). *Manual of instructions and interpretations for the Seashore Measures of Musical Talents.* San Antonio: The Psychological Corporation.

Thorndike, R. L., Hagen, E. P., and Sattler, J. M. (1986). *Stanford-Binet Intelligence Scale 4th Edition.* Chicago: Riverside Pub. Co.

Wechsler, D. (1974). *Wechsler intelligence scale for children*—Revised. New York: Psychological Corporation.

18

Extraordinary Visual Memory and Pattern Perception in an Autistic Boy

Lynn Waterhouse

This is the case study of J. D., a white male right-handed 18-year-old boy currently attending a day school for autistic children. J. D. was first diagnosed as autistic at the age of 5. At about that time he also exhibited in prominent fashion extraordinary abilities and interests in visual memory and perceptual pursuits that are the focus of this chapter.

Family History

The family history of J. D. is of interest. J. D.'s father has five cousins, and four of the five had extremely delayed language acquisition. Furthermore, all four now have some impairment in speech function—described by J. D.'s father as "slurred" and "not properly developed." According to family members, J. D.'s laugh sounds identical to the laugh of the paternal cousin whose speech is most impaired. J. D.'s mother's sister is mildly retarded, and one of her children has a seizure disorder that began in early childhood (approximately age 4). J. D.'s maternal grandmother had suffered from Saint Vitus dance (Sydenham chorea), a neurological disorder.

Interviews with J. D.'s mother and father concerning family histories revealed that neither had knowledge of anyone in either of their families having had a major or minor affective disorder, schizophrenia, or even a personality disorder. Though such disorders are typically underreported, J. D.'s parents were very open and frank—they have become accustomed to answering questions about their families put to them by the various professionals who have seen J. D. over the years.

J. D.'s siblings, two sisters and a brother, are all functioning successfully in jobs or college. None of the three had any difficulty in school; none had any special problems in language acquisition or in the development of social skills. They appear to be caring and concerned about J. D. Moreover, they all show significant respect for J. D.'s special abilities.

Lynn Waterhouse. Child Behavior Study, Trenton State College, Trenton, New Jersey.

J. D.'s parents love him and cope with his social withdrawal and developmental delays extremely well. J. D.'s mother is open, friendly, and gregarious, as is his father. His mother finished high school, and his father completed grade school (eighth grade). J. D.'s father works as a skilled manual laborer, and his mother is a clerical worker. At present both parents are in generally good health, although J. D.'s mother is overweight and suffers from high blood pressure. Both parents drink alcohol moderately. J. D.'s mother seems to be addicted to caffeine; she drinks two full pots of coffee plus caffeinated colas and iced tea every day.

J. D.'s Early History

J. D. was the fourth child born in 4 years in the family. He was the product of an uneventful, full-term pregnancy and 3-hour labor; at birth he weighed a little over 8 lb. The only complication of note was that his mother had had a uterine staph infection. J. D. was born with a staph skin infection and, because of this, was kept in isolation in the newborn nursery.

J. D.'s mother has good recall for the events surrounding J. D.'s birth. She reported his Apgar scores as 9 at 1 minute and 10 at 5 minutes. She remembers the birth as having been fairly easy. She was concerned about the staph rash, but other than that, J. D. presented no notable problems as a newborn. At birth he had no breathing problems, no jaundice, no seizures, and no problems with heartbeat or motor functions. J. D. was neither limp nor rigid, and he seemed to his mother to be a perfectly normal baby. He was bottle fed and had no problems sucking. J. D.'s mother didn't notice any abnormality in J. D.'s ability to see her or to see objects. In fact, his divergent strabismus was not picked up until he was evaluated by the school district's child study team when he was 5 years old.

J. D. crawled at 6 months, sat up at approximately 7 months, and walked unsupported at the age of 1 year. He had no abnormalities in motor behavior and was a normally affectionate child. He was toilet trained before the age of 2 and was competent at feeding himself. However, he never babbled or cooed, and began making sounds only at about $2\frac{1}{2}$. He developed a pattern of single-word speech at the age of 3 which has persisted to the present.

When J. D. was between $2\frac{1}{2}$ and 3 years old, his mother and father felt that a sharp change occurred in his behavior. They report that a switch seemed to be turned off in him, and he became withdrawn and socially unresponsive. They noticed a number of specific changes, and J. D.'s mother has at times attributed these changes to a fall he had at around age 3. J. D.'s father, however, believes that many of J. D.'s symptoms and behaviors were present before the fall.

The specific behaviors that J. D.'s parents began to notice included toe walking, hand flapping, making squawking noises and what they refer to as "horse" noises in a high-pitched voice, and having what seemed to be totally unprovoked temper tantrums, which would last for up to an hour. They also noticed that J. D. would be excessively "sweaty" when he hadn't been engaged in any vigorous activity. He began to rock back and forth for long periods of time. Furthermore, J. D. had an extremely narrow range of food preferences, which was quite rigid.

J. D.'s parents also noticed that he seemed to look right through them, avoiding their gaze. Most salient to them was the fact that J. D. didn't progress in speaking at a time at which they expected him to be progressing. Also salient was the fact that J. D. showed no interest in playing with his brother and sisters.

Sometime between $2\frac{1}{2}$ and 4 years, J. D. developed a pattern of echolalia, which he has continued into the present. He now repeats "That's old Sue" many times and also will often say "Pow, sock in the head." J. D.'s parents think the former phrase comes from something on MTV, and the latter phrase, from the *Laverne and Shirley* TV show. J. D. also often exhibits immediate echolalia— repeating exactly what has just been said to him. He has been trained to say "Hi, how are you?," "What's the weather like?," and "Have a pleasant day." J. D. does use these phrases but cannot sustain anything like a conversation. He does not have normal pitch or rhythm in speaking, and he states his learned phrases abruptly.

In toddlerhood J. D. had no trouble going to sleep or getting up at normal hours, but during the night, he would wake for several periods of body rocking—a practice that he has continued into the present.

J. D.'s mother kept him at home until he was 5 and could attend kindergarten. Although he avoided eye contact, was echolalic, and had only begun to develop a single-word vocabulary at age 4, his mother believed that his problems were developmental in nature. She hoped that he would outgrow his social isolation and would ultimately develop a more normal ability to communicate. The kindergarten teacher in public school found J. D. disruptive, not because he was aggressive or uncontrollable, but because he could not communicate, socialize, or participate in the activities of the class. At age 5 he was seen by his local school district's child study team and was given a complete neurological examination, which yielded no significant findings except divergent strabismus. An EEG, a CT scan, and a skull X-ray indicated nothing abnormal. Hearing was also normal.

Current Behavior of J. D.

In addition to solitaire, jigsaw puzzles, and connect-the-dot books (described in more detail later), J. D. is currently absorbed by MTV, a cable music video television channel. According to his siblings and parents, J. D. knows all the top 100 songs, can sing most of each song, and knows nearly all the songs written or sung by a large set of currently popular rock musicians. In a recent interview he demonstrated a very impressive knowledge in this area, but cataloging his memory accurately would require some *a priori* charting of musicians and their songs.

J. D. currently has a variety of rituals, mostly associated with TV. One major ritual is simply that when he watches the TV show, *The A-Team*, J. D. must have his Mr. T doll positioned on top of the TV set exactly in the center, facing front. J. D. will have a tantrum if this is not done.

Other than *The A-Team* and MTV, J. D. is not interested in TV. He used to watch *Laverne and Shirley*, but several years ago his parents stopped him from watching it because it usually upset him—at the conclusion of an episode, J. D. would have a full-blown tantrum. The tantrum would involve screaming, crying, hand flapping, toe walking, the "horse" noises, and excessive sweating. J. D.'s parents believe that the silly slapstick violence (Laverne and Shirley playfully punching each other, etc.) is what would trigger J. D.'s tantrums. However, there is a great deal of violence shown, some in a slapstick fashion, but most in a serious, active and aggressive manner, on the show, *The A-Team*, and yet J. D. has never had a tantrum in response to any of its episodes.

One other TV show has disturbed J. D., and that is a Bugs Bunny cartoon series. Although J. D. has had tantrums immediately after watching Bugs Bunny cartoons, he has consistently sought to watch them again and again, unlike his response to *Laverne and Shirley*. This has disturbed J. D.'s father, who is greatly upset by J. D.'s tantrum behavior. The father has tried to control TV access for J. D. but on occasion his son will nonetheless somehow get a chance to watch one of the cartoons and have the inevitable tantrum. At one point several years ago, J. D. had a TV set in his bedroom, but his father was so afraid that J. D. would watch another Bugs Bunny cartoon that he took the set out of J. D.'s room.

In the absence of Bugs Bunny cartoons and *Laverne and Shirley*, J. D.'s parents estimate that J. D. would have only two or three tantrum episodes a year. J. D. does make "horse" noises often, both at school and at home, despite many years of behavior modification programs instituted by the school in order to eliminate J. D.'s production of such noise. There has been no systematic analysis of the types of situations in which J. D. makes "horse" noises, but in test sessions he makes them when he appears to be slightly frustrated by his own inability to complete test items. School staff members believe that J. D. makes such noises when he is frustrated or angry. They have attempted to train him to make a statement of his feelings ("I'm angry") rather than make the noises.

Only two of the other elements of tantrum behavior (toe walking and hand flapping—but not screaming, crying, or excessive sweating) appear separately in J. D.'s day-to-day behavior at home or at school. J. D. will stop the toe walking once he has been reminded that he shouldn't walk on his toes, but he continues to engage in hand flapping in response to most questions that do not have a "yes" or "no" answer (i.e., open-ended questions). Although the school has had some success in getting J. D. to stop hand flapping, when he does not hand flap in response to open-ended questions, he will rub his hand up and down his legs. The school staff feels that J. D.'s hand flapping and leg rubbing are both signs of anxiety produced by the pressure he feels when he is asked to generate speech. Despite these recurring moments of apparent extreme stress, however, J. D. works very hard in school (a school for autistic children). In fact, he has been a model student, winning awards for improvement in academic skills and skill in sociability. His sociability is "trained"—that is, he has learned a variety of set phrases and greetings that he can use with cuing.

Social relations are empty; for example, when he is introduced to someone, one of the things he is interested in is the birthday of that person. Once someone tells him his or her birthdate, he will tell that person the names of all the people he knows who have birthdays in the same year. J. D.'s parents can't remember when he first started doing this, nor do they have any idea why. However, interest in others' birthdays represents J. D.'s main social focus of attention to other people.

History and Current Status of J. D.'s Special Ability

To the present, J. D.'s parents have maintained the belief that J. D. is extremely intelligent and that he "has the best memory of anyone in the family." They first noticed his special skills when he was between 4 and 5 years old. J. D. would watch TV at home and would then spell out words he saw on the screen (such as names of TV shows) using alphabet blocks, which were part of his set of playthings. When J. D. was first seen by the child study team, he took blocks during the test session and spontaneously spelled *DAKTARI*, the name of a TV show. He was also able to recognize written product names that had been advertised on TV. Though these anecdotes suggest that J. D. may have been hyperlexic, he was not given any formal test of his reading ability until much later, after several years of reading instruction.

Another aspect of behavior that J. D.'s parents thought remarkable was J. D.'s ability to remember routes they had traveled. When his parents took him someplace in the car and told him where they were going, J. D. would be very upset and agitated if the driver took a route different from the one taken before. And the reverse was true as well: If the family started its trip on a familiar route, J. D. would say the name of the place the route led to and would have difficulty if the driver altered that route and ended up at a different destination.

His parents also noted that J. D. was very good at certain sorts of games— jigsaw puzzles, connect-the-dots, and MATCH II, a matching game using national flags. Early on they noticed that he could complete a 500-piece jigsaw puzzle in about 2 minutes. Their solution to this "problem" was to buy him puzzles with 5,000 pieces, so that he could have a reasonable time to play with the game.

J. D. "cheated" at MATCH II, the flag-matching game. The game consists of 32 pairs of plastic tiles, blank on one side and imprinted with a national flag on the other. The board has 64 tile cradles, holding the pieces upside down in an 8 × 8 grid. In sequence each player gets a chance to turn over two tiles. When a match of two identical country flags is made, the player gets a point. J. D. would look at the tiles as he set up the board before the game and then, during the game, would continue to turn over pairs (the player who makes a successful match immediately gets another turn), so that the other players (his sisters and brother) would never even get to have a turn.

In a similar fashion J. D. "cheats" at solitaire—currently one of his favorite pastimes. Other packaged games that were of interest to J. D. and whose elements he memorized quickly were Concentration and Superheros. From early on J. D. has shown intense interest in connect-the-dot drawings. If his parents bring him a new connect-the-dot book, he will stay up past midnight filling in every outlined picture in the book. He makes no mistakes but takes a bit of time to draw in the lines; J. D.'s parents attribute his slowness to motor limitations and not to limitations in perception.

Results of Tests Given to J. D.

To provide more detailed and objective evidence of his visual talents, J. D. was given a set of standard and experimental tests. As a contrast to these visual tests, he was given the Peabody Picture Vocabulary Test and a sentence-repetition test; a spontaneous language sample was also recorded.

J. D.'s performance in language areas has not improved at all during the past 9 years. His mean length of utterance at age 9 was 2.25 words and at present has been indexed at between 2.00 and 2.75 (including trained phrases). His scores on the Peabody Picture Vocabulary Test have gone from a mental age equivalent of 3 years 9 months at age 9, to 5 years 7 months at age 12, and to 6 years 1 month at age 17. J. D.'s three scores on a standard sentence-repetition task have stayed the same: a score of 1 out of 16 at ages 9, 12, and 17.

In very marked contrast, J. D. shows remarkable skill on most visuo-spatial tasks involving complex pattern recognition and visual memory. He was given the WISC-R Object Assembly task. In this task an individual must take cut-apart pieces of a schematic picture of an object and assemble the complete picture from the pieces. J. D. had no trouble assembling a girl and an adult face. Furthermore, he was very fast in doing so.

J. D. was also given the Benton Judgment of Line Orientation Form (1983). Two lines are presented as the model; they may form an angle of between 10 and 180 degrees. The test subject identifies the target angle by calling out numbers on a full, fanlike array of lines. J. D. got a perfect score of 30, with no errors or hesitations. His only problem was a perseverative tendency to add the line numbers together as part of his answer (5 plus 12 makes 17, 6 plus 7 makes 13).

J. D. also did very well on a test of visual gestalt closure. This task involves verbal labeling of partially complete sketches of objects. Out of 26 items, J. D. rapidly labeled the correct object in 24 cases. The incomplete gestalt of a person playing a guitar was labeled "mom baby" by J. D., and the final item, a teapot, was labeled "fish" by J. D. J. D.'s performance on this test showed him to be good at determining what these schemas were—that is his ability to interpret full visual forms from sketchy information is intact. Since his score on the Peabody Picture Vocabulary Test is currently around the 6-year level, he has a very limited vocabulary to work with.

Visuo-Spatial Tests with Exceptional Performance

J. D.'s two most phenomenal performances were on the WISC-R Block Design task and on an experimental test of gestalt memory for object location, developed from the work of Brenda Spiegler (Spiegler & Waterhouse, 1985; Spiegler & Mishkin, 1981).

J. D. has been given the WISC-R Block Design subtest three times in his life. He was first tested in 1976, when he was 9. In the test there are eight complex figures to copy using four or nine blocks, and of these the average child of 9 should be able to complete about three. J. D. completed all the figures with great rapidity, getting the highest scores for the greatest speed in all but the last two of the eight items. J. D. took this test again when he was 12. Again, he got all of the items right, but this time he got the highest score possible on the test: He took a total of 113 seconds to assemble all eight complex designs. On a final retest at age 17, J. D.

completed the eight figures (each presented separately, as in all previous administrations) in 41 seconds. As a yardstick for J. D.'s performance, a normal boy of the same age, tested both at 9 and at 17, completed 4 items and 7 items, respectively. The total number of seconds for the normal control at age 9 to complete 4 items and attempt a few others was 241. The total number of seconds for the normal control at age 17 to complete 7 items was 437. The normal control took an average of 60 seconds per completed block design at age 9, and an average of 62 seconds per completed item at age 17. J. D., however, took an average of 29 seconds per completed item (8/232) at age 9, but only 5 seconds per completed item at age 17.

Though there has to be some effect from learning, it seems unlikely that J. D. would benefit so much more from an extra administration of the test over the course of 9 years. (Three tests were given to J. D. and only two to the normal control.) Furthermore, the normal control showed no increase in average speed per item over the course of two administrations of the test, whereas J. D. went from an average of 29 seconds to 14 seconds to 5 seconds per item.

The second test on which J. D. performed phenomenally well was the experimental test of gestalt short-term visual memory cited earlier. Based on a test developed by Brenda Spiegler (1984), whose work, in turn, was based on work done by Mishkin and colleagues, the task consists of having to replace on a board in their original positions "junk objects" such as bolts or sponges. The experimenter places the junk objects in unique positions on a large black plywood board. The subject sees each of ten or more objects for 2 seconds in position. At the end of the serial presentation, the subject is given the objects one by one, in the order in which they were originally placed on the board. It is the subject's job to place each junk object exactly where it had been placed originally (for 2 seconds) by the experimenter. At zero delay J. D. replaced ten objects correctly; at 1-minute delay J. D. got nine out of ten correct; and at a 2-minute delay, with still another set of objects placed in different positions, J. D. got ten out of ten correct. In addition, after a full board of ten objects placed in random positions was shown to J. D. for 10 seconds, with zero delay he replaced all objects correctly. When J. D. was shown another gestalt display of ten objects but was given a delay time of 3 minutes, he placed five of the ten objects perfectly and the remaining five next to, but not on, the exact positions.

The performance of J. D. on these tasks may not seem remarkable; however, the testing of normal controls from ages 4 to 67 ($N = 13$ subjects) has not yielded a single subject who could replace all ten items correctly. The best score among normal subjects tested to date is nine objects on the zero-delay one-by-one presentation task. The range of scores for adults on the serial presentation tasks is four to six objects correct in any delay condition. The range of scores for adults on the gestalt presentation tasks is one to four objects for the 3-minute-delay condition and one to six objects for the zero-delay condition. We have been searching for a normal subject who can do any of the five tasks without a mistake.

J. D. may be helped by the fact that he might not be providing verbal labels for the objects he sees. Verbal labels may provide a type of visual-memory interference for normal subjects. Furthermore, if a normal subject tries to encode verbal labels not only for objects but also for relative board positions, task performance may suffer double interference. Still another explanation may be that as we get older we lose the power of immediate storage of visual positions, as in the loss of ability for eidetic imagery. It may be that J. D. has not suffered this loss. Of course, that would not explain why we cannot find any young normal children who can get a perfect score on the task, and yet J. D. has done so in three trials and has had a nearly perfect score in two others. There is no question of rehearsal in J. D.'s performance on the five object-placement tasks. He performed effortlessly and perfectly throughout, without ever having seen the task before.

Raven's Progressive Matrices

J. D. was given another test of pattern perception and recognition—Raven's Progressive Matrices, Sets A, B, C, D, and E. This is a standard test of nonverbal intelligence, which consists of five sets of 12 test items each. Each of the sets operates similarly—subjects must select one of eight little squares of pattern that appear at the bottom of a test page as representing the missing piece of the larger picture above. J. D. completed the test of 60 items in a little over 5 minutes. His responses to all items on Sets A, B, and C were correct, and he got the first 8 items of Set D correct. The last 4 items in set D and all the items in Set E were incorrect. All of J. D.'s 12 D and E error choices represent the same strategy: he selected a small piece of pattern which was identical to the part of the pattern of the large picture adjacent to the missing target section.

The puzzle is why J. D. suddenly stopped for a few seconds on the 9th item of Set D and then, switching strategies, essentially gave up on the task. There was some disturbance in the room next door when the test was being administered, but that cannot be the whole explanation for the sudden shift. Both Item D8 and Item D9 require mental manipulation of the same number of feature shifts in order to come up with the correct answer. It may be that with D9, J. D. was not able to "see" the complete pattern as it could be completed and therefore could not quickly select the correct missing pattern piece.

What is of interest in J. D.'s performance on Raven's matrices is the incredible speed with which he selected the correct patterns. Though his correct responses averaged about 4 to 5 seconds per item, this time included the time that the experimenter took to turn the pages of the test booklet and to record each response. J. D.'s selection time was between 1 and 2 seconds per item. His total time of 5 minutes, amounting to a selection time of 1–2 seconds per item, appeared to be so fast that it didn't even look as if scanning were taking place. The time limit on the whole test is 40 minutes, but administration of this test in a class of undergraduates showed a range of time from 13 minutes to 35 minutes—with some students not completing the task within the 40-minute time limit. If J. D. had only performed at chance levels on the remainder of the test after he gave up, this young man with an IQ of 58 would still have performed at the 75th percentile for the adult population.

Mazes Task

Given J. D.'s ability to recognize patterns, it might be assumed that he would be very good at pencil mazes. This proved not to be the case. J. D. could complete only the first four mazes of the WISC-R mazes task. For Mazes 5, 6, 7, 8, and 9—mazes that are significantly and increasingly more complex—J. D. could not work through them, perhaps because they require complex planning and foresight in organizing the motor response rather than "merely" apperception of a complex pattern.

Facial Recognition Test

Surprisingly, despite his excellent visuo-spatial skills for certain tasks, J. D. seems to have trouble recognizing people. This inability is suggested by his questioning of someone he has just met as if he had never met him or her. J. D.'s inability to recognize people has been tested both clinically and by means of a neuropsychological test. In a clinical interview, J. D. was unable to state the names of individuals he had met five or six times before when they were brought into the interview room. He clearly understood the nature of the task because he went through a list of names of people, only once hitting on the name of the person in front of him. Despite this failing, J. D. does recognize his parents and siblings and his classroom teachers as well.

J. D. was given the Benton Facial Recognition Test. In this test, subjects attempt to match a target photograph of an individual with a photograph or photographs of that same individual placed in a set of six pictures. For the first set of items, J. D. had to match a target to an identical photograph placed among photographs of other individuals. He scored a perfect 6 out of 6 on this set. In the second set of seven items, J. D. scored only 5 out of a possible 21 points. His total adjusted score was 25 out of a possible adjusted total of 54. A score of less than 37 is coded nominally as "severely impaired." There was no difference in J. D.'s performance on the matching of faces that were presented turned and on those that were presented in shadow; he performed randomly on both these types of items. This was true even though he had performed perfectly on the first six items (identical matches).

Benton, Hamsher, Varney, and Spreen (1983) have not evaluated test findings for the first six items separately. They do argue that there may be two general sorts of problems in facial recognition: (1) impairment in ability to recognize familiar faces of family members and friends, and (2) impairment in ability to recognize unfamiliar faces, such as are presented in their test. J. D.'s performance on the test, combined with what we know of him through informal clinical testing, suggests a more complex deficit. He clearly has trouble recognizing people who fall into the acquaintance category, and yet he is able to recognize those with whom he is familiar—and he does this apparently by sight. (He does not have to touch them or hear the sound of their voices.) He is also able to pick out unfamiliar faces, as long as the face-matching tasks require matching identical photographs of the unfamiliar individuals. This suggests two possibilities, neither of which excludes the other.

First, it may be that J. D. is specifically impaired in his ability to recognize unfamiliar faces but *only* in context involving either three-dimensional presentations (i.e., the live people) or transformations (the test's positional shifts, and shifts of lighting on the face). Second, in the task of recognizing identical pictures of strange faces, J. D. may be employing skill in complex gestalt perception, which could be functioning completely independently of the normal human "special" ability to recognize faces.

How J. D. recognizes those around him is not understood. He does not sniff them or touch them, and he can identify teachers and family members without having to hear their voices. Perhaps he has learned to recognize them visually by means of understanding their images in some gestalt that doesn't require clear recognition of their faces.

Conclusion

By any of the usual definitions of what it is to be an idiot savant, J. D. could be so classified. He exhibits the social withdrawal, echolalia, perseveration, obsessive interests, rituals, and repetitive motor behaviors that characterize the syndrome of autism, and yet in certain areas his skills are beyond those of all other normal individuals tested.

What exactly are J. D.'s special abilities? Essentially, J. D. is able to recognize and store in short-term memory vastly more visual images than can the average person. He is also able to deal with the components of a visual image of great complexity with great rapidity. In particular, he has the unusual ability to quickly discern a large-scale pattern and its subcomponents (as evidenced by his speed and accuracy on the WISC-R Block Design subtest and on Raven's Matrices as well as by his ability to do 5,000-piece jigsaw puzzles in a very short period. He also has an ability to remember the positions of objects on a board (over a brief period) that exceeds any ability yet shown by normal controls. His special abilities to perceive and remember visual patterns are in stark contrast to his particularly extreme impairments in linguistic development. Though J. D. seems to understand most verbal communications, and though he can read at the eighth-grade level, he cannot follow a series of verbal commands with accuracy. He seems to have difficulty with a sequence of different commands or requests if they have to be processed at the same time. More important, J. D.'s speaking is limited to two- and three-word utterances. He has been trained to say a few set phrases, but even these are short.

The striking pattern of extraordinary ability and deficit in J. D. has implications for three important theoretical questions about savant skill and about giftedness in general. First is the question of innate differences versus practice (see Ericsson and Faivre, Chapter 24, this volume, for an extended discussion). Hill (1975), Smith (1983), and Hoffman (1971) have all argued that social isolation and intense practice are the wellspring for the special abilities of idiot savants. Sacks (1985), LaFontaine and Benjamin (1971), Brink (1980), and others have argued that special abilities arise from special and prodigious memory skills. In particular, LaFontaine and Benjamin (1971) have argued that if social isolation were the main cause of savant skills, then there should be a significantly greater number of savant individuals.

J. D.'s skill (in games and puzzles) is one in which he has engaged since early childhood. Could this be enough, given his social isolation, to allow him to develop such speed and accuracy? I would argue in the negative, for two reasons. First, the ability to reconstruct visual patterns is likely to have been present in J. D. from an early age. He showed his skill in discerning patterns in his very early awareness of routes and in his reconstructing of complex words by means of alphabet blocks. Of course, practice must have improved his skills. But it may be that J. D. engaged in those activities that were rewarding for him—rewarding precisely because he was good at them. Second, and more importantly, he showed outstanding performance on visual-perceptual and memory tasks that were novel to him.

The second general theoretical question—whether J. D. and savants in general show abilities beyond those of normal individuals—can be answered partially in the positive. Although a normal person might, with practice, develop to J. D.'s level of performance on, say, the object memory task, J. D.'s naive performance was beyond that of any normal person's naive performance. Moreover, individual variation in some aspects of skill at visualizing appears to be based in categorical strategy/style differences and not in vast differences across a single continuum of skill (Just & Carpenter, 1985).

In general, published reports suggest that some idiot–savant skills are well within the normal range of functioning (Steel, Gorman, & Flexman, 1984), whereas others appear to be quite beyond the normal range of skills (Sacks, 1985). Rapid ascertainment of prime numbers—an apparent skill of the famous twins described by Sacks—is, on the face of it, phenomenal (see Matthysse & Greenberg, Chapter 23, this volume). If the observable skill does rest on some endowed fundamental ability, what might that ability be?

Luria (1968), Sacks (1985), and Brink (1980) all have offered arguments about special abilities, claiming that idiot savants have a special type of visualizing memory. Sacks argues that "seeing" or "visualizing" of extraordinary intensity, limitless range, and perfect fidelity seems to be the key to the savant memory. Sacks further argues that the idiot–savant twins he saw who generated prime numbers are actually working with a special kind of imagination—an imagination that only admits numbers. He believes that their minds are a landscape only of numbers. Brink believes that the basis for the phenomenal memory is eidetic imagery. Luria's S. reported that he saw everything in his mind's eye; S's memory failure, in fact, seemed to him to be confusions in internal perception and not impairment of memory.

The case of J. D. would appear to support the notions of Brink, Sacks, and Luria. He has the ability to visualize and reconstruct images that seems to be beyond that of any normal subjects tested. The speed and accuracy of his performances suggest a visual memory power beyond normal and beyond that of superior and talented normal adults and children. Sacks's twins told him they see numbers, but J. D. cannot report on his mental processes.

The third and most difficult theoretical question is relating these observations and speculations to underlying brain function. I would like to suggest four speculative possibilities about what might be different about J. D.'s brain and the brains of other savants.

1. Face-recognition areas and object/pattern-recognition systems may occupy related, overlapping, or adjacent tissue areas. The "use" of such tissue exclusively for object recognition, without an ability to perform face-recognition tasks, may confer special abilities in visual pattern perception. One skill "crowds out" another skill.

2. Geshwind and Galaburda (1985) have argued that there may be a hereditary tendency for fetal testosterone to slow the development of the left hemisphere of the brain to the point of pathology, while allowing the right hemisphere to develop beyond its original (genetic) plan. J. D.'s skill at pattern recognition as well as his skill in music memory may be a functional expression of greater development of his right hemisphere—at the expense of the development of his left, or language, hemisphere. J. D. has four second cousins who have severe language impairments; the possibility that they may have special abilities has not yet been explored.

Reviews of cases of idiot savants (Hill, 1975; Rimland & Fein, Chapter 25, this volume; Rimland & Hill, 1984) show a wide variety of expressions of special abilities in them. These abilities include music, memory, mathematics, mechanical skills, calculation, route-finding, and art. Although these savant skills appear to be governed by right-hemisphere functions, and although the "idiot" label in most cases derives from the individual's impairment in language skills, nonetheless it is not so clear that special abilities in the idiot–savant syndrome spring from right-hemisphere functions alone.

Burling, Sappington, and Mead (1983) have reported on lateralization of skills in a calendar calculator. Using an admittedly rather weak inferential method (eye gaze), the researchers found that results indicated strong evidence for left-hemisphere specialization of calendar calculation. Albeit that one calendar calculator looking to the right 15 out of 16 times when asked questions pertaining to calendar calculating does not constitute a conclusive finding against the right-hemisphere hypothesis, the question remains open.

Putative left-hemisphere impairment may boost visual memory in a more indirect way as well. It may be that J. D.'s language impairment, perhaps stemming from an impaired left hemisphere, in some sense has freed his memory from the "bonds" of labeling. It may be that the natural process of mentally labeling objects, figures, and pattern elements actually slows people down and interferes with pattern memory. Studies of eidetic memory skills suggest that children perform better than adults on a variety of immediate visual memory tasks. Perhaps one reason for the decline in visual memory skills in normal teens and adults is that language and complex serial analytical skills are present and thus blocking or interfering with visual memory. Wallace (1984) has found that simple increases in visual complexity were not processed better by older normal children (where the age range was from 6 years to $9\frac{1}{2}$ years). Older children were significantly faster and more accurate when visuo-spatial tasks had a good deal of visual redundancy that could be used in solving the task, but 9-year-olds were no better than 6-year-olds at tasks in which complexity of the visual patterns increased. This research, too, suggests that analyzable components are more helpful to older children, while visual memory skills may not be improving developmentally.

3. The third possibility regarding brain function in savants is raised in a theoretical chapter in this volume (Waterhouse, Chapter 26). The argument presented there suggests the possibility that savant skills may arise from a novel form of neural tissue dedication. In this model it is argued that the genetically determined pattern of neural organization found in the visual cortex is reduplicated outside, but adjacent to, the visual cortex. The reduplicated visual-cortex-type tissue organization is hypothesized to confer the advantages of increased memory storage for visuo-spatial information and increased ability to perform complex pattern-recognition tasks. The model also outlines the possibility that a simple but novel spread of visual cortex areas beyond "normal" limits would be likely to have pathological effect. It may be that such a spread or reduplication would "crowd out" dedicated tissue areas for controlling language or face-recognition functions, thus significantly impairing the individual in whom this happened.

4. Still another possibility is that some impairment in interhemispheric connections combined with some unknown dysfunction in language processing has freed J. D.'s visuo-spatial processing.

The generation of savant skills is a crucial question: If answers can be found, we may be better able to understand not only the talents of "idiot" savants but why such marvelous talents are yoked to such tragic impairments.

References

Benton, A. L., Hamsher K. de S., Varney, N. R., & Spreen, O. (1983). *Contributions to Neuropsychological Assessment.* New York. Oxford University Press.

Brink, T. L. (1980). Idiot savant with unusual mechanical ability: An organic explanation. *American Journal of Psychiatry, 123,* 250–251.

Burling, T. A., Sappington, J. T., & Mead, A. M. (1983). Lateral specialization of a perpetual calendar task by a moderately mentally retarded adult. *American Journal of Mental Deficiency, 88,* 326–328.

Geschwind, N., & Galaburda, A. M. (1985). Cerebral lateralization, biological mechanisms, associations and pathology. A hypothesis and a program for research. *Archives of Neurology, 42,* 428–459.

Hill, A. L. (1975). An investigation of calendar calculating by an idiot savant. *American Journal of Psychiatry, 132,* 557–560.

Hoffman, E. (1971). The idiot savant: A case report and a review of explanations. *Mental Retardation, 9,* 18–21.

Just, M. A., & Carpenter, P. A., (1985). Cognitive coordinate systems; Accounts of mental rotation and individual differences in spatial ability. *Psychological Review, 92,* 137–171.

LaFontaine, L., & Benjamin, G. E., (1971). Idiot savants: Another view. *Mental Retardation. 9,* 41–42.

Luria, A. R. (1968). *The mind of a mnemonist.* New York: Basic Books.

Rimland, B., & Hill, A. L. (1984). Idiot savants. In J. Wortis (Ed.), *Mental retardation and developmental disabilities* (Vol. 13, pp. 155–169). NY: Plenum.

Sacks, O. (1985). Sublime idiot geniuses. In *The man who mistook his wife for a hat*. New York: Summit Books.

Smith, S. (1983). *The great mental calculators: The psychology, methods, and lives of calculating prodigies, past and present*. New York: Columbia University Press.

Spiegler, B. J., & Mishkin, M. (1981). Evidence for the sequential participation of inferior temporal cortex and amygdala in the acquisition of stimulus reward associations. *Behavioral Brain Research, 3*, 303–317.

Spiegler, B. J., & Waterhouse, L. (1985). A test of visual place memory. Unpublished manuscript.

Steel, J. G., Gorman, R., & Flexman, J. E. (1984). Neuropsychiatric testing in an autistic mathematical idiot–savant: Evidence for nonverbal abstract capacity. *Journal of the American Academy of Child Psychiatry, 23*, 704–707.

Wallace, J. R. (1984). Visual-motor processing: Relationships among age dimensional variation and use of information redundancy. *Journal of Genetic Psychology, 145*, 133–136.

IV
GROUP STUDIES

19

Is Superior Visual Memory a Component of Superior Drawing Ability?

ELIZABETH ROSENBLATT
ELLEN WINNER

A well-known pianist once confessed to insomnia whenever he happened to think of the opening bars of a piece of music while trying to fall asleep. Once the opening bars came to mind, he could not fall asleep until he had played the entire piece in his mind. It did not matter whether the piece was one that he had recently mastered or one that he had only heard once and had never tried to learn: In both cases, he could not get the piece "out of his mind" until he had completed it in his mind. This inability to forget musical patterns—even pieces not deliberately committed to memory—is a phenomenon that has been reported by many musicians (Gardner, 1983).

An analogous phenomenon may characterize visual artists. Those who are drawn to the visual arts may be individuals who cannot forget visual patterns, even those they do not strive to encode in memory. This inability to forget a pattern (which we call here "incidental" visual memory) is not necessarily the characteristic that *causes* a person to become an artist or a musician. No claim is made here that artists are driven to draw what they cannot get out of their minds. Rather, the inability to forget visual information may be a perceptual correlate of ability in the visual arts, just as the inability to forget music may be a correlate of musical proclivity.

In what follows, we raise three questions. First, is superior incidental memory for visual information characteristic of either adults gifted in the visual arts or children who show promise of achievement in the visual arts? Second, if so, does it make a difference if the visual information is aesthetic or nonaesthetic, and pictorial or three-dimensional? Third, if visual giftedness and superior visual

Elizabeth Rosenblatt. Harvard Project Zero, Harvard University, Cambridge, Massachusetts.
Ellen Winner. Psychology Department, Boston College, Chestnut Hill, Massachusetts; and Harvard Project Zero, Harvard University, Cambridge, Massachusetts.

memory can be identified, is there any evidence that these traits are related to sex and/or to laterality (Geschwind & Galaburda, 1987)?

There is evidence that adults who are skilled in the visual arts possess superior perceptual abilities in the visual and spatial domains. The most thorough study of cognitive and perceptual correlates of visual artists was carried out by Getzels and Csikszentmihalyi (1976), who found that students at the School of the Art Institute of Chicago performed above the norm of the population on two perceptual tests: a test of aesthetic judgment (the Welsh Figure Preference Test) and a spatial test of the ability to rotate a figure mentally (from the Guilford-Zimmerman Aptitude Survey). Getzels and Csikszentmihalyi also reported that superior "perceptual memory" correlated with achievement in art (as measured by teachers' ratings on originality and artistic potential and by grades in studio art classes). However, this correlation was found only for females. For males, it was personality but not perceptual variables that were correlated with these measures of achievement in the arts.

Our studies differ from the research of Getzels and Csikszentmihalyi (1976) in two respects. First, the perceptual memory test used by Getzels and Csikszentmihalyi was not a test of incidental visual memory—that is, the ability to remember without deliberately trying to remember, or the inability to forget what one does not try to store in memory. Rather, these researchers used a test of the ability to commit a picture to memory *deliberately*. In our studies we examined only incidental visual memory. While individuals who are not visually gifted may commit a pattern to memory if asked to do so, they may not spontaneously encode the pattern in memory.

Second, Getzels and Csikszentmihalyi examined the relationship between visual memory and level of artistic achievement within a population whose members had demonstrated ability in the visual arts: All of the subjects were art students. Their findings demonstrate that one's level of artistic ability is not necessarily correlated with level of visual memory, since the correlation held only for females. However, because Getzels and Csikszentmihalyi compared "better" versus "worse" artists rather than artists versus nonartists, their findings do not reveal whether artists of any caliber tend to possess visual memories that are superior to the baseline of those possessed by the general population. In our studies we examined whether superior visual memory distinguishes those individuals with some ability in the visual arts from those with no special ability.

We examined incidental visual memory in both adults (Study 1) and children (Study 2). If adult artists are shown to have superior visual memories, this finding could be attributed to their greater amount of practice in the visual domain. Superior visual memory could be a result of constant training of the eye. However, if children who demonstrate ability in the visual arts exhibit superior visual memory, a stronger argument can be made that this ability is not a result of performance in the visual domain but rather a prior (and necessary) component of such performance.

Visual memory ought not to be treated as a unitary skill. It includes memory for properties of two-dimensional arrays, such as pictures, as well as memory for properties of three-dimensional arrays of objects. Moreover, it may prove to be important to distinguish among types of properties remembered. Just as memory for two-dimensional arrays may be a different skill from memory for three-dimensional scenes, so also memory for "nonaesthetic" properties (content) may be different from memory for aesthetic properties (such as line quality, composition, form, and color). We examined memory for different kinds of visually specified properties in both two- and three-dimensional arrays.

We hypothesized that memory for two-dimensional (but not three-dimensional) arrays would be predictive of ability in drawing (a two-dimensional medium). We made this prediction because drawing does not necessarily involve three-dimensional perceptual skills.

In addition to examining the relationship of visual memory to giftedness in the visual arts, we examined, in Study 2, the relationship between visual giftedness and both sex and handedness. We examined whether children identified as gifted in the visual arts were more likely to be left-handed and/or male than children not so identified (as would follow from Geschwind & Galaburda, 1987). We also examined the relationship between visual memory and sex and handedness.

Study 1: Superior Visual Memory in Adult Artists

The first study we conducted served as a preliminary pilot study for our second investigation. In the first study we developed a test of incidental visual memory for both two- and three-dimensional arrays. We administered the test individually to two groups of college undergraduates: ten students majoring in studio art (our measure of giftedness in drawing) and ten majoring in other fields (not including fine arts).

The Tasks

Our test of two-dimensional memory consisted of a set of eight pairs of 9-inch × 12-inch black-and-white line drawings, which subjects were asked to look at, pair by pair, and from which they were to select the one they preferred. (The test of memory came later, as a surprise.) Subjects were allowed 45 seconds to study each pair. The members of each pair were similar to one another, so that subjects had to look carefully at both in order to select the preferred one.

After choosing the ones they preferred, subjects were taken out of the room for a brief break. During this time, the experimenter substituted a new picture for one member of each pair. Half of the substitutions were identical in all respects except line quality. For example, a drawing with thin lines was substituted for the "same" drawing with thick lines, scratchy lines were changed to smooth lines, dark lines were changed to light lines, and so forth. The remaining substitutions were identical in all respects except composition. For example, an abstract design with geometric shapes dispersed all over the page was altered so that the same shapes were clustered about the center of the page. Pairs were presented in the same random order during the preference task and the memory test. Lateral placement of the target pictures was also randomly determined.

Subjects were then brought back into the testing room and were shown each pair again. It was not until this point that they realized that their memory was to be tested. They were told that in each case one picture had been altered. They were asked to decide which picture had been altered and to indicate what had been changed. Because in the initial presentation of the pairs subjects believed that we were studying only their preferences, this test measured the information that was encoded in memory spontaneously rather than deliberately.

A test of three-dimensional incidental memory was also devised, which consisted of altering objects in the testing room and determining whether subjects noticed the alterations. When subjects were first brought into the room, before being given the visual preference task, they were given a camera and asked to decide on the most informative angle from which to photograph the objects in the room. These instructions served to ensure that subjects actually looked at the layout of the room. After the two-dimensional memory task was completed, subjects were again taken out of the room. The experimenter then altered several aspects of the room: A blue letter tray on a desk was replaced by a red one (a color change); a window shade was put up over the window in the door (a content change); three Coke cans (which originally formed a diagonal pattern) were moved so that they formed a triangular pattern, a tape recorder was moved from one side of the table to another, and a newspaper was moved from the corner to the side of the table (composition changes).

Subjects were then brought back into the room and were asked to note anything that looked different. After they pointed out the items that seemed different, they were asked to recall how the item had looked previously.

The Results

We performed T-tests on the various tasks in order to compare the scores of the art majors and those of the other students (nonartists). Art majors outperformed the nonartists on the two-dimensional test on both measures. Art majors detected which picture had been altered an average of 5 times (out of 8); the nonartists detected the altered picture an average of 3.2 times. This difference was significant at $p < .05$. Art majors were also more frequently able to recall what had been changed about each picture ($\bar{x} = 4.3$ vs. 1.9, respectively), a difference significant at $p < .01$. The differences between the two groups occurred only for the line-quality items; the composition items proved so difficult that they yielded a floor effect for both groups.

On the object task, art majors outperformed the nonartists on only one of the two measures. The nonartists performed as well as the art majors in detecting which objects were different; however, the art majors were better able to recall how the objects had been before ($\bar{x} = 2.3$ vs. 1.2 out of 4.0, significant at $p < .01$).

This preliminary study suggested that individuals who have ability in the visual arts have superior incidental visual memories and that this superiority is more marked when the information to be encoded is from two-dimensional, pictorial, and aesthetic arrays than from three-dimensional arrays of nonaesthetic objects. In the next study we revised the two-dimensional task to include more properties of pictures; we administered the task to children (rather than adults) who had been identified as showing a proclivity for the visual arts; and we examined the roles of sex and handedness in both artistic giftedness and incidental visual memory.

Study 2: Superior Visual Memory in Child Artists

Our first problem in Study 2 was to identify visually gifted children. The task of identifying visually gifted adults, though difficult, is less daunting, for one can rely on criteria such as grades in studio art courses (a measure used by Getzels and Csikszentmihalyi), success in the art world, or even simply the decision to major in studio art in college (the measure used in our first study). The criteria that one can use to identify visually gifted children are less obvious. One cannot rely on grades in school art classes because work in such classes is often ungraded or because the grades are based primarily on effort. Tests have been developed to identify visually gifted children (see Wilson & Wilson, 1981, for a review). However, many artists and art teachers feel that one can readily spot a visually gifted child without relying on a standardized test (Winner & Pariser, 1985). Thus, as a first cut, we relied on art teachers' identification of children who showed "talent" or "unusual ability" in drawing.

We gave no quotas to the art teachers because we did not want our sample to be filled with marginally talented children. Art teachers were told that they should identify only their most gifted children, even if this meant giving us only one or two (or not any) names. We also did not ask for an equal number of males and females, for we wished to determine whether males were more likely to be identified as visually gifted (Geschwind & Galaburda, 1987). By contacting a number of art teachers in local schools, both public and private, and the coordinator of Saturday drawing classes at a major art museum, we obtained a sample of 38 children (21 males, 17 females) identified by their teachers as gifted in the visual arts. The children ranged in age from 9 to 13 years.

Teachers also identified 26 children in the same age range who displayed no special talent in the visual arts: Teachers were asked to select children who were simply average (not outstandingly poor) in drawing ability. These children were used as a comparison group. The teacher of the museum class was not asked to provide names of nongifted children. We felt that children enrolled in an extracurricular art class were likely to possess more ability than the average child, and hence we chose not to include such children in our control group. However, we did not assume that all of the children enrolled in the museum class were gifted; we included in our study only those whom the museum teacher selected as showing special ability. All of the teachers were able to distinguish between gifted and average children on the basis of their performance in art class.

We did not give the art teachers a list of criteria by which to separate the gifted from the average children. We did not presume to know what these criteria are or how to define the cutoff point. We decided, instead, to rely on teachers' intuitions, intuitions that are, of course, based on implicit criteria that may well differ from teacher to teacher. Some may select children on the basis of technical skill, others on the basis of novelty, imaginativeness, creativity, expressiveness, and so forth. A child who might count as gifted in the eyes of one teacher might qualify as only average for another teacher using a stricter cutoff point. In particular, we felt that the teacher of the extracurricular group was likely to have children with a higher mean level of skill and hence may have selected gifted children who were more outstanding than those selected by school art teachers.

Because teachers may differ in their judgments of giftedness, we used teachers' identification only as a first cut of our sample. We then selected a subsample of the gifted children on the basis of a drawing produced by each child and evaluated as outstanding by a group of judges familiar with children's drawings. Further details on the selection of the subsample are given later.

The Tasks

As in Study 1, two types of incidental visual memory tests were administered: a test of memory for pictures, assessing memory for two-dimensional arrays, and a test of memory for objects located in three-dimensional space. The tests were administered to the children individually.

MEMORY FOR PICTURES

This two-dimensional test was constructed in the same way as the one used in Study 1. The children were shown 20 pairs of pictures. As in Study 1, in order to disguise the fact that this was a memory test, we first asked the children simply to decide which picture they preferred in each pair. To ensure that the children looked at each picture rather than only or primarily at the one they preferred, each picture was presented alone for 10 seconds, and then the two were presented side by side. The pairs were constructed so that their members were quite similar. For instance, both were abstract color designs, both were representational line drawings, and so forth. As in Study 1, this was done so that subjects would have to look carefully at both pictures before deciding on a preference.

Again, the preference task was used only as a way of getting the children to look at the picture without at the same time suggesting that this was part of a memory task. Had we simply presented pictures and asked the children to look at them, they might have guessed that they were being asked to remember what they were shown.

After selecting their preferred pictures, the children were taken into a separate room (or, in some cases, into the school hallway) and were seated at a table. They were given a 9-inch × 11-inch sheet of white paper and a black marking pen and were asked to draw a picture. The children were told that they could draw anything they wished. All children completed their drawings within 10 minutes.

While the children were out of the testing room drawing, the 20 pairs of pictures were altered. In each pair one member was replaced by a slightly altered version of the original picture. The children were then brought back into the room and shown the pairs again, but this time with the altered versions. They were told that one member of each pair had been changed and to point out all of the changes

FIGURE 19-1. Sample composition item. Changes in the altered version of the original picture are as follows: (1) One circle is moved inside the large circle. (2) One circle is moved up. (3) One small white circle is moved to the left. (This change was rated as subtle.)

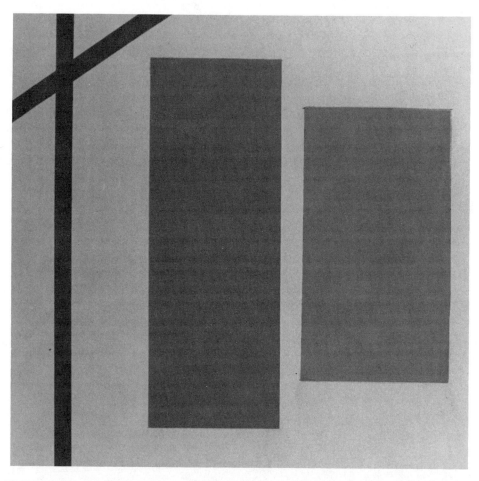

FIGURE 19-2. Sample color item. Changes made in the altered version of the original picture are as follows: (1) The right rectangle is purple on the original and yellow on the altered version. (2) The cross is blue on the original and purple on the altered version. (3) The left rectangle is royal blue on the original and turquoise on the altered version. (This change was rated as subtle.)

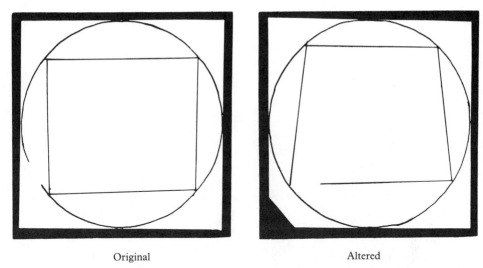

Original   Altered

FIGURE 19-3. Sample form item. Changes in the altered version of the original picture are as follows: (1) The square is changed to a trapezoid, which is broken. (2) The break in the circle is connected. (3) There is a wedge in the bottom left corner. (This change was rated as subtle.)

they noticed. Only at this point did it become clear to the children that this was a memory test. No time limit was placed on this task.

To investigate the relationship between pictorial memory and the type of pictured property recalled, we included changes not only in line quality and composition, as in Study 1, but also in content, color, and form. We also made the composition changes less subtle, so that the floor effect found in the first study would not recur. Figures 19-1 through 19-5 present samples of each of the five types of alterations. Each figure shows the original and altered versions of a picture and details the changes that were made. Four exemplars of each type of alteration were shown to the children.

We selected these five categories of changes for two reasons. First, they represent the major properties of drawings and paintings. Second, they differ in the extent to which they capture properties specific to pictures functioning aesthetically (e.g., drawings) as opposed to pictures functioning nonaesthetically (e.g., diagrams, maps, and graphs). Distinctions between properties that are important to notice when a picture is functioning aesthetically versus nonaesthetically have been articulated by philosophers such as Goodman (1976) and Langer (1953). For example, when a picture is functioning aesthetically, it commands "thick" attention: We are meant to attend to its line quality, color, form, and composition as well as, of course, its representational content (Arnheim, 1973). In contrast, when a picture is functioning nonaesthetically (e.g., a graph), we need not attend to so many of its properties: All that is important to note is what the line represents, that is the *content* of the picture (see Winner, Rosenblatt, Windmueller, Davidson, and Gardner (1986) for information on the development of the ability to perceive aesthetic properties, and Gardner (1982) and Gardner and Winner (1981) for information on the breakdown of such capacities). This distinction allowed us to

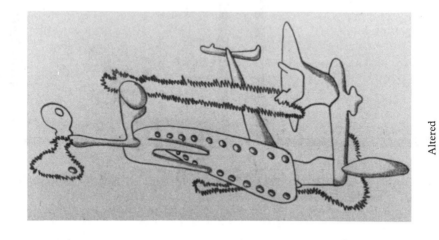

Original

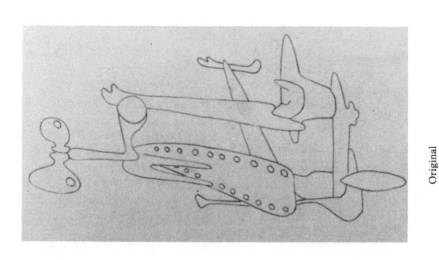

Altered

FIGURE 19-4. Sample line-quality item. Changes in the altered version of the original picture are as follows: (1) The lines are changed from light to dark. (2) The lines in some places are changed from smooth to scratchy. (3) The lines are changed from uniform in width to variable in width. (This change was rated as subtle.)

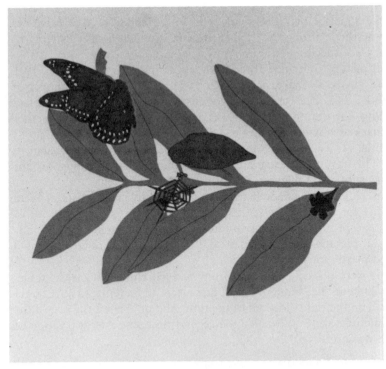

Altered

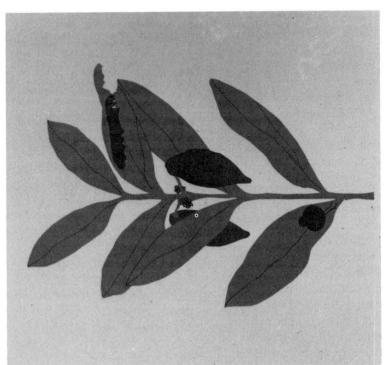

Original

FIGURE 19-5. Sample content item. Changes in the altered version of the original picture are as follows: (1) The caterpillar is changed to a butterfly. (2) The pod is changed to a spider web. (3) The ladybug on the bottom left leaf is changed to a small flower. (This change was rated as subtle.) The reproductions here are black and white. In the pictures shown to the children, both the caterpillar and butterfly were orange, the pod and spider web were gray, and the ladybug and flower were red. (From *Sally's Caterpillar* by Anne and Harlow Rockwell. Courtesy of MacMillan Publishing Company.)

examine whether a superior pictorial memory in gifted children (if it exists) is restricted to the aesthetic properties of pictures or whether it also extends to content, a property not specific to pictures functioning aesthetically.

Each altered picture contained three changes, as indicated in Figures 19-1 through 19-5. We strove to make one change obvious and the remaining two changes more subtle. As a check on the subjectivity of such distinctions, we asked 14 adults (including 7 artists) to look at the original and altered versions together and rate the changes as obvious or subtle. Of the 14 judges, 11 agreed that 12 changes were subtle. (In each of Figures 19-1 through 19-5, the third change is rated as subtle.) This distinction enabled us to dintinguish between memory for alterations rated as subtle and memory for more blatant alterations.

The pictures either were adapted from works by published artists or were created by an artist for the purposes of this study. All were constructed out of Color-Aid paper, except for the line-quality items, which consisted of black-and-white drawings. All pictures were 9 inches × 12 inches and were covered by a sheet of laminated plastic for protection.

The pictures were placed directly in front of each child, flat on the table. The order of the 20 items was randomized. The picture to be replaced (the target picture) was placed on the right side half of the time, and on the left the rest of the time. When the pictures were shown for the second time, the lateral position of the target picture was preserved.

MEMORY FOR OBJECTS IN THREE-DIMENSIONAL SPACE

To investigate memory for properties of objects located in three-dimensional space, we devised a test of incidental memory for objects located in the testing room. During the administration of the picture-preference task, each child was seated next to a chair that held two books (one to the left of the other), a pencil, a Coke can, and a blue shirt. Over the chair was slung a beige plaid wool scarf, and under the chair was a pair of sneakers with white socks rolled up and stuffed in one of the shoes. The arrangement looked natural: It appeared to be a chair on and around which some objects had been casually left (see Figure 19-6).

To ensure that the children looked at the scene, we asked them to look at all of the objects on the chair and then to guess the price of three of the items: the chair, the sneakers, and one of the books. This pricing task was simply a ruse, like the picture-preference task, to make sure that the children looked at the stimuli whose recall from memory was later to be tested.

While the children were out of the room drawing, several changes were made. There were three color changes: a gray plaid scarf was substituted for the beige one, black socks were substituted for the white ones, and a purple shirt replaced the blue one. There were also two content changes: a Diet Coke can replaced the Coke can, and a pen replaced the pencil. Finally, there was one change in composition: the two books were originally placed at a 45-degree angle to one another; this angle was changed to 90 degrees (see Figure 19-6). After the children had completed the two-dimensional picture task, they were told to look at the chair again and to describe whether anything had been changed, and if so, what.

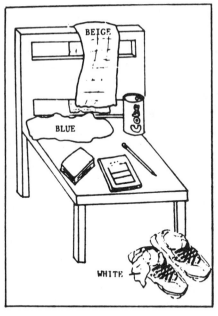 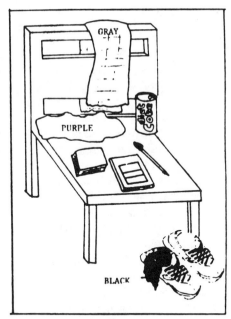

Original   Altered

FIGURE 19-6. Original and altered layout in the testing room. In the pictures shown to the children the three color changes in the altered version were as follows: (1) The beige scarf was changed to gray. (2) The blue shirt was changed to purple. (3) The white socks were changed to black. One change was made in the composition: The angle of the book on the left was changed. The two content changes were as follows: (1) The Coke can was changed to a Diet Coke can. (2) The pencil was changed to a pen.

Scoring

PICTURE TASK

Children received three scores for each item in the two-dimensional task: (1) a score of one point for correct identification of the altered picture; (2) a latency score (in seconds) for selections of the versions perceived as altered; (3) a score of one point for each of the three changes noticed. Sometimes children gave responses that were only partially correct—for example, a child might notice that a color had been changed but be unable to recall what the color was originally. Such responses received a half point. The latency score was determined by the experimenter, who counted to herself.

OBJECT TASK

On the object task, children received one point for each of the six changes noticed. Again, partially correct responses, in which, for example, subjects noticed that the scarf was a different color but could not recall what color scarf had been replaced, received a half point. Thus a score of a half point was equivalent to the first measure used in Study 1—the ability to note that an object had been altered; a score of one point was equivalent to the second measure used in Study 1—the ability to recall the original object.

Selection of Subsample

We selected a subsample of children who were identified as gifted not only by their teachers but also by judges on the basis of the one drawing that each child made. We asked seven judges to categorize the drawings as indicative of exceptional giftedness, possible giftedness, or nongiftednesss. The judges consisted of two art educators, two graduate students in art education, and three psychologists whose research focuses on children's drawings. Four of these judges were also artists. When the drawings were presented to the judges, they were identified only by the age of the child. Drawings from each age group were presented separately, so that judges would not select superior drawings simply on the basis of age. Each group of drawings included those done by the children identified as gifted and those identified as nongifted.

We selected a subset of 21 of the original 38 children on the basis of the judges' ratings of the drawings. These 21 children were ones who were rated as either "definitely gifted" or "somewhat gifted" by four of the seven judges. As these figures show, the judges did not always agree on whether a drawing was indicative of giftedness. However, all but two of the disagreements related to whether the children identified by their teachers as gifted were in fact gifted rather than to whether a child not identified as gifted ought to be considered gifted. Thus it was easier to recognize and agree on the lack of talent than to agree on the presence of talent. That disagreements occurred almost always with respect to the gifted children's drawings indicates that judges distinguished at some level between the two groups of subjects. We think that the disagreements occurred because the judges (inevitably) used different baselines to separate the gifted from the average. The agreement level would most likely have been higher had the judges been shown more than one drawing by each child, in more than one medium. The judges had

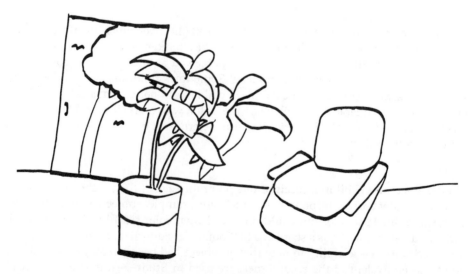

FIGURE 19-7. Drawing by a 9-year-old identified as gifted by teacher and judges.

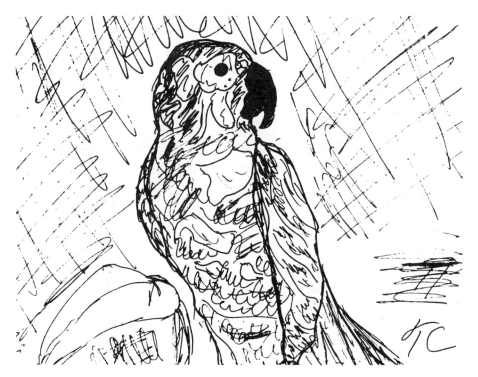

FIGURE 19-8. Drawing by an 11-year-old identified as gifted by teacher and judges.

to make their selections on the basis of only one drawing done in black marker on white paper and completed in an unusual situation within 10 minutes. Considered in this light, it is perhaps surprising (and reassuring) that the judges could make such classifications with any degree of agreement. Drawings by a 9-year-old and an 11-year-old child in the subset of 21 gifted children are shown in Figures 19-7 and 19-8, respectively; a drawing by an 11-year-old nongifted child is shown in Figure 19-9.

Handedness

Children were asked if they were left- or right-handed. As a check on the child's answer, we noted the hand with which the child drew. There were no discrepancies between children's self-reports of handedness and demonstrated hand preference.

The Results

Analyses of variance were conducted in order to determine in what ways, if any, gifted children performed differently from average children. Each of these analyses was performed twice. Our first analyses included in the gifted group all children identified by their teachers as gifted. We next relied on a more stringent criterion—teacher identification *plus* agreement by four of the seven judges that the drawing

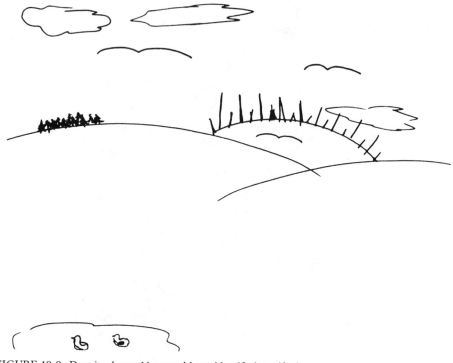

FIGURE 19-9. Drawing by an 11-year-old not identified as gifted.

produced should be classified as either definitely or somewhat indicative of gifted-ness. The results of the second set of ANOVAs were identical to those of the first, indicating that the judges selected a representative sample of children identified as gifted by their teachers. Thus we report only the analyses based on teacher identification of giftedness.

PICTURE TASK

A two-way ANOVA, Group (gifted vs. nongifted) × Item Type (color vs. compo-sition vs. line quality vs. form vs. content), was performed once for each of four dependent variables: (1) number of pictures correctly identified as having been altered; (2) latency for correct choice of picture identified as having been altered; (3) number of alterations noticed; and (4) number of subtle alterations noticed. (The mean scores for each of these dependent variables are given in Tables 19-1 through 19-3.)

Number of Altered Pictures Correctly Noted. Out of a total possible score of 20, the mean number of pictures correctly noted as having been altered was 18.1 for the gifted group and 17 for the nongifted group (see Table 19-1). Athough, as can be seen from these scores, both groups performed close to ceiling on this task, the difference between the two groups was significant, $F(1, 62) = 5.375$, $p = .024$. There was also a main effect of Item Type, $F(1, 62) = 4744.904$, $p < .001$. This occurred because for both groups of subjects, line-quality and content changes

TABLE 19-1. Mean Number of Pictures Correctly Identified as Altered

	Item type					
Group	Line (out of 4)	Form (out of 4)	Composition (out of 4)	Color (out of 4)	Content (out of 4)	Total (out of 20)
Gifted	3.9	3.3	3.7	3.1	4.0	18.1
Non gifted	3.7	3.2	3.5	2.8	3.8	17.0
Total	3.8	3.2	3.6	3.0	3.9	

proved the easiest to detect, composition changes were intermediate in difficulty, and color and form changes were the most difficult. There was no interaction of Group and Item Type.

Latency to Note Altered Pictures. As shown in Table 19-2, the gifted children noted the altered pictures somewhat more quickly that the nongifted children ($\bar{x} = 3.3$ vs. 4.2 seconds, respectively), but this difference did not prove significant. There was a main effect of item type, $F(1, 62) = 124.361$, $p < .001$: The two types of alteration that yielded the highest correct scores, line quality and content, also yielded the shortest latencies to respond. There was no interaction of Group and Item Type.

Number of Alterations Noted. Gifted children recalled an average of 26.4 properties (out of 60) that had been altered; nongifted children recalled an average of 21.9 (see Table 19-3). Although the difference between these means is small, the difference was highly significant, $F(1, 62) = 7.599$, $p = .008$. There was also a main effect of item type, $F(1, 62) = 866.164$, $p < .001$. This occurred because children in both groups recalled the most changes in content and line-quality items (the two easiest types of items on both of the previously discussed measures). There was no interaction of Group and Item Type.

Number of Subtle Alterations Noted. Gifted children recalled an average of 3.9 of the 12 properties rated by judges as subtle; nongifted children recalled an average of 2.8 of these properties (see Table 19-3). Again, this difference was significant, $F(1, 62) = 10.25$, $p = .002$. We did not examine effects of, or interactions with, item type, since item type was confounded with subtlety (twice as many alterations in the content items were rated as subtle than in the other items).

TABLE 19-2. Mean Latency (in Seconds) to Identify Altered Pictures Correctly

	Item type					
Group	Line	Form	Composition	Color	Content	Total
Gifted	2.1	4.5	4.2	3.8	2.0	3.3
Nongifted	3.6	4.9	4.8	5.1	3.3	4.2
Total	2.7	4.7	4.4	4.3	2.5	

TABLE 19-3. Mean Number of Pictorial Alterations Noted

	Item type						
Group	Line (out of 12)	Form (out of 12)	Composition (out of 12)	Color (out of 12)	Content (out of 12)	Total (out of 60)	Subtle alterations (out of 12)
Gifted	6.3	4.5	4.5	3.8	7.3	26.4	3.9
Nongifted	4.8	4.0	3.8	3.0	6.2	21.9	2.8
Total	5.7	4.3	4.2	3.5	6.9		

OBJECT TASK

A two-way ANOVA, Group × Item Type (color, composition, content), was performed on the number of alterations noted in the object task. In contrast to the results of the picture task, there were no significant effects. Although gifted children noted an average of 3.4 changes out of 6, and nongifted children noted 2.8, this difference did not prove significant. There was a main effect of Item Type, $F(1, 62) = 344.892$, $p < .001$. Content changes were noted most often, color changes were intermediate in difficulty, and composition changes were noted least often (see Table 19-4).

HANDEDNESS

There were striking differences in the frequency of left-handers in the two groups of children. Among the 38 children identified as gifted by their teachers, 6 boys and 3 girls of the 38 were left-handed (24%); among the 26 identified as nongifted by their teachers, none were left-handed. Among the 21 children in the more stringently defined gifted subgroup, 5 were left-handed (again, 24%). Given that the percentage of left-handers in the general population is between 5% and 12% (Segalowitz, 1983), our gifted sample, selected either loosely or stringently, was populated by more than twice as many left-handers as one would expect from a random selection. These findings replicate those reported by Mebert and Michel (1980), who compared art students at the Massachusetts College of Art and the Boston University School of Fine Arts with undergraduate liberal arts students at Boston University and found that 20% of the artists were left-handed in contrast to only 7% of the nonartists.

TABLE 19-4. Mean Number (and Percentage) of Alterations Identified on Object Task

	Item type			
Group	Content (out of 2)	Color (out of 3)	Composition (out of 1)	Total (out of 6)
Gifted	1.4 (70%)	1.7 (56%)	0.3 (26%)	3.4 (57%)
Nongifted	1.2 (59%)	1.3 (44%)	0.3 (26%)	2.8 (47%)
Total	1.3 (65%)	1.5 (51%)	0.3 (26%)	

A t-test was performed to compare the mean scores of left- and right-handers within the gifted group on each of the dependent variables discussed previously. There were no differences between the two groups on any measure. Thus, although our gifted sample contained a disproportionate number of left-handers, and the gifted children overall showed superior visual memory, handedness did not prove to be related to level of visual memory among children already identified as gifted.

SEX

There was no difference in the frequency of males and females betweeen the two groups. In the group identified by teachers only, roughly half (21 of the 38 gifted children and 14 of the 26 nongifted children) were male. In the group identified as gifted by both teachers and judges, again about half (12 of the 21) were male.

A t-test compared mean scores for males and females within each group. No sex differences were found in the nongifted group on any measure. However, females outperformed males on several measures in the gifted group. Girls detected more altered pictures than did boys ($\bar{x} = 18.9$ vs. 17.6, respectively, out of 20), $t = 2.616$, $p = .013$; they detected the altered picture more quickly than did boys ($\bar{x} = 2.2$ vs. 4.2 seconds, respectively), $t = 3.611$, $p < .001$; and they recalled more color changes in the picture task ($\bar{x} = 4.6$ vs. 3.2 out of 12), $t = 2.239$, $p = .031$. This superior performance on the part of females is consistent with the sex differences on perceptual memory reported by Getzels and Csikszentmihalyi: There seems to be a moderately stronger association between visual memory and giftedness in females than in males, even though in our sample, females were no more likely to be selected as visually gifted than were males.

Discussion

Our results shed some light on the three questions raised by our studies.

1. Do gifted artists have superior visual memory? Our investigations suggest that both adults gifted in the visual arts and children who show promise of achievement in the visual arts possess superior incidental visual memory. Just as musical information "sticks" in the minds of musicians, visual information seems to stick in the minds of visual artists. Information from one's domain of ability appears to be effortlessly encoded and stored, and easily recalled.

2. For what kind of visual information do artists show superior memory? Our visually gifted subjects showed superior visual memory more consistently for pictures than for objects. In Study 1 the art majors outperformed the nonartists on both measures used in the picture task: They recalled which pictures had been altered and what had been changed about them more often than did the nonartists. However, on the object task, the art majors performed at a superior level only on the more sensitive measure: They were more likely than the nonartists to recall how an altered object had been before it was altered; they did not outperform nonartists on the easier task of indicating which objects were different. In Study 2 the gifted children showed superior memory on the picture task but performed no better than the control group on the object task (which was scored to capture both the ability to note which objects had been altered and the ability to recall the original objects).

How can we explain the fact that it was the picture task but not the object task that most consistently distinguished the gifted from the control subjects? We suggest two possibilities. One is that the picture task assessed the ability to encode two-dimensional information, whereas the object task assessed the ability to encode three-dimensional information. It is possible that an exceptional ability to encode two-dimensional information leads an individual to excel in drawing, a two-dimensional medium. In contrast, an ability to encode three-dimensional information may lead an individual to excel in any number of domains that call upon spatial skill—for example, athletics, engineering, architecture, or mathematics as well as the visual arts. If so, there would be no reason to expect performance on the object task to distinguish individuals identified as gifted in the visual arts.

There is, however, an alternative explanation that cannot be ruled out. In our studies the medium of presentation was confounded with whether the stimuli were presented as works of art or as ordinary, nonaesthetic objects. In the picture task, subjects saw stimuli that were presented as works of art, that is, as aesthetic objects (Goodman, 1976). The stimuli were clearly paintings or drawings rather than nonaesthetic pictures such as graphs, diagrams, or maps. In contrast, in the object task, subjects were tested for recall of ordinary household objects that were not presented as works of art. Had we used sculptures instead, or had we displayed the objects as if they were works of art (e.g., mounting a Coke can on a pedestal), our gifted children might have shown superior recall.

We are currently conducting studies of memory for visual and verbal information in children who are gifted in drawing and writing, in which we disentangle medium from aesthetics. If gifted individuals demonstrate superior memory only for properties of aesthetic stimuli, and only in their domain of giftedness (e.g., visual for the artists, verbal for the writers), then we will be able to conclude that what distinguishes gifted individuals is a superior ability to encode information from stimuli in their domain of giftedness that are perceived with the kind of "thick" attention called for by aesthetic objects. In other words, a visually gifted individual may be more likely than an individual who is not visually gifted to encode visual information, but only for stimuli perceived to be functioning as art.

In the second study described in this chapter, some attempt was made to distinguish memory for aesthetic versus nonaesthetic properties. In the picture task we compared memory for content (a property important to notice in pictures functioning nonaesthetically as well as aesthetically) with memory for properties important to notice *only* in pictures functioning as art. As we reported, gifted children showed superior memory for all types of properties, including content. However, we have come to the conclusion that our study does not adequately test the hypothesis that it is aesthetic properties particularly that are recalled by the visually gifted. When pictures are perceived as works of art, *all* of their properties command our attention, even a property such as content, which we attend to in maps or diagrams. Thus individuals skilled in the visual arts may encode visual information of *any* sort better than do ordinary individuals, but only when that information comes from an object perceived to be a work of art. What artists may do better than nonartists, then, is to pay "thick" attention to visual stimuli perceived as works of art.

3. Are visual giftedness and superior visual memory related to laterality and/or sex? A clear relation between visual giftedness and left-handedness was revealed in our second study. Children identified as gifted either by their teachers alone or by their teachers and our judges were much more likely to be left-handed than were the children in our control group (all of whom turned out to be right-handed). This finding is not new. It has been noted anecdotally and in a systematic study (Mebert & Michel, 1980) that visual artists are often left-handed; in addition, Nadia, an autistic child who had exceptional drawing ability, was left-handed and showed superior right-hemisphere abilities (Selfe, 1977). Our study replicates the handedness finding and extends it to children who show some proclivity in the visual arts but who may or may not go on to pursue the arts as adults. Thus even a modest proclivity in the visual arts (our gifted children were not Leonardos!) may be related to superior right-hemisphere development (Geschwind & Galaburda, 1987). Whether such individuals show superior ability on other visuo-spatial tasks besides drawing is a question worthy of future investigation.

In contrast to the suggested relationship to laterality, we found no relationship between visual giftedness and sex. Thus, although Geschwind and Galaburda's (1987) theory would predict more males in the visually gifted group (because males are more likely to have superior right-hemisphere development), males were not more likely to be identified as gifted either by their teachers (who, of course, might have tried to equalize the number of males and females selected) or by our judges (who were blind to sex).

What about the relationship of superior visual memory to laterality and/or sex? When we compared left- and right-handers from the gifted group in Study 2, we found no differences on any measure. Thus, while left-handedness seems to be related to giftedness in the visual arts, it is clearly not a *necessary* component. This need not surprise us: Although artists as a group are disproportionately left-handed, the majority of great artists have been right-handed.

As for sex, we found some relationship to visual memory, but a relationship in the direction of that reported by Getzels and Csikszentmihalyi (1976) and not in the direction that would follow from Geschwind and Galaburda (1987). That is, it was the females identified as gifted in Study 2, not the males, who demonstrated superior visual memory on some measures. This may reflect any number of factors: a greater willingness on the part of girls to attend to the task at hand, more seriousness on their part about the task, the earlier maturation of girls, a different relationship between visual memory and visual giftedness in males versus females, and so forth.

The Nature of Talent in the Visual Arts

A proclivity in the visual arts seems to be detectable even in the preschool years (Winner & Pariser, 1985) and clearly by the elementary school years, as shown in our second study. One of the first signs of such ability in children is a precocious ability to draw with representational accuracy: Even when drawing from memory, such children surprise their parents and teachers by an ability to encode spatial relationships (both two- and three-dimensional) as well as details of form and content. Such children tend to make drawings filled with decorative, aesthetic detail and to create unusual compositions (Clark & Winner, 1986). These children also tend to focus on a particular aspect of the drawing medium (such as linearity) and to exploit the various properties of this aspect in one drawing after another; they spend much more time intensively involved in drawing than do "average" children (Clark & Winner, 1986).

The amount of time and attention given to an activity is a clear indicator and predictor of exceptional ability in a particular domain (Hurwitz, 1983; Renzuli, 1978; Robinson, 1985). Thus visually gifted children show a wide variety of abilities—the visuo-motor mastery necessary for representational accuracy, the aesthetic inclination leading to decorative detail, the creativity resulting in the making of unusual compositions, and the focused attentiveness necessary for mastery in any domain. The present research shows that these children possess an unusual ability to encode pictorial and/or aesthetic information and may possess superior right-hemisphere development as indexed in some instances by left-handedness.

Children who show ability in the visual arts are likely to be encouraged by the praise of teachers, parents, and peers. (The phenomenon of the "class artist"—the child recognized as best in the class at drawing—is a commmon one). However, those children who also show strong gifts in other, more academic areas (such as mathematics or English) may, we speculate, be at risk for dropping out the arts by adolescence (Gardner, 1980). Although skill in the arts is certainly respected in our society, ability in academic areas is more highly prized by teachers and parents, since it is ability in these areas that leads to college acceptances and hence to high-paying jobs. Thus, because of the priorities our society focuses on, children who go on in the visual arts may be ones who do not excel in academic domains. Indeed, artists often report that they did poorly in academics but took refuge—and flourished—in the arts (Winner & Pariser, 1985). Thus it is not only giftedness that determines whether a child goes on to master a domain but also social forces that conspire in the "winnowing" process. Certain individuals may be selected by brain maturation and laterality to be at promise in the arts, but if society conspires against them, they may drop out. For a child to succeed in the arts, it is helpful if art is the only domain of school performance in which that child excels—at least as long as society continues to signal that academic pursuits are more highly valued than the arts.

Acknowledgments

The two studies reported here grew out of research supported by a grant to one of us (E. W.) from The Spencer Foundation. We thank Howard Gardner for help in designing the studies. We are grateful to the following individuals for helping to select gifted children and for allowing us to conduct our research in their institutions: Lorri Berenberg, Coordinator of Workshop Programs, Boston Museum of Fine Arts; Mary Alice Brennan-Crosby, Principal, Buckingham, Browne and Nichols Lower School; William Burback, Director, Department of Education, Boston Museum of Fine Arts; Clifford Card, Principal, Acton Junior High

School; Parker Damon, Principal, McCarthy-Towne School, Acton; Gloria Fitzgerald, Art Teacher, Clarke Junior High School, Lexington; Margot Grallert, Humanities Instructional Consultant, McCarthy-Towne School, Acton; John Hibbard, Principal, Clarke Junior High School; Nancy Howard, Head, School and Community Programs, Boston Museum of Fine Arts; Miriam Kronish, Principal, Hillside School, Needham; and James Palavrous, Principal, Gates School, Acton. We thank Patricia Hoerth, Margaret Clark and Kathy Deuschle for help in constructing the pictures used in the pictorial memory test, and Joseph Walters for help in analyzing the data. Karen Earle and Mark Caterini conducted the first study reported here, as part of a research practicum taught by one of us (E.W.) in the Psychology Department of Boston College.

References

Arnheim, R. (1973). *Art and visual perception*. Berkeley: University of California Press.

Clark, M., & Winner, E. (1986). *Early signs of giftedness in drawing: Two case studies*. Unpublished manuscript.

Gardner, H. (1980). *Artful scribbles: The significance of children's drawings*. New York: Basic Books.

Gardner, H. (1982). Artistry following damage to the human brain. In A. Ellis (Ed.), *Normality and pathology in cognitive functions*. New York: Academic Press.

Gardner, H. (1983). *Frames of mind: The theory of multiple intelligences*. New York: Basic Books.

Gardner, H., & Winner, E. (1981). Artistry and aphasia. In M. Sarno (Ed.), *Acquired aphasia*. New York: Academic Press.

Geschwind, N., & Galaburda, A. (1987). *Cerebral lateralization: Biological mechanisms, associations, and pathology*. Cambridge, MA: Bradford Books.

Getzels, J., & Csikszentmihalyi, M. (1976). *The creative vision: A longitudinal study of problem finding in art*. New York: Wiley.

Goodman, N. (1976). *Languages of art*. Indianapolis: Hackett.

Hurwitz, A. (1983). *The gifted and talented: A guide to program planning*. Worcester, MA: Davis Publications.

Langer, S. (1953). *Feeling and form*. New York: Scribner.

Mebert, C., & Michel, G. (1980). Handedness in artists. In J. Herron (Ed.), *Neuropsychology of left-handedness*. New York: Academic Press.

Renzuli, J. (1978). What makes giftedness: A redefinition. *Phi Delta Kappan, 60*, 3.

Robinson, R. (1985, April). *The daily experience of giftedness in adolescence: Sex differences and achievement*. Paper presented at the meeting of the American Educational Research Association, Toronto.

Segalowitz, S. (1983). *Two sides of the brain*. Englewood Cliffs, NJ: Prentice-Hall.

Selfe, L. (1977). *Nadia: A case of extraordinary drawing ability in an autistic child*. London: Academic Press.

Wilson, B., & Wilson, M. (1981). *Instruments for the identification of artistic giftedness*. Unpublished manuscript, Pennsylvania State Univeristy, Psychology Department, University Park, PA.

Winner, E., & Pariser, D. (1985). Giftedness in the visual arts. *Items, 39(4)*, 65–69.

Winner, E., Rosenblatt, E., Windmueller, G., Davidson. L., & Gardner, H. (1986). Children's perception of aesthetic properties of the arts: Domain-specific or pan-artistic? *British Journal of Developmental Psychology, 4*, 149–160.

20

The Special Talent of Grammar Acquisition

SUSAN CURTISS

How could language development (acquisition of the knowledge to speak and understand one's native language) be considered a talent; that is, why should it be considered appropriate for this volume on the neuropsychology of talent? After all, language is an ordinary ability. All normal children acquire language and do so without overt instruction (in contrast, for example, to reading, writing, or arithmetic operations). In this sense it is unlike all of the other abilities covered in this volume, for in these other domains, either there is great variability within the normal population as to the degree of talent possessed or the ability normally requires overt instruction (e.g., reading), or both (e.g., chess, music). Although there are certainly differences in verbal talent, there is remarkable uniformity in the ability to acquire one's native language and in the developmental period and rate at which language acquisition occurs.

This special or unique status of language learning has led some to consider language acquisition as akin to physical growth, in that it is viewed as a fixed, genetically determined and maturationally constrained process, independent in important respects from other aspects of social and cognitive development. Language development is not typically thought of in these terms, however. Language acquisition does not take place in isolation from the rest of development. It normally occurs within the context of development in many areas, and its ties to and roots in nonlinguistic social and cognitive development are the focus of most theoretical models of language acquisition.

This chapter describes instances in which language acquisition nonetheless "behaves" as if it were a specialized talent. First, I present cases in which language acquisition stands apart as an area of developmental impairment. I then present cases of selectively intact language acquisition, that is, instances in which language acquisition proceeds in the absence of the social and cognitive developmental support that are concomitants to language acquisition in normal development. Through these data I attempt to build a case for the existence of specialized neuropsychological mechanisms for language acquisition, especially with respect to the

Susan Curtiss. Department of Linguistics, University of California at Los Angeles, Los Angeles, California.

acquisition of grammar. In doing so, I provide empirical support for the view that in certain important respects, the mechanisms underlying language acquisition may be different from, and may operate independently of, development in other domains. Finally, I attempt to fit this material into the larger context of the neuropsychology of talent.

Before proceeding, it may be useful to define what I mean by "grammar." "Grammar" refers to the system of knowledge comprising the structural principles, constraints, and rules constituting both those facts true of every language (Universal Grammar) and those true only of particular languages, such as English. Here "grammar" does not encompass the "communicative" component of language—that is, the system of rules and constraints governing the use of language in communicative contexts—or the "conceptual" or "semantic" component—that is, the system of rules for mapping the conceptual knowledge system onto linguistic forms, and rules for deciding the truth value or logical well-formedness of propositions or their component parts. This is not to say that these other areas are not part of language, or even what makes language most interesting to some individuals. They are nevertheless being separated from grammar here, and some empirical justfication for doing so will emerge as the cases are presented.

Methodology

Except where noted, the subjects of the cases discussed in this chapter were studied by our laboratory via in-depth investigation of their linguistic and nonlinguistic abilities. Our methodological aim was to obtain a detailed mental profile for each subject, which would then enable us to delimit and compare functioning within and across a substantial range of mental abilities.

In these investigations we examined in detail both receptive and expressive language abilities, including lexical and phrasal semantics, morphology, syntax, conversational pragmatics, and, to a lesser extent, phonology. Comprehension was analyzed by means of formal comprehension tests and observation of comprehension in spontaneous conversation. Production was examined through analysis of imitated, elicited, and spontaneous speech. Our examination of nonlinguistic function included (where appropriate) sensorimotor tasks; preoperational tasks of classification and number; examination of visuo-constructive ability, including drawing, copying, nesting, and hierarchical construction; observation of structured and spontaneous play; memory tests, including tests of short-term auditory and visual memory, examination of visual and spatial skills, including disembedding and visual closure; tests of temporal and logical sequencing; a variety of concrete operational tasks, including those of conservation, classification, reversibility, and perspective; and a variety of tasks involving number concepts and operations. A list of tests used is presented in Table 20-1. (For specific task descriptions and other methodological details, see Curtiss, Kempler, & Yamada, 1981).

Where possible, we attempted to (1) utilize tests of nonlinguistic function that require only nonverbal presentation and responses, (2) utilize tests that tap

TABLE 20-1.   Test Used in Assessing Abilities of Case Subjects

Language tests	
Curtiss-Yamada Comprehensive Language Evaluation—R	Curtiss-Yamada Comprehensive Language Evaluation—E
Token Test	Curtiss-Yamada Comprehensive Language Evaluation—S
Peabody Picture Vocabulary Test—Revised	
Sentence Imitation (Yamada)	Developmental Sentence Scoring

Nonlanguage tests	
Uzgiris-Hunt Scales	Hierarchial construction
Classification (Sugarman, 1981)	Logical sequencing
Copying (Piaget & Inhelder, 1967)	Drawing
Object Nesting	Play
Seriation	Wepman-Morency Auditory Memory Span Test
Number battery (adapted from Gelman & Gallistel, 1978)	Knox Cubes Test
Conservation	ITPA[a] Visual Sequential Memory Test
Classification (Curtiss & Yamada, 1970)	Mooney Faces
Localization of topographical stimuli (Laurendeau & Pinard, 1970)	Witkin Children's Embedded Figures Test
Stereognosis	Southern California Figure–Ground Perception Test (Ayres, 1966)

[a]Illinois Test of Psycholinguistic Abilities

one ability at a time and (3) select tasks that would enable us to evaluate abilities on the basis of age level and cognitive-stage norms.

The Selective Impairment of Grammar Acquisition

The seemingly obvious choice of populations to include here would be developmentally aphasic children—children who are traditionally defined as manifesting impaired language development alongside normal nonverbal intelligence, normal peripheral hearing, no (obvious) central nervous system damage, and no significant emotional disturbance, that is, children having a selective language-learning impairment. Recent research on this population indicates, however, that it evidences nonlinguistic as well as linguistic deficits and, moreover, that it is heterogeneous, probably for etiology as well as for actual neuropsychological and linguistic dysfunction (e.g., Johnston & Kamhi, 1984; Johnston & Weismer, 1983; Kamhi, 1981; Kamhi, Catts, Koenig, & Lewis, 1984; Tallal & Piercy, 1975; Tallal, Stark, & Mellits, 1983). Thus, while it may yet turn out to be the case that a subgroup of children identified as developmentally aphasic do have only specifically linguistic deficits, this population currently presents too unclear and varied a picture to be included here.

The subjects I include here represent three cases of linguistic and social isolation, in which otherwise across-the-board successful postisolation development is limited by impaired grammar acquisition. These three cases are of Kaspar Hauser, Genie, and Chelsea.

Kaspar Hauser

Although there is some disagreement as to the validity of the case of Kaspar Hauser I feel comfortable including his case for several reasons. First, there are more than 2,000 documents regarding this case, and the vast majority of them substantiate its validity and provide interesting and detailed information about K. H.'s postisolation progress. Second, the key sources of information on this case were highly regarded professionals in their time, with undisputed credentials (von Feuerbach, 1832; Daumer, 1832; Pietler-Ley, 1927), and additional careful research and examination of the case has been conducted more recently (e.g., Heyer, 1964; Pies, 1966). Third, it is difficult to imagine that authors living in another century could or would have conspired to invent a case that presents such an unpredictable developmental story, one that, when turned upside down, illustrates the special talent of grammar acquisition. So, on to the facts of the case.

K. H. was isolated from the approximate age of 3 or 4 years until he was about 16. During these years, he was kept in a small, cell-like room, totally isolated, and was supplied with food and otherwise cared for while he was asleep (or, perhaps, drugged). The limited size of the room prohibited him from standing erect or lying flat, and during his imprisonment he neither stood nor walked, and he never spoke or was spoken to.

Upon his release and subsequent discovery in 1882, K. H.'s impressive intellectual capacity began to be revealed (and documented and described in numerous writings). He made strikingly rapid progress in almost every area. Within months of his discovery he displayed remarkable ability in drawing, memory, reasoning capacity, and even less expected areas, such as horsemanship. He lived only 5 years after he was found, but during that time was noted for his astonishing intellect. For example, he was consistently reputed to have philosophized about life in general, and his own peculiar circumstances in particular. Within that short 5 years after his discovery, he learned to read and write (within limits as noted below) and became competent in mathematics and several other academic areas.

His linguistic progress, however, reportedly stood alone as the single area of mental function that remained problematic. His language abilities were interestingly uneven: rapid and impressive in certain respects, notably deficient in others. Conceptual (or "semantic") aspects of language (German) were those he apparently mastered readily. Upon entering society he immediately began learning words, and within a few months he acquired a sizable vocabulary and began combining words into short "sentences." The vocabulary he mastered and the logical well-formedness and complexity of the propositions he evidently comprehended and produced as time went on were sufficiently sophisticated to allow him to participate actively in philosophical and intellectual discussions. In contrast, however, he apparently displayed consistent and persistent difficulties with the grammar of German, producing what might be described as both agrammatical and ungrammatical output.

> To the astonishment of all . . . he . . . very soon learned to speak, sufficiently, at least, in some degree to express his thoughts. Yet, his attempts to speak remained for a long time a mere chopping of words, so miserably defective . . . that it was seldom possible

to ascertain . . . what he meant to express by the fragments of speech which he jumbled together. (Von Feuerbach, 1832, translated by Simpkin and Marshall.)

From a later description:

His enunciation of words which he knew, was plain and determinate, without hesitating or stammering. But, in all that he said, the conjunctions, participles and adverbs were still almost entirely wanting; his conjugation embraced little more than the infinitive; and he was most of all deficient in respect to his syntax, which was in a state of miserable confusion. The pronoun I occurred very rarely; he . . . spoke of himself in the third person, calling himself Caspar. (Von Feuerbach, 1832, translated by Simpkin and Marshall.)

K. H. reportedly never mastered German syntax or morphology, evidencing a selective deficit in acquiring grammar. This grammar-learning impairment stood in marked contrast to his impressive intellectual development in all other areas written about, including conceptual or "semantic" aspects of language. It is testimony to his remarkable cognitive gifts that he could communicate so effectively and at such a high level, given his linguistic deficiencies.

Genie

The second case of impaired grammar acquisition is that of Genie. There are a number of published reports on the case (e.g., Curtiss, 1977, 1979; Curtiss, Fromkin, & Krashen, 1978; Curtiss, Fromkin, Krashen, Rigler, & Rigler, 1974; Fromkin, Krashen, Curtiss, Rigler, & Rigler, 1974), and the reader is referred to these for more information. Although certain details about Genie's early life remain unknown, there is considerable information on both the case history and her life subsequent to her discovery.

Genie was isolated for a period of 12 years, from the age of 20 months to 13 years, 7 months. Little is known about her life prior to her enforced isolation at 20 months, but during her first year, she had to wear a physically restraining Frejka splint for 7 months to correct a congenital hip dislocation. Other facts regarding her infant development raise the possibility of malnutrition and neglect.

Beginning at 20 months, Genie was confined to a small bedroom in the back of the family home, where she was harnessed to an infant potty seat. Isolated in this room for 12 years, she was fed only infant food and received practically no visual, tactile, or auditory stimulation of any kind. She received little linguistic input; there was no TV or radio in the home, and because of her father's extreme intolerance for noise, all speech in the home was kept to a nearly inaudible volume. Genie's brother and father were her primary caretakers, and by design, neither spoke to her.

Shortly after she was $13\frac{1}{2}$ years of age, Genie was discovered. She could barely walk, could not chew or bite, understood only a few individual words, and spoke not at all. Like K. H., Genie's intellectual development was uneven in intriguing ways. In large part her progress was rapid and impressive. From the time of her discovery on, Genie avidly explored her surroundings and began to show clear conceptual and intellectual gains. She quickly began organizing and classifying her environment (evidenced by her play activities and, a little later, by her language) and followed a course of steady growth and development. Her mental age (as measured by standard psychological measures such as the Leiter International Performance Scale, the WISC, and Raven's Progressive Matrices) increased 1 year for each year postdiscovery. Within 4 years of her discovery, she had clearly attained most aspects of concrete operational intelligence, including both operational and figurative thought (e.g., reversibility, decentrism), and had demonstrated not only fully developed but superior abilities in the domain of visual and spatial function (e.g., Gestalt and part/whole abilities; spatial rotation; spatial location; conservation of spatial features; and knowledge about visual and spatial features, such as size, shape, and color). Table 20-2 presents some details of relevant task performance.

In marked contrast, Genie showed persistent impairments in verbal short-term memory and language acquisition. Like K. H., language acquisition was not an all-or-none affair for Genie. Rather, her language development was marked most notably by a large discrepancy between her acquisition of referential/lexical and propositional knowledge on one hand (semantics) and her acquisition of grammatical rules on the other.

TABLE 20-2. Profile

Test/task	Genie's Performance level
Drawing (spontaneous)[a]	Approximate 6- to 7-year-old level
Logical sequencing (Curtiss & Yamada, 1980)	$8\frac{1}{2}$- to 9-year-old level; at ceiling of test presented
Conservation[b]	6- to 7-year-old level (conserves area and length; number questionable)
Classification (Curtiss & Yamada, 1980)	8-year-old level; at ceiling
Spatial operations (Laurendeau & Pinard, 1970)	12-year-old level; appears to have all concrete operational spatial operations
Nesting (Greenfield, Nelson, & Saltzman, 1972)	At ceiling
Hierarchical construction (Greenfield, 1976, 1978; Greenfield & Schneider, 1977)	Able to copy all models, regardless of internal complexity; at least 11- to 12-year-old level
Auditory short-term memory (ITPA; Kirk, McCarthy, & Kirk, 1968)	3-year-old level
Visual sequential memory (Knox Cubes Test)	6- to 7-year-old level
Disembedding (Southern California Figure–Ground Perception Test)	10- to 11-year-old level

[a]Drawing assessed by criteria per Goodenough (1926), Kellogg (1970), and Goodnow (1977).

[b]Conservation assessed by a series of tasks modeled after Beard (1963); Goldschmid & Bentler (1968); Elkind (1961); Elkind (1966); Lovell, Healey, & Rowland (1962); Wallach, Wall, & Anderson (1967); Wohlwill & Lowe (1962).

Within a few months after her discovery, Genie began to produce single words and then acquired vocabulary rapidly. Within 3 to 4 months of her first single-word utterances, she had acquired an expressive vocabulary of 100–200 words and had begun to combine words. Her early vocabulary was quite rich and included words of color concepts, numbers, emotional states, and all levels of category membership (superordinate, basic, subordinate), including some rather subtle distinctions (e.g. "pen" vs. "marker," "jumper" vs. "dress"). Her acquisition of lexicon and the expression of meaning relations, including multipropositionality, steadily progressed and increased (see Curtiss, 1977, 1979, 1981, & 1982 for more details). However, her ability to produce "sentences" developed *only* insofar as she was able to produce increasingly longer strings and strings that increased in propositional complexity. In contrast, her utterances remained largely agrammatic and hierachically flat, as seen in Examples 1a–j.

(1) (a) I like hear music ice cream truck.
    (b) After dinner use mixmaster.
    (c) Like kick tire Curtiss car.
    (d) Ball belong hospital.
    (e) Genie Mama have father long time ago.
    (f) Think about Mama love Genie.
    (g) Dark blue, light blue surprise square and rectangle.
    (h) Teacher say Genie have temper tantrum outside.
    (i) Father hit Genie cry longtime ago.
    (j) Genie have Mama have baby grow up.

Her speech, even after 8 years, was devoid of almost all bound and freestanding grammatical morphology and of most syntactic devices and operations. Her major achievement in the acquisition of syntax was the acquisition of categorical information, including some subcategorization facts. This knowledge was evidenced, for example, by her ability to answer WH questions with the correct constituent category (usually) and by her frequent, although not exceptionless adherence to subcategorization facts and constraints of many verbs, as, for example, in producing strings like "Put car [in] garage" or "Mr. W say put face in big swimming pool" or "Genie want buy nother shoe box" but not "Put car," "Mr. W say," or "Genie want buy." It appeared for a time that she also had learned English phrasal and clausal word order constraints. However, over the years there were persistent, even increasing, violations of such constraints in production and persistent miscomprehension of word order (e.g., in reversible actives). The dissociation between acquisition of "conceptual" aspects of language and acquisition of grammatical forms and rules reported in K. H.'s case, then, was a hallmark of Genie's language, too.

Genie's linguistic limitations extended to the use of language for effective interactive purposes. Despite the fact that her utterances were usually well formed with regard to their logical structure and were generally truthful, relevant, brief, and on topic, especially in response to questions or in conversational turns directed by others, as illustrated in Example 2, her means of initiating, participating in, and controlling or regulating verbal interaction on her own were greatly restricted. She possessed an impoverished set of linguistic-pragmatic devices and relied heavily on simple statements of a proposition or on repetition of a proposition to perform a variety of pragmatic functions—introducing topics; continuing topics; acknowledging or responding to comments, requests or questions; making comments or requests; and asking questions—as illustrated in Example 3. Moreover, she failed to use social rituals (e.g., "Hi," "How are you?") or conversational operators (e.g., "Well," "O.K.")—the trappings that help to make a conversation fluid and interactively normal.

We see, then, that the rules underlying the use of language for communicative purposes were not uniformly affected by Genie's adverse language-learning circumstances. Those aspects of effective communication depending on an appreciation of conversational content and the communicative intent and needs of one's listener were least impaired, whereas those aspects of effective communicative interaction depending on socially conditioned skills of conversational participation were sorely deficient or absent altogether.

(2) (a) *G*: Neal come.

M: Yes, Neal is going to come tomorrow. Neal makes you happy. He's a friend of yours.

G: Neal not come happy. Neal come sad.

(b) *C*: Why aren't you singing?

G: Very sad.

C: Why are you feeling sad?

G: Lisa sick.

(3) (a) *G*: Think about Mama bus.

C: Did you see Mama on Saturday?

G: Saturday.

C: I need a "yes" or "no."

G: Yes. I want think about Mama riding bus. Think about Mama bus.

(b) (*Touching yellow crepe paper that a gift for her—a picture frame— received at school was wrapped in*)

G: At school. Paper at school. Picture at school.

C: The picture is from school, too?

G: From school.

C: That's a picture frame, actually.

G: At school. (*An interruption*; *then . . .*) Big present.

Chelsea

A third case showing the same general pattern as that of K. H. and Genie has only recently begun to be investigated. Brought to light by P. Glusker, it involves a hearing-impaired adult, Chelsea, who is attempting first-language acquisition in her 30s. No systematic investigation of Chelsea's language development has yet been carried out; thus the data are largely preliminary and anecdotal (Curtiss, unpublished data; P. Glusker, C. O'Connor, V. Yancy, J. Watters, & N. Dronkers, personal communication 1982–1987). Nonetheless, they reveal a profile characterized by marked scatter in abilities, parallel in many respects to those seen in K. H. and Genie.

Although little testing of Chelsea's nonlinguistic intellectual function has been carried out, her performance on the Raven's Progressive Matrices and several Piagetian tasks demonstrates a sufficient intellect to support grammar acquisition. Yet, there is a clear and striking disparity between Chelsea's lexical knowledge and her ability to manipulate that knowledge on the one hand, and her ability to combine vocabulary into appropriate and grammatical utterances on the other. Her lexical knowledge has steadily progressed and is quite substantial. For example, in 1984 Chelsea scored above the 12th-grade level on the Producing Word Associations subtest of the Clinical Evaluation of Language Functions (CELF; Semel & Wiig, 1980), the highest norms for the test. In contrast, her multiword utterances are, almost without exception, unacceptable grammatically at the level of the phrase and the clause and are quite often propositionally unclear or ill-formed as well, as illustrated in Examples 4a–g.

(4) (a) The they.
    (b) Breakfast eating girl.
    (c) Orange Bill car in.
    (d) The man is walking [unintelligible] truck car truck walking.
    (e) The woman is bus the going.
    (f) Daddy are be were to the work.
    (g) They are is car in the Bill.

Thus her lexical knowledge seems limited to (denotative) definitional cores and does not appear to encompass either subcategorization information or logical structure constraints. Likewise, her expressive language, in violation of constituent structure, subcategorization constraints, phrasal and clausal word order, agreement phenomena, and so forth appears, at its best, to be limited to the production of combinations of semantically relevant substantives.

Chelsea's discourse skills appear, at least superficially, to be almost the reverse of Genie's. It is Chelsea's topic-related skills that are limited, but these limitations may reflect her comprehension difficulties as well as propositional limitations. Other discourse abilities seem remarkably developed (e.g., speech act range, use of social rituals, use of conversational operators) and enable Chelsea to engage in conversation that in some respects is interactively appropriate.

Summary

Taken together, the cases of K. H., Genie, and Chelsea suggest that there is a critical difference between acquisition of the conceptual and communicative aspects of language and acquisition of rules of grammar (here, syntax and morphology). This critical difference has two potential explanations. First, the learning capacity displayed by K. H., Genie and Chelsea and the mechanisms they utilized for growth in other intellectual domains, including conceptual and communicative aspects of language, were insufficient and/or inappropriate for learning grammar. In K. H.'s case, even apparently extraordinary intellect was not sufficient. Second, either the learning principles governing acquisition of grammar were selectively impaired from birth, or Chelsea, Genie, and K. H. had passed the age at which they were still functional. Both explanations point to a task-specific grammar-acquisition ability, that is, a special talent for grammar acquisition.

Selectively Preserved Grammar Acquisition

If grammar acquisition is indeed a special and neuropsychologically independent talent, it should, in principle, be possible to identify individuals who are otherwise cognitively deficient but who show intact grammar-learning ability. Such individuals have been alluded to in the literature for some time. For example, a subpopulation of hydrocephalic children has been described as "hyperverbal" and as mentally retarded, with a "cocktail party syndrome" (Dennis, Lovett, & Wiegel-Crump, 1981; Swisher & Pinsker, 1971; Tew, 1977). Children with Williams syndrome have been similarly described (Jones & Smith, 1975; von Armin & Engel, 1965), as have children with Turner syndrome and Noonan syndrome (Silbert, Wolff, & Lilienthal, 1977). Detailed examination of the language-acquisition capacity and patterns of these populations has yet to be undertaken, however.

In our own lab, the extent to which language acquisition may be based on task-specific mechanisms has been the focus of research for some time (e.g., Curtiss, Fromkin, & Yamada, 1979; Curtiss et al. 1981). In the course of our work we have studied in detail several subjects who, although not part of any of the previously mentioned populations, illustrate the profile of an intact island of talent—that of grammar acquisition. These case studies involve children who are mentally retarded but who have surprisingly intact grammars, despite their pervasive cognitive deficits. Though we have data from several such cases,[1] we discuss just three of them here. In two of the three cases the etiology of the retardation is unknown.

Antony

The first case is that of Antony, a child of 6–7 years when we studied him (see Curtiss & Yamada, 1981 for a detailed description of the case). Antony's IQ estimates ranged from 50 to 56. At chronological age 5 year 6 months, his mental age was 2 years 9 months. Parental reports indicate speech onset at 1 year and full sentences at 3 years, despite numerous professional reports of pervasive developmental delays in many areas.

---

1. The data discussed in this section were collected jointly with Jeni Yamada or Daniel Kempler, with the exception of some of Marta's data, which were collected solely by J. Yamada and were drawn from Yamada (1983).

We found in Antony's language a profile quite the opposite of Genie's. Antony's language was well formed phonologically and syntactically and was structurally rich. It was fully elaborated with inflectional and derivational bound morphology and "free" grammatical morphemes, and it included syntactic structures involving movement, embedding, and complementation, although Antony made errors not atypical for his age, suggesting that he was still mastering some grammatical rules. Examples 5a–l illustrate Antony's abilities.

(5) (a) The wolf is not here.
    (b) Are you Miss W.?
    (c) Could I take this home?
    (d) Jeni, what'd you touch?
    (e) Why don't you fly?
    (f) Jeni, will you help me draw pictures of Susie?
    (g) I got my brother named David.
    (h) That clock says it's time to get some prizes.
    (i) I don't want Bonnie coming in here.
    (j) I don't know who he gots.
    (k) He eats carrot.
    (l) A stick, that we hit peoples with.

Antony's linguistic strengths, therefore, lay in phonology, morphology, and syntax—that is, in the grammar.

Antony's language was semantically quite deficient, however. First, his lexical specifications were incomplete and sometimes inaccurate. This resulted in incorrect word usage, a problem frequently leading to miscommunication with others. Notably, none of Antony's lexical errors involved violations of syntactic class, subcategorization features, grammatical case, or word order. Almost all of his errors were errors in semantic feature specification. Errors with lexical substantives involved confusions or inadequate definitional differentiation between words within a particular semantic area (e.g., "birthday" for "cake," "cutting" for "pasting"). Errors with prepositions involved errors in marking direction, location, or semantic case or function (e.g., "to" for "from," "in" for "with"). Pronoun errors involved errors in gender or animacy (e.g., "who" for "what," "that" for "he"). At times, Antony exploited his grammatical knowledge to compensate for deficient lexicon, creating a different kind of error. These errors involved creating nouns from verbs in his vocabulary for words that already have a derivationally simple noun form (e.g., "sweeper" for "broom," "sewing" for "spool"). These latter errors reveal a productive knowledge of derivational morphology and the syntactic class such morphology creates.

A second area of semantic deficiency lay in Antony's formulation of propositions. Propositional content, unless quite simple, was often confusing and incompletely expressed. He frequently failed to grasp the intent or full meaning (including presupposition and implicature) of his own and others' utterances, causing consistent communication failures, as illustrated in Examples in 6 and 7.

(6) (*Anthony's library teacher, Miss C, has just walked into the room and is standing in full view of Antony, rather close to him.*)

A: You guys, lookit who's in our class. I want to see who's in that class.

E: Who's in what class?

A: No, in ours.

E: Everyody's here!

A: Not Miss C.

(7) *A*: I watch *Bewitched.*

E: But what does your daddy do, Antony? What does your daddy do all day?

A: Nothing.

E: Nothing! I don't believe it. Does your daddy stay at home all day and cook?

A: Nope.

E: Make supper and . . .

A: He was not comin' home.

Antony's conversational abilities included a wide range of pragmatic functions and intentions (e.g., naming, turn taking, commenting, requesting, protesting, responding to requests and questions, and acknowledging), and he had learned the conventional means for expressing them (rejoinders, words and phrases of acknowledgment, request phrases, etc). However, he was not sensitive to the needs of his listener, his topic-maintenance skills were poorly developed, and he rarely appeared to be concerned with being relevant or informative (again, see Curtiss, 1981, for details).

Given his semantic and communicative deficiencies, Antony's language was well formed generally only out of context (see Curtiss, 1981, 1982, for details). It thus appears that Antony acquired the grammatical system separate from the semantic structures that are mapped onto sentences by means of the grammar and separate from the rules guiding the use of grammar for effective communication. To the extent that this is true, he may be said to have acquired an autonomous syntax, and his case illustrates the separability of grammar acquisition from the development of other aspects of language.

Antony's nonlinguistic profile reveals a further dissociation of grammar from other abilities. In structured and unstructured situations his attention span was markedly short. Many tasks we successfully administered to normal 2-year-old children proved too difficult for him to grasp. On those tasks for which he was able to give a measurable performance, he showed substantial deficiencies in every area except auditory-verbal short-term memory, as illustrated in Table 20-3. His drawings were prerepresentational, his play was at the 1- to 2-year-old level, he was unable to perform any of the classification tasks, and his logical reasoning abilities were at the 2-year-old level. His nonlinguistic cognitive level appeared to be at or just beyond sensorimotor stage VI (normally attained at approximately 20–24 months), with nonlinguistic symbolic abilities (e.g., play, drawing, copying) below that. His one area of nonlinguistic

TABLE 20-3. Antony's Nonlanguage Performance Profile

Ability	Antony's performance level
Auditory short-term memory	7-year-old level
Drawing	Prerepresentational
Copying	Prerepresentational
Nesting	28- to 32-month-old level
Hierarchical construction	Less than a 2-year-old level
Conservation	Couldn't administer, even via "Magic Show"[a]
Logical sequencing	2-year-old level
Classification	Unable to perform at all; below 2-year-old level
Play	1 to 2 year-old level

[a]Gelman and Gallistel (1978).

strength was auditory-verbal short-term memory, in which he performed above age level.

Antony thus showed a dissociation of grammar acquisition not only from development in other areas of language but from development in nonlanguage areas as well. In other words, he displayed a selective talent for grammar acquisition.

Marta

The second case is that of Marta, a teenager studied from the age of 16–18 years (Curtiss, 1982; Yamada, 1981). Marta's IQ estimates ranged from 41 to 44. All developmental milestones are reported to have been delayed, including speech onset and other linguistic developments. From the age of about 4–5 years, however, language clearly stood apart as Marta's area of greatest strength.

Marta's linguistic profile was much like Antony's. Her speech was well formed phonologically and fully elaborated morphologically, and it embodied rich, complex, and well-formed syntactic structures. Like Antony, Marta produced errors demonstrating that her utterances were not merely (delayed) repetitions of someone else's speech; her utterances, however, were generally much longer and propositionally more complex and convoluted than Antony's, as illustrated in Examples 8a–h. In addition, her lexicon was much richer and contained many more quantifiers and adverbs than Antony's, as is also illustrated in these examples.

(8) (a) Last year at [name of school], when I first went there, three tickets were gave out by a police last year.
(b) That's where my sister, J, lives!
(c) I don't want to get eaten by one.
(d) We're really excited about school starting, and I love it myself.
(e) She, does paintings, this really good friend of the kids who I went to school with last year and really loved.

    (f) He was saying that I lost my battery-powered watch that I loved.

    (g) The cook who does it, um sometimes give us these good enchiladas an' oh, they're so good!

    (h) He's my third principal I've had since I've been here.

Although Marta had a larger vocabulary than Antony, their lexical semantic abilities were quite parallel. Much of Marta's lexicon was incompletely specified, not for grammatical features, but for semantic features. Thus she, too, often misused words, most frequently words referring to number, time, manner, and dimensionality (see Examples 9a–f). The propositional content of her utterances, though apparently rich and varied when only a small sample of her speech is considered, was largely repetitious of a small repertoire of themes and, at its best, was loosely structured.

    (9) (a) It [her watch] was broken, desperately broken.

        (b) *J*: How many nights did you stay there?
            [at the hotel with the family]
         M: Oh, about four out of one.

        (c) "Jack," that's my father's last name, "Jack."

        (d) (*M has just turned 16.*)
         I was 16 last year and now I'm 19 this year.

        (e) It's very soon that they asked us to fly out.

        (f) (*J. Y. had just given M two pennies*)
         J: How many pennies do you have now?
         M: Five.

Marta's conversational performance was strongest in those areas incorporating conventionalized social routines and early developed (Dore, 1978) pragmatic functions and was weakest in the areas of topic maintenance, relevance, informativeness, and truthfulness as illustrated in (10). Marta, too, then, appears to have an advanced level of grammatical knowledge alongside dramatically less developed semantic and pragmatic ability.

    (10) (*J. is explaining to M what they're going to do in their session that day. M just begins talking.*)

        M: I might get my bangs [unintelligible] trimmed, 'cause this friend of my mom's is away, my mom's haircutting, go to the airport, 'n my haircutting came in! An' so we haven't made one yet. Just to get (*gesturing cutting at back of head*) back [unintelligible] here, 'n one [k]! y'know, [k] [unintelligible] really get the, thing, the what do you call it.

        S: The hair, the scissors?

        J: The scissors?

        M: I was goin' there, cross the street from where I live it's right across from, [unintelligible] this is . . .

        S: From your new, from where you live now?

M: Yeah, an' it's really nice, me 'n this friend went there, an' I went there an' I'm (*sort of sings*) grad-du-a-ting from it! I'm [unintelligible] (*slaps self as if in rhythm*) . . .

S: You're now what?

J: What are you?

M: [I think it's, they] go up to fifty an hour, a dollar an hour an' um,

S: Hm. A new class you mean, or a new place?

M: It's no, the place where I get my hair cut, pays an hour if it's a woman, I think, if it's a man it pays, he pays, five hours, I think, of work he pays, five hours, I think, of work he pays. He's out of town, so the woman works by herself, she knows where the phone is. An' this new girl my mother [as] got was so upset, an' she didn't know any kind of work. She was brand new, an' she didn't know, she didn't even , . . .

Marta's nonlinguistic performance showed further dissociations between her knowledge of grammar and other domains of knowledge, as illustrated in Table 20-4. She lacked almost all number concepts, including basic counting principles; her drawing was perseverative and at a preschool level; her play behavior was limited (symbolic play was noted on one occasion); her auditory-verbal memory span appeared to have an upper limit of three units; and logical reasoning and operational thought were at an early preschool level (preoperational). Unlike Antony, Marta did not appear to have any area of strength or well-developed ability in her nonlinguistic profile. Unlike Antony, however, Marta appeared to have some conscious cognitive appreciation of language as an object of contemplation in its own right, that is, metalinguistic ability. On imitation tasks, she was able both to detect and to correct surface syntactic and morphological errors and at times to detect semantic anomalies as well. In addition, she was sensitive to foreign accents and often made comments about such accents or the use of a foreign language (e.g., "They're speaking Spanish, can you hear it?"; "The mother's accent spits right out

TABLE 20-4. Marta's Nonlanguage Performance Profile

Ability	Marta's performance level
Auditory short-term memory	3-year-old level
Drawing	Preschool level
Copying	$3\frac{1}{2}$- to 4-year-old level
Nesting	28-month-old level
Hierarchical construction	2-year-old level
Counting	Unable to count to 5; did not have one-to-one principle
Conservation	Did not conserve
Seriation	Failed all aspects of task
Stereognosis	$3\frac{1}{2}$- to 4-year-old level

the mouth"). Thus not only did Marta acquire remarkably developed grammatical knowledge in contrast to all other aspects of mental ability examined but that knowledge developed beyond the stage of unconscious acquisition to a stage allowing for some conscious awareness and manipulation.

Rick

The third case is that of Rick, a mentally retarded 15-year-old who suffered anoxia at birth and evidenced pervasive developmental problems throughout his childhood. Rick was institutionalized most of his life in a state hospital for the severely retarded. His case is described in detail in Curtiss and Kempler (1987).

Rick's language profile is quite parallel to that of Antony and of Marta—well-developed phonological, morphological, and syntactic ability alongside poorly developed lexical and propositional semantic ability. He made frequent lexical errors and occasional morphological errors, both indicating that at least much of his speech was novel and productive. However, he also made frequent use of a small set of phrases in combination with novel phrases, giving his speech, over extended discourse periods, a somewhat repetitious quality. Some illustrations of his speech are presented in Examples in 11a–i.

(11) (a) He's the one that plays around like a turkey.
    (b) You already got it working.
    (c) If they get in trouble, they'd have a pillow fight.
    (d) She's the one that walks back and forth to school.
    (e) She can get a ponytail from someone else.
    (f) It was hitten by a road; but one car stopped and the other came.
    (g) She must've got me up and thrown me out of bed.
    (h) I find pictures that are gone.
    (i) Would you please give me the trash can?

Rick was an extremely social child and had well-developed interactive linguistic skills. He made appropriate use of social rituals and other conventionalized conversational forms. His semantic deficiencies impeded his communicative effectiveness, however, since he often misinterpreted or failed to understand the meaning of utterances directed to him and often made lexical and propositional errors of his own (see Examples 12 and 13).

(12) *R*: She looks like she has blonde hair.
    Ex: What color is blonde?
    R: Black.

(13) *Ex*: Who gets up first in the morning?
    R: Me.
    Ex: And then what?
    R: Cindy gets up third.
    Ex: Third?! Is there someone else getting up?
    R: No.

TABLE 20-5. Rick's Nonlanguage Performance Profile

Ability	Performance level
Auditory short-term memory	6-to 7-year-old level
Visual short-term memory	Below basal (below 2.1 years)
Seriation	Preoperational
Drawing	Prerepresentational
Copying	Prerepresentational
Classification	2-to 3-year-old level

Rick thus showed a linguistic profile similar to that of Antony and of Marta in that he evidenced a highly developed grammatical system alongside impaired semantic knowledge; however, he showed more pragmatic competence that they.

Rick's nonlanguage profile (highlights are presented in Table 20-5) was most similar to Antony's, although Rick was more readily testable. Rick's drawing and copying were prerepresentational, and his logical reasoning and operative thought performance were also at an early preschool level. He could rote count to 20 and knew some of the basic counting principles, but he could count correctly only sets of five items or fewer, and his number reasoning was primitive (e.g., "What is the biggest number you can thing of?" Rick: "3"). His classification abilities were difficult to assess in that, with one exception, his manipulation of separate classes of objects appeared to be random and indifferent to object classes or category, even on tasks designed for use with children under 2 years (Sugarman, 1981). However, in every case he readily labeled each separate class of objects; in one instance, given four cups and four small cars, he placed one car in each cup, calling his product "car-cups," then first removed all of the cars and stacked the four cups. Still, even his best performance was at about a 2-year-old level. In contrast, he performed at the 6- to 7-year-old level on auditory-verbal short-term memory tasks.

Discussion

The cases presented here all share two common properties: (1) grammar acquisition was dissociated from other aspects of language learning—conceptual aspects, communicative aspects, or both, and (2) grammar acquisition was dissociated from nonlinguistic development. Moreover, the cases illustrate a double dissociation between grammar acquisition and development in other components within the domain of language as well as between grammar acquisition and development in other, nonlinguistic cognitive domains. This double, double dissociation marks grammar acquisition as a separate area of neuropsychological function and therefore a not unreasonable candidate for a specialized neuropsychological talent.

There is other evidence consistent with this possibility. Data on children with left hemispherectomy or hemidecortication have shown in some cases substantial, and in other cases rather subtle but persistent, deficits in grammar acquisition alongside relatively normal or at least significantly better nonlinguistic abilities and abilities in noncomputational aspects of language (Day & Ulatowska, 1979; Dennis, 1980a, 1980b, 1981; Dennis & Whitaker, 1976; Zaidel, 1973, 1981). The marked deficits in cases of left hemispherectomy after at least early stages of language acquisition involve severe limitations in both comprehension and production of morphology and syntax. Specific deficits in the acquisition of linguistic structural knowledge in cases of hemidecortication *before* language acquisition include impairments involving phonological manipulations and recodings, processing and/or representation of certain nonlexical grammatical markers, and the assignment of noun phrase function and negative scope on the basis of syntactic structure. Recent research on adult dyslexics (Kean, 1984) shows similar deficiencies in this population in processing nonlexical grammatical formatives and in the assignment of referential relations between noun phrases (nouns or pronouns) based on syntactic structure. These deficiencies may appear remarkably limited compared to the gaping lacunae in grammar acquisition in the cases of K. H., Genie, and Chelsea. Yet, these cases, involving clear-cut neurological impairment as they do, provide strong evidence to support the existence of neuropsychological mechanisms specialized for grammar acquisition in the normal brain.

These data also suggest a tie between specialized grammar-learning mechanisms and the left cerebral hemisphere. Such a tie is supported by the results of neurolinguistic experiments with Genie, which indicated that she was using her right hemisphere for language representation and processing (Curtiss, 1977; Curtiss et al., 1978; Fromkin et al., 1974). This finding and the childhood hemispherectomy and hemidecortication data suggest only that the left hemisphere as a whole is functionally specialized for grammar acquisition. Data from a case report of stroke in childhood (Dennis, 1980c) and emerging data on dyslexia (Galaburda, 1983; Galaburda & Kemper, 1979; Galaburda, Sherman & Geschwind, 1983) suggest that certain areas *within* the left hemisphere are especially important for normal and complete mastery of the grammar. This possibility is, of course, consistent with the data on adult acquired aphasia, which impute special importance to certain areas of the left hemisphere for the maintenance of normal linguistic capacity.

Still other data suggest a critical period for the operation or utilization of grammar-learning mechanisms. The cases of K. H., Genie, and Chelsea all involve language acquisition after the proposed critical period for such acquisition (Lenneberg, 1967). In addition, age of acquisition has been shown to impinge critically on the character and extent of sign language acquisition. Mayberry, Fischer, and Hatfield (1983) demonstrated experimentally that individuals who acquired American Sign Language (ASL) in the teenage years performed worse on a variety of tasks testing competence in ASL grammar than those who acquired ASL in childhood. What is more, the later sign language was learned, the worse the performance. In additional work Mayberry (1984) reports that the signers who had learned ASL later (from 8 years up) not only performed more poorly but also performed differently. Similar findings are reported by Newport (1984). She investigated the relative effects of number of years signing versus age at acquisition on production and comprehension of ASL utterances involving grammatically complex verbs of motion. There was a small effect such that the later sign language was acquired, the worse the performance. However, the main effect found was between native and early acquirers on the one hand and "late" learners (those learning sign language between the age of 12 and 21) on the other, with only native signers and early learners demonstrating mastery of the complex grammatical structure of verbs of motion. Moreover, the structural analyses and hypotheses entertained by the late learners were very different from those of the native and early learners (for related findings, see Fischer, 1978; Newport, 1981, 1982; and Woodward, 1973).

Conclusion

I have argued for the existence of specialized neuropsychological mechanisms for grammar acquisition, mechanisms that appear to be tied to the hemisphere prepotent for language at birth (usually the left) and to function within strong maturational constraints. There is good reason to expect that if there are specialized mechanisms required for its acquisition, grammar must rest on domain-specific organizational principles (i.e., principles of Universal Grammar). Therefore, having marshaled evidence for such mechanisms, I have also built a case for grammar being a distinct faculty or module of the mind, a module that, there is reason to believe, may in itself be modular (cf. Chomsky, 1981). In turn, if grammar is a separate module of the mind, one may assume that the mind is more generally modular in character, with different knowledge domains governed by distinct modules of mind, each of which embodies its own structural constraints and principles and is uniquely responsive to information that meets its structural specifications. It thus becomes possible in development and in mature function to exhibit selectively intact or impaired modules, even selectively enhanced or precociously developing modules of mind. Where the latter situation exists, we see domains of talent. Not surprisingly, then, since there appears to be a separate faculty of mind for grammar and specialized mechanisms for its acquisition, there appears to be a talent for grammar acquisition. Fortunately for us, it is a talent all normal individuals have.

References

Ayres, J. (1966) Southern California Figure–Ground Visual Perception Test. Western Psychological Services. Los Angeles.

Beard, R. M. (1963). The order of concept development studies in two fields. *Educational Review, 15*,(3) 228–237.

Chomsky, N. (1981). *Lectures on government and binding: The Pisa lectures.* Dordrecht: Foris Publications.

Curtiss, S. (1977). *Genie: A psycholinguistic study of a modern-day "wild child."* New York: Academic Press.

Curtiss, S. (1979). "Genie: Language and cognition." *UCLA Working Papers in Cognitive Linguistics, 1,* 15–62.

Curtiss, S. (1981). Dissociations between language and cognition. *Journal of Autism and Developmental Disorders, 11,* 15–30.

Curtiss, S. (1982). Developmental dissociations of language and cognition. In L. Obler & L. Menn (Eds.), *Exceptional language and linguistics* (pp. 285–312). New York: Academic Press.

Curtiss, S. (1982-1986). Chelsea's language development. Unpublished raw data.

Curtiss, S., Fromkin, V., & Krashen, S. (1978). Language development in the mature (minor) right hemisphere. *ITL: Journal of Applied Linguistics, 39–40,* 23–27.

Curtiss, S., Fromkin, V., Krashen, S., Rigler, D., & Rigler, M. (1974). The linguistic development of Genie. *Language, 50,* 528–554.

Curtiss, S., Fromkin, V. & Yamada, J. (1979). *The independence of language as a cognitive system.* Unpublished manuscript.

Curtiss, S., & Kempler, D. (1987). *Syntactic and pragmatic development without a semantic base.* Unpublished manuscript.

Curtiss, S., Kempler, D., & Yamada, J. (1981). The relationship between language and cognition in development. Theoretical framework and research design. *UCLA Working Papers in Cognitive Linguistics, 3,* 1–59.

Curtiss, S., & Yamada, J. (1981). Selectively intact grammatical development in a retarded child. *UCLA Working Papers in Cognitive Linguistics, 3,* 61–91.

Curtiss, S., & Yamada, J. (1980). Tests of classification and logical sequencing. Unpublished.

Daumer, G. (1832). *Mittheilungen über Kaspar Hauser.* Nürnberg.

Day, P., & Ulatowska, H. (1979). Perceptual, cognitive, and linguistic development after early hemispherectomy: Two cases studies. *Brain and Language, 7,* 17–33.

Dennis, M. (1980a). Capacity and strategy for syntactic comprehension after left or right hemidecortication. *Brain and Language, 10,* 287–317.

Dennis, M. (1980b). Language acquisition in a single hemisphere: Semantic organization. In D. Caplan (Ed.), *Biological studies of mental processes.* Cambridge: The MIT Press.

Dennis, M. (1980c). Strokes in childhood 1: Communicative intent, expression, and comprehension after left hemisphere arteriopathy in a right-handed nine-year-old. In R. Rieber (Ed.), *Language development and aphasia in children* (pp. 45–67). New York: Academic Press.

Dennis, M. (1981). Language in a congenitally acallosal brain. *Brain and Language, 12,* 33–53.

Dennis, M., Lovett, M., & Wiegel-Crump, C. (1981). Written language acquisition after left or right hemidecortication in infancy. *Brain and Language, 12,* 54–91.

Dennis, M., & Whitaker, H. (1976). Language acquisition following hemidecortication: Linguistic superiority of the left over the right hemisphere. *Brain and Language, 3,* 404–433.

Dore, J. (1978). Variations in preschool children's conversational performances. In K. Nelson (Ed.), *Children's Language* (Vol. 1, pp. 397–444). New York. Gardner Press.

Elkind, D. (1961). Children's discovery of the conservation of mass, weight, and volume: Piaget replication study II. *Journal of Genetic Psychology, 98,*(2), 219–227.

Elkind, D. (1966). Conservation across illusory transformation in young children. *Acta Psychologica, 25(*4), 389–400.

Fischer, S. (1978). Sign language and creoles. In P. Siple (Ed.), *Understanding language through sign language research.* New York: Academic Press.

Fromkin, V. A., Krashen, S., Curtiss, S., Rigler, D., & Rigler, M. (1974). The development of language in Genie: A case of language acquisition beyond the "critical period." *Brain and Language, 1,* 81–107.

Galaburda, A. (1983). Neuroanatomical aspects of language and dyslexia. In Y. Zotterman (Ed.), *Dyslexia: Neural, cognitive and linguistic aspects*. Oxford: Pergamon Press.

Galaburda, A, & Kemper, T. (1979). Cytoarchitectonic abnormalities in developmental dyslexia: A case study. *Annals of Neurology, 6*, 94–100.

Galaburda, A., Sherman, G., Rosen, E., Aboitiz, F., & Geschwind, N. (1985). *Developmental dyslexia: Four consecutive patients with cortical anomalies. Annals of Neurology, 18*, 222–233.

Gelman, R., & Gallistel, C. (1978). *The child's understanding of number*. Cambridge, MA: Harvard University Press.

Goldschmid, M. L., & Bentler, P. (1968). *Concept assessment kit—Conservation*. Educational and Industrial Testing Service. San Francisco.

Goodenough, F. (1926). *Measurement of intelligence by drawing*. New York: Harcourt, Brace, and World.

Goodnow, J. (1977). *Children's drawing*. Cambridge MA: Harvard University Press.

Greenfield, P. (1976). The grammar of action in cognitive development. In C. O. Walter, L. Rogers, & J. Finzinred (Eds.), *Conference on human brain function*, Los Angeles: Brain Research Institute. Publications Office.

Greenfield, P. M. (1978). Structural parallels between language and action in development. In A. Lock (Ed.), *Action, symbol, and gesture: The emergence of language*. London: Academic Press.

Greenfield, P., Nelson, K. & Saltzman, F. (1972). The development of rulebound strategies for manipulating seriated cups: A parallel between action and grammar. *Cognitive Psychology, 3*, 291–310.

Greenfield, P., & Schneider, L. (1977). Building a tree structure: The development of hierarchical complexity and interrupted strategies in children's constructive activity. *Developmental Psychology, 13*(4), 299–313.

Heyer, K. (1964). *Kaspar Hauser und das Schicksal Mitteleuropas in 19 Jahrhundert*. Stuttgart: Verlag Freies Geistesleben.

Johnston, J., & Kamhi, A. (1984). *The same can be less: Syntactic and semantic aspects of the utterances of language-impaired children*. Merrill-Palmer manuscript. *Quarterly, 30*, 65–85.

Johnston, J., & Weismer, S. (1983). Mental rotation abilities in language disordered children. *Journal of Speech and Hearing Research, 26*, 397–403.

Jones, K., & Smith, D. (1975). The Williams facies syndrome: A new perspective. *Journal of Pediatrics, 86*, 718–823.

Kamhi, A. (1981). Nonlinguistic symbolic and conceptual abilities of language-impaired and normally developing children. *Journal of Speech and Hearing Research, 24*, 446–453.

Kamhi, A., Catts, H., Koenig, L., & Lewis, B. (1984). Hypothesis testing and nonlinguistic symbolic abilities in language-impaired children. *Journal of Speech and Hearing Research, 49*, 162–176.

Kean, M.-L., (1984). The question of linguistic anomaly in developmental dyslexia. *Annals of Dyslexia, 34*, 137–151.

Kellogg, R. (1970). *Analyzing children's art*. Palo Alto, CA: Mayfield.

Kirk, S. A., McCarthy, J. J., & Kirk, W. D. (1968). *The Illinois Test of Psycholinguistic Abilities* (rev. ed.). Urbana: University of Illinois Press.

Laurendeau, M., & Pinard, A. (1970). *The development of the concept of space in the child*. New York: International University Press.

Lenneberg, E. (1967). *Biological foundations of language*. New York: Wiley.

Lovell, K., Healey, D., & Rowland, A. D. (1962). Growth of some geometrical concepts. *Child Development, 33*(4), 741–757.

Mayberry, R. (1984, November). *Early and late learning of sign language: Processing patterns.* Paper presented at American Speech-Language-Hearing Association Convention, San Francisco, CA.

Mayberry, R., Fischer, S., & Hatfield, N., (1983). Sentence repetition in American Sign Language. In J. Kyle & B. Woll (Eds.), *Language in sign: International perspectives on sign language* (pp. 206–214). London: Groom Helm.

Newport, E. (1981). Constraints on structure: Evidence from American Sign Language and language learning. In W. Collins (Ed.), *Aspects of the development of competence* (Minnesota Symposia on Child Psychology, Vol. 14, pp. 93–124). Hillsdale, NJ: Erlbaum.

Newport, E. (1982). Task specificity in language learning? Evidence from speech perception and American Sign Language. In E. Wanner & L. Gleitman (Eds.), *Language acquisition: The state of the art* (pp. 450–486). New York: Cambridge University Press.

Newport, E. (1984). Constraints on learning. Studies in the acquisition of ASL [Keynote address]. *Papers and reports on child language development,* Stanford University, (Vol. 23, pp. 1–22). Stanford, CA.

Piaget, J., & Inhelder, B. (1967). *The child's conception of space.* Translation of *La représentation de l'espace chez l'enfant.* New York: W. W. Norton.

Pies, H. (1966). *Kaspar Hauser, Eine Dokumentation.* Ansbach: Brueghel Verlag.

Pietler-Ley, L. (1927) *Kaspar Hauser Bibliographie.* Ansbach: Brueghel Verlag.

Semel, E., & Wiig, E. (1980). *Clinical evaluation of language functions (CELF).* Columbus, OH: Charles E. Merrill.

Silbert, A., Wolff, P. H., & Lilienthal, J. A. (1977). Spatial and temporal processing in patients with Turner's Syndrome. *Behavior Genetics, 7,* 11–21.

Sugarman, S. (1981). The cognitive basis of classification in very young children: An analysis of object-ordering trends. *Child Development, 52,* 1172–1178.

Swisher, L., & Pinsker, E. (1971). The language characteristics of hyperverbal hydrocephalic children. *Developmental Medicine and Child Neurology, 13,* 746–755.

Tallal, P., & Piercy, M. (1975). Developmental aphasia: The perception of brief vowels and extended stop consonants. *Neuropsychologia, 13,* 69–74.

Tallal, P., Stark, R., & Mellits, D. (1983). Identification of language-impaired children on the basis of rapid perception and production skills. *Brain and Language, 25,* 314–322.

Tew, B. (1977). The cocktail party syndrome in children with hydrocephalus and spina bifida. *British Journal of Disorders of Communication, 14,* 89–101.

von Armin, G., & Engel, P. (1965). Mental retardation related to hypercalcemia. *Developmental Medicine and Child Neurology, 6.*

von Feuerbach, A. (1832). *Example of a crime on the intellectual life of man.* Ansbach.

Wallach, L., Wall, A. J., & Anderson, L. (1967). Number conservation: The roles of reversibility, addition, subtraction, and misleading perceptual cues. *Child Development, 38*(2), 425–442.

Wohlwill, J. F., & Lowe, R. C. (1962). Experimental analysis of development of conservation of number. *Child Development, 33*(1), 153–167.

Woodward, J. (1973). Inter-rule implication in American Sign Language. *Sign Language Studies, 3,* 47–56.

Yamada, J. (1981). Evidence for the independence of language and cognition: Case study of a "hyperlinguistic" adolescent. *UCLA Working Papers in Cognitive Linguistics, 3,* 121–160.

Yamada, J. (1983). *The independence of language: A case study.* Unpublished doctoral dissertation, University of California, Los Angeles.

Zaidel, E. (1973). *Linguistic competence and related functions in the right cerebral hemisphere of man following commissurotomy and hemispherectomy.* Unpublished doctoral dissertation, California Institute of Technology, Pasadena.

Zaidel, E. (1981). Reading in the disconnected right hemisphere: An aphasiological perspective. In Y. Zotterman (Ed.), *Dyslexia: Neural, cognitive, and linguistic aspects* (pp. 67–91). Oxford: Pergamon Press.

21

An Association of Special Abilities
with Juvenile Manic-Depressive Illness

G. ROBERT DELONG
ANN L. ALDERSHOF

Special abilities, such as hyperlexia or calendar calculating, have been reported in several populations: autistics, the mentally retarded, and children of psychotic mothers (Kauffman, Grunebaum, Choler, & Gamer, 1979). Our experience brings to light another population in which special abilities exist: children with bipolar affective disorder, or manic-depressive illness.

We define such special ability as an area of ability above that of other children the same age, exceptional in relation to the child's other areas of functioning, and not formally developed (i.e., by training). This ability might show itself in one or several areas and might be very narrow or broad. Our definition, which is similar to Hill's (1979), allows for the inclusion of children with rather different presentations. Some of them are idiot savants; their IQs fall in the defective range, yet they possess an ability that is exceptional both in comparison to the level of their other functions as well as to the ability of normal children. Others are of at least average intelligence and resemble the children of psychotic mothers described by Kauffman (Kauffman et al., 1979), who referred to them as "superkids." These are colorful, creative children with sophisticated interests and talents.

R. R. is an example of the idiot–savant type. He is able to perform calendar calculations, giving the correct day for any past or present date, despite his inferior IQ. He is also able to do some arithmetic calculations in his head, although he does not understand simple mathematical concepts.

He has required residential treatment because of his unmanageable behavior, which has the features of childhood manic–depressive illness, including disturbed sleep pattern, excessive eating, crying jags, withdrawal, agitation, irritability ("loses control and becomes violent due to momentary frustration"), press of speech ("sometimes he is a radio, jabberwocky talk"), and flight of ideas. A psychologist reported that the Rorschach projective test revealed extraordinarily intense emotions and emotional lability.

G. Robert DeLong. Massachusetts General Hospital and Harvard Medical School, Boston, Massachusetts.
Ann L. Aldershof. Boston University School of Medicine, Boston, Massachusetts.

His other abnormal behaviors are more characteristic of the developmental disorders. He did not like being held when young and, at that time, used single words once and never again. There has been self-abuse in the form of face scratching. His language now, as a teenager, is slow and stilted. He exhibits many obsessions, such as airplanes, math, time, the drawing of clocks and calendars, and light switches. Also possibly associated with his autism are his interest in music and his memory for topography.

Additional clinical features of interest are hyperdipsia, enuresis, extreme salt craving (eats bouillon cubes), and fits of rage. Both his mother and maternal grandmother are manic–depressives.

J. H. is an example of the second type of patient we have seen. He has a full-scale IQ of 147 (99.9th percentile) but is failing most of his subjects in school because of low motivation and poor conduct. His teacher reports, however, that he has a "great thirst for knowledge, much inquisitiveness." This is reflected in his engrossment in subjects of his choice. At one office visit these were Hamlet, Liberace, concerts, history, and astronomy. Another skill he displays is drawing of very detailed pictures (see Figure 21-1).

His mother describes phasic highs and lows in his behavior. His high phases are associated with manic silliness, overconfidence, inability to sit still, anorexia, and overactive excitement. At other times he acknowledges feeling very depressed, withdraws, either "starves or gorges," cannot concentrate, and feels badly about himself.

Other behavior problems include explosiveness, aggressiveness, and violence (e.g., threatening his mother with scissors and knives). This conduct has reached

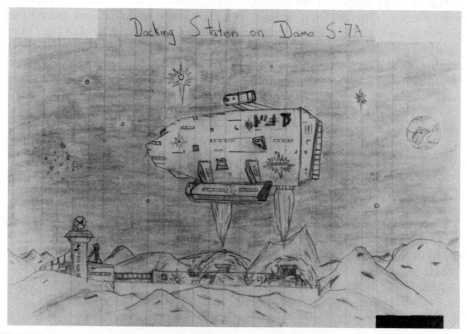

FIGURE 21-1. Sample detailed picture drawn by J. H., a juvenile manic-depressive.

obsessive proportions; he is obsessed with blowing things up and other sadistic acts. The patient's father was manic–depressive and alcoholic, and yet was described as a brilliant electronics technician. His paternal grandfather is thought to be similar to the father in these respects.

A Study of Special Abilities in Juvenile Manic–Depressives

Clinically, we were impressed by the coincidence of special ability and manic–depressive illness. We set out to try to verify this impression by examining the records of a large sample of children for the presence of special abilities. Groups of patients were as follows: (1) all manic-depressive children seen in the practice ($n = 42$); (2) all patients with pervasive developmental disorder (including pervasive developmental disorder and autism with onset in childhood) and developmental language disorder ($n = 23$); and groups of behavior-disordered patients randomly chosen, consisting of (3) children with the diagnosis of unipolar depression ($n = 61$) and (4) children with attention deficit disorder ($n = 35$).

Special abilities had to fit our previously stated criteria and be demonstrable to the examiners; we did not accept parents' reports of exceptional performances that we did not witness. The types of special abilities and representative vignettes may be seen in Table 21-1. Behavioral and psychiatric diagnoses were made according to DSM-III (American Psychiatric Association, 1980) by an experienced rater. The diagnosis of childhood manic–depressive illness was made using the same criteria as for adults, a procedure used by others (Puig-Antich & Gittelman, 1980), which we have found satisfactory. The diagnosis of bipolar affective disorder was further verified by the K-SADS (Schedule of Affective Disorders of Children; Puig-Antich & Chambers, 1978). Family history data were obtained from detailed interviews with parents concerning the child's first- and second-degree relatives. In the majority of cases these reports were verified in an interview by another examiner using the Family History–Research Diagnostic Criteria (Endicott, Andreasen, & Spitzer, 1975). Clinical features of the children were assessed by extensive interviews with parents and by examination of the child.

We found special skills to exist in only two of the diagnostic groups examined: manic–depressives and developmentally disordered children (see Tables 21-1 and 21-2). Specifically, of the 25 children identified as having special abilities, 17 met the criteria for manic–depressive illness, 6 were autistic or had childhood onset pervasive developmental disorder, and 2 had developmental language disorder. None of the children with special abilities were diagnosed as having conduct disorder, attention deficit disorder–hyperactivity, or unipolar depression.

The incidence of special abilities among all the children with manic–depressive illness and among those with developmental disabilities in our sample is striking; 40% of the manic–depressive and 35% of the developmentally disordered children seen exhibited some form of special talent. When the group of manic–depressives with positive lithium response and a family history of affective disorder is isolated, the percentage with special abilities is 42% (See Table 21-2).

TABLE 21-1. Types of Special Abilities in Our Patients

Hyperlexia	All of the hyperlexics taught themselves to read between the ages of 3 and 4 years. The majority showed sophisticated preferences in subject matter, reading about topics such as history, politics, and science at an early age. Lack of comprehension is a universal feature of the hyperlexics.
Precocious categorization and writing	This feature was characterized by an early ability to classify and precisely name categories of objects, for example, types of boats or trucks. These children also learned to write their names and the letters of the alphabet by 2–3 years of age.
Calendar calculation	In spite of low IQs, these children were able to perform calendar calculation, that is, giving the date for any day, and vice versa. In all cases, scores on the Digit Span subtest of the WISC-R were significantly higher than those on any other. Each of these children was also obsessed with numbers, calendars, and clocks.
Art	This group produced works exceptional in the degree of detail and the sophistication of the lines. The subjects tend to be technological—spaceships, robots, and the like.
Music	The one patient with this skill taught himself to play piano by ear at the age of 11.
Poetry	This patient exhibited advanced word usage, especially in comparison to his failing grades in school.
Superior memory	This group demonstrated superb memory ability for topography or verbal material. These children, often with low intellect, could remember long, complicated television commercials, routes traveled once many years prior, and so forth.

Special Abilities in Children with MDI^a ($n = 17$)

Hyperlexia	6	Music	1
Precocious categorization and writing	3	Poetry	1
Calendar trick	3	Superior memory	1
Art	2		

Special Abilities in Children with Developmental Disorders without MDI ($n = 8$)

Superior memory	4	Hyperlexia	4

^{a}Manic–depressive illness.

TABLE 21-2. Incidence of Special Abilities in Our Patients

Diagnostic group	Number of patients	Number with special abilities	Percentage with special abilities
Manic-depressive illness	42	17	40
Manic-depressive illness plus lithium response plus positive family history	31	13	42
Developmental disorder	23	8	35
Depression	61	0	0
Attention deficit disorder	35	0	0
Conduct disorder	40	0	0

The next step in our strategy was to search for factors that distinguished these children with special abilities from those other manic–depressive and developmentally disordered children without special abilities as well as from children with other psychiatric disorders without special abilities. Of the parameters we compared (somatic complaints, neurovegetative function, EEG, family history, attention, and drug response), significant differences emerged only in family history and in the incidence of obsessive interests. Although we did not have data for a systematic comparison, it appears that there was not an increased incidence of left-handedness in our children with special abilities.

Family History

All of the manic–depressive children with special abilities had a family history of affective disorder (manic–depressive illness or depression), as opposed to 84% of the manic–depressive children without special abilities (see Table 21-3). In 76% of the families of manic–depressive children with special abilities, this included specifically manic–depressive illness. In contrast, the incidence of bipolar disease in families of manic–depressive children without special abilities was much lower, only 16% (4 of 25). The familial psychiatric disorder found in manic–depressive children with special abilities involved the patient's mother in 6 cases, the father in 3 cases, and a sibling of the mother in 2 cases. Major affective disorder was present in two generations, excluding the index case, in 6 of the 17 children; in 4 of these families manic–depressive illness was found in two generations, and sociopathy in 1 case.

Neither of the children with developmental language disorders and special abilities had a family history of affective disorders. Of the 6 with a diagnosis of pervasive developmental disorder, 4 had a family history of affective disorder, of which 2 were manic–depressive illness (1 in the mother, 1 in the mother's sister).

TABLE 21-3. Incidence of Affective Disorder in the Family History of Our Patients

Diagnostic group	Number of patients	Number of patients (percentage) with family history of affective disorder	Number of patients (percentage) with family history of MDI
Manic–depressive illness	42	37(88)	17(40)
Manic–depressive illness with special abilities	17	17(100)	13(76)
Manic–depressive illness without special abilities	25	21(84)	4(16)
Developmental disorders with special abilities	8	4(50)	2(25)
Developmental disorders without special abilities	15	6(40)	3(20)
Attention deficit disorder	35	7(20)	1(2)

The incidence of a family history of affective disorder in other diagnostic groups is given in Table 21-3; it is notably low in the group with attention deficit disorder (20%).

Obsessive Interests

The incidence of obsessive interests unrelated to the specific area of special ability was examined (Table 21-4). Of the manic–depressive children with special abilities, 82% had definable obsessive interests, compared to 100% of the developmentally disordered children with special abilities. The content and nature of obsessive interests were notably different between the affective group and the group with developmental disorders. In the affective group the obsessive interests concerned violent, sexual, antisocial, and death themes, whereas those of the children with developmental disorders concerned objects. The incidence of obsessive interests is shown in Table 21-4: The occurrence in the group with attention deficit disorder is small, 5%. Other significant differences in the profiles of children with special abilities emerged when the group of manic–depressive children with special abilities was compared to a group of manic–depressive children without these skills. A total of 12 manic–depressive children with special abilities were able to be matched by age to 12 manic–depressive patients without such abilities. They were compared on all of the previously stated points. In addition to the differences in incidence of family history of affective disorders and obsessions that we mentioned, the group with special abilities showed a considerably higher frequency of autistic characteristics, such as stereotypies, rigidity, and self-abuse; these features are virtually absent in the bipolar patients without special abilities (see Table 21-5). These observations suggest that the group with special abilities is more severely abnormal and qualitatively different from manic–depressive children without special abilities.

TABLE 21-4. Incidence of Obsessive Interests in Our Patients

Diagnostic group	Number of patients	Number of patients with obsessive interests	Percentage with obsessive interests
Manic–depressive illness with special abilities	17	14	82
Developmental disorders with special abilities	8	8	100
Manic–depressive illness without special abilities	25	7	28
Developmental disorders without special abilities	15	12	75
Attention deficit disorder	35	1	5

TABLE 21-5. Features of Manic–Depressive Children with and without Special Abilities

Feature	Manic–depressive illness with special abilities ($n = 12$)	Manic–depressive illness without special abilities ($n = 12$)	χ^2
Family history of affective disorder	10	6	3.0
Family history of manic–depressive illness	8	1	8.6
Obsessive interests	9	2	7.0
Stereotypy	3	0	3.44
Rigidity	5	1	4.88
Self-abuse	4	0	4.8

$p < 0.05$.

Conclusions

We draw several conclusions from this study:

1. There is a high incidence of special abilities associated with childhood manic–depressive illness (bipolar affective disease).

2. There is a spectrum of special abilities and special interests, ranging from those children with generally normal intellectual abilities and complex high-level areas of special interest to those with severe developmental disorders and extremely narrow and bizarre special abilities and interests. Whether this represents a true continuum of severity or a unitary process is a question for further study. Despite this variability, we believe there is an element common to all the cases, with a gradient or continuum of breadth and intensity of this feature among the group of children showing special abilities.

3. The children with special abilities uniformly show obsessive interests in addition to their area of special ability. We believe these two features are closely related, both reflecting an intense, highly focused, and perhaps perseverative intellectual style. This is opposite in essential respects to the attention deficit disorder and might be characterized an an "attention excess disorder" similar to Kinsbourne's conception of the overfocused child (Kinsbourne & Caplan, 1979).

4. The occurrence of special abilities appears to be associated with a more severe degree of childhood manic–depressive illness in this population. This is shown not only by the clinical severity of mental illness in these children but also by their heavy genetic loading for affective disease: Of the manic–depressive children with special abilities, 86% had a family history of bipolar illness, as opposed to 16% of those manic–depressive children without special abilities. It is known that individuals with manic–depressive illness have heavier genetic loading (i.e., stronger family histories of affective disease) than those with unipolar depression and that those with earlier age of onset of manic–depressive illness have heavier genetic loading than those with later onset. Children with manic–depressive illness

have even heavier genetic loading than adult manic–depressive patients, especially for bipolar disease (Dwyer & DeLong, 1987). As the culmination of this intensification, our data suggest that the heaviest genetic loading, and presumably the most severe expression of bipolar illness, may result in early childhood onset of symptoms and a peculiarly intense emotional and intellectual style manifesting itself in special hyperfocused interests and abilities.

5. This same process may apply in some cases of infantile autism or pervasive developmental disorder, those that are marked by strong affective symptoms, obsessiveness, perseveration, and special abilities. That is, we raise the possibility that some cases of autism and pervasive developmental disorder may represent an extreme expression of manic–depressive disease. Our anecdotal experience, encompassing approximately a score of patients in whom pervasive developmental disorder (including autism) with marked affective features occurs in families with bipolar illness, supports this suggestion. We are currently carrying out family history studies of such children to determine whether they have a strong genetic loading for affective, particularly bipolar, disease.

The nature of the special abilities and obsessive interests seen in these children varies widely; in some cases they are broad, including an entire area of knowledge, and are pursued with creativity and imagination; in other cases they are narrow, rote, and perseverative, such as the calendar trick. The basis of these differences is unclear: They may reflect a single process with a spectrum of severity, the more narrow forms reflecting greater severity. Certainly the special abilities and obsessions in the autistics are narrower and more stereotyped than those in the manic–depressives. There is also a notable tendency for the focus of the autistic's interest to be on inanimate, neutral objects, but it is uncertain whether this relates to the autistic child's difficulty in dealing with human or interpersonal matters or simply reflects the more severe and constricted field of attention of the autistic child. We find it hard to escape the impression that we are observing a spectrum showing all gradations in the expression of special abilities and obsessions between the manic–depressive and the autistic children.

Acknowledgments

We gratefully acknowledge support by grants from the Jessie B. Cox Charitable Trust and the Charles and Sara Goldberg Charitable Trust.

References

American Psychiatric Association (1980). *Diagnostic and statistical manual of mental disorders* (3rd ed.). Washington, DC: APA.

Dwyer, J., & DeLong, G. R. (1987). *A family history study of twenty probands with childhood manic–depressive illness. Journal of the American Academy of Child and Adolescent Psychiatry*, 26, 176–180.

Endicott, J., Andreasen, N., & Spitzer, R. L. (1975). Family history–Research diagnostic criteria. New York Biometrics Research. New York: New York State Psychiatric Institute. Unpublished manuscript.

Hill, A. L. (1979). Savants: Mentally retarded individuals with special skills. In *International review of research in mental retardation* (Vol. 9, pp. 277-298). New York: Academic Press.

Kauffman, C., Grunebaum, H., Choler, B., & Gamer, E. (1979). Superkids: Competent children of psychotic mothers. *American Journal of Psychiatry, 136*(11), 1398–1402.

Kinsbourne, M., & Caplan, P. J. (1979). *Children's learning and attention problems.* Boston: Little, Brown.

Puig-Antich, J., & Chambers, W. (1978). *Schedule of affective disorders and schizophrenia of school-age children (K–SADS).* New York: New York State Psychiatric Institute.

Puig-Antich, J., & Gittelman, R. (1980). Depression in childhood and adolescence. In E. S. Payhel (Ed.), *Handbook of affective disorders.* London: Churchill.

Rimland, B. (1978, August). Inside the mind of the autistic savant. *Psychology Today, 12,* 69–74.

V

OVERVIEW

22

Expertise in Chess, Music, and Physics: A Cognitive Perspective

NEIL CHARNESS

A Framework for Understanding Expert Performance

The goal of this chapter is to suggest a general framework for examining expert performance, particularly for what Simon (1979) has termed "semantically rich domains"—those domains that require a large knowledge base for superior performance. What constitutes a semantically rich, as opposed to a nonrich, domain is open to debate. A useful distinction might be that expertise in the former requires knowledge of more than 100 "facts" about the domain, whereas expertise in the latter does not. Thus to play a skillful game of tic-tac-toe, the player needs to know a very few critical configurations, mainly those that represent threats and double threats, and their associated moves (what moves produce or avoid them), whereas to play a skillful game of chess, many thousands of configurations must be accessible. Also being assumed is that the expert possesses general problem-solving skills, general programs for making physical responses, and a language system for communication, although each of these capabilities undoubtedly represents a semantically rich domain in its own right.

The domains examined in detail in this chapter are chess, music, and physics. An outline of the proposed framework is given in Table 22-1.

Performance on complex tasks like playing chess, solving physics problems, and composing or performing music is multidimensional. For example, a person may be able to "read" music perfectly (perform masterfully on the piano) but be unable to play it on a guitar. Evidently, there are competent performing musicians who are very poor sight readers but other, equally competent performers who are quite good at this task (Bean, 1938; Wolf, 1976).

The business of understanding expertise demands that several tasks related to the skill be performed in order to assess some of the dimensions along which performance can vary. Much of the current work has failed to employ a rich-enough network of tasks. Thus a critical issue is to classify the nature of the expected differences. A crude, though useful, distinction is "hardware" versus "software."

Neil Charness. Psychology Department, University of Waterloo, Waterloo, Ontario, Canada.

TABLE 22-1. Sources of Differences in Skilled Performance

Software	Hardware
Process Differences	

Speed of elementary processes
  Encoding, comparison, response execution
	Asymptotic speed
	  Speed after much practice

Size of information units
  Number of elements per unit
	Working memory capacity
	  Number of units (chunks)

	Long-term memory consolidation rate e.g., learning rate
Data Structure Differences **(Semantic memory characteristics)**	

Mode
  Declarative, procedural, spatial, verbal, motoric
	Preference for mode
	  e.g., visualization vs. verbalization

Size Number of nodes or productions	
Element types Facts, evaluations, operators	
Organization Linear, hierarchical, matrix	
Strategy Differences	

Search characteristics
  Type
    Generate and test
    Heuristic search
      Forward, backward, means–ends
      Breadth-first, depth-first, best-first
  Extent
    Width, depth, cutoff by motivation, level of aspiration
    Node-generator constraints
    Node-evaluation constraints
    Working memory constraints	

People may differ because their eyes, ears, and brains have structural differences that are due to genetics or to maturational-hormonal (Geschwind & Galaburda, 1985a, 1985b) or other influences. Although it may be a depressing possibility, experts may be born different—that is, they may see more acutely, have faster neural conduction times, or have brain circuits specialized for encoding the "grammar" of the domain. Most of the evidence is inconsistent with this "hardware" hypothesis, though each investigation of a new domain must take this idea into account. The simplest way to rule out hardware differences as an explanation is to demonstrate with parallel tasks that no skill differences exist between expert and novice.

The classical example of demonstrating an Expertise × Task interaction can be found in the domain of chess. If you show a structured game position to a chess player for a few seconds, his or her recall varies directly with skill level (Chase & Simon, 1973a, 1973b; de Groot, 1966, 1978). If the same pieces are randomly arranged on the board, however, there is no relation between skill level and recall score, with everyone remembering only a few pieces (five or so) correctly (Chase & Simon, 1973a, 1973b; de Groot, 1966). Better chess players do not have better eyes or visual-perceptual memory capacity. It should be noted in passing that reproducing a structured chess position after a brief glance is not a task that chess players practice. Thus reconstructing both structured and random positions is a novel task.

There is some recent evidence that better chess players can *recognize* a single chess piece, or an attack relation between two pieces, more quickly (Saariluoma, 1984). This would fit with some of the work by Hunt and his colleagues (e.g., Hunt, 1978) showing that certain elementary information processes, such as abstracting the name of a visually presented letter, are carried out more quickly by more highly verbal people. It may also represent another case of the well-known word-frequency effect, where words occurring more frequently have lower visual recognition thresholds. In Saariluoma's case, better chess players may see chess pieces more frequently than less skilled players.

The demonstration of an interaction (skill effects on one task, or at one level, but not at another) makes hardware explanations of skill difficult to defend. There does remain the possibility of hardware differences in certain classes of component processes. For instance, Jackson (1980) has shown that skilled readers seem to have a *generalized* speed advantage in accessing name codes from visual symbols. Also, some people may be able to acquire domain-specific skills more quickly than others because of a general hardware advantage in learning speed (memory consolidation rate) or possibly because of a domain-specific learning-rate advantage, one peculiar to certain classes of symbols.

"Software" explanations, for example, the learning of task-specific component skills, do become favored when an interaction effect is observed. Only domains with large intellectual problem-solving aspects are discussed in this chapter, though the proposed framework may prove quite useful for other domains, for instance, skill in sports (Allard & Burnett, 1985).

At the molar level, experts typically outperform novices both in speed and in accuracy of performance. Molar differences can emerge from differences in process, structure, and strategy. Admittedly, it is difficult to differentiate process from structure, since, as was made clear in the early conceptualizations of declarative versus procedural representations (Winograd, 1975), it is easy to rearrange your model to weight one dimension more heavily than the other. That is, knowledge can be seen either as a set of complex processes operating on a nonactive declarative data base (e.g., a large list of facts) or as a relatively simple set of ordering rules interacting with a very complex procedural representation of information (a large list of condition–action rules).

Nonetheless, the distinction between declarative and procedural representations has heuristic value, as seen in the neuropsychological literature that deals with amnesic patients. Such patients have great difficulty learning new information when that information consists of facts to be recalled, yet they evidently can learn new procedures, as evidenced by improved performance on psychomotor tasks, such as pursuit rotor tracking and mirror tracing, and on cognitive perceptual procedures, such as inducing a Fibonacci series (Wood, Ebert, & Kinsbourne, 1982) and solving the Tower of Hanoi disk transfer problem (Cohen, 1984).

Process Differences

Process variables refer to both the size of the unit capable of entering into an operation and the time it takes for an operation to go to completion. Thus an expert may carry out the encoding of a stimulus array more quickly, may compare two encoded structures for identity or nonidentity more quickly, or may organize and execute a response more quickly. These are all conceptualized as software differences, in that they depend on experience. (Processes that are practiced are executed more quickly.) It is likely that asymptotic speed for any operation is hardware limited and that hardware differences do exist between individuals.

It is also quite likely that when a sequence of operations is executed, if there are differences in the size of the unit that can be processed—for example, experts can process larger chunks in a single step—overall speed will also favor the expert. Thus, if it takes about 10 seconds to fixate or consolidate a chunk in long-term memory (Simon, 1974), someone whose chunk consists of four elements will learn more quickly than someone whose chunk consists of one element. The number of elements constituting a chunk is seen as a software, or learning-related, effect.

Conversely, the number of units, or chunks, that can be activated in short-term memory (working memory capacity) is considered to be a function of individual differences in hardware. That is, even when optimal strategies are defined for a task and familiarity with the elements is equivalent, individual differences in performance can remain (e.g., in serial span, Lyon, 1977). Thus experts may have larger chunks, or more units of working memory capacity, or some combination of the two. Nonetheless, even here there is the possibility that differences in working memory capacity may be due to software factors such as the development of domain-dependent retrieval structures that allow the expert to keep track of more information (Ericsson, 1985; Ericsson & Faivre, Chapter 24, this volume). Finally, learning rate, the rate at which new information becomes consolidated in long-term memory, can be seen to vary between individuals, enabling some people to acquire novel skills more quickly than others.

Data Structure Differences

The permanent data structures that skilled performers tap may differ from those of the less skilled on a number of dimensions. One viewpoint is that experts are more likely to represent their knowledge as a set of highly differentiated procedures, whereas novices represent their more general information in a declarative format (Anderson, 1982; Larkin, 1981; Neves & Anderson, 1981).

Somewhat related to the declarative–procedural debate is whether the information is tied to a particular mode of representation. That is, are there code-type distinctions (e.g., Posner, 1978, Chapter 3) between experts and novices? It may be possible to demonstrate through modality-specific interference paradigms, for instance, that experts represent information spatially, whereas less skilled individuals rely on a verbal, or motoric, representation (for example, Hatano, Miyake & Binks, 1977). Alternatively, preference for a given mode (e.g., spatial versus verbal) may be hardware determined.

If you assume that there is a uniform format for information in long-term memory, for example, memory nodes (declarative) or productions (procedural), a potentially important individual difference is the number of such pieces of information, or the size of the knowledge base. Experts may be able to match or recognize more patterns than novices by virtue of a superior vocabulary of patterns.

Even if the size of a knowledge base were the same for experts and novices, it is possible that there would be differences in retrieval performance due to differences in the organization of the knowledge base. Information may be organized as a linear sequence (e.g., for adults, the numbers 1–10 in counting) or hierarchically (Chase & Chi, 1981). For instance, novices solving problems in domains where equations represent important relationships may have a linear order of equations that they evoke for every problem, followed by an examination and a selection of relevant equations. Experts may nest the equations under principles of applicability for the equations (Chi, Glaser, & Rees, 1982). The indexing system for semantic information may also take the form of a matrix rather than a hierarchy (Broadbent, Cooper, & Broadbent, 1978).

There is also the issue of determining what mix of information composes the knowledge base, that is, what types of elements reside in the base. Aside from *facts* (e.g., "A" is the first element of the alphabet), a knowledge base may contain *evaluations* (e.g., "good" versus "bad" nodes in a search space). For instance, chess players at low levels of skill may not have an evaluation stored with a given pattern description, whereas an expert player may know that the position described is a theoretical win ("good") for one side. Similarly, appended to a pattern description may be a *generator process* that automatically provides a new element, as in the case of patterns triggering legal moves in a search task. It may be more parsimonious to call all these elements "facts," but a better elaborated description of expertise should result when elements are partitioned into these types or classes, particularly if the number of elements is the same across skill levels while proportion of types changes.

Strategy Differences

Strategy differences refer to choice about program construction or selection for the purpose of problem solving in a given domain. An exemplary case is seen when search through a set of alternatives takes place, as in theorem proving or game playing (Newell & Simon, 1972).

Apart from the case of simple recognition, search methods fall into two broad classes: (1) generate and test and (2) heuristic search (Newell & Simon, 1972). The former method is exemplified by the game "Guess my number; it's between 1 and 10," when the player can elicit only yes-or-no answers to whole numbers in that range. Generate and test is a very general procedure that is available to novices. One simply proposes an element and tests if it is the solution.

Heuristic search represents the case in which generator and test components are permitted to interact, resulting in selective search through a set of alternatives. There are a number of variants within heuristic search that result in characteristic search paths. Forward search involves starting from the givens and applying operators to generate new nodes until the solution is obtained. Backward search takes the opposite approach, starting from the goal node and applying operators to chain back to the initial node. Means–ends analysis is a very general search strategy that makes use of both types of search. Adoption of a particular search strategy depends on the perceived nature of the problem space, which in turn depends on the searcher's level of skill for representing a problem.

The extent of search depends on rules for stopping search (width or depth), which in turn may depend on skill level (e.g., Charness, 1981b). Search can be carried out basically in a depth-first manner, which, to oversimplify, involves generating all descendants of a top node to a given depth and backing up the evaluation before generating the descendants of alternate top nodes. An alternate approach is breadth-first search, where, again to oversimplify, all top nodes are evaluated before descendants at the next ply are generated for evaluation, with some depth cutoff applied. Usually some hybrid of these two approaches is adopted, for example, best-first search (Berliner, 1979), where more effort is allocated to bounding the value of a given node (ensuring its promise) before analysis nodes are generated.

These search strategies are constrained by a number of skill-sensitive parameters: memory for evaluations of nodes, node-generation capabilities, node-evaluation functions, and search-cutoff rules. Search is obviously constrained by limitations in remembering and backing up evaluations. Even if it were possible for humans to generate several thousand terminal nodes in, say, a 15-minute search episode, it would be impossible to keep track of them.

It is also not obvious that node-generation processes can be assumed to be uniform across skill levels, either for speed or for completeness. Similarly, different individuals having identical generation and evaluation functions could vary in terms of the cutoffs they select. Perhaps what we mean by motivational terms such as "persistence" is captured by variations in willingness to search more widely or more deeply. It is also possible that variations exist in the individual's "level of aspiration," the person's expectation of what should be found from an initial node.

In summary, what the framework in Table 22-1 provides is a taxonomy of sources of individual differences in performance in semantically rich domains, based primarily on an information-processing analysis. This first approximation can undoubtedly be elaborated and extended.

This analysis suggest one way of looking at differences between experts and novices, namely, finding micro tasks to measure or dissect out components (e.g., Sternberg's 1977 componential analysis) or elementary information-process differences (Chase, 1978; Newell & Simon, 1972). If you ensure that expert and novice use the same algorithm for a task, algorithm execution speed may be expected to vary. If the novice is missing a data structure, providing it may allow a solution to a previously insoluble problem.

There are several other dimensions to understanding expert performance. Development seems a major issue. Are there critical periods for developing expertise? Do some training techniques result in better or faster learning than others (e.g., in reading, phonics versus whole-word techniques)? On the far side of lifespan development, the issue of the effects of aging arise. As experts grow old, does their skill diminish? Does it diminish at different rates for different skill levels? What does it take to maintain performance?

Within neuropsychology these same questions have important counterparts. Does brain injury affect specialized skills differently than general problem-solving ability? Are processes more impaired than data? What are effective techniques for reacquiring skill? In fact, the issue of how to separate hardware from software seems best attacked in brain-damaged populations when dissociations can be obtained.

In the remaining sections of this chapter, I attempt to apply this framework to understanding expert performance in the domains of chess, music, and physics. Other domains could probably serve equally well (as long as they have the characteristic of being semantically rich, e.g., reading), but these particular domains have recently attracted fairly concerted research efforts.

Chess

Chess has continued to attract the interest of psychologists over the last century. One of the earliest English-language analyses was a paper by Cleveland (1907) entitled "The Psychology of Chess and of Learning to Play It."[1] Although the analysis was mostly descriptive, based on interviews with players and on Cleveland's intuitions about the game, Cleveland identified many of the dimensions of expertise:

> The mental qualities most utilized in chess playing are: a strong *chess* memory, power of accurate analysis, quickness of perception, strong constructive imagination and a power of far reaching combination. These are *chess* qualities, however, and skill at chess is not a universally valid index of high mental endowment. . . . The most important psychological feature in the learning of chess (and it seems equally true of all learning) is the *progressive organization of knowledge*, making possible the direction of the player's attention to the relations of larger and more complex units. (p. 305; italics added)

Experimental investigations by the many researchers who followed Cleveland have borne out most of his speculations. Perhaps the most elegant investigation was completed by de Groot (1966, 1978) when he managed to get access to some of the world's finest chess players in the late 1930s. He uncovered two major principles about skill in chess. First, chess masters do not differ much from less expert players

1. Binet, 1894, is cited in Cleveland for an untranslated book, *Psychologie des grands calculateurs et joueurs d'échecs*. The flavor of his work is conveyed well in a translation of an early monograph (Binet, 1893/1966).

in the breadth or depth of their search process through the tree of move possibilities—they merely look at the better continuations. Second, chess masters can retain more information about a structured chess position from a brief glance than can less skilled players. This is true only for structured positions; when pieces are randomly placed on the board, the master is no better than the novice. The master's perceptual memory advantage is chess-specific.

As is often the case in psychology, these generalizations have been extended and modified by further research (see Cranberg & Albert, Chapter 7, this volume, and the recent book by Holding, 1985.) The first principle, that the search process proceeds to the same depth and extent regardless of skill, has been demonstrated to break down with players at more moderate skill levels (experts to novice range; Charness, 1981b.) Virtually all studies have shown an immediate perceptual or later short-term or long-term memory advantage for more skilled players *only with structured chess positions or chess-related processing activities.*

Current models of chess skill, for example, that of Chase & Simon (1973b), Simon and Gilmartin (1973), and Simon and Chase (1973), attribute superior performane to a large repertoire of recognizable chess patterns (50,000) in long-term memory that are associated with production of plausible moves or plans. Grand master intuition, which Cleveland (1907) commented on, is seen today as the result of the automatic indexing of moves, plans, or evaluations through a powerful pattern-recognition system, which takes about a decade of practice to develop.

The expert is better than the less expert individual on a multiplicity of tasks: choosing the best move, evaluating middle-game and end-game positions (Charness, 1981a; Holding, 1979; Holding & Reynolds, 1982; Holding & Pfau, 1985), doing a knight tour, remembering sequences of moves (Chase & Simon, 1973a), remembering incidentally learned positions (e.g., Lane & Robertson, 1979), remembering intentionally learned positions, and even recalling names of standard opening positions (Winkelman, 1975). Better performance usually includes advantages in both speed and accuracy.

Using the framework outlined earlier, how does work on chess skill fare? Are there hardware differences between master and nonmaster? The brief-exposure intentional memory task with random board positions rules out the view that the master has better immediate memory capacity, as does the incidental memory study by Lane and Robertson (1979), which showed that memory for chess positions presented under instructions to count the number of black and white pieces was unrelated to chess skill ($r = -.15$), whereas memory for chess positions presented under instructions to choose a move and evaluate the position was strongly related to skill level ($r = .82$). Hence it is worth considering software differences.

Process Differences

The speed with which the skilled player can recognize a chess pattern has been investigated directly by Ellis (1973) and Saariluoma (1984). Ellis demonstrated that when positions are shown for 50 milliseconds, the stronger player reproduces more pieces correctly than the weaker player. Furthermore, in a same–different judgment, the slope of reaction time as a function of number of pieces in the two diagrams (three to seven pieces) is virtually flat for strong players (6 milliseconds) while showing a strong linear relationship for weak players (160 milliseconds). This result supports the idea that for strong players a large cluster of pieces is the basic unit for matching, whereas for weaker players single pieces may be the basic unit. (The slope for both strong and weak players on dot comparison resembles that of weak players on chess diagram comparison.)

Saariluoma (1984) showed that more skilled players took less time to decide whether a king or knight was present in a slide consisting of a single piece on one of the four central squares. He also showed that stronger players were faster to detect the color of a king that appeared in either expected or unexpected chess formations. Better players were also faster in counting minor pieces (knights or bishops) in structured and random chess positions and at detecting whether a king was in check and whether a one-move mate was possible.

All these studies indicate that the expert extracts information more quickly from game-related displays, probably by matching clusters or chunks of chess pieces to their long-term memory representations. That more skilled players are faster even at simple discrimination of a king from a knight—that is, at single-piece identification—could be taken as evidence for a hardware advantage. Nonetheless, experience with chess diagrams is probably correlated with chess experience and chess skill level, and it is *asymptotic* identification performance that is needed to establish a hardware advantage.

Examination of the speed of the search process (when players choose a move) has provided mixed results. On the whole there are few differences in the speed of search (Charness, 1981b; de Groot, 1978), though de Groot found grand masters somewhat faster than experts at generating unique base moves (first moves), whereas Charness found more skilled players (in the intermediate skill range) slower at generating unique base moves. Chances of detecting small differences in search speed are relatively poor given the time scale (minutes) for the thinking-aloud process.

Data Structure Differences

Although it is almost impossible to separate process from structure, it may be useful to view skill in chess as partly attributable to the greater knowledge store of the expert. Certainly, as discussed earlier under matching processes, the expert has a larger repertoire of patterns in long-term memory, perhaps as many as 50,000 (similar to the size of the word vocabulary of college undergraduates; Oldfield, 1963). It is critical to note that not only does the expert have more patterns, but the patterns are also larger (Chase & Simon, 1973b). Assuming that people build chunks by concatenating smaller basic units, it is likely that only the expert possesses very large clusters of pieces (four to five pieces per chunk).

Whether the patterns are indexed more efficiently for the expert is an unanswered question that could be examined experimentally. As Chase and Chi (1981) have pointed out, although local patterns may be linearly organized, the entire position may have a hierarchical structure, with single pieces embedded in several chunks.

It is also the case that experts have better evaluation functions associated with pattern descriptions (Charness, 1981a; Holding, 1979; Holding & Reynolds, 1982). As skill increases, accuracy of static evaluation increases for classical end-game positions, as does dynamic evaluation for middle-game positions.

It seems highly likely that better players also have more precise move generators associated with their repertoire of patterns; otherwise, it is difficult to account for their greater success in the choice-of-move task, given only marginal search differences (considering the size of the problem space, sometimes estimated as 10^{120} nodes).

On the other hand, it seems that differences in knowledge structures between experts and those less skilled are more a matter of quantity than quality—that is, the representations of the problem space are quite similar, as opposed to, for instance, the case in physics or music.

Strategy Differences

There are very few differences in the nature of the search strategy between experts and novices. All players proceed through forward search, generating new nodes from the starting position. They all progressively extend search by returning to the base position and deepening a few more plies, or branch for one or two plies within a given line of moves. There are exceptions to this forward-search strategy. When players are told to look for checkmates in problems, more of a means–ends search can be adopted (Baylor, 1965; Newell & Simon, 1972).

Although the broad outline of the general search algorithm is similar for players at all skill levels, the microstructure of search does vary (Charness, 1981b). Stronger players search more extensively and push their search to a greater depth than do weaker players, at least at moderate skill levels. Whether this increased search depth with skill is due to greater memory limitations of weaker players for keeping track of changes in the base position or to faulty evaluation by less skilled players of low-ply nodes as not tactically active is not yet known. The best bet at this point is that depth of search is limited by a skill-sensitive memory span for changes in piece positions. Daneman and Carpenter (1980) have shown a similar difference in working memory between skilled and less skilled readers; Salthouse (1984) has shown a comparable eye–hand span advantage for skilled typists.

Metamemory

There is also some evidence that more skilled players can predict their memory performance more accurately than less skilled players. Chi (1978) had low-, medium-, and high-skill players predict (based on a 5-second look) the number of pieces they could recall from structured and random positions, and the number of trials they would need for perfect recall. They were given a different set of four positions, two random, two structured. As skill level increased, players predicted a greater difference in learning for structured versus random positions. Their predictions also tended to correspond more accurately to their performance as skill increased.

Summary of Chess Skill

Although a large list of differences between expert and less skilled players has been developed, the differences seem to be more a matter of degree than of kind. Experts in this domain encode and match input patterns more quickly because of their larger knowledge base of patterns. Speed may also be the result of faster execution of elementary information processes through a practice or exposure advantage. The knowledge store contains more information about what relevant actions can be carried out and about what evaluations can be assigned to the outcome of a series of actions. It does not seem necessary to invoke hardware explanations for skill in chess, but until measures of asymptotic speed for basic matching operations are gathered, "mechanistic" differences (Hunt, 1978) in elementary information processes may remain unnoticed.

Neuropsychological cases, such as those outlined by Cranberg and Albert (Chapter 7, this volume), will also prove useful in determining hardware constraints. For instance, if specific dissociations can be found following brain damage, such as an inability to perceive chess positions as meaningful coupled with intact perception of other symbol systems (e.g., perceiving words, or faces), this would argue for a privileged "module" for processing chess relations in the cortex.

My own bias is to view the cortex as providing general symbol-manipulation capabilities rather than specialized domain-specific ones, though it is very clear that there is specialized processing for language and possibly also for the manipulation of spatial representations. Linguistic and spatial processing are all activities that have evolutionary significance. It is doubtful that there were significant pressures to select for traits underlying skill in music, physics, or chess. Nonetheless, there is always the possibility that traits (specialized neural circuitry) that provide an individual with survival or mating advantage in one niche also provide unexpected benefits in another. (Could there be ironic truth to the humorous slogan "Chess players mate better?")

There are a number of weaknesses in chess research. Most of the studies reviewed dealt with very small samples: Chase and Simon (1973a, 1973b), for example, based many of their comparisons on one novice, one class A (intermediate) player, and one master. The range of skill sampled in any one study has also been restricted—only de Groot (1978) has studied the very top of the scale, and no one has studied rank beginners. As recent research has demonstrated, the relation between skill (chess rating) and performance on component tasks (e.g., search depth) may be approximately linear within narrow ranges of skill and then reach an asymptote at higher ranges. Thus inferences across studies that deal with different skill ranges may be suspect.

Age of the player is a relevant concern, since the same mechanism may not support equivalent performance across different ages (Charness, 1981a, 1981b, 1981c). In particular, encoding ability seems to decline with age across the range of 16–64 years. There is also good evidence that tournament performance of Grand masters undergoes a decline of about half a standard deviation from a peak at 35 years of age to the mid-60s (Elo, 1966, 1978).

Studies have shed light on development of skill only indirectly, as is usually the case with cross-sectional research, though Goldin and Herstein (1979) have documented the progress of one player over a period of a year and have found the expected increase in chunking ability. Probably because of the frequent tests, the absolute level of recall performance rose to that of a class A player, though the subject was still rated three standard deviation units below this skill level. Though difficult and expensive to do, longitudinal research could provide a much more detailed analysis of skill development.

Little if anything is known about whether there are critical periods for learning to play chess well, though both anecdotal evidence and retrospective analysis suggest that this issue should be pursued (Elo, 1978, p. 100; Krogius, 1976, pp. 234–243). Reanalysis of data cited by Krogius reveals that the length of a player's optimal period of tournament performances is related to the age at which he or she learned to play chess. Early learners have longer peak productive careers. Similarly, Elo has shown that players who were to reach very high performance levels (e.g., World Championship candidates) hit earlier levels, such as Master and International Master, at younger ages than did those who leveled off at lesser performance levels.

Virtually nothing is known about how motivational or emotional factors influence performance in chess—for example, how effort or affect influence processing—though one study suggest they can be important. Tikhomirov and Vinogradov (1970) present evidence that when players attempt to maintain a flat galvanic skin response (GSR) indicative of stable affect or arousal, they are unable to solve complex problems; conversely, when they achieve insight into a problem solution, their GSR shows a pronounced change. There are other explanations for this result. One is that attention or capacity is required for monitoring emotion; another is that skilled chess players are less able to divide attention between two tasks (Britton & Tesser, 1982). Nonetheless, anecdotes supporting the importance of emotional involvement are widespread in the chess subculture.

Future research aimed at establishing whether there are critical periods for skill acquisition and whether the degree of emotional and motivational involvement is important could address the hardware versus software issue of skilled performance. It is conceivable that achievement motivation has a genetic origin, though cultural factors would seem to be stronger mediators. Further, critical periods are well-established for biological processes such as the development of secondary sexual characteristics (phenotypic sex differentiation). It is uncertain whether a similar developmental process governs the formation of neural structures underlying cognitive processes. Work by Waber (1979) suggests that asynchronies in the onset of puberty may influence spatial abilities. Geschwind and Galaburda (1985a,b) have theorized that variations in intrauterine hormone levels are a major factor in brain lateralization, and thereby in both handedness and developmental disorders.

Music

Music is a domain in which the mystique of innate talent (hardware differences) is probably the strongest. One can point to a child prodigy such as Mozart, who not only achieved early expert performances on a musical instrument but also composed musical masterpieces by the age of 15. Equally mysterious is the ability termed "absolute pitch," which some musically talented individuals possess. It is often alleged that one must be born with such abilities, that they cannot be developed (Bachem, 1940).

Nonetheless, software explanations of such differences in expertise seems quite viable. Absolute-pitch judgments can be developed or improved with sufficient training, as Brady (1970) and Cuddy (1970) have shown (see Judd , Chapter 6, and Ericsson & Faivre, Chapter 24, this volume, and Ward & Burns, 1982, for further discussion). Even relative pitch, the ability to identify standard tonal intervals on an absolute basis (e.g., tones as being a perfect fifth, tritone, or major third), which most musicians, though few nonmusicians, seem to possess, is categorical, in the same sense that speech sounds are categorical (Siegel & Siegel, 1977a). For skilled Western listeners, music is categorically defined as a function of experience with the Western diatonic scale system. Even highly skilled musicians experience difficulties when making judgments within categories: They cannot tell "sharp" from "flat" (Siegel & Siegel, 1977b).

It is possible that absolute-pitch ability involves hardware differences. According to Klein, Coles, and Donchin (1984), those musicians who reported that they had absolute pitch (and who were very much superior to musicians who did not report absolute pitch on such judgments) did not show a P300 evoked potential for auditory probes when asked to count instances of an infrequent stimulus. Since P300 is normally associated with updating working memory, the authors suggest that those possessing absolute pitch have a set of internal standards that allow them to compare a current tone directly, eliminating the need to remember the comparison stimulus. Those without absolute pitch needed to remember the standard. Both those with and those without absolute pitch showed equivalent P300 responses when the task was to count instances of a visual stimulus. It would be very interesting to see if those who develop absolute pitch (e.g., Brady, 1970) show similar evoked response patterns.

A further argument for the software explanation is that even in the case of a child prodigy such as Mozart, it is probable that 10 years of composition experience is necessary for the production of excellent musical works. Hayes (1981) has reviewed the histories of noted musical composers and found that the "10-year rule" holds in most cases. Mozart began composing around age 5.

As was the case with chess, a multitude of tasks show musicians to be superior to nonmusicians. These can again be broken into the three categories of process, structure, and strategy differences.

Process Differences

Musicians can make same–different judgments of pitches (as well as absolute judgments) more quickly and accurately than nonmusicians, both with and without tonal contexts (Cuddy, 1971; Dewar, Cuddy, & Mewhort, 1977). Frances (1972) has also shown that musicians can recognize transpositions of a melodic pattern more accurately, can recognize changed chords in a melody more accurately, and can pick out the subjects (voices) in a fugue more quickly and accurately than can nonmusicians.

Does this mean that musicians have better "ears"? A dissertation by Beal (1980, 1985) is inconsistent with this hardware explanation. She asked skilled musicians (defined as having at least 8 years of music conservatory training) and nonmusicians (less than 4 years of such training) to discriminate whether two successive chords were the same or different. Chords were played either on the same or on different instruments—that is, there were timbre differences (differences in the overtones or harmonics of the notes) on half the trials. Only musicians could accurately recognize when the same chord was repeated on a different instrument. But when the chords were unlawful collections of notes (unlawful according to Western tonal conventions), musicians and nonmusicians were equally poor in the same-chord–different-instrument condition. The "hearing" advantage for musicians disappeared much like the "seeing" or "memory" advantage for chess masters when they were confronted with randomly configured chess positions. As a further check, Beal tested instrument (timbre) discrimination ability and found equal proficiency for musicians and nonmusicians.

There are other checks in the literature that assess chunking or capacity differences between musicians and nonmusicians. Gordon (1917) found that the number of trials to criterion to learn to hum a note sequence depended heavily on musical skill. This advantage could not be attributed to general memory capacity (number of chunks of short-term memory). When nonsense syllables were substituted for notes in the same criterion-learning situation, there was no relation between musical ability and learning time.

More evidence concerning an advantage for musicians in the speed of matching operations can be found in the case of reading musical notation. In a classic study Bean (1938) presented short selections of music notation for 190 milliseconds to people varying in skill (international concert performers to those with 6 months of training) and had them play the tune on the piano. In this eye–hand span task, the span for professional musicians was about 4.8 notes for melodies and 3.6 notes for chords, whereas for moderately experienced musicians the figures were about 2.4 and 3.1, respectively. A group with no music-reading training, whose members were allowed to write the notes, rarely recalled more than 1 note correctly.

Sloboda (1976) has also shown with quasi-musical patterns that recall accuracy for briefly presented notes on a musical staff varies with skill in music only for relatively long exposure durations; at 20 milliseconds there is no difference (1 note correct), but at 2 seconds musicians recalled 5 of 6 notes compared with 1 of 6 notes for nonmusicians. Sloboda (1978) also found that even at 50 milliseconds, musicians show an advantage in coding the absolute contour of a set of pitch-symbol stimuli, although their absolute note accuracy was no better than that of nonmusicians.

It is interesting to observe that when Sloboda presented three randomly chosen pitch symbols for 150 milliseconds, his musicians averaged 1.7 notes correct compared with 2.4 notes correct for similarly skilled musicians who had to play the notes in Bean's (1938) study—possibly implying that musicians code best when presented with real music and decrease in recall as the stimulus departs from standard musical schemata. Chase and Simon (1973b) obtained such an effect when they presented handwritten symbols of chess pieces for recall. It is also possible that the representation evoked when reading music is motoric for playing and that an additional recoding step is needed to prepare a *writing* response.

Other studies by Halpern and Bower (1982) and by Clifton (1986) have also found a perceptual-memory advantage for more skilled musicians. Halpern and Bower showed that "good" 10-note visually presented melodies were remembered better than "bad" ones by musicians but not by nonmusicians. When random melodies were included, the musicians showed steady decline from good to bad to random, whereas the nonmusicians performed equivalently on good and bad ones (though worse than the musicians) but worse on the random ones.

Clifton (1986) has shown that sight-reading ability specifically is predicted by recall of briefly presented musical scores. She chose pianists of comparable training and performance ability who differed broadly on sight-reading speed and accuracy. She showed that a 2-second recall task was predictive of sight-reading performance even more highly than a 5-second recall task. She also employed a reaction-time task involving physical identity and name identity in which the pianists had to decide whether two notes, an alphabetic character and a note, or two alphabetic characters had the same name. Again, the time to abstract a name code, or, more precisely, the difference between the time to make a physical-identity judgment and the time to make a name-identity judgment, was predictive of sight-reading performance. More skilled sight readers obtained a smaller difference score. This is strong evidence for Hunt's (1978) view that elementary, or "mechanical," information processes differ as a function of ability.

We can probably take these studies to indicate that musicians differ from nonmusicians in the size and type of unit that they can match to incoming information. Also, matching or encoding is performed more quickly. Sloboda's study showing an advantage for musicians in coding contour presents a result similar to that found by Chase and Simon (1973b) for placement errors by chess players. When players placed pieces incorrectly, they still maintained information about the relative positions of the pieces—their errors preserved functional relations. Frances (1972) also stresses the importance of being able to perceive large clusters or patterns of notes: "thus conceived, global perception should not be confused with a mechanical registration of the flow of information. It is conditioned, undoubtedly, by the number of sensory elements which the listener can grasp at once, and by their degree of presence or salience" (p. 247; author's colloquial translation).

Data Structure Differences

It seems evident from the preceding discussion that musicians and nonmusicians map their inputs to different musical structures. Multivariate techniques have uncovered some of the dimensions to these structures. Krumhansl and Shepard (1979) showed, through cluster analysis, that judgments of the goodness of a final tone in a tone-sequence-completion task differed as a function of musical skill. Pitch height was attended to more closely by less skilled listeners, whereas octave equivalence and tonal function within the major scale were dimensions most salient to skilled musicians.

Beal (1980; 1985) demonstrated that different factor structures emerged for musicians and nonmusicians when rating the similarity of chords played on different instruments. Features of chord identity (e.g., number of chord notes) played a more important role for musicians, but timbre seemed more salient for nonmusicians. Similarly, Miller and Carterette (1975) also found differences between music-major and nonmusic students with cluster analysis of similarity judgments for complex tones when fundamental frequency was held constant while number of harmonics, envelope structure, and onset times varied between tone pairs.

Even earlier than these studies, Allen (1967) demonstrated that the octave effect—judging tones an octave apart as highly similar—did not hold for nonmusicians. Such differences in internal representation seem to be best characterized as qualitative differences, though it is possible to see them as differential weighting of the same acoustic dimensions as a function of musical skill.

Search Strategy Differences

Musical problem solving has not been well investigated, particularly with respect to skill differences. Reitman (1965) describes a study where he investigated the ill-structured problem of composing a fugue, but no formal model has evolved yet, and in particular, no model of possible skill differences. A questionnaire study by Gross and Seashore (1941) seems to downplay the idea that composition takes place through inspiration. More skilled composers were less likely to work from inspiration and more likely to check their ideas by playing themes on an instrument. The importance of hard work and training was also stressed by Whitaker, Hutchinson, and Pickford (1942).

If the polishing of the performance of a piece of music (practicing behavior) is considered problem solving, work by Gruson (1981; in press) may be relevant. She observed and coded practicing behavior (for up to ten sessions) over a wide skill range (amateurs to professionals) for three short pieces of music (the pieces varied over skill level). The one practicing category (aside from error frequency) that discriminated groups quite consistently was the frequency of repeating a section of music rather than repeating the note or measure (smaller musical units). This difference very much appears to be a chunk-size difference, and it is carried along across practice sessions as well as between groups.

Acquisition of Skill

As was mentioned earlier, retrospective accounts of musical composition suggest that 10 years are necessary in order to reach the height of competence, and apparently it does not much matter when you start (Hayes, 1981). The case for instrumental performance may be different. Most famous instrumental performers seem to have started when quite young, but this may be attributable to cultural constraints dictating that children start their music lessons quite early in life, if necessary, with miniature musical instruments. Whether there is a critical period physiologically or psychologically, as opposed to culturally, remains to be researched. It does seem clear that the basic perceptual and cognitive apparatus to code pitch sequences and to recognize the equivalence of transposed sequences is present very early. In a review of the development of pitch perception, Dowling (1982) concludes that infants as young as 6 months can notice contour changes and match pitches.

From the perspective of training techniques, it is again unclear whether one or another method leads to faster development of skill, though Cuddy's (1970) work on teaching absolute pitch suggests that certain techniques (e.g., providing pitch anchor points) may be more effective than others. (Ericsson and Faivre, Chapter 24, this volume, demonstrate rather convincingly that the development of anchors is critical to improving absolute judgments of hue.) What is clear is that universally, whether for sight reading or for instrumental performance, everyone extols the virtues of practice (see also Judd, Chapter 6, this volume).

Weaknesses of Music Research

One major problem in music is quantifying skill, though using music-conservatory training level is helpful. As a result, particularly because musical skill is so difficult to quantify, generalizations across studies are tentative at best. Aside from Beal's (1980) study, few investigations can be said to rule out "hearing" or "seeing" differences between groups at different skill levels. There are enough cases of no differences being observed between people of different skill levels (e.g., Sloboda's 1976 and 1978 recognition studies) to warrant the argument that hardware hypotheses of musical skill are less likely than software hypotheses.

Most musicians, music critics aside, do not make their living by listening. On the performance end we know all too little about the development of skill or its maintenance, except that constant practice is important. Anecdotal evidence suggests that, barring physical disabilities, a very high level of skill can be maintained well into old age, as those of us who have been privileged to hear late-life performances of Pablo Casals or Arthur Rubinstein can readily attest, but more specific information relating age and other musical abilities remains to be discovered.

Musical performance probably has much in common with typing, telegraphy, and other well-researched motor domains (see MacKenzie & Marteniuk, 1985); music as an alternative language system is a rich source for investigation, as previous researchers and Judd (Chapter 6, this volume) have pointed out.

As some critics have argued, for example, Davies (1979), the tasks presented in order to study the coding of music (e.g., same–different judgments on tone sequences) are often too limited to provide sound inferences about coding dimensions for real melodies. They suit the goals of internal validity for experimental design much better than those concerning external validity. In sum, creative experimentation could provide a much more penetrating insight into skill in music.

Physics

Claims of hardware differences between physicists and nonphysicists do not seem to be very frequent. As opposed to music or chess, child prodigies in physics do not appear very often; physicists' earliest contributions usually do not precede age 20 (Lehman, 1953, p. 187).

Process Differences

Recent investigations of problem solving in physics have dealt with problems that typically appear in high school or university undergraduate texts. An investigation by Simon and Simon (1978) of a novice and an expert problem solver working on high-school-level problems revealed some striking differences. At the molar level, there were vast differences in solution time between the two people—a ratio of about 4:1. There was little difference in accuracy, though the novice made two arithmetic errors in the set of 25 problems.[2]

Major differences appeared in the search paths of the two problem solvers. Although the basic structure of search was well mapped for both as Find Equation → Instantiate Equation → Solve Equation, the two diverged in which equations they invoked. As a result, the novice's search could be characterized as working backward (a form of means–ends search), that is, setting subgoals of finding unknowns in equations from knowns. Surprisingly, the expert could best be characterized as working forward, that is, operating on givens and solving equations until the solution was reached, an apparently less goal-directed approach.

Simon and Simon (1978) hypothesized that because the domain is so simple for the expert, he or she can launch straight into solving equations, knowing that the solution will soon be generated. A very similar observation has been made for the performance of mathematicians doing algebra (Lewis, 1981). Lewis noted that the probable reason why the skilled algebra problem solver often failed to notice direct ways of simplifying the structure of the equations was that arithmetic operations were so automatic and easy that it was not cost effective to "problem solve" the structure of the problem. It was cheaper to work with relatively automatic arithmetic procedures than to proceed interpretively on structural descriptions.

Data Structure Differences

Simon and Simon (1978) suggest that one difference between novice and expert in physics is that the expert represents problems using "physical intuition." That is, the problem is initially translated into a physical representation, and then that representation is used to select the proper equations. The novices went straight from the problem statements to equations; that is, he or she adopted an algebraic representation only.

---

2. Faster solution times by experts are not always the rule. Chi *et al.* (1982) noted that two novices were faster than two experts for college-level problems, though there was the confound that the novices made three times as many errors, and solution times were based only on correctly solved problems.

Compelling evidence for this assertion of differing representations of the problem statements appears in articles by Chi, Feltovich, and Glaser (1981) and Chi *et al.* (1982). In a number of studies they showed that experts group mechanics problems into very different categories than novices. Experts categorize on the basis of physics principles (e.g., Newton's second law, energy and momentum conservation), whereas novices do so on the basis of surface features, such as the fact that there is an inclined plane, a spring, or a velocity being mentioned. As an experiment on rating problem difficulty showed, it was *not* the case that novices picked out different features in the problem statements. Rather, the experts drew better inferences. Surprisingly, Chi *et al.* (1982) found few quantitative differences between novices and experts in their analysis of protocols taken during the solution of mechanics problems; aside from the expected difference in accuracy as a function of skill, large individual differences seemed to be the rule.

Thus the expert appears to evoke a very sophisticated problem schema, which differs quite radically from that of the novices (with intermediate solvers falling somewhere in between). This work helps to explain why the expert can afford to work forward. He or she can restrict the selection of equations by letting higher order principles guide the search process. The novice is forced to apply very general (but less powerful, for this domain) means–ends analysis, to bootstrap his or her way from unknowns to knowns.

This explanation still does not totally account for the differences in speed between expert and novice. Larkin, McDermott, Simon, and Simon (1980) speculate that experts can carry out sequences of problem-solving steps quickly because their production-system representations are in a ready-to-execute format, whereas novices must interpret theirs, that is, take each statement and translate it into an executable one. Larkin (1981) reported that major time differences occurred between novices and experts in condition testing and search for principles with mechanics problems.

The physics area is also noteworthy because the first steps have been taken in simulating skill acquisition: for example, Larkin's (1981) model. Adaptive production systems have been developed to simulate the process of becoming expert (see also Neves & Anderson, 1981; Pirolli & Anderson, 1985). These systems contain a learning component that possesses rules that modify the current performance component, based on working out examples and generalizing the result. In effect, they generate productions that have very complex conditions, which are concatenations and modifications of previous productions. Knowledge changes from a general "declarative" or fact form to a very specific "procedural" or action form. To some extent this mirrors the view that chess masters have very specific knowledge about many thousands of patterns, whereas novices know only a few very general things that have broad, but inexact, applicability.

Summary of Skill in Physics

In terms of the general framework, some interesting features appear to differentiate experts and novices in physics. There are process differences, particularly in the time to read and interpret problem statements. As well, experts can carry out sequences of problem steps much more quickly. A chunking demonstration (as in the chess or music domains) has yet to be run, but we can speculate that in subjects given 5 seconds to reconstruct a diagram of a physics situation, the usual differences will emerge. Egan and Schwartz (1979) have produced precisely this result with skilled electronics technicians observing circuit diagrams.

In physics the semantic structures of expert and novice differ quite drastically. Experts have access to a physical representation, which in turn enables an equation representation to be formed. Novices apparently have only an algebraic representation. The schema that experts can activate also seems to have embedded information about which of a set of possible search paths is the more promising. As a result of differences in the efficiency of their respective problem representations, the search strategies of experts and novices diverge.

Research on physics expertise also speaks to the issue of skill development. The knowledge representation does seem to change, becoming increasingly proceduralized as skill is acquired. Indirectly, the sufficiency claims of simulations would seem to imply that working out many physics problems is all that is necessary to achieve more expert performance. As a counter to that argument, one could also claim that specifying the conditions of applicability of actions (production rules) more explicitly might well speed the learning process along.

Problems in Physics Research

In the physics domain it is difficult to quantify skill. Few studies have attempted directly to rule out hardware explanations. Although it is certainly a long shot, perhaps those who can easily generate and manipulate physical representations are destined to succeed more easily at physics: Their "mind's eye" may have greater acuity. It is easy to think of studies to test this interpretation.

Very few subjects have been investigated, and only a very few problem types (undergraduate-level textbook ones) have been used in physics research. A skilled physicist undoubtedly knows much more than how to solve kinematics and mechanics problems. Some of the speed with which problems are dispatched by the expert is probably attributable to greater facility with algebra and arithmetic-like operations. Chronometric studies on these component processes are worth pursuing.

Summary

The proposed framework for understanding expert performance represents a first step in partitioning a rather vast behavioral domain. Real skills are very rich and complex. Experts overshadow novices on many dimensions. This has led one theorist to suggest that "the expert is quantitatively and qualitatively different than the non-expert" (Norman, 1980). This chapter has tried to suggest a number of ways to quantify the differences.

Although there are many differences among the domains of chess, physics, and music, some similarities in the description of expertise have emerged. In all three domains experts map incoming information faster and more efficiently than novices. The bigger (faster) chunk or pattern hypothesis has received support from many other domains: GO (Reitman, 1976), bridge (Charness, 1979, 1983; Engle & Bukstel, 1978), electronics (Egan & Schwartz, 1979), serial span (Ericsson, 1985; Ericsson, Chase, & Falcon, 1980), and even sports (Allard & Burnett, 1985; Spilich, Vesonder, Chiesi, & Voss, 1979). Hunt's (1978) work on verbal ability also suggests that certain mechanistic encoding operations operate faster for the more verbal person.

When experts solve problems, the structure of the search process seems to depend a great deal on the nature of the problem space. In some cases the powerful pattern-recognition system of the expert virtually solves the problem with minimal search. In other cases the knowledge base constrains the search to manageable proportions, but novice and expert alike must search in the same way because they face the same kind of immediate memory limitations. Experts in one field may appear very different from experts in another in terms of search strategy.

Experts have evidently worked a tremendous number of hours building up their knowledge bases. The 10,000-hour (or 10-year) rule seems a good approximation for mastering chess and music as well as telegraphy, even for the prodigies. Lindsay and Norman (1977, p. 563) cite similar estimates for becoming proficient at reading, racing an automobile, singing, playing soccer, juggling, and becoming a professional psychologist. Unanswered is what keeps individuals in contact with a domain for the number of hours necessary to achieve high skill levels. Ericsson and Faivre (Chapter 24) and others in this volume speculate about possible personality traits as well as environmental pressures that may produce the high drive levels needed to achieve mastery.

Certain caveats should be raised even about these broad conclusions. Age is a relatively unexplored variable in skill. The work in chess has demonstrated that a given level of expertise may be attained by different performance systems at different ages. Another issue worth considering, in that same vein of individual differences, is whether the relationship between skill and various indices of semantic memory size is linear (e.g., the linear relationship between chess skill and memory for structured chess positions). Too few subjects and tasks have been explored to answer this question.

Issues revolving around skill acquisition are virtually untouched, though more in vogue (Ericsson & Faivre, Chapter 24, this volume; Pirolli & Anderson, 1985). The impression conveyed is that if you practice (how?) for 10 years, you will become an expert in a semantically rich domain. It is doubtful that we can convince either a granting agency or a subject to undertake that longitudinal study. Certainly, anecdotal data suggest that trying hard for a long time is not sufficient for making it into the upper echelons. Perhaps some people can use feedback about their efforts more effectively than others. Many hours of practice may be *necessary but not sufficient* for mastery of a semantically rich domain.

This speculation leads quite naturally to further speculation about the role of motivation and emotion in skill acquisition and even in performance. We probably all know one or two individuals who set out quite young to become physicians, hockey players, or simply "wealthy," and whose drive and determination finally paid off. We also probably know of others with similar drive levels who met with less success. Some work on search in chess suggests the importance of emotion (Tikhomirov & Vinogradov, 1970).

We can also wonder whether it is necessary to start off young and learn a given domain as your "mother tongue." There are certainly enough counterexamples around to suggest that this is not strictly true (e.g., Miguel de Cervantes, who published his first novel in his 40s and his masterpiece, *Don Quixote*, in his 60s). Even the literature on language learning suggests that a second language can be acquired quite successfully in later life, though it is possible that a first language must be acquired early.

Very little has been learned about how practice (current or past) and its spacing (e.g., massed vs. spaced) relate to performance levels in semantically rich domains (see Annett, 1979, for a review). Semantic memory performance seems to be quite sensitive to practice (Bahrick, 1979). Bahrick's work suggests that maintaining easy access to a rich knowledge base (e.g., spatial layout of a college town) depends on periodically accessing the information. Perhaps the fact that subjects in my chess studies reported spending an average of 6 hours a week studying or playing chess is related to their successful problem-solving performance (no age decrement). An interesting hypothesis is that lack of practice results in procedural knowledge reverting back to the declarative format, where it must again be interpretively executed. The old excuse for poor performance that "I'm out of practice" may have some validity.

Finally, we can speculate on the relationship between psychometric intelligence and expert performance. The survey of these skill domains has one strong implication: If you want to become an expert, it will take many hours to do so. That is, you can become an excellent chess player and remain a musical illiterate. The interaction effects reviewed earlier suggest that people are not generally good at nominally isomorphic tasks, for example, reproducing structured and random chess positions. Chase and Simon's (1973a) novice and master players stood more than five standard deviations apart in chess skill, yet their intelligence test scores are unlikely to be that far apart since both are PhD scientists who are highly renowned in their respective fields. In fact, even spatial ability as measured by the Guilford-Zimmerman Spatial Visualization Subtest is quite insensitive to chess skill. Lane (personal communication, May 26, 1980) and Lane and Robertson, 1979) reported a nonsignificant correlation with both chess rating (− .09) and intentional recall of chess positions (.06) in a small sample ($N = 16$) whose chess-rating range was about four standard deviations.

There are many examples of people who achieved excellent performance in domains like chess and mental calculation but who would have been almost unmeasurably low on intelligence tests (for the latter, see examples in Ericsson & Faivre, Chapter 24, this volume). Tom Fuller, the "Virginia calculator," was an illiterate slave who, at age 70, could, in less than 2 minutes, tell you how many seconds a 70-year-old man had lived, including an adjustment for leap years (Scripture,

1891). Mir Sultan Khan reached the grandmaster level in chess ability yet was uneducated and virtually illiterate (Coles, 1977; Golombek, 1966).[3]

In short, one would expect, on theoretical grounds, little relationship between psychometric intelligence and expert performance in semantically rich domains. At the very top levels of expert performance, it may be necessary to have some innate advantages, of the sort that also permit excellent performance on psychometric tests of intelligence. Speed of thinking may be such a component. Sheer speed in searching the game tree in chess is, of course, what allows current computer programs to beat 90% of human chess players, so "brute force" is sometimes sufficient for masterful performance. Nonetheless, knowledge of chess enables current human grandmasters to defeat the best programs by doing a selective search of the chess game tree, looking at only about 100 positions, compared to the computer's search of a million positions. Acquired knowledge can overcome innate raw processing speed.

Finally, there is impressive neuropsychological data supporting the view that functions such as language and spatial abilities are mediated by localized cerebral regions. The challenge for investigators is to see whether a finer mapping can be made between the current theoretical framework of information-processing psychology, with its emphasis on software explanations, and the rich case studies of individuals with specific hardware deficits.

Acknowledgments

This project was supported by a grant to the author by the Natural Sciences and Engineering Research Council of Canada (NSERC A0790) and was written while the author was supported by a Leave Fellowship from the Social Sciences and Humanities Research Council of Canada (SSHRC 451-84-8284) at the Mental Performance and Aging Lab, VA Outpatient Clinic, Boston. This chapter is based on a paper delivered at the meeting of the Canadian Psychological Association in Calgary, Alberta, June 18, 1980. I am grateful to Fran Allard and Derek Besner for comments on an earlier draft, and to Deborah Fein and Loraine Obler for comments on this draft.

References

Allard, F., & Burnett, N. (1985). Skill in sports. *Canadian Journal of Psychology, 39,* 294–312.

Allen, D. (1967). Octave discriminability of musical and non-musical subjects. *Psychonomic Science, 7,* 421–422.

Anderson, J. R. (1982). Acquisition of cognitive skill. *Psychological Review, 89,* 369–406.

3. He perhaps represents the one exception to the 10-year rule for becoming a grandmaster. He reached this level within 5 years of learning the rules of Western chess, though he had previously attained the highest levels of play for Indian chess, which differed only in the laws of promotion and stalemate and in prohibiting castling and two-square pawn moves. His sponsor also hired the very best players in India to instruct him.

Annett, J. (1979). Memory for skill. In M. M. Gruneberg & P. E. Morris (Eds.), *Applied problems in memory* (pp. 215–247). London. Academic Press.

Bachem, A. (1940). The genesis of absolute pitch. *Journal of the Acoustical Society of America, 11,* 434–439.

Bahrick, H. P. (1979). Maintenance of knowledge: Questions about memory we forgot to ask. *Journal of Experimental Psychology: General, 108,* 296–308.

Baylor, G. W., Jr. (1965). *Report on a mating combinations program. SP-2150.* Santa Monica, CA: System Development Corporation. Cited in Newell & Simon, 1972.

Beal, A. L. (1980). *Musical judgements and musical skill: Overtones in auditory memory.* Unpublished doctoral dissertation, University of Waterloo, Waterloo, Ontario.

Beal, A. L. (1985). The skill of recognizing musical structures. *Memory and Cognition, 5,* 405–412.

Bean, K. L. (1938). An approach to the reading of music. *Psychological Monographs, 226,* 1–80.

Berliner, H. (1979). The B* tree search algorithm: A best-first proof procedure. *Artificial Intelligence, 12,* 23–40.

Binet, A. (1894). *Psychologie des grands calculateurs et joueurs d'echecs.* Paris: Hachette.

Binet, A. (1966). Mnemonic virtuosity: A study of chess players. *Journal of Genetic Psychology, 74,* 127–162. (Translated from *Revue des Deux Mondes,* 1893, *117,* 826–859).

Brady, P. T. (1970). Fixed scale mechanism of absolute pitch. *Journal of the Acoustical Society of America, 4,* 883–887.

Britton, B. K., & Tesser, A. (1982). Effects of prior knowledge on use of cognitive capacity in three complex cognitive tasks. *Journal of Verbal Learning and Verbal Behavior, 21,* 421–436.

Broadbent, D. E., Cooper, P. J., & Broadbent, M. H. P. (1978). A comparison of hierarchical and matrix retrieval schemes in recall. *Journal of Experimental Psychology: Human Perception and Performance, 4,* 486–497.

Charness, N. (1979). Components of skill in bridge. *Canadian Journal of Psychology, 33,* 1–16.

Charness, N. (1981a). Aging and skilled problem solving. *Journal of Experimental Psychology: General, 110,* 21–38.

Charness, N. (1981b). Search in chess: Age and skill differences. *Journal of Experimental Psychology: Human Perception and Performance, 7,* 467–476.

Charness, N. (1981c). Visual short-term memory and aging in chess players. *Journal of Gerontology, 36,* 615–619.

Charness, N. (1983). Age, skill, and bridge bidding: A chronometric analysis. *Journal of Verbal Learning and Verbal Behavior, 22,* 406–416.

Chase, W. G. (1978). Elementary information processes. In W. K. Estes (Ed.), *Handbook of learning and cognitive processes* (Vol. 5, pp. 19–90). Hillsdale, NJ: Erlbaum.

Chase, W. G., & Chi, M. T. H. (1981). Cognitive skill: Implications for spatial skill in large-scale environments. In J. Harvey (Ed.), *Cognition, social behavior and the environment* (pp. 111–136). Potomac, MD: Erlbaum.

Chase, W. G., & Simon, H. A. (1973a) The mind's eye in chess. In W. G. Chase (Ed.), *Visual information processing* (pp. 215–281). New York: Academic Press.

Chase, W. G., & Simon, H. A. (1973b). Perception in chess. *Cognitive Psychology, 4,* 55–81.

Chi, M. T. H. (1978). Knowledge structures and memory development. In R. S. Siegler (Ed.), *Children's thinking: What develops?* (pp. 73–96). Hillsdale, NJ: Erlbaum.

Chi, M. T. H., Feltovich, P. J., & Glaser, R. (1981). Categorization and representation of physics problems by experts and novices. *Cognitive Science, 5,* 121–152.

Chi, M. T. H., Glaser, R., & Rees, E. (1982). Expertise in problem solving. In R. J. Sternberg (Ed.), *Advances in the psychology of human intelligence* (pp. 7–75). Hillsdale, NJ: Erlbaum.

Cleveland, A. A. (1907). The psychology of chess and of learning to play it. *American Journal of Psychology, 18,* 269–308.

Clifton, J. V. (1986). Cognitive components in music reading and sight reading performance. Unpublished doctoral dissertation. University of Waterloo, Psychology Department, Waterloo, Ontario.

Cohen, N. J. (1984). Preserved learning capacity in amnesia; Evidence for multiple memory systems. In L. R. Squire & N. Butters (Ed.), *Neuropsychology of memory* (pp. 83–103). New York: Guilford Press.

Coles, R. N. (1977). *Mir Sultan Khan.* St. Leonard's on Sea, East Sussex, UK: British Chess Magazine Ltd.

Cuddy, L. L. (1970). Training the absolute identification of pitch. *Perception and Psychophysics, 8,* 265–269.

Cuddy, L. L. (1971). Absolute judgment of musically related pure tones. *Canadian Journal of Psychology, 25,* 42–55.

Daneman, M., & Carpenter, P. A. (1980). Individual differences in working memory and reading. *Journal of Verbal Learning and Verbal Behavior, 19,* 450–466.

Davies, J. (1979). Memory for melodies and tonal sequences: A theoretical note. *British Journal of Psychology, 70,* 205–210.

de Groot, A. D. (1966). Perception and memory versus thought: Some old ideas and recent findings. In B. Kleinmuntz (Ed.), *Problem solving: Research, method and theory,* (pp. 19–50). New York: Wiley.

de Groot, A. D. (1978). *Thought and choice in chess.* (2nd ed.) The Hague: Mouton.

Dewar, K. M., Cuddy, L. L., & Mewhort, D. J. K. (1977). Recognition memory for single tones with and without context. *Journal of Experimental Psychology: Human Learning and Memory, 3,* 60–67.

Dowling, W. J. (1982). Melodic information processing and its development. In D. Deutsch (Ed.), *The psychology of music* (pp. 413–429). New York: Academic Press.

Egan, D. E., & Schwartz, B. J. (1979). Chunking in recall of symbolic drawings. *Memory and Cognition, 7,* 149–158.

Ellis, S. H. (1973). Structure and experience in the matching and reproduction of chess patterns. Unpublished doctoral dissertation, Carnegie-Mellon University Pittsburgh.

Elo, A. E. (1966). Age changes in master chess performance. *Journal of Gerontology, 20,* 289–299.

Elo. A. E. (1978). *The rating of chessplayers, past and present.* New York: Arco.

Engle, R. W., & Bukstel, L. (1978). Memory processes among bridge players of differing expertise. *American Journal of Psychology, 91,* 673–689.

Ericsson, K. A. (1985). Memory skill. *Canadian Journal of Psychology, 39,* 188–231.

Ericsson, K. A., Chase, W. G., & Faloon, S. (1980). Acquisition of a memory skill. *Science, 208,* 1181–1182.

Frances, R. (1972). *La perception de la musique.* Paris: Librairie Philosophique J. Vrin.

Geschwind, N., & Galaburda, A. M. (1985a). Cerebral lateralization: Biological mechanisms, associations, and pathology: 2. A hypothesis and a program for research. *Archives of Neurology, 42,* 521–552.

Geschwind, N., & Galaburda, A. M. (1985b). Cerebral lateralization: Biological mechanisms, associations, and pathology: 3. A hypothesis and a program for research. *Archives of Neurology, 42,* 634–654.

Goldin, S. E., & Herstein, J. A. (1979). *Longitudinal development of chess memory: A case study*. Unpublished manuscript, Carnegie-Mellon University, Psychology Department, Pittsburgh.

Golombek, H. (1966). Personalities of modern chess: Mir Sultan Khan. In T. Tiller (Ed.,) *Chess treasury of the air* (pp. 61–65). Baltimore: Penguin Books.

Gordon, K. (1917). Some tests on the memorizing of musical themes. *Journal of Experimental Psychology*, 2, 93–99.

Gross, B., & Seashore, R. H. (1941). Psychological characteristics of student and professional musical composers. *Journal of Applied Psychology*, 25, 159–170.

Gruson, L. (1981). *What distinguishes competence? An investigation of piano practicing*. Unpublished doctoral dissertation, University of Waterloo, Waterloo, Ontario.

Gruson, L. (in press). Rehearsal skill and musical competence: Does practice make perfect? In J. Sloboda (Ed.), *Generative processes in music*: Oxford, Oxford University Press.

Halpern, A. R., & Bower, G. H. (1982). Musical expertise and melodic structure in memory for musical notation. *American Journal of Psychology*, 95, 31–50.

Hatano, G., Miyake, Y., & Binks, M. G. (1977). Performance of expert abacus operators. *Cognition*, 5, 47–55.

Hayes, J. R. (1981). *The complete problem solver*. Philadelphia: Franklin Institute Press.

Holding, D. H. (1979). The evaluation of chess positions. *Simulation and Games*, 10, 207–221.

Holding, D. H. (1985). *The psychology of chess skill*. Hillsdale, NJ: Erlbaum.

Holding, D. H., & Pfau, H. D. (1984). Thinking ahead in chess. *American Journal of Psychology*, 98, 271–282.

Holding, D. H., & Reynolds, R. I. (1982). Recall or evaluation of chess positions as determinants of chess skill. *Memory and Cognition*, 10, 237–242.

Hunt, E. (1978). Mechanics of verbal ability. *Psychological Review*, 85, 109–130.

Jackson, M. D. (1980). Further evidence for a relationship between memory access and reading ability. *Journal of Verbal Learning and Verbal Behavior*, 19, 683–694.

Klein, M., Coles, M. G., & Donchin, E. (1984). People with absolute pitch process tones without producing a P300. *Science*, 223, 1306–1308.

Krogius, N. (1976). *Psychology in chess*. New York: RHM Press.

Krumhansl, C. L., & Shepard, R. N. (1979). Quantification of the hierarchy of tonal functions within a diatonic context. *Journal of Experimental Psychology: Human Perception and Performance*, 5, 579–594.

Lane, D. M., & Robertson, L. (1979). The generality of the levels of processing hypothesis: An applications to memory for chess positions. *Memory and Cognition*, 7, 253–256.

Larkin, J. H. (1981). Enriching formal knowledge: A model for learning to solve textbook physics problems. In J. R. Anderson (Ed.), *Cognitive skills and their acquisition* (pp. 311–334). Hillsdale, NJ: Erlbaum.

Larkin, J. H., McDermott, J., Simon, D. P., & Simon, H. A. (1980). Expert and novice performance in solving physics problems. *Science*, 108, 1335–1342.

Lehman, H. C. (1953). *Age and achievement*. Princeton, NJ: Princeton University Press.

Lewis, C. H. (1981). Skill in algebra. In J. R. Anderson (Ed.), *Cognitive skills and their acquisition* (pp. 85–110). Hillsdale, NJ: Erlbaum.

Lindsay, P. H., & Norman, D. A. (1977). *Human information processing* (2nd ed.). New York: Academic Press.

Lyon, D. R. (1977). Individual differences in immediate serial recall: A matter of mnemonics? *Cognitive Psychology*, 9, 403–411.

MacKenzie, C. L., & Marteniuk, R. G. (1985). Motor skill: Feedback, knowledge and structural issues. *Canadian Journal of Psychology*, 39, 313–337.

Miller, J. R., & Carterette, E. C. (1975). Perceptual space for musical structures. *Journal of the Acoustical Society of America*, *58*, 711–720.

Neves, D. M., & Anderson, J. R. (1981). Knowledge compilation: Mechanisms for the automatization of cognitive skills. In J. R. Anderson (Ed.), *Cognitive skills and their acquisition* (pp. 57–84). Hillsdale, NJ: Erlbaum.

Newell, A., & Simon, H. A. (1972). *Human problem solving*. Englewood Cliffs, NJ: Prentice-Hall.

Norman, D. A. (1980). Twelve issues for cognitive science. *Cognitive Science*, *4*, 1–32.

Oldfield, R. C. (1963). Individual vocabulary and semantic currency: A preliminary study. *British Journal of Social and Clinical Psychology*, *2*, 122–130.

Pirolli, P. L., & Anderson, J. R. (1985). The role of learning from examples in the acquisition of recursive programming skills. *Canadian Journal of Psychology*, *39*, 240–272.

Posner, M. I. (1978). *Chronometric explorations of mind*. Hillsdale, NJ: Erlbaum.

Reitman, W. R. (1965). *Cognition and thought: An information processing approach*. New York: Wiley.

Reitman, J. S. (1976). Skilled perception in GO: Deducing memory structures from inter-response times. *Cognitive Psychology*, *8*, 336–356.

Saariluoma, P. (1984). Coding problem spaces in chess. *Commentationes Scientiarum Socialium*, *23*, 1–121. (Published by the Finnish Society of Sciences and Letters).

Salthouse, T. A. (1984). Effects of age and skill in typing. *Journal of Experimental Psychology: General*, *13*, 345–371.

Scripture, E. W. (1891). Arithmetical prodigies. *American Journal of Psychology*, *4*, 1–59.

Siegel, J. A., & Siegel, W. (1977a). Absolute identification of notes and intervals by musicians. *Perception and Psychophysics*, *21*, 399–407.

Siegel, J. A., & Siegel, W. (1977b). Categorical perception of tonal intervals: Musicians can't tell *sharp* from *flat*. *Perception and Psychophysics*, *21*, 143–152.

Simon, H. A. (1974). How big is a chunk? *Science*, *183*, 482–488.

Simon, H. A. (1979). Information-processing models of cognition. *Annual Review of Psychology*, *30*, 363–396.

Simon, H. A., & Barenfeld, M. (1969). Information-processing analysis of perceptual processes in problem solving. *Psychological Review*, *76*, 473–483.

Simon, H. A., & Chase, W. G. (1973). Skill in chess. *American Scientist*, *61*, 394–403.

Simon, H. A., & Gilmartin, K. (1973). A simulation of memory for chess positions. *Cognitive Psychology*, *5*, 29–46.

Simon, D. P., & Simon, H. A. (1978). Individual differences in solving physics problems. In R. Siegler (Ed.), *Children's thinking: What develops?* (pp. 325–348). Hillsdale, NJ: Erlbaum.

Sloboda, J. A. (1976). Visual perception of musical notation: Registering pitch symbols in memory. *Quarterly Journal of Experimental Psychology*, *28*, 1–16.

Sloboda, J. A. (1978). Perception of contour in music reading. *Perception*, *7*, 323–331.

Spilich, G. J., Vesonder, G. T., Chiesi, H. L., & Voss, J. F. (1979). Text processing of domain related information for individuals with high and low domain knowledge. *Journal of Verbal Learning and Verbal Behavior*, *18*, 275–290.

Sternberg, R. J. (1977). *Intelligence, information processing, and analogical reasoning: The componential analysis of human abilities*. Hillsdale, NJ: Erlbaum.

Tikhomirov, O. K., & Vinogradov, Yu. E. (1970). Emotions in the heuristic function. *Soviet Psychology*, *8*, 198–203.

Waber, D. P. (1979). Cognitive abilities and sex-related variations in the maturation of cerebral cortical functions. In M. A. Wittig & A. C. Peterson (Eds.), *Sex-related differences in cognitive functioning* (pp. 161–186), New York: Academic Press.

Ward, W. D., & Burns, E. M. (1982). Absolute pitch. In D. Deutsch (Ed.), *The psychology of music* (pp. 431–451). New York: Academic Press.

Whitaker, W. G., Hutchinson, W. O., & Pickford, R. W. (1942). Symposium on the psychology of music and painting. *British Journal of Psychology, 33*, 40–57.

Winkelman, J. H. (1975). *Tests of chess skill.* Unpublished manuscript, Psychology Department, University of Oregon.

Winograd, T. (1975). Frame representations and the declarative/procedural controversy. In D. G. Bobrow & A. Collins (Eds.), *Representation and understanding. Studies in cognitive science* (pp. 185–210). New York: Academic Press.

Wolf, T. (1976). A cognitive model of musical sight-reading. *Journal of Psycholinguistic Research, 5*, 143–171.

Wood, F., Ebert, V., & Kinsbourne, M. (1982). The episodic-semantic memory distinction in memory and amnesia: Clinical and experimental observations. In L. Cermak (Ed.), *Human memory and amnesia* (pp. 167–193). Hillsdale, NJ: Erlbaum.

23

Anomalous Calculating Abilities and the Computer Architecture of the Brain

STEVEN MATTHYSSE
STEVEN GREENBERG

Individuals with special abilities far outside the normal range, like lightning calculators, pose tantalizing problems for psychology and neurobiology. In the rare cases in which the special ability appears in the context of general mental retardation, the mystery is profound indeed. A possible explanation of these anomalous abilities is that a substitution has taken place: Cerebral architecture normally used for general intellectual activity has become dedicated to a specialized function. The substitution accounts both for the unusual ability and for the general intellectul deficit. We will show that a more systematic and quantitative analysis leads essentially back to this "naive" interpretation. Substitution in cerebral architecture (either structural or functional) seems to us the most plausible interpretation, at least for the instance that we have studied (see Waterhouse, Chapter 26 this volume).

The case that we discuss in this chapter is that of John and Michael, mentally retarded twins with prodigious calculating abilities, especially with respect to prime numbers. We have not had the opportunity to see the twins in person; all of our information comes from the report by Sacks (1985), to which the reader is referred for more detail. Sacks is both a respected neurologist and a gifted writer; it was his compelling and provocative description of the twins that first attracted our interest.

Sacks (1985) reports that the twins spontaneously exchanged 6-digit prime numbers: "John would say a number—a six-figure number [which turned out to be a prime]. Michael would catch the number, nod, smile, and seem to savor it. Then he, in turn, would say another six-figure number [also a prime], and now it was John who received, and appreciated it richly" (p. 17). Sacks then entered into the dialogue (bringing a table of prime numbers with him), naming an 8-digit prime. "There was a long pause—the longest I have ever known them to make, it must have lasted a half-minute or more—and then suddenly, simultaneously, they both broke into smiles" (p. 18). John proposed a 9-digit number, Sacks, a prime with 10 digits, and after an hour's time, the twins were exchanging numbers with 20 digits, which Sacks assumed to be prime but did not have the means to verify.

Steven Matthysse. Mailman Research Center, McLean Hospital, Belmont, Massachusetts.
Steven Greenberg. Harvard Medical School, Cambridge, Massachusetts.

There are two different abilities described in this account: generating prime numbers and testing for primality numbers that are proposed. In principle, the ability to test implies the ability to generate, since numbers can be tested one by one in ascending sequence until a prime is found. (The procedure will always work eventually, since there is no largest prime.) It does not follow, however, that the twins generate primes by sequentially testing candidate numbers; they may use other strategies. The ability to generate primes does not imply the ability to test any proposed candidate number. For example, the sequence of "Mersenne numbers," $2^n - 1$, is rich in primes (although not every Mersenne number is prime; take $n = 4$) and would be an aid to generating, but it would not be of much use in testing since most primes are not Mersenne numbers. We assume, based on Sack's account, that the twins can correctly test the primality of at least most numbers with up to six digits and that they can carry out the test in half a minute or less with numbers of this size. Judging from the narrative, that would be a very conservative estimate of their abilities.

Methods of Primality Testing

There are many known methods for testing the primality of a number, i.e., deciding whether a given number is prime or composite (composed of factors). A simple and straightforward way might be called the "brute-force" method. In this method one divides n, in sequence, by every number up to the square root of n. If none of them divide into n evenly, then n is a prime; if one of them divides n, then n is composite. This method is guaranteed to work but is quite slow. The time it takes depends sharply on the size of the number being tested. For example, suppose we used a computer that could perform 1 million of the trial divisions at n per second. With such a device, a 20-digit prime number would take about 3 hours to prove prime, while a 40-digit number would take about 1 million years.

Because of the theoretical and practical interest in primality testing (e.g., primes are useful in cryptography), and because of the shortcomings of the brute-force method for large numbers, mathematicians have sought more sophisticated techniques. Most are only partially satisfactory. One of these methods is not hard to understand and is a good example of how higher mathematics can be used to test primality.

The concept involved is that of modular groups and rings; it is sometimes referred to as "modular" or "clock" arithmetic. The idea in a modular system is that ordinary integers take on new meaning and new laws for adding and multiplying and that other operations on these integers are defined.[1] A simple example will demonstrate a modular arithmetic. Suppose we take a system based on the number 7, so that we imagine the seven digits 0, 1, 2, 3, 4, 5, and 6 arranged (clockwise) around the perimeter of a clock. If we start at 0 and go 10 spaces clockwise, we will

1. A note in Sacks's article (p. 18) refers to a suggestion by Israel Rosenfield that the twins might be using modular arithmetic for prime number calculations. Details are not given, but it is true that all sophisticated algorithms for prime number calculation do make use of modular arithmetic in some form (see Sacks, 1985).

end up at 3. Thus, in this system of modulo 7 arithmetic, 10 is equivalent to 3, and we write $10 \equiv 3 \bmod 7$. Similarly, 9 is equivalent to 2 ($9 \equiv 2 \bmod 7$), 7 is equivalent to 0 ($7 \equiv 0 \bmod 7$), and $36 \equiv 1 \bmod 7$. In other words, if we start at 0 and go clockwise around the clock 36 numbers, we will stop at 1. There is a simple way to do the calculations in the preceding examples. To reduce (find a small number equivalent to) a number n in a modulo m system, divide n by m as many times as it will go and take the remainder. The remainder is the answer. Thus we reduce 36 modulo 7 by dividing 7 into 36 as many times as possible (5) and taking the remainder (1), so $36 \equiv 1 \bmod 7$. In a modular system an ordinary integer is classified by its remainder after dividing it within the system. Clocks keep time in the same way, repeating every 12 hours.

In addition to defining a new system of numbers, a modular system has laws for addition, subtraction, multiplication, and (sometimes) division. Operations are carried out on numbers as if they were ordinary integers, and then the result is reduced in the modular system. For example, in modulo 5 arithmetic, we compute 3×4 as follows: As integers, $3 \times 4 = 12$; reducing 12 modulo 5 gives remainder 2. Therefore $3 \times 4 \equiv 2 \bmod 5$. Another example: $2^4 = 16$, and 16 reduced modulo 5 is 1, so $2^4 \equiv 1 \bmod 5$.

Modular arithmetic is useful in primality testing because modular systems based on prime numbers have special properties not possessed by modular systems based on composite numbers. One property that almost provides a successful test is Fermat's Little Theorem, which is stated as follows: Let p be a prime number and construct a modular system based on p (in the preceding examples, the systems were based on 5 and 7, both primes). If a is any number less than p (other than 0), $a^{p-1} \equiv 1 \bmod p$. We have already seen an example of this with $p = 5$ and $a = 2$:

$$a^{p-1} = 2^4 = 16 \equiv 1 \bmod 5$$

Other examples with $p = 5$:

$$3^{5-1} = 3^4 = 81 \equiv 1 \bmod 5$$

$$4^{5-1} = 4^4 = 256 \equiv 1 \bmod 5$$

The primality test suggested by Fermat's theorem is as follows: Suppose n is a number to be tested for primality. Pick a small number a, for example, $a = 2$, and then calculate a^{n-1} and reduce it modulo n. If a^{n-1} does not reduce to 1 modulo n, then n is not prime, since if it were prime, then $a^{n-1} \equiv 1 \bmod n$. If a^{n-1} does reduce to 1, try another a, say $a = 3$, and see what this a^{n-1} reduces to. If we ever find an a such that a^{n-1} does not reduce to 1 modulo n, then we have demonstrated that n is not prime. For example, here is a proof that 6 is not prime based on this idea. Take $n = 6$ and $a = 2$.

$$2^{n-1} = 2^{6-1} = 2^5 = 32 \equiv 2 \bmod 6$$

The number 6 is not prime; otherwise $2^{6-1} \equiv 1 \bmod 6$ would be true.
A proof that 9 is not prime:

$$2^{9-1} = 2^8 = 256 \equiv 4 \bmod 9$$

As a test for primality, the method based on Fermat's theorem has a major drawback. It can never declare for certain that a number *is* prime; it is only good at catching numbers that are not prime. For example, suppose we were given $n = 561$. We might test 561 for primality first by taking $a = 2$ and computing 2^{560}. We would find that $2^{560} \equiv 1 \bmod 561$. Then we might try $a = 3$ and find that $3^{560} \equiv 1 \bmod 561$. We could try $a = 4, 5, 6$, and so forth, and we would always find that $a^{560} \equiv 1 \bmod 561$. Could we conclude that 561 is prime? The answer is no—561 is not prime $(561 = 3 \times 187)$. It is an example of a "Carmichael number", defined as any number that satisfies Fermat's Little Theorem but is not prime. Fermat's method is not satisfactory because it fails to reject some composite numbers. It is not known whether the number of Carmichael numbers is finite or infinite, but they are uncommon (561 is the smallest one). However, as a practical test that demonstrates, for most composite numbers, that they are composite, the Fermat method is excellent.

There are other mathematical techniques based on properties of modular arithmetic that are more complicated but also more successful. One such technique, the strong pseudoprime method[2], has similarities to the method based on Fermat's theorem. Although still not adequate theoretically, as a practical test the strong pseudoprime method has been shown to be effective for determining the primality of numbers up to nine digits in length.

A primality-testing algorithm that has received much attention in the last 5 years is the "APR" algorithm discovered by Adelman, Pomerance, and Rumely and modified by Cohen and Lenstra. It is of interest to mathematicians because it is theoretically more satisfactory than most other primality algorithms; although complicated, it is fast and rigorous. The APR algorithm is not well suited for mental calculation. It would require sophisticated mathematical training in addition to prodigious calculating abilities.

2. The idea of a "strong pseudoprime" is typical of many approaches to primality testing. Let n be an odd composite number and write $n - 1 = 2^s u$ with u odd and $s \geq 1$. Thus we separate $n - 1$ into an odd part (n) and an even part (2^s). Now let a be any number such that a and n have no common factors except the number 1. Consider the following two conditions: (i) $a^u \equiv 1 \bmod n$; (ii) $a^{(2^r)u} \equiv -1 \bmod n$ for some r with $0 \leq r < s$. We say that n is a strong pseudoprime to the base a if n is odd and composite and satisfies either (i) or (ii). If n is a prime number, then it satisfies either (i) or (ii) for every a with $a < n$. It can be proved that if n is composite, then the number of a's for which $a < n$ and n is a strong pseudoprime to the base a is less than $\frac{1}{4}(n - 1)$. Thus the number of numbers for which composite numbers and primes "appear" the same (with respect to the given criteria) is sparse. Given an n, we can pick an a and test conditions (i) and (ii). If we find neither condition satisfied, we conclude that n is composite. Otherwise, we try another a. If n is composite, there is a high probability that we will quickly find an a for which n is not a strong pseudoprime to the base a. However, if n is prime, we would have to try too many a's to give a strict proof. Thus, theoretically, the strong pseudoprime test is not efficient. Practically, though, it has been shown that there are only four numbers n less than 2×10^9 for which n is a strong pseudoprime to bases 2, 3, and 5. Thus we can test any given number $< 2 \times 10^9$ with just these bases; if it passes the test and is not one of four special numbers, we can conclude that n is prime (see Lenstra, 1982).

Serial and Parallel Computation Strategies

The major innovation in computer hardware today is the development of parallel machines and algorithms to replace the serial devices that have dominated the field until the present. Serial machines carry out their computations in sequence; parallel machines do many computations at once. Parallelism is faster but requires more units of computing hardware, since the problem is divided up among them.

Despite the elegance of primality tests based on Fermat's theorem, they require an essentially serial computation strategy. A small number, for example 3, must be raised to a large power, $p - 1$, modulo p:

$$3^{p-1} \bmod p$$

must be computed. For certain special values of p, for example, $p = 129$, the task admits a substantial shortcut

$$3^{p-1} = 3^{128} = 3^{2^7} = (((((((3^2)^2)^2)^2)^2)^2)^2$$

so only seven squarings–modulo-129 are required. These must be carried out in sequence, so parallel hardware is of no help. For other values of p the same kind of shortcut can be used, but it is less timesaving.

Consider, for example, the prime $p_0 = 524,287$. This number is called a "Mersenne prime" because it is one less than a power of two ($2^{19} - 1$). The number p_0 is well within the range of primes that the twins were reported to exchange. Because p_0 is one less than a power of two, the calculation of the Fermat expression

$$a^{p_0-1} \bmod p_0$$

(where a is a small prime) requires more steps than would be needed for numbers just larger than certain powers of two, for example, $2^{16} + 1$. Knuth's (1981) argument shows that 19 serial steps are required for p_0. Twelve of these require squaring a six-digit number, modulo p_0. Each such step certainly requires at least twice as long as two ordinary multiplications, so a time at least equal to 24 six-digit multiplications is needed. To test primality properly, several values of n must be used; but the calculations for each n could be done in parallel, so there would be no further increases in time.

Sacks observed that the twins seemed to recognize an eight-digit prime in about half a minute. We can compare this time with the records of lightning calculators who have been tested (most of whom have had normal or superior IQs). The best, although still fragmentary, compilation of calculation times is Steven Smith's (see Chapter 2, this volume, and references therein). He reports the following times for mental multiplication of numbers in the five- to six-digit range: Jacques Inaudi—32,978 × 62,834 in 40 seconds; 729,856 × 297,143 in 4 minutes; Wim Klein—57,825 × 13,489 in 44 seconds. Twenty-four multiplications could not be carried out, even by these lightning calculators, in the time that Sacks reports for numbers much larger than $p_0{}^3$.

The brute-force primality-testing strategy, although far less sophisticated than the method based on Fermat's theorem, has the advantage of permitting complete parallelism. A proposed number can be simultaneously divided by each of a previously memorized list of primes.[4] If none divides it, the candidate is prime, providing it does not exceed the square of the largest memorized prime. One can imagine the twins continually testing numbers, even unconsciously, and adding each new prime that they discover to the memorized list. Thus larger and larger candidates could be tested, in the course of time. A total of 168 memorized primes would suffice to test all six-digit numbers, 1,229 for all eight-digit numbers, and 9,592 for all ten-digit numbers.

A. C. Aitken, who was an excellent mathematician as well as a lightning calculator, once said that numbers "felt prime" to him (Smith, 1983). If parallel divisions were being carried out as the brute-force theory suggests, the conscious experience would be likely to be an intuition, a global appreciation of primality, rather than awareness of all the separate divisions.

Each of the two theories of primality-testing strategy makes different predictions about performance.[5]

---

3. We are speaking here of the observed limits on speed of performance, not about theoretical limits. Raising a number to a high power (the exponent having N digits), and division of N-digit numbers, can be carried out by suitably designed logic circuits in time proportional to log N, when N is very large (Beame, Cook, & Hoover, in press). In other words, doubling the length of the number to be tested for primality does not double the time required to test it. Estimates of this type are relative (proportional to the processing time of the actual hardware used) and asymptotic (valid for large N), so their relevance for understanding the twins is limited. Moreover, a "suitably designed" logic circuit may be too complex a structure to be a likely product of brain development. Beame et al. (in press) show that the powering circuit is simple to construct in the sense that a Turing machine (the most elementary form of computer) could specify its construction in less than N^k steps, where k is some fixed integer. Since, however, there is no Turing machine in the embryonic brain, which, like a homunculus, can oversee the laying down of connections, a still simpler architecture is necessary, for example, one in which a regular blueprint is stamped out in repeating modules with only near-neighbor connections. Remarkably, Atrubin (1965) has shown that multiplication (he did not study raising to a high power) can be carried out by an array of identical modules, with simple nearest-neighbor connections, in time linearly proportional to the number of digits. Thus the information needed to specify the array does not increase with the number of digits it can handle, although its size does. The fact remains that human calculators, so far as is known, take substantial amounts of time to carry out these operations, far more than contemporary computing machines.

4. The term "brute force," as we have used it, has two different meanings. Numbers can be tested for primality by dividing by every *integer* up to their square root, or by dividing by every *prime* up to the square root. The first method has the advantage of not requiring any memorized list of primes; the second has the advantage of making far fewer divisions. The two strategies might be called "crude brute force" and "refined brute force," respectively. Since it is easy to imagine the twins memorizing small prime numbers and adding each newly discovered prime to the list, we will take "brute force" to mean the "refined" method.

5. The editors called our attention to the possibility that the twins might be using spatial imagery to test numbers for being prime. Smith, in this volume, points out that whenever a number is composite, a collection of objects representing that number can be arranged in a rectangle, whereas if the number of

1. Carmichael numbers (discussed earlier) are numbers that pass Fermat's test for all *a* but that are not actually prime. The example previously discussed is 561 (3 × 187). Anyone testing primality by the Fermat formula alone will get this number, and others like it, wrong. Carmichael numbers would pose no problem for the brute-force strategy.

2. As mentioned before, numbers just under a power of two will take longer to test for primality by the Fermat method than numbers of similar length just over certain powers of two. For example, the numbers 65,537 (a so-called Fermat prime, because it is one more than 2 raised to an exponent, which is itself a power of two, namely, 16) can be tested in 18 steps, whereas 65,521, also a prime, and very similar in size, would require 28 steps. These irregular time requirements would not be characteristic of the brute-force strategy.

3. The brute-force strategy fails as soon as a candidate composite number has no prime factors as small as the largest that has been memorized. For example, suppose the subject has memorized the 550 primes up to 4,000 and can divide in parallel by them. If the eight-digit number 24,681,023 is proposed, he or she will fail, because it is not a prime, but no memorized prime divides it. (Its factors are 4,967 and 4,969, so-called twin primes because they are consecutive odd numbers.) If the number 24,786,259, of very similar size, is proposed, however, the subject will succeed easily, because its factors are 307 and 80,737, and 307 is well within his or her list. This kind of irregular failure would not be characteristic of the Fermat-theorem strategy.

Parallelism and Brain Physiology

The brute-force or parallel-computation theory makes predictions about brain physiology as well as about the types of numbers that the calculator will find easy or difficult to test. The model presupposes that, in the brains of persons with anomalous calculating abilities, large numbers of neuronal assemblies have been entrained to function in parallel to solve problems more quickly than is possible in serial mode. The entrainment may not be voluntary; it may even be determined genetically. If large numbers of neuronal assemblies are recruited to solve a problem, it is likely that the volume of brain tissue activated during the calculation will be larger than in persons who do not use parallel strategies.

The volume of brain tissue activated by a mental task can, in principle, be

---

the objects is prime, they cannot be arranged in a rectangle except as a single row. In order to use the rectangle method with numbers of the order the twins are reported to produce, enormous collections of objects would be required. For example, taking two specific composite numbers that we discuss, in order to spatialize 24,681,023 the twins would have to count up to 4,969 on a side; to handle 24,787,259 they would have to count up to 80,737 on the long side. It is interesting that the predictions of relative task difficulty using the rectangle method are, in this case, just the opposite of the 'brute force' method. The second of these two numbers has a small factor, 307, which would be readily discovered by a parallel division algorithm, but it also has a large factor, which would have to be counted off as one side of the rectangle. The spatial theory, like the others that we have discussed, can be tested because of the unique predictions it makes about speed and accuracy of performance in testing specific numbers.

estimated in two ways: (1) by study of the spatiotemporal pattern of EEG activity associated with the task and (2) by measurement of regional cerebral metabolism by PET scanning.[6]

Topographical mapping techniques have been developed for processing EEG signals recorded from multiple electrodes in order to display the spatiotemporal distribution of waves of electrical activity across the surface of the brain. In dyslexia this technique was able to reveal functional activation of several areas involved in speech and reading, especially under conditions requiring sound–symbol association and phonetic discrimination (Duffy, Denckla, Bartels, & Sandini, 1980).

The volume of cerebral tissue activated by a psychological task can also, under favorable circumstances, be estimated by PET scanning. An elegant example is the work of Mazziotta, Phelps, Carson, and Kuhl (1982) on differences between the responses of the left and right hemispheres in subjects listening to a Sherlock Holmes story. The activated area of the left hemisphere was larger than the right, in accordance with the anatomical asymmetries known to exist in the areas of the temporal lobe concerned with speech.

It is conceivable that cytoarchitectonic study of brain tissue from individuals with anomalous calculating abilities, obtained postmortem, would reveal connectivity differences corresponding to a high degree of functional parallelism. On the other hand, it is important to recognize that a network of logic units can be converted from serial to parallel processing mode by "software" alone, without any change in the observable connections between units. Devices of this type, called "reconfigurable processor arrays," already exist in prototype form (Snyder, 1982). The problem that the reconfigurable array is designed to solve is flexibly adapting the data flow pattern within the array to the needs of the computation. Some tasks are best handled by processing elements arranged as a rectangular mesh, and others, by an arrangement like a binary tree. If these patterns were hard wired, the array might be highly efficient for one phase of a calculation but not for others. By including within the chip a programmable switch lattice, the effective geometry of the array can be changed from the outside. If analogous systems exist in the brain, parallel entrainment might be unobservable anatomically, but it might still be detected physiologically, or inferred from the detailed analysis of calculating performance.

References

Atrubin, A. J. (1965). A one-dimensional real-time iterative multiplier. *Institute of Electrical and Electronic Engineers Transactions–Electronic Computers–14*, 394–399.

Beame, P. W., Cook, S. A., & Hoover, H. J. (1986). Log depth circuits for division and related problems. *Society for Industrial and Applied Mathematics Journal of Computing, 15*, 994–1003.

---

6. When special calculating abilities occur in the context of general mental retardation, the subjects may not be able to give legally and ethically appropriate informed consent, if consent implies judging and accepting invasiveness or risk.

Duffy, F. H., Denckla, M. B., Bartels, P. H., & Sandini, G. (1980). Dyslexia: Regional differences in brain electrical activity by topographic mapping. *Annals of Neurology*, *7*, 412–420.

Knuth, D. E. (1981). Seminumerical algorithms. In *The art of computer programming* (2nd ed., pp. 442–443). Reading, MA: Addison-Wesley.

Lenstra, H. W., Jr. (1982). Primality testing. In H. W. Lenstra, Jr., & R. Tijdeman (Eds.), *Computational methods in number theory* (pp. 55–77). Amsterdam: Mathematics Centrum.

Mazziotta, J. C., Phelps, M. E., Carson, R. E., & Kuhl, D. E. (1982). Tomographic mapping of human cerebral metabolism: Auditory stimulation. *Neurology*, *32*, 921–937.

Sacks, O. (1985). The twins. In *The man who mistook his wife for a hat*. New York: Summit Books.

Smith, S. B. (1983). The great mental calculators: *The psychology, methods, and lives of calculating prodigies, past and present*. New York: Columbia University Press.

Snyder, L. (1982). Introduction of the configurable, highly parallel computer. *Computer*, *15*, 47–56.

24

What's Exceptional About Exceptional Abilities?

K. ANDERS ERICSSON
IRENE A. FAIVRE

Exceptional Ability

The last decade has seen a renewed interest among psychologists in attempting to define the structures and mechanisms underlying skilled performance. One reason for this revival is that recent developments in cognitive psychology have provided models for describing complex cognitive systems and methods for testing the validity of such models. The predominant theoretical framework of cognitive psychology is the information-processing model, in which all cognitive activity is explicated in terms of processes that operate on information stored in different memory systems. This framework has been successfully used in analyzing and describing such skills as reading, mathematics, and physics. Of particular interest are studies of persons with below-average performance or even disability in these areas. The goal of these studies has been to identify the faulty processes or inferior memory systems that could be responsible for the observed disabilities.

Other studies have taken the opposite tack, analyzing superior performance and seeking to discover the source of differences between novices and experts in chess (Chase & Simon, 1973a, 1973b; de Groot, 1965, 1966) and in physics (Chi, Feltovich, & Glaser, 1981; Larkin, McDermott, Simon, & Simon, 1980). These studies have shown that the superior performance can be attributed to the experts' vast knowledge about the task domain. For example, the knowledge of chess masters consists of a very large number of similar chess games from their own experience and from the chess literature as well as aquired higher level concepts relating to the interaction of groups of chess pieces, which are automatically accessed in the analysis of unfamiliar chess-board configurations. No available evidence indicates that their memory systems *per se* are better. Neither do experts in one domain consistently show superior performance on tasks outside their fields of expertise. Whether extensive periods of practice are sufficient to attain expert-level

K. Anders Ericsson and Irene A. Faivre. Department of Psychology, University of Colorado, Boulder, Colorado.

performance in a task is currently unknown, but the necessity of such practice is uncontroversial. In chess, for example, it appears that around 10 years of dedicated study are required to attain the level of a chess master (Chase & Simon, 1973a, 1973b). For many skills there is strong evidence that extensive practice can result in performance which is so far above average that we are forced to call the final performance exceptional.

The controversy over the relative importance of environmental and genetic influences on skills and performance is older than psychology itself. Studies of heritability of mental and personality traits have demonstrated clearly the significance of genetic factors (Plomin & DeFries, 1980; Plomin & Rowe, 1978). Similarly, studies of skill acquisition have shown the remarkable improvements possible through extensive practice (Newell & Rosenbloom, 1981). The current issue is how genetic and practice effects interact to determine individual performance, particularly when that performance is exceptional. In this chapter we explore the nature and locus of both genetic and environmental factors.

We have been able to identify two rather different loci for genetic effects on performance. The most commonly held view is that genetic factors determine the degree and extent of basic abilities. This means that persons endowed with greater capacity or specialized capability are able to achieve a specified level of performance more easily than normal persons. In some cases these gifted individuals appear to be able to display levels of mastery that normal persons would never be able to attain, regardless of amount of practice invested. A different, but not incompatible view, is that genetic factors influence subjects' motivation and drive for acquiring skills. This approach implies that some persons possess the ability to maintain intense, focused attention on some task for weeks, months, and even years. It is important to distinguish this long-term motivation or drive from the short-term motivation that allows persons to do well during hour-long tests of different types. Later in this chapter we will try to develop this account of individual differences in terms of drive, but let us first turn to the more common view of genetic mediation through inherited basic aptitudes.

Given that any cognitive process mediating the expression of an ability must be embodied in the neurophysiology of the brain, it is very plausible that the proficiency of that ability is determined to a large extent by the corresponding neurophysiological structure. The recent indications that many abilities (or skills) are localized in certain areas of the brain make such an account even more convincing (cf. Kolb & Whishaw, 1980). However, there is little understanding of the relationship between cognitive processes described by psychological studies and underlying neurophysiology beyond the sensory analysis in the cortex. Several investigators have proposed that the difference between psychological and neurophysiological analysis can be understood in terms of an analogy with computers. The neurophysiological aspects, such as size of short-term memory and speed of thinking, correspond to the computer's hardware (i.e., storage capacity and efficiency of operation); the psychological aspects, such as strategies and knowledge, are analogous to the computer's software (i.e., programs and data stored in the memories). Within such a framework one would expect that ability differences between individuals would correspond to the combined differences in their "hardware" and "software." Somewhat facetiously, a genetically well endowed person could be compared to a high-performance mainframe computer, whereas a genetically less well endowed individual would be analogous to a stripped-down personal computer. To make the analogy reasonably complete, we can add the possibility of hard-wired programs, which would correspond to the inherited predispositions to perform well on certain tasks involving particular sensory domains, such as vision and audition.

When we talk about *exceptional aptitude*, we will assume that some hardware or wired-in program is necessary for that aptitude and that subjects born without this basic capacity cannot acquire it, regardless of the amount of practice invested. It is important to distinguish between this assumed underlying aptitude, which we cannot actually "see," and the performance itself. Therefore we will refer to the observable behavior as "extraordinary performance." The latter term we wish to keep free of implications about its underlying cause.

Extraordinary performance has been observed in various domains, such as music, chess, and mathematics. Identifying the locus of extraordinary performance in such complex skills is, at least, very difficult. Many have assumed a genetic predisposition. In musical performance, for example, absolute-pitch ability has been cited as a talent that is not trainable and hence indicative of an inherited basic aptitude or capacity. However, since mastery in each of these areas requires a vast amount of experience, an alternative explanation would look to the parameters that relate to practice. It is possible that a general mechanism regulating sustained interest in and concentration on a topic for a period of several years may provide a better account of extraordinary performance than any structural predisposition for a particular ability. At a first step in determining the relative contribution of aptitude and practice, we will critically examine the empirical evidence for the basic aptitude view.

To avoid the problems associated with the necessity of extensive practice in complex skills, some have sought evidence for exceptional aptitude in areas where practice would seem to contribute relatively little. This is most evident in the area of very basic human functions, such as memory or perception. Often, the performance of some subjects on tests of these basic functions is so *vastly superior* that it seems that no amount of learning or practice could yield such differences (cf. Kolb & Wishaw, 1980, Luria, 1968). In some cases the extraordinary performance is not just more accurate than that of normal subjects but has *different characteristics* (types of errors, speed, etc.). Accepted learning mechanisms seem unable to account for such differences, so it has been assumed that special capabilities, rather than learning, must be involved. Thus the first type of evidence favoring the aptitude view is not empirical but intuitive and is based on the default acceptance of an alternative to an explanation in terms of learning.

A second kind of support comes from reports provided by the extraordinary performers themselves. Often, these individuals are unable to describe the cognitive processes used in the skill. They sometimes claim that the ability has always been with them, from their earliest memories. In addition, the parents or other people who knew the exceptional person as a child can attest to the sudden emergence of the extraordinary performance.

The third type of converging evidence for exceptional aptitude comes from observations that children and mentally retarded persons demonstrate instances of extraordinary performance in the same or similar tasks. At face value the evidence for exceptional aptitudes in these cases may appear very strong, but the poor scientific quality of this evidence makes any reliable conclusions questionable.

Framework for Our Discussion

The remainder of our chapter is organized in three major parts; each part addresses some evidence that has been offered as clear support for the involvement of basic aptitudes in extraordinary performance. The first part investigates the allegation that the performance of exceptional persons is outside the range of performance for normal persons, even when such persons are given extensive practice. A critical study of the evidence for such a claim shows that it is primarily inferential and indirect rather than strictly empirically based. The *observed* fact is simply that a given performance is outside the range of normal persons. It is then *inferred* that normal persons could not improve their performance to the same level. The argument against improvement appears to be based largely on the belief that very basic cognitive and perceptual processes cannot be influenced by learning. This conclusion derives from the linear extrapolation of disappointingly small (or nonexistent) improvements in these functions after short periods of practice. We will argue that these theoretical assumptions are incorrect. Our own research as well as that of others shows that with extensive practice cognitive processes emerge that result in performance that is structurally different from performance with little or no practice.

The second part of the chapter contains a critical review of the evidence on the sudden emergence of extraordinary performance. We will try to show that the available evidence is much less conclusive than it is often thought to be. We will also discuss the feasibility of attaining extraordinary performance with minimum instruction and address the issue of how or why these persons could maintain motivation to persist in long-term practice. The third part extends our analyses to extraordinary performance displayed by mentally retarded persons.

In concluding the chapter we summarize the weak, or totally lacking, evidence that individual differences in performance are due to inherited basic aptitudes. Then we expand on an alternative possibility—the effects of genetic factors as contributors to drive and sustained concentration during extensive practice.

The Improvability of Basic Perception and Memory Processes

Perception

PERCEPTUAL JUDGMENTS OF SENSATIONS

One area in which it may seem surprising to find improvement with practice is in basic perceptual skills. One might think that by adulthood we would have learned all that is possible about how to gather information from our various sensory receptors. Of course, we would expect to learn new associations for certain perceptual stimuli, such as learning the names of musical notes. But actually learning to *perceive* differences between two stimuli that previously were indistinguishable from one another may appear to be far less likely. Even a brief introspective look at our own experiences demonstrates that such perceptual learning does seem to occur. Wine-tasting classes, for example, are designed to improve olfactory and taste discrimination for a particular type of stimuli. The empirical evidence clearly supports improvement in perception with practice. Gibson (1969) reviewed the literature and listed an impressive array of documented evidence. The effects of practice are found for all the major types of preceptual judgment paradigms and for several different modalities. Absolute threshold (the ability to detect very faint stimuli) was clearly improved by practice, whether the modality was auditory (Zwislocki, Maire, Feldman, & Rubin, 1958) or olfactory (Engen, 1960). Discrimination (the ability to detect differences between similar stimuli) was likewise improved with practice (Baker & Osgood, 1954).

One type of perceptual task that has proved very difficult, though not impossible, to improve is that known as absolute judgment (Engen, 1961; Hanes & Rhoades, 1959; Hartman, 1954). In making an absolute judgment one is required to assign labels to stimuli as they are presented one by one, in isolation from one another. Subjects normally find this task extremely difficult, particularly when stimuli are very simple, varying along, perhaps, a single dimension. In fact, George Miller (1956) reported that five to nine unidimensional stimuli were about all that could be kept straight when absolute judgments were required. There is a well-known exception to this rule, however, in the case of musicians possessing absolute pitch. These persons can easily identify as many as ten times the number of notes identified by the average subject in an absolute-judgment task.

Does such phenomenal performance require an inherited basic aptitude, or is it a learned skill? One argument in favor of the skill position would be a demonstration that equivalent performance can be achieved through practice. It would also be interesting to show that highly accurate absolute judgment is not limited to the auditory domain. If such improvement is possible, we should like to know what mechanisms underlie the learning. In the following section we describe an attempt to trace the course of perceptual learning for one subject, A. F., as she achieved a fourfold increase in her ability to identify simple color stimuli.

A CASE STUDY OF EXTENSIVE PRACTICE ON IDENTIFICATION OF HUES

The ability of humans to identify and name colors is often assumed to be far superior to other perceptual identification skills (e.g., Costall, Platt, & Macrae, 1981, Ward, 1963). This belief probably arises from our subjective experience with color naming. But such experience is deceiving. In fact, the number of hues that can be identified in an absolute-judgment task has been calculated to be as low as three or as high as ten (Halsey & Chapanis, 1951). Even the higher estimate is surprisingly low compared to our estimated ability to differentiate thousands of colors in comparative judgments (Halsey & Chapanis, 1951). The study of hue is further complicated by the fact that colors can vary in saturation and brightness as well as in hue. Halsey & Chapanis (1951) attempted to improve a subject's absolute judgment of color using stimuli that varied on all three dimensions and spacing the stimuli for maximum discriminability. Their subject succeeded in identifying 50 colors after several months of daily practice. However, the spacing and the complexity of their stimuli makes it difficult to compare their result to the item limit of five to nine reported for undimensional stimuli.

We have reported on a training study of absolute identification using very simple color stimuli (Ericsson & Faivre, 1982). We chose a subset of colors from a test of color vision known as the Munsell Hundred Hue Test. The color samples used in the test are equated for saturation and brightness but vary in hue by a few just noticeable differences. The color chips forming the Munsell test change very gradually in hue from one chip to the next, so that the entire set of 85 chips forms a complete color circle in which each color gradually grades into the next, with no apparent boundaries. From this set we chose a subset of 21 consecutive chips, ranging in color from pink to yellowish green. The difficulty of this absolute-judgment task was substantial, both because of the number of chips involved and because of their similarity. In fact, subjects with normal color vision often misorder about three chips when their task is simply to rank order them from the pinkest to the greenest chip, with all chips simultaneously available. Our goal was for the subject, A. F., to learn to identify quickly and reliably by number all 21 chips when presented individually. More important, we wanted to observe and record the course of improvement, to understand how perceptual learning occurs.

Our subject engaged in the hue-identification task for about 2 hours per day, 2 to 5 days per week, for more than a year. Feedback was given only after all 21 chips had been judged, which took 30–40 minutes. In her first session A. F. judged only 5 of the 21 stimuli correctly (an average performance). After 80 sessions subject A. F. was able to identify an average of 18 colors correctly, a remarkable increase. It is not surprising that improvement beyond that level was small or nonexistent, since she had reached the limit of discrimination for subjects with normal color vision.

Two interesting findings emerged from our data. First, we could show that practice did not simply reduce the general "noise level" associated with the perception of the stimuli, but that it also made it possible to judge certain stimuli (later classified as "anchors") more accurately than others. Second, the mechanism of learning was not one of gradual improvement, with performance on some chips increasing somewhat faster than on others. Instead, identification improved suddenly to virtually perfect recognition of particular stimuli (anchors) at different stages of training.

It appeared that A. F. was comparing nearby chips to the anchors. But we wanted to know what made such a comparison possible. Retrospective verbal reports by the subject after each judgment provided evidence for a possible mechanism. The improvement in performance on a chip tended to correspond with verbalized changes in features observed in the chip. One dramatic example was the sudden recognition and verbalization in Session 9 that Chip 16 appeared bright. After this recognition, Chip 16 was correctly identified in 33 of the next 35 sessions, as compared to only once in the preceding 8 sessions. Similarly, A. F. noticed "orange" in Chip 8 and "gold" in Chip 12, with corresponding improvement in identification as a result. Although these new additional features almost invariably emerged with respect to a single color chip, they gradually came to be elicited by adjacent chips as well. At the same time, accuracy for these related chips tended to improve.

A. F.'s verbal protocols revealed a noticeable change in verbal description with practice. For example, three chips (19, 20, and 21) were all described simply as "green" in Session 3. By the end of training, Chip 19 was described as "green with a lot of gold, brighter than 18." Chip 20 was "green and a little blue, doesn't glow as 21, greener than 19," and Chip 21 was "green and blue, bright, frosty, glowing." Initially, most verbalizations were single-word color descriptions (13 color chips were described by a single color name). But by the end of training, all but 1 chip were described by up to three or four features that were often related to each other in terms of magnitude. A total of 6 different descriptors were used in the first session, whereas 15 different terms were used to describe the set of 21 colors at the end of the training.

A learning mechanism that consists of the recognition of new features would predict that the improvement is restricted to the stimuli in the training set and hence would not transfer to stimuli from a different part of the stimulus continuum. To test the generalizability of A. F.'s developing skill, we chose another subset of 21 colors, ranging from bluish green to violet. On three different occasions—at the beginning, at the middle, and at the end of the training period—A. F. followed the same familiarization procedure as our control subjects and then attempted to iden- tify the color chips. Her performance on this subtest was no different from control subjects' performance on the training chips. So it appears that the skill is not a generalized "learning-to-attend" phenomenon but is limited to performance on the training materials. This is in agreement with other researchers' findings of no transfer to different stimuli in absolute judgments of pitch (Wyatt, 1945) and for absolute detection threshold of auditory frequencies (Zwislocki et al., 1958).

It may seem surprising that A. F. was able to improve her performance, given that nearly all her practice time was spent looking at the color chips for which she didn't know the correct labels. Other investigators have found the same phe- nomenon (Campbell & Small, 1963). Improvements of perceptual judgment can occur without feedback on the correctness of judgments. This is reasonable if we distinguish between the process of learning to recognize features and that of attach- ing labels. The process leading to the emergence of the distinguishing aspects is the time-consuming one. Linking the stimulus to the identifying label can be achieved in a comparatively short time.

A RECONSIDERATION OF ABSOLUTE PITCH

The skill view would suggest that absolute pitch is *not* an all-or-none phenomenon. In fact, studies of large groups of subjects, particularly musically trained subjects, show that pitch-identification performance varies essentially continuously from poor identification to perfect. Even among subjects alleging to have absolute pitch, there are great performance differences when they are tested (Bachem, 1937; Ward & Burns, 1982), and performance often depends on the instrument used (Baird,

1919). Only a very small number can identify perfectly all notes from the musical scale, and an even smaller number of subjects are able to identify the full range of pure tones produced by a tone generator. These facts are consistent with our findings just discussed.

At least three findings about absolute-pitch performance appear to be inconsistent with a skill view. First, it is unclear why most musicians seem unable to attain absolute pitch, even though they may exhibit very good relative pitch (identifying a tone when given a reference tone). It has been suggested that relative pitch involves completely different aspects of tones and that attending to these aspects may actually counteract perception of those relevant to absolute pitch (Abraham, 1901; Brady, 1970). In the only documented case of a subject achieving a level of pitch performance equivalent to that of absolute pitch, the training emphasized learning to identify a single tone (Brady, 1970). Once that tone was established as an internal referent, the subject was able to identify other tones quickly and easily, drawing on his previously developed relative pitch. Brady reported that once developed, the identification task required little effort and that no conscious practice was necessary in order to maintain the skill. (As a musician, he was, of course, exposed to the stimuli.) He reported no decrement in his ability after 6 months without practice, and even after 13 years, he found only a small decrease (Costall, 1985).

The second finding about absolute pitch that seems inconsistent with a skill view is the early emergence of absolute pitch in children, but that finding is confounded by the fact that early training in music is also highly correlated with absolute-pitch ability (Sergeant, 1969). Further, Sergeant & Roche (1973) found that absolute-pitch ability judgments are, in general, made for notes produced on the first instrument on which the child received training. They suggested that absolute pitch involves attending to musical notes as individual entities and that such piecemeal perception is typical of very young children. In their study young children (aged 3–4) were more likely than older children (aged 6–7) to sing songs in the pitch originally used to teach the song. From these and other data, they concluded that absolute pitch usually disappears as the child develops the ability to perceive the notes as parts of a coherent whole that has a character of its own.

Finally, the pattern of errors of pitch identification given by subjects with absolute pitch is quite different from that of untrained subjects. Those with absolute pitch tend to confuse tones with the same location in different subscales rather than tones having the smallest difference in fundamental frequencies. Thus an average subject might confuse C with B, whereas a subject with absolute pitch would confuse C in one octave with C in a different octave (Ward & Burns, 1982). These differences in errors are consistent with our argument that with increased performance, different perceptual aspects of the stimulus are used, as was clearly evidenced in our training study with colors.

A particularly interesting study that relates to differences in patterns of errors as a result of training was conducted by Shepard (1963). He analyzed the perceptual similarity of Morse code signals as a function of level of practice with naive, trained, and advanced subjects. Naive subjects discriminated different Morse code signals on the basis of the number of elements (dots and dashes) and the relative preponderance of dots versus dashes in each signal. Subjects who had memorized each of the different 36 signals also used a number of elements for discrimination. However, these trained subjects also distinguished between homogeneous signals (composed of all dots or all dashes) and signals composed of a mixture of the dots and dashes. Hence these subjects were likely to confuse signals composed of all dots with those composed of all dashes, whereas naive subjects did not make this error. Finally, the advanced subjects appeared to have the most difficulty in distinguishing the number of elements in homogeneous signals, in direct contrast to the naive subjects. We can conclude from this that with practice the structure of the perceptual identification of signal changes.

Exceptional Memory

Basic memorial processes have been the focus of psychological reasearch in memory since Ebbinghaus (1964/1885) introduced the nonsense syllable in 1885. His goal was to discover and measure those processes involved in forming new memory traces. To do so he created a pool of items that would be uncontaminated by past experiences and memories. Since that time, studies using nonsense syllables and other essentially meaningless materials have provided a vast body of experimental evidence that reveals many generalizable aspects of basic memory processes. These studies have also uniformly shown that memorization of such materials is remarkably difficult. With fast presentation rates of around one item per second, it appears impossible to retain more than a very few such items for any length of time. In current terminology we say the subjects fail to transfer information about the material to long-term memory (LTM). It is possible, however, to keep some of the information in short-term memory (STM). In fact, a basic test of STM capacity consists of having subjects recall a list of items that have been presented one at a time. Miller (1956) showed that people are quite similar in their performance of this task and can correctly recall around seven to ten pieces of information. Further, the type of items presented did not appear to change that estimate much. Memory performance was approximately the same for digits, consonants, geometric shapes, and unrelated words. Miller summarized this research by saying that STM has the capacity to retain seven plus or minus two symbols, or familiar units, which he called "chunks." The distinction we have made here between STM and LTM is one that psychologists have found very useful. Short-term memory is seen as a temporary store with very limited capacity but very fast access. In contrast, LTM has virtually unlimited capacity, but storage of unrelated bits of information and access to it, is very slow.

These characteristics are assumed to be basic parameters of the human information-processing system. Thus they are limits shared by all normal humans and are not easily changed, if they can be changed at all. Given this presumed immutability, it is surprising to find well-documented reports of individuals who have dramatically exceeded these limits by memorizing long lists of digits and other essentially meaningless materials in a single, fast-paced presentation. Around the turn of the century, Binet (1894) published a study of the exceptional memory of mental calculators and chess masters. More recently, Luria (1968) examined the memory of a newspaper reporter (S.), who showed an exceptional ability to memorize information such as digits, nonsense syllables, and poems in unfamiliar languages. Luria suggested that S.'s memory was based on storing visual images, which were retained in memory after careful visual inspection of the material. He believed that S.'s exceptional memory was different from that of normal people and was based on noncognitive, sensory processes (for a more complete review of exceptional memory feats, see Ericsson, 1985, and Brown & Deffenbacher, Chapter 8, this volume).

We would like to argue that exceptional memory feats can be achieved without postulating exceptional physiological structure. But if we restrict ourselves to improvements of existing memory systems, we must assume either that the capacity of STM is increased or that techniques for rapid storage of information in LTM are developed. We will start with a discussion of how the amount of information held in STM could be extended through practice.

The primary learning mechanism allowing for improvements in the amount of information stored in STM involves forming chunks, or higher level groups of items, from previously unrelated items. Miller (1956) used the concept of chunks to reconcile the fact that subjects remember about the same number of words and consonants. By expressing the memory limit in terms of chunks, four six-letter words would take the same storage capacity as four unrelated letters. Thus the limit was measured in terms of chunks of information, not individual bits of data. Defining a chunk is somewhat intuitive. In sequences of unrelated words the largest familiar unit is a word. If scrambled consonants are presented, the unit size is a single consonant. Chunking strategies can be learned that transform unrelated symbols into familiar units. For example, through extensive practice immediate memory for sequences of binary numbers can be improved by learning to recode inputs of binary digits into octal numbers (e.g., $010 = 2$), as shown by a study by Sidney Smith described in Miller (1956). In sum, vast differences in immediate memory for presented elements can be obtained without violating the number of chunks or familiar units stored in memory.

The real constraint on improvement in memory span comes from the time required to memorize the large number of chunks necessary to acquire really superior memory performance. If one remembered binary-digit sequences as seven 2-digit numbers, it would be necessary to have 100 different chunks corresponding to each possible number between 00 and 99. Remembering the digit sequence as 3-digit numbers would require 1,000 different chunks, and remembering in terms of 4-digit numbers, 10,000 different chunks. How likely is it that such a feat could be achieved?

The evidence from group studies is not very promising. Given the extensive exposure to different numbers during their lives, it seems likely that normal adults would acquire a large number of meaningful associations that could be used in chunking. Laboratory studies have shown statistically reliable effects of recall from STM for repeated presentation of the same digit string. However, the effects found are remarkably small and consistent with only very limited learning of unique digit combinations (Bower & Winzenz, 1969; Hebb, 1961). Mere opportunity to practice on digit span has been repeatedly found to improve performance, but the size of the increase varies dramatically from study to study. Gates and Taylor (1925) showed that after 78 days of practice, kindergarten children had improved their digit spans by about 50% (from 4.3 to 6.4 digits). Martin and Fernberger (1929) found an improvement of digit span from 8–11 digits to 15–16 digits with 50 sessions of practice. Finally, Pollack, Johnson, and Knaff (1959) found an improvement from 7 digits to 11.6 digits with over a hundred hours of practice on a memory task similar to regular digit span. These improvements are sizable, but they don't result in performance that could be termed exceptional.

A CASE STUDY OF THE ACQUISITION OF EXCEPTIONAL MEMORY

The preceding studies, though interesting, provide very limited insight into the mechanisms that underlie the observed improvement (Ericsson, 1985). Further, none of the studies provided really extensive practice for their subjects. To explore these questions, Chase and Ericsson initiated a study of long-term practice on digit span with a single subject. An undergraduate (S. F.) with average memory abilities, and average intelligence for a college student, engaged in the memory-span task for about an hour a day, several days a week, for more than 2 years. S. F. read random digits at the rate of 1 digit per second; he then recalled the sequence. If the sequence was reported correctly, the next sequence was increased by one digit; otherwise, it was decreased by one digit. During the course of 30 months of practice (more than 250 hours of laboratory testing), S. F.'s digit span steadily improved, from 7 to over 80 digits (Figure 24-1). This more than tenfold increase of digit span was not due to an expansion of STM. During a postsession recall period at the end of each session, we tested S. F.'s LTM storage of digits by asking him to recall as much as he could about any of the large number of digits sequences that had been presented to him. Usually, subjects can remember almost nothing from the presented sequences during postsession recall (Ericsson & Karat, 1981). This indicates that they used only STM during the session. For S. F., the amount of postsession recall increased along with improvement of his digit span. Iin the beginning he could recall virtually nothing at the end of an hour-long session; after 20 months of practice he could recall more than 80% of the digits presented to him.

What were the mechanisms that enabled S. F. to use LTM despite the rapid presentation rates used in memory-span testing? Our primary understanding of the strategy he used was obtained from retrospective verbal reports, which he gave after his recall of the presented digits. In these reports he described his thoughts as they occurred during the presentation and recall of the digits. Two general techniques described in the verbal reports were also supported by specially designed experiments, which are reported in detail elsewhere (Chase & Ericsson, 1981, 1982; Ericsson, Chase & Faloon, 1980).

The first mechanism we uncovered was a process used by S. F. to encode, or store, the presented digits in LTM. The key principle for storing information in LTM is to make associations to familiar elements already there. By definition, material like random digits is not meaningful specifically because it lacks these associations. The improvement of S. F.'s digit span did not start until he realized that he could generate meaningful associations to groups of 3 and 4 digits each. This was possible because he had been an excellent long-distance runner for several years and had acquired an extensive knowledge of running times for a wide range

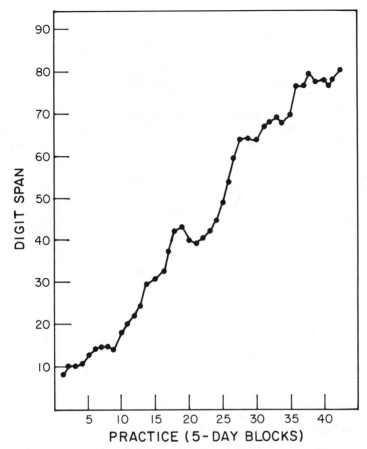

FIGURE 24-1. Average digit span as a function of practice for subject S. F. Each data point corresponds to the mean digit span based on five training sessions of around 1 hour each.

of races (half mile to marathon). This knowledge base was used to form meaningful associations to the presented digits. For example, 3,492 was recoded as "3 minutes and 49 point 2 seconds, near world-record mile time." During the first 4 months, S. F. gradually constructed an elaborate set of associations based initially on running times and later supplemented with ages (893 was "89 point 3 years old, very old man") and dates (1,944 was "near the end of World War II") for those sequences that could not be categorized as times. In Chase and Ericsson (1982) we have explicated the complete series of encoding processes necessary for storing all the information contained in 4-digit groups.

The second mechanism we found enabled S. F. to recall and report all these 3- and 4-digit groups in the correct order. To locate some specific information among the immense amount already stored in LTM, it is necessary to attend to retrieval cues, which were associated with the stored digit groups. When S. F. started to store digits in the LTM, he would recode the first 3 digits as a running time and keep the remaining 4 to 6 digits in an STM rehearsal buffer. Once he had memorized the digits in the rehearsal buffer, he would recall the digit group in LTM and report the digit sequence. When S. F. started to store two and more digit groups in LTM, he had to associate each digit group with information about its location in the series (first, middle, last).

S. F. began to experience real difficulty in keeping the order straight for more than three or four groups of digits in LTM. Eventually he was able to keep the order of more digit groups straight by segmenting the digit groups into super-groups, with no more than four digit groups ever included in a single supergroup. A series of 80 digits was stored as 22 digit groups organized in a hierarchical fashion. The systematic association of certain retrieval cues (retrieval structures) to information stored in LTM allowed him to rapidly retrieve this information on demand—at rates approaching retrieval times for information in STM. Informa-tion stored with the appropriate retrieval structure in LTM can be viewed as being functionally equivalent to storage in STM.

Not only was S. F. able to remember more digits when they were presented at a constant rate, but his speed of storing a fixed number of digits increased as well. When S. F. could determine the speed of presentation himself, we found that he could memorize 15–50 digits at less than half of the original presentation rate of 1 digit per second. We called this continuous reduction of the time required to store a fixed amount of information the "speed-up principle." It is important because it shows that with sufficient practice, storage of information in LTM can be as rapid as that normally assumed possible only in STM.

After all this practice, can we conclude that S. F. increased his STM capacity? There are several reasons to think not. (1) The sizes of S. F.'s groups were almost always 3 and 4 digits, and he never generated a mnemonic association for more than 5 digits. (2) He almost never allowed his rehearsal group to exceed 6 digits. (3) He generally used three groups supergroups and, after some initial difficulty with five groups, never allowed more than four groups in a supergroup. (4) In one experi-mental session after 3 months of practice, S. F. was switched from digits to letters of the alphabet and exhibited no transfer: His memory span dropped back to about 6 consonants.

These effects of practice on digit-span performance have been replicated several times by Chase & Ericsson (1981, 1982). Three additional subjects have acquired digit spans of over 20 digits after more than 100 hours of practice. One of these subjects (D. D.) was also a long-distance runner and was given training in the use of S. F.'s system. Currently, his digit span is well over 100 digits and is still improving. Although the subjects show individual differences in the kind of mnemonic associations used and in the grouping pattern used for the retrieval structure, an analysis of their performance gave support for the principles we have described.

A RECONSIDERATION OF EXCEPTIONAL MEMORY

The research on our trained subjects shows that normal adults can, with practice, dramatically improve their memory for briefly presented information. We argue that the memory feats of exceptional persons reported in the literature could be accounted for in the same way. Apparently, "exceptional" memory may be acquired through extensive practice by persons with normal memory. Of course, from equality of memory performance we cannot directly infer equivalence of the structure of memory. Neither is it sound practice simply to trust the reports of the mnemonists themselves. The mnemonist S. claimed that he did not use LTM associations to encode digits into memory. Instead, he said he was able to store them directly as visual images, an unusual ability that he had always possessed (Luria, 1968). It is, of course, difficult to determine empirically the truth or falsity or his claim.

As Brown and Deffenbacher (Chapter 8, this volume) report, Binet (1894) analyzed the digit memory of two mental calculators and a mnemonist. The emphasis on memory for digits was fortunate for us because it provided an interesting test for our trained subjects (S. F. and D. D.). One of the tasks Binet used was memorization of a 25-digit matrix. Luria (1968) reported on memorization of a 50-digit matrix by his subject; S. Ericsson and Chase (1982) had their trained subjects memorize each of the two matrices and compared the time they required to that reported for the exceptional performers of Luria and Binet. They found that their trained subjects could memorize the matrices as fast as, or faster than, the exceptional subjects. They then had their trained subjects recall the digits from the matrix in a wide range of different orders (backward and forward recall of rows, recalling columns of digits starting at the bottom, etc.). It had been argued by Binet (1894) that the observed recall times could differentiate between auditory and visual memory representations. A reanalysis of these recall times showed a remarkable similarity between all exceptional subjects and our trained subjects. In fact, the only difference between normal *untrained* subjects and memory experts appears to be the length of time required to memorize the matrix. Once stored in LTM, the pattern of recall times was not reliably different (Ericsson & Chase, 1982).

When Luria (1968) argued that his subject, S., had an exceptional memory, his belief was based on a combination of performance data and S.'s verbal descriptions of how he memorized information. A review of a surprisingly large number of case studies of memory experts shows that the subjects showing the most exceptional memory performance do *not* claim to have structurally different memories (Ericsson, 1985). Professor Rückle (Müller, 1911, 1913, 1917) and a professional mnemonist, Isihara (Susukita, 1933, 1934), provide detailed accounts of their methods for memorization, which are directly consistent with the attributes of acquired memory skill discussed above (Chase & Ericsson, 1982). The empirical evidence indicates that the extraordinary memory performance is due to acquired memory skill, regardless of claims for exceptional ability (Ericsson, 1985). Their superior memory is primarily limited to a single type of material, such as digits. The digit spans of several memory experts drop back to normal if the rate of presentation is increased and hence is insufficient for making associations to knowledge in LTM. A few memory experts have had their memory tested after several years of practice. In spite of the extraordinary memory performance displayed at the initial testing, further significant improvement is shown at the subsequent tests. The pattern of memory performance is so similar between subjects alleging exceptional abilities and subjects with acquired memory skill that the same basic mechanisms in both cases can be inferred (Ericsson, 1985).

There is no reason to believe that exceptional memory performance is possible only for a small number of special individuals. In addition to the several case studies just described, we have more direct evidence from group studies in which a large number of subjects were given 5 or more hours of practice (for an extensive review see Ericsson, 1985). After practice without any instruction, subjects were able to memorize meaningless and unrelated material two to five times faster than before. Hence practice is a much more important determiner of memory performance than initial differences between individuals. The evidence for mechanisms underlying the improvement in memory performance in these "average" subjects is directly consistent with that identified in our earlier analysis of people with exceptional memory (Ericsson, 1985).

Acquired exceptional memory skill for digits and other "meaningless" materials appears to rely on the same mechanisms that average subjects use for sentences and other meaningful materials (Ericsson & Chase, 1982). With extensive practice, subjects can acquire and use knowledge to store information about digits in LTM at rapid presentation rates. In fact, their rate for digits equals that of normal subjects for storing information about sentences. With fast presentation rates skilled subjects can remember more digits than subjects can remember words in meaningful sentences (Ericsson & Karat, 1981), and skilled subjects can memorize lists of more than 2,000 digits as fast as, or faster than, normal subjects can memorize a text with a comparable number of words (Susukita, 1933). Other converging evidence regarding the effects on memory of practice and experience with unfamiliar materials comes from a series of studies comparing the memory performance of experts and novices in chess (Chase & Simon, 1973b) and on other tasks (Charness, 1979; Egan & Schwartz, 1979; Engle & Bukstel, 1978). Chess experts, who have acquired a vast knowledge of chess positions, can store all the information in a chess configuration in LTM after only a brief exposure. In contrast, novices are forced to rely on STM, where they can hold only a small fraction of the information (Charness, 1976; Chase & Simon, 1973b). In sum, extensive practice and experience with a given type of material yields cognitive structures and processes that allow for a qualitatively different memory performance with that material.

The observation that the performance of subjects with exceptional ability is qualitatively different from the performance of unpracticed people is quite consistent with the skill hypothesis. With extensive practice the absolute identification of several color chips occurred rapidly through automatized recognition. Extensive practice allowed our trained digit experts to store information in LTM, whereas normal subjects had to rely on STM and rehearsal of the presented digits. Such qualitative changes of performance are well known from the study of many skills. For unskilled subjects many cognitive processes require conscious attention to a sequence of individual steps, but with extensive practice the same processes in a skilled subject can occur automatically in a single step with a minimum of conscious attention (Schneider & Shiffrin, 1977; Shiffrin & Schneider, 1977). The types of errors in perception (Shepard, 1963) and in the production of responses (Grudin, 1983) are quite different between skilled and unskilled subjects and suggest different cognitive representations emerging with the higher levels of expertise in many tasks. Hence the skill hypothesis can also account for structural differences in exceptional ability.

A Reconsideration of Aspects of Exceptional Aptitude in Basic Skills

For exceptional ability in memory and perception assumed to reflect basic processes, we have shown that practice can lead to dramatic improvements. Normal subjects can, with extensive practice, attain memory performance that exceeds that of subjects with alleged exceptional memory. The claim that the subjects with exceptional abilities perform at a level unobtainable by normal subjects with extensive practice is shown to be incorrect when data from appropriate training studies are collected. Data on improvement with extensive practice are available for a wide range of other cognitive and perceptual tasks (Newell & Rosenbloom, 1981). The results from all these studies show uniformly that performance improves with practice and that with extensive practice, the improvement in performance is dramatic. The improvability of human performance with practice is so great and well documented that the burden of empirical evidence to the contrary ought to lie with anyone who wishes to claim that a certain performance reflects exceptional aptitude or capacity. We are not aware of any empirical evidence providing such support for any exceptional ability.

The Emergence of Extraordinary Performance

In the preceding section we tried to demonstrate that current empirical evidence cannot differentiate between performance due to exceptional aptitude and that which can be attained with extensive practice. The developmental course of extraordinary performance may provide another means of distinguishing between the two causes. Inherent in the idea of performance due to exceptional aptitude is the assumption that the ability can appear suddenly, even at a very early age, with no apparent period of learning. What is the evidence that supports the sudden emergence of aptitudes? How certain can we be that such sudden achievements cannot be due to gradual improvement through practice?

At least three criteria need to be met in order to show that extraordinary performance was not acquired through practice. These criteria refer to different prerequisites for learning. First, it is necessary to have *sufficient time to practice the skill*. Second, nearly any skill requires some *instruction and access to whatever tools are needed*. (For example, to acquire perfect pitch one would need to be told the names of the notes and to hear them produced on some musical instrument.) It may also be necessary to gain feedback about the correctness of the actions performed. In cases of claimed exceptional ability, required instruction must be minimal; otherwise, the instructor would be aware of the gradual improvement in the pupil's performance. Finally, but most important, persons having a special aptitude for the task must demonstrate *a level of performance that is "exceptional."* If we are to argue that all normal individuals are potentially capable of such performance, we must explain why so few persons invest the time and effort required to become extraordinary. We have already mentioned the possibility of a genetic contribution to a generalized drive mechanism. Now we will also argue, on the basis of some suggestive evidence, that certain combinations of environmental and psychological conditions can generate sufficient drive for the sustained practice needed to develop extraordinary levels of performance in a given skill. To make our review task more manageable, we will limit our discussion to exceptional aptitudes assumed to reflect basic capacities and hence will not discuss talent for music, drawing, and other complex aptitudes.

We might expect to find reports of people displaying gifted performance on any imaginable task. However, it appears that the exceptionality of a performance lies in the eyes of the beholder. That is, we attribute to special gifts that which is rare and therefore seems beyond the reach of the average individual. The ability to interpret instantaneously very complex abstract symbols would seem to be an amazing accomplishment in a culture that had not developed written language. Likewise, the ability to navigate across miles of open water during daytime, with no instruments, seems almost miraculous to us but is not regarded as the least bit unusual in the Puluwat culture (Gladwin, 1970). What are the abilities in our culture that are considered "exceptional"? There are surprisingly few. Those for which systematic studies have been conducted are limited to mental calculation, absolute pitch, speaking backwards, and memory for verbatim information and meaningless facts. It appears to us that these are all likely candidates for acquisition through practice, without such practice being obvious to other persons in the immediate environment. They are all *mental*, and hence only the end product is observable, that is, the process by which they are performed cannot be observed. They all require considerable *effort* and *concentration*. In the remainder of this section we argue that the special characteristics of these tasks are directly related to the perception and assessment of them as exceptional.

Evaluation of the case for exceptionality is made more difficult by possible bias in the available evidence. This is probable particularly with respect to the allegation that emergence of the special talent is quite sudden and without practice. What we may actually have is a biased sample of cases in which the observers failed to find, or were unwilling to search for, evidence of prior practice. The sudden discovery that a person in one's immediate environment can perform some task at an exceptional level does not necessarily mean that the ability *developed* suddenly, only that it was *first observed* at a high level of proficiency. The ideal evidence for sudden emergence would consist of two tests separated by only a few days. In the first test of the ability, normal performance would be recorded. In the second, performance would be exceptional. It is not surprising that such evidence does not exist. Tests of a skill are generally administered to check the progress of expected improvement. Yet it is the unexpectedness of the ability that causes it to be noticed at all. All the same, it is important to realize the lack of conclusive evidence for the suddenness of emergence. In situations in which evidence for practice and a gradual acquisition of the skill is readily available, people would not be likely to claim exceptionality.

To complicate matters further, we can find evidence suggesting that people who discover apparently gifted performance are less likely to seek evidence for practice. Parents of mentally retarded children may view the discovered ability as a gift from God to compensate for their child's other handicaps (Horwitz, Kestenbaum, Person, & Jarvik, 1965). Parents of otherwise normal children have often profited, financially or otherwise, from demonstrating the child's exceptionality (Brill, 1940). There are some truly absurd anecdotal reports, such as the claim that one child was able to speak fluently only 2 hours after delivery (Barlow, 1952). Thus we need to be aware of the all-too-human temptation to exaggerate and even intentionally make up evidence for innate exceptionality of the individual. In sum, the evidence for the sudden emergence of ability is weak and is based on anecdotal reports.

The Availability of Time for Practice

How likely is it that one could practice to the extent required for extraordinary performance without drawing the attention of persons in one's immediate environment? First, we address the issue of how practice could go unnoticed and then we derive some estimates of how much practice would be required for extraordinary performance.

Unlike learning physical skills or playing musical instruments, many mental skills can be performed in complete silence and in nearly any physical environment. Furthermore, it is almost impossible for an observer to discriminate the more frequent daydreaming from the practice of a mental skill. It is perhaps no accident that the only skills for which sudden gifted performance has been reported are exactly those for which practice is particularly difficult to observe. In sum, it is quite possible that people in the immediate environment who observe and report the apparent sudden emergence of a mental skill are simply unaware of the prior practice.

The length of time required for the improvement of a skill to exceptional levels is less than what one would expect. For both memory and perceptual skills we have already found that a normal adult can attain an exceptional level of performance after *less than* 50 *hours of practice.* Even if we allow for a duration ten times longer, it would total only 500 hours. This would correspond to a little more than an hour a day for only 1 year. Such a regular investment of time would be much less than half of the time spent by people seriously interested in chess, sports, and music. Ironically, persons investing such long hours in observable practice are rarely considered exceptional by those around them. Although their actual performance may be extraordinary compared to that of untrained persons, they are compared to other musicians, chess players, and athletes who have invested similar amounts of effort and so achieved similar levels of accomplishment. Later we will discuss the rare case of "talented" individuals whose improvements are remarkably rapid and significant even relative to other subjects with comparable practice.

During childhood and adolescence, any person would have at least 30 minutes per day when he or she is alone and free to practice mental skills. During long periods of sickness and in some living circumstances, the availability of time would be far greater.

The Feasibility of Skill Acquisition with Minimal Instruction

Only a very few of the skills we have mentioned (i.e., memorization of various kinds of information) require no instruction at all. Even when ability is claimed to be innate, some instruction must be given before the subjects can display their skilled performance. For absolute pitch the subject needs to learn the names of the notes and possibly which key on a piano they correspond to. To be able to do mental calculation, the subject must learn to count and must also be taught addition, subtraction, multiplication, and division.

The issue is whether such *minimal initial instruction* is sufficient for attaining exceptional levels of performance through practice. Certainly, the instruction needed to acquire absolute pitch would be minimal. From our own work (Chase & Ericsson, 1981, 1982) in the digit-span training study, we know that both of our initial subjects acquired their skill without any coaching or instruction. Large-scale group studies of the effectiveness of teaching good memorization strategies (mnemonics) have repeatedly found that a fair proportion of the subjects use related methods spontaneously (Bower, 1972).

The only reported exceptional skill that would appear to require extensive instruction is that of mental calculation. We will return to this topic in our discussion of mental calculation by mentally retarded subjects. For now we will simply make two brief comments. There is evidence that novices initially do multiplication and division by successive additions and subtractions. With sufficient practice, subjects may be able to do the corresponding operations with direct retrieval from memory, if so, they have internalized a multiplication table (for a detailed analysis of this extrapolation process, see Mitchell, 1907). In sum, for tasks with observed extraordinary performance, it appears to be possible to acquire the skills needed with a minimal amount of instruction.

Drive

The question of drive is possibly the most difficult one to answer. Why would anyone devote time and energy to acquiring levels of performance in such "useless" skills as mental calculation? Given the state of the art of research on motivation, a definite answer may not be possible. In this section we argue that such interests are common among children. Extraordinary performance results when the interest persists for a longer time, and in a more intense form, than for most. An analysis of the physical and psychological environment of exceptional children will show that preoccupation with a mental skill may be an adaptive response to their circumstances. Finally, we argue that similar levels of performance have been attained with external pressure from teachers and parents.

Most children experience periods of time during which they thoroughly enjoy memorizing lists of names and other verbatim information. Virtually the only games involving skill in which children are competitive with adults involve memory (e.g., the commercially available game Memory). Many children are also interested in acquiring other skills (chess, speaking backwards, etc.) in which, for the first time, they can successfully compete with average adults. Virtually all children spend countless hours acquiring motor skills in games, sports, and/or music. We must account for why such spontaneous interest in skill acquisition might be channeled into unusual mental skills, and why the interest and motivation could be maintained without external reward and pressure.

It is important to realize that a very large proportion of all children who show exceptional mental skills grew up in very sterile environments, without toys or attention from adults. In many families children were required to sit silently for long periods of time. Mitchell (1907) described as follows the specific background of a majority of mental calculators known to him:

> Several of the calculators—Mondeux, Mangiamele, Pierini, Inaudi—were shepherd-boys, an occupation which, since it requires an ability to count and affords ample leisure, is peculiarly favorable for practicing calculation; several, again,—Grandmange (born without arms or legs), Safford, Pierini, the present writer,—were sick or otherwise incapacitated for active play to a greater or less extent, and thus enjoyed an equally good opportunity to practice calculation. (pp. 98–99).

Although Mitchell's (1907) analysis does not capture conditions peculiar to all mental calculators, it convincingly demonstrates plausible preconditions for the development of exceptional ability in most of them. A psychoanalyst, Brill (1940), published a case study of a mental calculator named Jungreis and demonstrated a possible link between the subject's social and psychological isolation and his exceptional performance. The emergence of Jungreis's ability occurred 2 months after the death of his mother and the simultaneous departure of his sister, who was the only sibling he had significant contact with. Hence psychological isolation, which is more difficult to document than physical isolation, may be another possible factor in the development of exceptional ability.

What might underlie this link between isolation and motivation? From the literature on skill acquisition in general, it appears clear that for major improvement in performance, full concentration and focused attention are necessary. Casual and intermittent engagement in an activity appears to lead to slight, if any, improvement. Judging from the general interests in skill acquisition by children and adults, brief periods of concentration appear to be motivating and rewarding, whereas longer periods are fatiguing and aversive. Based on some rather tentative evidence, we suggest that there might be situations in which the opposite becomes true. Under normal conditions daydreaming and nondirected thinking might be pleasant and rewarding. However, in fearful situations, with the intrusion of anxiety-provoking thoughts, such relaxed states would be aversive. Focusing attention as required in the practice of a mental skill would serve to block out such thoughts. As continued practice makes the activity easier and less absorbing, it would be necessary to constantly increase the complexity of the tasks. As a result, an impressive skill would develop, given sufficient time. This account, while admittedly speculative, is consistent with the preceding reports about psychological turmoil and social isolation.

Some evidence of various kinds supports our fanciful account. One contemporary mental calculator reported in an interview with one of us (K.A.E.) that he used to engage in calculation when he felt lonely. Schaefer (cited in Kubek, 1969) has demonstrated that the biochemical indicators of stress during exposure to prolonged sensory deprivation could be almost completely eliminated by preisolation training in mental geometric construction. Hence focused mental activity appears to suppress the normal stress reaction to sensory deprivation. From accounts of the existence in concentration camps, it is clear that suppression of anxiety-provoking thought was often accomplished by focused attention on other tasks (Des Pres, 1976). Thus we can say that exceptional ability is the result of a focused attention during extensive practice of the skill, but the motivational cause of this focus is still uncertain.

We argued earlier that the requirement of instruction for the development of these mental skills is secondary to practice. This means that we can compare skills acquired in isolation to skills acquired in schools and under the supervision of a teacher. Although not much is known about the motivational mechanisms for skills gained in isolation, the recent attempts to give early training to young children in a wide range of sports and arts show that a large proportion of children can sustain such focused and extensive training. Few results are available for purposes of comparing the performance levels attained in isolation with those acquired in school systems. A young mental calculator (Mondeux) was compared to students in a school in which mental multiplication was actually taught and exercised. One quarter of the best students equaled or surpassed Mondeux's mental calculation performance (Leaning, 1927).

One of the widely cited examples of extreme pressure in the development of early extraordinary performance concerns the famous British philosopher John Stuart Mill. His reading lessons began when he was 2 years old, and at 3 he studied Greek.

> When he was still only seven, he had read the whole of Herodotus, and of Xenophon's "Cyropaedia" and "Memoria's of Socrates"; some of the lives of the philosophers by Diogenes Laertius; parts of Lucian, and Isocrates ad Demonicum and Ad Nicolem. (Elliot, 1910, p. xiv)

These accomplishments were achieved under extreme pressure from his father, James Mill, as shown by the following quote:

> James Mill not only heard his son's recital of what he had been set to learn: he also required written summaries and comments, which were discussed between them at home or on the long walks which they took together. He always demanded more than his son was capable of giving, and his reproofs for premature opinions were immediate and crushing. (Britton, 1953, p. 12)

What is more remarkable than the extraordinary performances of John Stuart Mill is the fact that he was able emotionally to survive such enormous pressure and demands. He was 14 years old when he was allowed contact for the *first* time with the outside world and with children other than his siblings (Britton, 1953).

In the traditional schools of the past, students were required to memorize extensive amounts of material by rote. Although most improvement in memorization due to practice appears to be specific to the particular material memorized, it is possible to acquire general methods for memorization, which can be relatively easy to extend to other materials. Hunt and Love (1972) proposed that the extensive memorization required by two mnemonists, S. and V. P., might have provided the necessary learning and practice for the acquisition of their memory skills.

Extraordinary Performance in Mentally Retarded Persons

Some particularly illuminating information about exceptional ability comes from studies that have investigated extraordinary performance by persons of very low mental achievement. It has been assumed that because of their low IQ's, these persons were unable to learn to perform mental tasks in the same way in which those with average IQs would do them. Yet, there are reports of idiot savants who excel in mental tasks such as memory for meaningless information (numbers, names, etc), mental calculation, and calendar calculation.

The last two tasks are particularly interesting because of the enormous number of individual facts that would be required if one relied on memory alone. A mental calculator able to multiply any two 3-digit numbers would require a million pieces of information. A date calculator who can correctly name the day of the week of an arbitrary date until the date A.D. 40,400 would require storage of more than 10 million individual facts. In view of the difficulty normal children experience in learning the multiplication table, which contains only 100 such relations, memorization of such a large number of facts would be truly incredible.

How can we account for such retarded persons' skill without resorting to the assumption that they simply have an unusually large memory capacity for these kinds of information? If we accept the assumption that persons with low IQ could not learn the rules and shortcuts employed by their counterparts with normal IQ, then we indeed have no choice. If, however we could find empirical evidence regarding cognitive mechanisms mediating performance in the retarded person's area of expertise, we could compare these mechanisms to those acquired by normal subjects in the same or related tasks. A close relation between the mechanisms of mentally retarded and normal subjects would provide strong evidence for the acquired-skill hypothesis.

In this section we review studies of extraordinary performance in three areas: memory for unrelated facts, mental calculation, and date calculation. We will look for mediating cognitive processes that could account for these abilities in persons who otherwise show little intellectual capacity. Then we will discuss the repeated observations that mentally retarded persons showing exceptional abilities are incapable of describing, or unwilling to describe, any methods underlying their extraordinary performance.

Exceptional Memory for Unrelated Facts

There have been many reports of mentally retarded persons showing a surprising ability to retain apparently unrelated bits of information. This includes persons who have exhibited extraordinary recall of dates, names of people and geographic places (Byrd, 1920; Otis, 1925), numbers of automobiles and freight cars (Downey, 1926), and demographic information (Jones, 1926). Two points must be kept in mind when considering their exceptional ability. First, extraordinary performance is not found under standardized conditions. Subjects who have been tested extensively, using standardized tests and rates of presentation, showed that under these conditions their memory performance was not superior to that of unexceptional persons of the same age and having normal IQ. Overall, their performance on the tests was far below average. When they achieved comparatively high scores on a particular part of the test, it was found that performance was linked to familiarity with the material. For example, subject L. (with ability in mental calculation and calendar calculation; Scheerer, Rothman, & Goldstein, 1945) had a memory span for digits that was much higher than his memory span as measured using other types of tests.

The second point that must be realized when considering the exceptional ability of these memory experts is that the ability to recall a large amount of information is not evidence that this information was stored more rapidly in memory. All the available evidence suggests that the rate of memorization for these subjects is slower than for normal subjects. Hence these subjects can memorize substantial amounts of information by concentrated effort for extended periods of time. Jones (1926) mentions a subject (with IQ of 75) who memorized, from the 1910 census, the population of all towns with populations over 2,000. To accomplish such a feat, he worked 6 to 8 hours per day for 3 weeks. Hamblin (1966) notes that the two calendar twins (with IQ's of 60–70) have memorized, from *The World Almanac*, the dates of Easter for all years between 1901 and 2100. For such extended practice, it is necessary that the information be readily available. Byrd (1920) noticed that the mentally retarded memory expert he studied used a notebook in which the facts were written down and thus were accessible for repeated practice.

How can such memory feats be attained, even with long periods of practice? Given the low IQ of these persons, it is tempting to believe that they must rely on rote memorization of these facts. Evidence for or against this belief is generally lacking, but there is some evidence that these retarded subjects are able to use mnemonics in a manner similar to that of trained memory experts. Jones (1926) analyzed subject K.'s memorization of digits under laboratory control. The following is a verbal protocol taken from the subject as he memorized the number 30,249,385,274. It bears a striking resemblance to those of our trained digit-span experts.

> 30 is the number of days in a month. 249—if there were 149 it would be the distance from Chicago to Peoria, Illinois. 385—I once paid $3.85 railroad fare going from Cheyenne, Wyoming to Wheatland, Wyoming. 274—I can remember that by putting a 6 in front of it for the time being. 6274 is the seating capacity of the Hippodrome. (Jones, 1926, p. 372)

Although the specific LTM associations he makes are different from those of our subjects, they share many similarities. The subject K. was not limited to making exact matches with known facts in memory, as would be expected if rote memorization were all he was capable of. Rather, he makes many partial matches, altering a number temporarily to make it more similar to known facts and relying on reinstituting the correct number when needed at recall.

Thus it isn't necessary to postulate larger memory capacities for exceptional performance in memorizing large bodies of information. Material to be memorized is acquired, if anything, at rates slower than normal. By using external memory aids, such as written lists, the mentally retarded subjects can study the material for extended periods of time. One should, of course, note that only extremely basic decoding skills are necessary for reading tables of numbers, calendars, and so forth.

Mental Calculation

Ability in mental calculation presents a somewhat different problem. Rarely reported are mentally retarded subjects who perform at levels similar to those of mental calculators with otherwise normal IQ. In fact, in reviews of mental calculators (Mitchell, 1907; Scripture, 1891; Smith, 1983 and Chapter 2, this volume) there is only a mention of two who might possibly be mentally retarded. The evidence is scanty, because both lived during the 18th century. It is clear that both were illiterate, but that was not uncommon during the 1700s. In addition, the fact that one was a slave makes it likely that the evaluation of his intelligence might be severely biased. In comparison with other mental calculators, these two appeared to be much slower in their calculations (Mitchell, 1907).

With the possible exception of these two cases, the reports of mental calculation in the mentally retarded do not place their performance outside the normal range. Their ability is exceptional only in comparison to the performance of the individual on other tasks. Scheerer *et al.* (1945) reported that the previously mentioned subject L. (with IQ of 50) could rapidly add a long series of 2-digit numbers. Wizel (1904) collected detailed data on his subject, Sabine, who was able to mentally multiply any two 2-digit numbers. With unusual patience, he tried to extract the methods she used. After each multiplication, Wizel asked her to explain how she calculated the multiplication. She did not give a normal explanation, but, as part of her incoherent speech, she mentioned numbers. For example, after giving the answer (4,096) to the multiplication of 64×64, she would say 256, 512, 1,024, 4,096. From these numbers Wizel reconstructed the process of calculation: $16 \times 16 = 256$; $256 \times 2 = 512$; $512 \times 2 = 1024$; $1024 \times 4 = 4096$. From the verbalization of such intermediate products for a large number of multiplications, he identified a bias towards factoring 2-digit numbers into two single-digit multiplications. For example, $49 \times 49 = 49 \times (7 \times 7) = 343 \times 7 = 2401$ and $17 \times 35 = 17 \times (7 \times 5) = 119 \times 5 = 595$. He found similar evidence for other, more complex methods for calculating products of numbers. The most interesting implication of his analysis is that a mentally retarded subject (Sabine's intelligence was at the level of a 3-year-old by Wizel's informal assessment) can use methods quite similar to those preferred by more advanced mental calculators of average intelligence.

Sabine also displayed a puzzling tendency to given a regular answer $(23 \times 23 = 529)$ and then tell the number of multiples of 16 it contained: $33 \times 16 + 1$. From extensive analysis it became clear that beyond the normal number system, Sabine encoded numbers as multiples of 16. She was particularly rapid in her multiplications and divisions involving 16. Hence, during her own study of counting and addition, she must have developed that idiosyncratic organization.

Calendar Calculation

Calendar calculation is the only skill for which there are reports of mentally retarded persons whose performance surpasses that of professional performers having normal IQ's. It involves rapidly answering two types of questions: the day of the week for arbitrary dates (Type 1) and the date that corresponds to some arbitrary day (e.g., the first Tuesday) in a given month and year (Type 2). Lafora (1934) reported one remarkable mentally retarded subject, Victoria (with IQ of 65), who was able to answer Type 1 questions in 1–4 seconds and Type 2 questions in about 5 seconds. This is two to four times faster than the average time for professional performers.

We know that memory plays an important role in such performance. Some subjects have been limited to naming dates in a restricted range, such as a single year or 1901–1920 (Byrd, 1920; Scheerer et al., 1945). However, it is unlikely that calendar calculation can be performed through sheer memorization alone. It is implausible not only because of the tremendous amount of memorization that would be required but also because many calendar calculators are able to name correctly the days of the week of dates far in the future (Horwitz et al., 1965; Jones, 1926). The most extensive range includes dates into the year A.D. 132,470 (Addis, 1968; Parsons, 1968). Hence calendar calculation is most likely best described as a combination of memory and calculation.

If calculation is involved, it may seem surprising that subjects are unable to describe the processes they are using as they are generating the answers. Yet this is one of the most reliable findings in investigations of calendar calculators (Byrd, 1920; Horwitz et al., 1965; Jones, 1926). Many researchers have interpreted this lack of self-awareness to imply that cognitive processes are simply not involved. However, several investigators have pursued this issue in much further depth and have found supporting and refuting evidence for likely mechanisms mediating the skill (Rimland, 1978; Scheerer et al., 1945).

Simple algorithms for calculating the day of the week for arbitrary dates are well known (Barlow, 1952). The simplicity of these mathematical methods clearly demonstrates the simple relations between dates and days of the week. For example, the day of the week of a given date (e.g., one's birthday) is one day earlier in the week the following year (except in leap years). However, using the algorithms for more complicated questions and for years far removed from the present year involves considerable simple mental arithmetic and methods unlikely to be used by date calculators for two reasons. First, some date calculators are unable to perform even simple mental arithmetic (Horwitz et al., 1965). Second, the rapidity of responses to questions about dates, and the wide range of questions answered correctly, such as "In what years will April 21st fall on a Sunday?," make application of such mathematical methods highly unlikely.

Three studies have attempted to uncover the methods of calendar calculators by intensive observation and experimentation (Lafora, 1934; Rimland, 1978; Scheerer et al., 1945). Sheerer et al. recorded the response time and the ordinarily silent verbalizations of subject L. as he named days of the week for specified dates. Most of the verbalizations were simply numbers. From their analyses of these data, they concluded that L. could directly recall the days of the week of a fairly large number of dates. To calculate the desired day, he found a date close to the one desired and "counted" his way there. Their proposal for a counting mechanism is plausible because L. had earlier shown great facility at "skipping numbers," that is jumping to numbers separated by a given integer. Furthermore, they showed that L. could correctly identify all leap years from 1898 to 1950.

Lafora (1934) is the only investigator who has been able to obtain extensive verbal reports on the process of date calculation from a mentally retarded subject. His subject, Victoria, showed an extensive knowledge of relations between months that start with the same day of the week in a given year. In the following retrospective report on her thoughts, Victoria shows several methods for generating the correct answer:

> Question: Which day of the week is the 5th of August 1934?
> Response: Sunday (two seconds).
> Retrospective report: Because August begins with the same week-day as November (in years that are not leap years) and I know that November begins on Wednesday and moreover July ends on Tuesday because it begins on Sunday (Tuesday plus five days equals Sunday). Moreover I know it because this year the 5th of August fell on a Saturday. And that I remember. (translated from Spanish; Lafora, 1934, p. 60)

Victoria demonstrated knowledge of deriving the desired day of the week from the day of the week of the same day on the preceding year, that is the day of the week plus 1 day (for years that are not leap years). She also showed how she could derive the day of the week of any date in a given month from the day of the week of the first day of that month. She did not calculate the day of the week by counting up from the first day but knew that the 1st, 8th, 15th, 22nd, and 29th of any month are all on the same day of the week, as is demonstrated by the following translated protocol:

> Question: What day of the week would be 22 July, 1934?
> Response: Sunday (two seconds)
> Explanation: July begins like April, for that reason the 1st of April, like the 1st of July, would be Sunday; because the days 8, 15, *22*, 29 of each month are the same as the first it means that the 22nd would be a Sunday. (translated from Spanish; Lafora, 1934, p. 60)

In a rather extensive analysis Lafora uncovered several shortcut methods and showed that the reported methods or thought sequences were consistent with the response latencies as well as with occasional errors. His analysis shows that Victoria's skill was based on memory for specific dates and a "mechanical" extrapolation to derive information about the desired date.

In a rare additional report on calendar-calculation ability in subjects with normal IQ's, Robertson (1958) describes a schizophrenic subject with several memory skills. This subject had, for example, memorized the squares of all numbers from 1 to 1,000 and the cubes of all numbers from 1 to 100. Robertson randomly selected 80 dates during a 16-year period, and the subject rapidly responded with the correct day of the week for over 90% of the dates (the errors were incorrect by a day only). A more detailed examination showed that the subject had the day of the week memorized for 118 dates and used these dates as starting points for calculation of the presented dates, using his knowledge of invariant calendar relations.

Addis (1968) and Parsons (1968) took it upon themselves to analyze the amazing skill of the two calendar-calculation twins (with IQs of 60–70; Hamblin, 1966). Within an average of 6 seconds, one of the twins could name the day of the week of any date ranging as far away in the future as the year 132,470. Through a task analysis Addis (1968) found that the calendar repeats itself completely every 400 years. Hence, by simple division by 400, any number year can be mapped onto the familiar range of years 1600–2000 (e.g., $2470 = 6 \times 400 + 70 \rightarrow 1600 + 70 = 1670$). The complexity of this conversion is remarkably reduced once one realizes that any multiple of 10,000 is perfectly divisible by 400, and hence only the last 4 digits need be considered (e.g., $132,470 \rightarrow 2,470 \rightarrow 1,670$). Rather than memorizing the days of the week of all these 400 years (1600–2000), Addis used a method of adding integers corresponding to the century, the year, the month, and the day of the month, and from the sum he derived the day of the week. To determine whether this would be a reasonable method, Addis gave training to a graduate student. Figure 24-2 gives the latency for reporting the days of the week for dates between year A.D. 1600 and year A.D. 2000 (solid line) and between year A.D. 0 and year A.D. 999,999 (dashed line). During the first part of training, Mr. Langdon, the graduate student, had the tables visually available, but at the 8th session, the tables were removed, and he performed the calculation completely mentally. Toward the end of the 16 sessions of practice, he reported that the calculations were becoming automatic, and his response latencies approached the speed of the fastest of the calendar-calculating twins.

From a detailed analysis of the best twin's calculating performance, Addis found support for initial conversion from the presented year to a year within the familiar 400-year range. The twin uttered the word "four" and mixed in "four" when he repeated the presented date. When asked the day of the week of a given date (July 19) in several different years, the twin responded much faster when the different years mapped onto the same year within the 400-year range (i.e., 132,470 and 6870 both correspond to 1670.) In a follow-up study Addis (personal communication, December 1984) compared the performance of Mr. Langdon to that of one of the twins on several hundred problems and concluded that Mr. Langdon was using the same system as the twin or a very similar one.

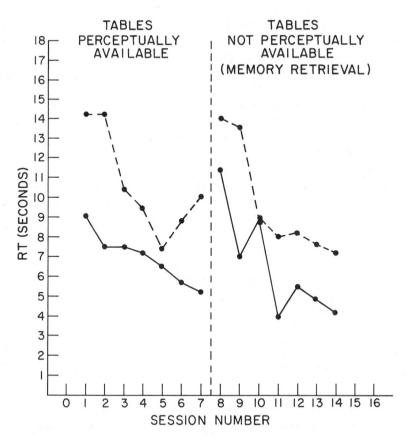

FIGURE 24-2. Average latency (RT = reaction time) to name the days of the week of two types of arbitrary dates as a function of training session. The dashed line corresponds to the average latency for any date between January 1 of A.D. 0 and December 31 of A.D. 999,999, and the solid line corresponds to the average latency for dates between January 1 of A.D. 1600 and December 31 of A.D. 2000. During the first seven sessions, the graduate student used available tables, but during the last seven sessions, he performed without access to the tables.

Summary

Both in memory for unrelated facts and in mental calculation, mentally retarded subjects are not exceptional in comparison to normal subjects. They are exceptionally good in these abilities in comparison to other subjects with comparable IQs as well as to their own performance on other tasks. The available data on the mediating mechanism are quite consistent with the general characteristics of skills acquired through practice. Wherever detailed information is available, we find a remarkable similarity between the structure of mentally retarded subjects' skill and that of normal subjects' skill. In sum, within the limited realm of their exceptional ability, the mentally retarded subjects rely on thoughts (intermediate steps) that are indistinguishable from those of normal subjects.

Before turning to our general discussion, we will briefly address the issue of the inability or unwillingness of mentally retarded subjects to describe their methods. The expectation that these subjects should be able to describe their methods is derived from the incorrect inference that normal subjects with the same skills could describe their methods. With extensive practice a skill is automatized, and the subject then relies on automatic retrieval of relevant knowledge and useful shortcuts (for an extensive discussion of what is verbally reportable during thinking for normal subjects, see Ericsson & Simon, 1984). Hence the mentally retarded subjects appear to be no less able than normal skilled subjects to report their methods. When the instruction is to *retrospectively* report one's thoughts during a calculation, both mentally retarded subjects and those with normal IQs are able to do the task. These verbal reports contain intermediate steps or thoughts in which the general methods are not explicitly stated but must be inferred by the investigator. Once again, the results from skilled subjects are remarkably similar, regardless of IQ level.

The reviewed evidence supports the notion that these exceptional abilities are skills acquired after substantial practice. The studies on mentally retarded subjects almost invariably comment on the gradual improvement of the ability and on the enormous amount of time that the subjects spend focused on the corresponding tasks (Parker, 1918; Scheerer *et al.*, 1945; Wizel, 1904). One reason for the apparent discrepancy with earlier research on normal children is probably the close monitoring of retarded children's development. It is likely that parents of retarded children will be worried about delayed development and be more attentive to any activity that might suggest improvement and a better diagnosis. Another piece of evidence supporting the skill view comes from the observation that a mentally retarded child may show proficiency in more than a single ability. A prime example is subject L. (Scheerer *et al.*, 1945), who, as noted before, was remarkable in terms of memory, mental calculation, and calendar calculation. Although his ability in any one of these tasks did not match that of most of the other exceptional subjects, his diversity was notable. According to our hypothesis, his less outstanding performance in any one task is explained by the lack of time and energy to devote to so many interests. In sum, the evidence on exceptional ability in mentally retarded subjects is remarkably well described by the acquired-skill interpretation.

Summary and Discussion

The purpose of this chapter was to identify the contributions of environmental and genetic factors in attaining extraordinary levels of performance in particular areas of endeavor. We have argued that there is weak evidence—and in some cases no evidence—that the genetic contribution consists of inherited differences in basic and unmodifiable aptitudes. Our reviews of empirical studies show that individuals who sustain a focus of attention and effort for extended periods can achieve a level of performance that is both qualitatively and quantitatively different from that of normal persons. The necessity (and sufficiency) of concentrated practice for attaining extraordinary performance is shown by three types of evidence:

1. Comparison of the performance of average subjects after training with that of supposedly gifted individuals.
2. The lack of evidence that gifted performance arises without practice.
3. Comparison of the performance of idiot savants with that of persons having average intelligence.

Let us summarize the evidence in each of these areas.

First, we showed that very basic cognitive and perceptual functions are amenable to improvement with practice. The improvement does not depend on any observable predisposition. Several seemingly average persons, after long periods of intensive practice, have achieved levels of performance on perceptual and memory tasks that match or even surpass those of persons credited with special gifts in the same area. Fine-grained analyses of strategies and error patterns showed that outstanding performance acquired by individuals through practice is qualitatively different from their own initial performance but not different from the performance of supposedly exceptional persons. In our training studies of digit span, we found that subjects were able to meaningfully encode and store unrelated digits at rates of presentation that allow untrained persons barely enough time to repeat or rehearse them.

We also found that trained subjects experience clear difficulties in verbally describing the nature and structure of their skill. Thus the fact that exceptional persons cannot explain how they manage their feats is not evidence for a structural explanation of extraordinary performance. The difficulty that both trained subjects and exceptional persons have in describing their skill can better be explained by automatization of a cognitive skill. With automatization of a skill, the substeps of the cognitive task are collapsed and are performed with little or no supervision from the higher level, conscious portion of the brain. As a result, the time required to execute the various encoding and decision steps is shortened dramatically, but awareness of the detailed cognitive process is lost. All adults have many automatized skills. If we had no records and no memory of our early efforts in automatizing our reading skills, it would be tempting to cite structural or innate sources for such an amazing ability. In sum, the characteristics of exceptional ability are completely consistent with the characteristics of skills acquired through extensive practice.

The second argument we presented in favor of a skill explanation for extraordinary performance was the lack of evidence that such ability arises without practice. We pointed out the crucial difference between lack of practice and lack of *observed* practice. Nearly all of the reported exceptional ability that was not dependent on practice involved mental skills. This practice is particularly difficult to observe. An analysis of the environmental circumstances of childhood for several exceptional persons, primarily mental calculators, revealed a number of factors that might encourage development of mental rather than other skills. It is not unusual for normal children and adolescents to practice a variety of skills, some of which are rather esoteric. We have argued that occasionally individuals will display an acquired skill that is sufficiently impressive that others in the environment will regard it as being beyond the reach of normal people. Given the natural human desire to be considered special, it is not surprising that early practice is not reported, and possibly not even remembered.

We believe that to prove exceptionality, the skill must be one that is not attainable by other persons through practice. This point can be illustrated by an example from the current literature. Coltheart and Glick (1974) investigated a woman who could visualize words and sentences and spell this material in reverse order. They argued for a structural account of her superior image ability by proposing that her internal visual representation was exceptionally vivid. Subsequently, Cowan and his associates (Cowan & Leavitt, 1982; Cowan, Leavitt, Massaro, & Kent, 1982) reported on several people who displayed very similar patterns of memory performance. These subjects all reported having practiced backwards spelling extensively during childhood and adolescence. Their achievement of the same skill casts doubt on the need for unusual basic capacities as prerequisites.

The third type of evidence we investigated involved reports of exceptional ability among mentally retarded children and adults. The existence of such idiot savants has been considered a strong argument against achievement of the skills through learning. Given the usual consistency of poor performance on mental tasks by mentally retarded persons, the outstanding performance in isolated areas by a few idiot savants has been attributed to some quirk of structural arrangements that endows a particular area with superior capacity. We have argued the opposite—that a general attention and drive mechanism provides a better explanation. We have shown that the exceptional ability of the mentally retarded person is generally exceptional only in comparison to the individual's performance in other areas. With the exception of calendar calculation, the performance of idiot savants is generally not outside the range displayed by normal persons. (Calendar calculation is a task at which normal subjects can become proficient after 20–30 hours of practice.) A detailed analysis revealed that the skills of exceptional mentally retarded persons display the general characteristics of skills acquired through practice by normal subjects (i.e., specificity of the skill, mediating cognitive processes, and a gradual improvement in performance). The most remarkable finding was that the cognitive processes of these mentally retarded subjects, as revealed by their verbal protocols while performing in their area of expertise, appear indistinguishable from those of normal subjects who had acquired the same skills.

In sum, our detailed review of cases reflecting "clear" evidence for gifted performance shows that these abilities are indistinguishable from those that are acquired through extensive practice. All the characteristics of exceptional performance known to us can be accounted for in terms of acquired skills. More recent neurophysiological studies have shown that even at the most basic level of the brain's organization, adaptations can be made as a result of experience. Edelman and Finkel (1984) have demonstrated such changes as a result of experience in the mapping of sensory input onto the primary projection area in the cortex. Hence there is now neurophysiological evidence for rejecting the notion of immutable neurological structures (cf. the notion of hardware discussed early in the chapter).

The evidence from these supposedly clear cases of gifted performance has often been used to support the more general notion that ability differences in normal subjects are due to similar basic differences. In light of our earlier analyses, we want to briefly review the evidence that individual differences in normal subjects can be described in terms of basic (neurological) capacities and processes of the human brain.

The studies we discussed that showed remarkable improvement in "basic" processes raise serious doubt regarding the validity of the assumption of inherited basic aptitudes. In fact, there is an almost complete lack of behavioral evidence for individual differences in such capacities. A century of intensive psychometric research failed to reveal any "basic" differences among individuals. Instead, studies of basic processes have found them to be unrelated to general ability or intelligence (Goodenough, 1949; Spearman & Jones, 1950). For example, general individual differences in ability to commit new information to memory have not been found. Neither is there evidence of significant correlation between memory for different materials in the same individual. Likewise, there is a lack of correlation among different methods of measuring memory (see Ericsson, 1985, for a discussion). Recent systematic attempts by Hunt (1978) to identify the locus of differences between people with high and low scores on IQ tests of verbal ability have been unable to find any "basic" differences. Hunt (1978) proposes that a more likely locus of individual differences is "general information processes, simple strategies that are used as steps in virtually every larger problem" (p. 128). These general information processes need to be acquired, but once they become automatized through extensive practice, they can serve as building blocks for a wide range of more complex cognitive processes. Systematic studies have shown that even between adults and children, differences can be better described in terms of acquired knowledge and strategies than in terms of differences in basic capacity or processes (Chi, 1978). Hence the evidence for a locus of individual differences in terms of inherited basic aptitudes is, at the least, weak or may even be lacking.

The reviewed evidence indicates that the contribution of genetic factors is unlikely to be in the area of heritable aptitudes or basic capabilities. An alternative locus for the genetic contribution involves the factors motivating the subject to sustain focused attention on the task during extensive periods. We have argued for a general mechanism, one akin to drive, which enables sustained, focused effort to be expended in practicing mental skills. We have purposely been vague about the origin of that drive, because so little is currently known about the physiological and environmental causes of sustained motivation. Most of the work done in that area is of a clinical nature, making conclusions tentative. Most laboratory studies of motivation concern short-term motivation, which is limited to improved performance for 1 or 2 hours (the normal duration of tests in college). We believe the ability to sustain concentration and interest for such a short period may be regulated by entirely different mechanisms than those involved in long-term motivation or drive. Long-term motivation is the willingness to invest time and intense effort in the same task on a regular basis over periods of weeks, months, and years. In clinical psychology there is considerable knowledge about idiosyncratic difficulties in sustaining long-term motivation or drive; however, we have found no directly applicable clinical research on the mechanisms underlying the sustained motivation exhibited by those persons who attain extraordinary performance in some domain.

In our own research we made some interesting observations. By chance, we started our research on memory training with long-distance runners. In retrospect, this group of subjects may be particularly well suited for study in training studies. They are accustomed to concentrated daily practice, and hence the motivational mechanisms supporting such practice could possibly be channeled into other tasks. Other subjects have been graduate students and other types of athletes. These groups have a similar history of successful long-term focus on developing exceptional ability in one or more task domains.

Within this framework of sustained motivation or drive, we would like to provide some hypotheses for the striking observation that some people appear to be more able than others, regardless of tasks. These subjects appear to be able to rapidly attain full concentration on a wide range of tasks (cf. Müller, 1911, 1913). With an additional investment of 20–30 hours, we know that it is possible to attain a performance level outside the normal range on many tasks. Hence such subjects could, for tasks deemed important, rapidly and easily attain such performance without disrupting their normal lives. Subjects who acquire skills in such a cumulative manner will have the additional advantage of relying on earlier developed skills when acquiring new ones. In support of this argument some investigators have pointed to the focus on specific domains for people making extraordinary achievements in the sciences and arts (Carroll, 1940).

The acquired-skill view is both good news and bad news for educators. On the one hand, it suggests that outstanding achievement need not be beyond the reach of any motivated student. On the other hand, even adequate levels of performance in such complex skills as reading, speaking a new language, or learning games such as chess or tennis require substantial periods of focused attention and practice. Children of average intelligence who are unable to focus attention adequately and sustain the effort early on are structurally handicapped in the sense that no short-term remedial effort can hope to succeed. Finding several hundred hours of free time for study would be hard enough, but in addition, the child needs to be able to concentrate and sustain motivation during all those hours. According to the hypothesis, remedial efforts should be aimed at helping the child develop long-term internal motivation and concentration rather than focus on teaching skills *per se.*

What we hoped to show in this chapter is that individual differences in inherited basic aptitudes need not be the *limiting* factor in human achievement. We believe that the role of genetic factors in determining the acquired level of skill and performance more likely concerns the motivation necessary for maintaining concentrated practice over extended periods. A number of physiological factors might be the mediating inherited factors. It is clear that many possibly relevant personality traits, such as anxiety level and temperament, are determined, at least in part, genetically (Plomin & Rowe, 1978). The amazing preponderance of male savants (three males to every female; Rimland, 1978) is probably also best understood in terms of differences in hormonal levels. A great deal of further research will be necessary in order to explicate the exact mechanisms underlying the genetic mediation.

By reconceptualizing what the *limiting* factor of human performance is most likely to be, we see several important implications. The kind of beneficial environmental support for fostering drive to maintain improvement throughout a person's life should be rather different from the attempts of many parents to push their children to acquire certain target behaviors. It is quite possible that such early pressures might hurt or even destroy the motivational factors or drive for later stages of development. From extensive analysis of persons displaying extraordinary performance, several necessary environmental factors have been identified. Bloom (1979) showed that persons who display extraordinary levels of achievement have inevitably benefited during childhood from an adult who supported the child's interest and very early expressed confidence in his or her ultimate success. The nature of the interaction between environmental and genetic factors in determining the performance and skill level attained by subjects is still almost unknown. With more knowledge about the prerequisites, we believe that appropriate environmental intervention and support will allow any individual to greatly increase his or her achievements.

Acknowledgments

First we want to acknowledge the support of the Office of Naval Research (Contract No. N00014-84-K-0250) to one of us (K. A. E.). We also want to acknowledge the helpful comments and suggestions given in response to earlier drafts of the chapter by Lyle Bourne, Bruce McNaughton, Dick Olson, Robert Plomin, and Michael Wertheimer.

References

Abraham, O. (1901). Das absolute Tonbewusstsein. Sammelbde. *International Musikges, 3,* 1–85.

Addis, B. (1968, April). *Resistance to parsimony: The evolution of a system for explaining the calendar calculating abilities of idiot savant twins.* Paper presented at the meeting of the Southwestern Psychological Association, New Orleans.

Bachem, A. (1937). Various types of absolute pitch. *Journal of the Acoustical Society of America, 9,* 146–151.

Baird, J. W. (1917). *Memory for absolute pitch in studies in psychology.* (Titchner Commemoration Volume). Worcester, MA: Wilson.

Baker, R. A., & Osgood, S. W. (1954). Discrimination transfer along a pitch continuum. *Journal of Experimental Psychology, 48,* 241–246.

Barlow, F. (1952). *Mental prodigies.* New York: Greenwood Press.

Binet, A. (1894). *Psychologie des grands calculateurs et joueurs d'échecs.* Paris: Librairie Hachette.

Bloom, B. (1979). A conversation with Benjamin Bloom. *Educational Leadership, 37,* 157–161.

Bower, G. H. (1972). Mental imagery and associative learning. In L. W. Gregg (Ed.), *Cognition in learning and memory* (pp. 51–88). New York: Wiley.

Bower, G. H., & Winzenz, D. (1969). Group structure, coding, and memory for digit series. *Journal of Experimental Psychology Monographs, 80* (2, Pt. 2).

Brady, P. T. (1970). The genesis of absolute pitch. *Journal of the Acoustical Society of America, 48,* 883–887.

Brill, A. A. (1940). Some peculiar manifestations of memory with special reference to lightning calculators. *Journal of Nervous and Mental Disease, 90,* 709–726.

Britton, K. (1953). *John Stuart Mill.* London: Penguin.

Byrd, H. (1920). A case of phenomenal memorizing by a feeble-minded negro. *Journal of Applied Psychology, 4,* 202–206.

Campbell, R. A., & Small, A. M. (1963). Effect of practice and feedback on frequency discrimination. *Journal of the Acoustical Society of America, 35,* 1511–1514.

Carroll, H. A. (1940). *Genius in the making.* New York: McGraw-Hill.

Charness, N. (1976). Memory for chess positions: Resistance to interference. *Journal of Experimental Psychology: Human Learning and Memory, 2,* 641–653.

Charness, N. (1979). Components of skill in bridge. *Canadian Journal of Psychology, 33,* 1–50.

Chase, W. G., & Ericsson, K. A. (1981). Skilled memory. In J. R. Anderson (Ed.), *Cognitive skills and their acquisition,* (pp. 141–189). Hillsdale, NJ: Erlbaum.

Chase, W. G., & Ericsson, K. A. (1981). Skill and working memory. In G. H. Bower (Ed.), *The psychology of learning and motivation* (Vol. 16, pp. 1–58). Academic Press.

Chase, W. G., & Simon, H. A. (1973a). Perception in chess. *Cognitive Psychology, 4,* 55–81.

Chase, W. G., & Simon, H. A. (1973b). The mind's eye in chess. In W. G. Chase (Ed.), *Visual information processing* (215–281). New York: Academic Press.

Chi, M. T. H. (1978). Knowledge structures and memory development. In R. S. Siegler (Ed.), *Children's thinking: What develops?* (pp. 73–96). Hillsdale, NJ: Erlbaum.

Chi, M. T. H., Feltovich, P. J., & Glaser, R. (1981). Categorization and representation of physics problems by experts and novices. *Cognitive Science, 5,* 121–152.

Coltheart, M., & Glick, M. J. (1974). Visual imagery: A case study. *Quarterly Journal of Experimental Psychology, 26,* 438–453.

Costall, A., (1985). The relativity of absolute pitch. In P. Howell, I. Cross, & R. West (Eds.), *Musical structure and cognition* (pp. 189–208). London: Academic Press.

Costall, A., Platt, S., & Macrae, A. (1981). Memory strategies in absolute identification of "circular" pitch. *Perception and Psychophysics, 29* (6), 589–593.

Cowan, N., & Leavitt, L. A., (1982). Talking backward: Exceptional speech play in late childhood. *Journal of Child Language, 9,* 481–495.

Cowan, N., & Leavitt, L. A., Massaro, D. W., & Kent, R. D. (1982). A fluent backward talker. *Journal of Speech and Hearing Research, 25,* 48–53.

de Groot, A. (1965). *Thought and choice in chess.* The Hague: Mouton.

de Groot, A. (1966). Perception and memory versus thought: Some old ideas and recent findings. In B. Kleinmuntz (Ed.), *Problem solving* (pp. 19–50). New York: Wiley.

Des Pres, T. (1976). *The survivor.* New York: Oxford University Press.

Downey, J. E. (1926). A case of special ability with below average intelligence. *Journal of Applied Psychology, 10,* 519–521.

Ebbinghaus, H. (1964). *Memory: A contribution to experimental psychology* (H. A. Ruger & C. E. Bussenius, Trans). New York: Dover. (Original work published 1885)

Edelman, G. M., & Finkel, L. H. (1984). Neuronal group selection in the cerebral cortex. In G. M. Edelman, W. E. Gale, & W. M. Cowan (Eds.), *Dynamic aspects of neocortical function* (pp. 653–697). New York: Wiley.

Egan, D. E., & Schwartz, B. J. (1979). Chunking in recall of symbolic drawings. *Memory and Cognition, 7,* 149–158.

Elliot, H. S. R. (1910). *The letters of John Stuart Mill* (Vol. 1). New York: Longmans, Green.

Engen, T. (1960). Effect of practice and instruction on olfactory thresholds. *Perceptual and Motor Skills, 10,* 195–198.

Engen, T. (1961). Identification of odors. *American Perfumer, 76,* 43–47.

Engen, R. W., & Bukstel, L. (1978). Memory processes among bridge players of differing expertise. *American Journal of Psychology, 91,* 673–690.

Ericsson, K. A. (1985). Memory skill. *Canadian Journal of Psychology, 39,* 188–231.

Ericsson, K. A., & Chase, W. G. (1982). Exceptional memory. *American Scientist, 70,* 607–615.

Ericsson, K. A., & Chase, W. G., & Faloon, S. (1980). Acquisition of a memory skill. *Science, 208,* 1181–1182.

Ericsson, K. A., & Faivre, I. A. (1982, November). *Acquiring "absolute pitch" for colors.* Paper presented at the meeting of the Psychonomic Society, Minneapolis.

Ericsson, K. A., & Karat, J. (1981, November). *Memory for words in sequences.* Paper presented at the meeting of the Psychonomic Society, Philadelphia.

Ericsson, K. A., & Simon, H. A. (1984). *Protocol analysis.* Cambridge, MA: The MIT Press/Bradford.

Gates, A. I., & Taylor, G. A. (1925). An experimental study of the nature of improvement resulting from practice in a mental function. *Journal of Educational Psychology, 16,* 583–592.

Gibson, E. J. (1969). *Principles of perceptual learning and development.* Englewood Cliffs, NJ: Prentice-Hall.

Gladwin, T. (1970). *East is a big bird.* Cambridge, MA: Harvard University Press.

Goodenough, F. L. (1949). *Mental testing.* New York: Rinehart & Company.

Grudin, J. R. (1983). Error patterns in novice and skilled transcription typing. In W. E. Cooper (Ed.), *Cognitive aspects of skilled typewriting* (pp. 121–143). New York: Springer-Verlag.

Hamblin, D. J. (1966, March 18). They are "idiot savants"—Wizards of the calendar. *Life,* p. 106.

Halsey, R. M., & Chapanis, A. (1951). On the number of absolutely identifiable spectral hues. *Journal of the Optical Society of America, 41,* 1057–1058.

Hanes, R. M., & Rhoades, M. V. (1959). Color identification as a function of extended practice. *Journal of the Optical Society of America, 49,* 1060–1064.

Hartman, E. M. (1954). The influence of practice and pitch distance between tones on the absolute identification of pitch. *American Journal of Psychology, 67,* 1–14.

Hebb, D. O. (1961). Distinctive features of learning in the higher animal. In J. F. Delafresnoye (Ed.), *Brain mechanisms and learning* (pp. 37–46). Oxford: Blackwell.

Horwitz, W. A., Kestenbaum, C., Person, E., & Jarvik, L. (1965). Identical twins—"Idiot savants"—Calendar calculators. *American Journal of Psychiatry, 121,* 1075–1079.

Hunt, E. (1978). Mechanics of verbal ability. *Psychological Review, 85,* 109–130.

Hunt, E., & Love, T. (1972). How good can memory be? In A. W. Melton & E. Martin (Eds.), *Coding processes in human memory,* New York: Holt, Rinehart & Winston.

Jones, H. E. (1926). Phenomenal memorizing as a special ability. *Journal of Applied Psychology, 10,* 367–377.

Kolb, B., & Whishaw, I. Q. (1980). *Fundamentals of human neuropsychology.* San Francisco: W. H. Freeman.

Lafora, G. R. (1934). Estudio psicologico de una debil mental calculadora del calendario. *Archivos de Neurobiologia, Psicologia, Fisiologia, Histologia Neurologia, y Psiquiatria, 14,* 45–70.

Larkin, J. H., McDermott, J., Simon, D. P., & Simon, H. A. (1980). Expert and novice performance in solving physics problems. *Science, 208,* 1335–1342.

Leaning, F. E. (1927). Calculating boys. *British Journal for Psychical Research*, *1*, 374–381.

Luria, A. R. (1968). *The mind of a mnemonist*. New York: Avon.

Martin, P. R., & Fernberger, S. W. (1929). Improvement in memory span. *American Journal of Psychology*, *41*, 91–94.

Miller, G. A. (1956). The magical number seven, plus or minus two. *Psychological Review*, *63*, 81–97.

Mitchell, F. D. (1907). Mathematical prodigies. *Amerian Journal of Psychology*, *18*, 61–143.

Müller, G. E. (1911). Zür Analyse der Gedachtnistätigkeit und des Vorstellungsverlaufes: Teil 1. *Zeitschrift für Psychologie, Erganzungsband 5.*

Müller, G. E. (1913). Neue Versuche mit Rueckle. *Zeitschrift für Psychologie und Physiologie der Sinnesorgane*, *67*, 193–213.

Müller, G. E. (1917). Zür Analyse der Gedachtnistätigkeit und des Vorstellungsverlaufes: Teil 2. *Zeitschrift für Psychologie, Erganzungsband 9.*

Newell, A., & Rosenbloom, P. S. (1981). Mechanisms of skill acquisition and the law of practice. In J. R. Anderson (Ed.), *Cognitive skills and their acquisition* (pp. 1–55). Hillsdale, NJ: Erlbaum.

Otis, F. E. (1925). Phenomenal memory in its bearing upon various mental tests. *Journal of Applied Psychology*, *9*, 311–318.

Parker, S. W. (1918). Orthogenic cases 12: Obadiah, a child with a numerical obsession. *The Psychological Clinic*, *12*, 105–131.

Parsons, O. A. (1968, April). *July 19, 132, 470 is a Saturday: Idiot–savant calendar-calculating twins.* Paper presented at the meeting of the Southwestern Psychological Association, New Orleans.

Plomin, R., & DeFries, J. C. (1980). Genetics and intelligence: Recent data. *Intelligence*, *4*, 15–24.

Plomin, R., & Rowe, D. C. (1978). A twin study of temperament in young children. *Annual Progress in Child Psychiatry and Child Development*, 216–222.

Pollack, I., Johnson, L. B., & Knaff, P. R. (1959). Running memory span. *Journal of Experimental Psychology*, *57*, 137–146.

Rimland, B. (1978, August). The autistic savant. *Psychology Today*, pp. 69–80.

Robertson, J. P. S. (1958). Exceptional memory for dates and weather in a schizoid psychopath. *Journal of General Psychology*, *58*, 37–39.

Scheerer, M., Rothman, E., & Goldstein, D. (1945). A case study of an "idiot savant": An experimental study of personality organization. *Psychological Monographs* (4, Whole No. 269).

Schneider, W., & Shiffrin, R. M. (1977). Controlled and automatic human information processing: 1. Detection, search, and attention. *Psychological Review*, *84*, 1–66.

Scripture, E. W. (1891). Arithmetical prodigies. *Journal of Psychology*, *4*, 1–59.

Sergeant, D. (1969). Experimental investigation of absolute pitch. *Journal of Research in Music Education*, *17*, 135–143.

Sergeant, D., & Roche, S. (1973). Perceptual shifts in the auditory information processing of young children. *Psychology of Music*, *1*(2), 39–48.

Shepard, R. N. (1963). Analyses of proximities as a technique for the study of information processing in man. *Human Factors*, *5*, 33–48.

Shiffrin, R. M., & Schneider, W. (1977). Controlled and automatic human information processing: 2. Perceptual learning, automatic attending and a general theory. *Psychological Review*, *84*, 127–189.

Smith, S. B. (1983). *The great mental calculators: The psychology, methods, and lives of calculating prodigies, past and present.* New York: Columbia University Press.

Spearman, C., & Jones, L. W. (1950). *Human ability.* London: Macmillan.

Susukita, T. (1933). Untersuchung eines ausserordentlichen Gedaechtnisses in Japan (1). *Tohoku Psychologica Folia, 1* 111–134.

Susukita, T. (1934). Untersuchung eines ausserordentlichen Gedaechtnisses in Japan (2). *Tohoku Psychologica Folia, 2,* 14–42.

Ward, W. D. (1963). Absolute pitch, Part 1. *Sound, 2*(3), 14–21.

Ward, W. D., & Burns, E. M. (1982). Absolute pitch. In D. Deutsch (Ed.), *The Psychology of music* (pp. 431–451). New York: Academic Press.

Wizel, A. (1904). Ein Fall von phaenomenalem Rechentalent bei einen Imbecillen. *Archiv für Psychiatrie und Nervenkrankheiten, 38,* 122–155.

Wyatt, R. F. (1945). Improvability of pitch discrimination. *Psychological Monographs, 58*(2, Whole No. 267).

Zubek, J. P. (1969). Physiological and biochemical effects. In J. P. Zubek (Ed.), *Sensory deprivation: Fifteen years of research* (pp. 254–288). New York: Appleton-Century-Crofts.

Zwislocki, J., Maire, F., Feldman, A. S., & Rubin, H. (1958). On the effect of practice and motivation on the threshold of audibility. *Journal of the Acoustical Society of America, 30,* 254–262.

25

Special Talents
of Autistic Savants

BERNARD RIMLAND
DEBORAH FEIN

Remarkable Savants

Autistic children present us with a a number of baffling mysteries. Their striking disinterest in interacting with others (even their parents), their preternatural good looks, and, perhaps above all, their relatively frequent manifestations of extraordinary mental powers seem almost designed to provoke bewilderment. In this chapter we report a taxonomy of the unusual abilities, primarily of autistic children, but also of mentally retarded idiot savants, and discuss several theoretical explanations for their extraordinary performances.

In his review of research on the idiot savant, Hill (1978) employed the following definition: "A savant is a mentally retarded person demonstrating one or more skills above the level expected of non-retarded individuals" (p. 281). For the most part, the special skills appear to fall within several areas: music, calendar calculating, mechanics, memory, sensory discrimination, and calculation. Let us begin with several recently described cases.

A savant who has attracted a good deal of attention in both the television and print media is Nadia, the subject of an excellent book by Lorna Selfe (*Nadia: A Case of Extraordinary Drawing Ability in an Autistic Child*, 1977). Nadia's mother had brought the child at age $6\frac{1}{2}$, to the Child Development Research Unit at Nottingham University because Nadia had almost no speech and was making no progress in the local school for severely abnormal children. The mother mentioned to the interviewing psychologist that Nadia liked to draw and showed her some of Nadia's drawings. One must see the drawings, which are reproduced in Lorna Selfe's book, in order to imagine their effect on the psychologist: A normal 6-year-old would have been hailed as a creative genius for producing such pictures. Nadia, however, was a clumsy, lethargic, and passive child who could not be counted upon to recognize her own name. Nadia's story, and of course her drawings, created

Bernard Rimland. Institute for Child Behavior Research, San Diego, California.
Deborah Fein. Laboratory of Neuropsychology, Boston University School of Medicine, Boston, Massachusetts; and Department of Psychology, University of Connecticut, Storrs, Connecticut.

somewhat of a furor in Great Britain and, later, in the United States, where her story was told both in national publications and on network television.

Some of the 146 drawings in the book are not very good, but others are truly excellent and would be a credit to a gifted adult artist. It is of special interest from the standpoint of this chapter that Nadia had started drawing at about $3\frac{1}{2}$ years of age and reportedly had not started by scribbling. Her mother reported that Nadia began drawing recognizable objects from "the moment she put pen to paper."

Nadia had reached 10 years of age when the book was written. She had not progressed very far socially or academically. She had developed a little speech, could count, and had a few social skills. By this time her drawing skills had deteriorated considerably.

Not surprisingly, the television and magazine writers concluded that it was the development of Nadia's social and academic skills, modest as they were, that had resulted in the decline of her artistic capabilities. It seemed plausible, and it may be true, that the structured learning that had caused her to begin to use more of her left hemisphere had taken its toll by making the creative drawing ability, presumably based largely in the right hemisphere, less potent. The hypothesis is an interesting one: regrettably, we are in no position to test it.

Another remarkable savant, who has autistic features but who cannot be called truly autistic, is Richard Wawro. Richard is a gifted artist, and his colorful renditions of scenes he has observed in the *National Geographic* Magazine or on television are brightly colored, beautifully composed, and, remarkably enough, the product of a person who has been declared legally blind (Blank, 1983)!

At age 30 Richard Wawro was just beginning to learn to write his name, and his speech was intelligible only to members of his own family and to others who were willing to listen to him carefully and patiently. Richard's "paintings" (actually produced with artist's crayons) have been displayed in one-man shows throughout Europe and the United States. Strangely, Richard, like Nadia, was born in Scotland of Polish parents. Also like Nadia, Richard showed his precocious artistic ability as a very young child.

The story of Alonzo Clemmons, a severely retarded young black man, has appeared on both national television and in *The New York Times*. Alonzo produces extraordinarily beautiful sculptures, primarily of animals. His skill in sculpting was discovered only when a worker at the institution where he resided chanced upon Alonzo's collection of tiny sculptures of various animals, composed of tar he had dug from the parking lot with his fingernails! His exceptional talent was quickly recognized, and bronze copies of his works now sell in art galleries for thousands of dollars.

Perhaps the most extraordinary of all the savants yet identified is Leslie Lemke. Leslie's story has been featured on the *That's Incredible* television show as well as in the *Reader's Digest* (Blank, 1982). His story also appeared in fictionalized form on television, and *May's Boy*, a full-length book, has been written about him (Monty, 1981). Leslie was born not only blind but totally without eyes, and was further severely crippled with cerebral palsy. His natural parents abandoned him soon after birth, feeling that the child, who appeared to be not only blind but also

deaf, and who did not even respond to touch, was totally beyond hope. Nevertheless, a kindly nurse, May Lemke, decided to adopt the infant and thereafter devoted
her life to caring for him. Not until he was 16 years old was May able to get Leslie
to stand by himself for the first time. He was utterly without speech and seemed to
have very few desires. He did not speak his first sentence until his mid-20s, but at
age 28 he "began talking in earnest."

When Leslie was about 20 years old, May and her husband were awakened at
3 A.M. on a winter morning to the sound of someone playing Tchaikovsky's Piano
Concerto No. 1. on their piano. The music was being played by Leslie, who had
never played the piano before or even shown any interest in the instrument. In a
short time Leslie turned out to be a remarkably good musician, both vocally and on
the piano.[1]

A different type of savant skill, calendar calculation, was the forte of the
well-known and widely described twin savants George and Charles, who were
residents of the Bronx State Hospital in New York. George and Charles have been
the subject of a number of articles in professional journals (e.g., Altshuler &
Brebbia, 1968; Horwitz, Kestenbaum, Person, & Jarvik, 1965). Both of them could
figure out virtually instantly on what day of the week a date would fall over a range
of thousands of years into the past or into the future. They could, in addition,
answer such difficult questions as "During what years between 1780 and 1795 did
the 7th of August fall on a Wednesday?" The twins could also remember, with
extraordinary accuracy, virtually every event that had happened to them during
most of their lives and could also tell with precision what the weather had been on
a certain day: "On April 15, 1956, Dr. Williams came to visit me and to ask me
questions about dates. It was rainy and windy in the morning, but the sun came out
in the middle of the afternoon." (personal visit, B. R. 1966).

Savant Abilities and Autism

Although savant abilities occur in the population of autistic children far more
frequently than in any other group, it is by no means true that all autistic children
exhibit these skills. Some idiot savants in the severely retarded population who
manifest unusual mental abilities may also exhibit a few of the signs of autism, but
many do not.

Several investigators have looked for cognitive correlates of special ability
using formal IQ measures. Hill (1982) found that retarded savants performed
better than nonsavant retarded controls on the Information, Arithmetic, Digit

---

1. (Added in press) The early published accounts of Leslie's background appear to be in error. D. A.
Treffert, in interviewing family members and reviewing medical records for his forthcoming book
Savant: Genius Among Us, Genius Within Us, Harper & Row (in press, 1988) learned that Leslie had
been exposed to the piano starting at age 7 or 8. He was able to play folk songs and religious songs before
the "miracle" night. May, his adoptive mother, already quite elderly at the time, and confused by the
extraordinary event of his playing classical music for the first time, without practice, overlooked his
prior piano work.

Span, and Block Design subtests of the WAIS. He further suggested that savants skilled in memory and calendar calculating did equally well on verbal and performance subtests, while those skilled in music had superior verbal skills, and those skilled in art had superior performance skills. Spitz and LaFontaine (1973) also found that savants had a higher digit span than nonsavant retarded controls; in fact, they were at normal levels. Duckett (1976), on the other hand, using tasks drawn from the Guilford Structure of Intellect Model, found no striking differences between retarded savants and nonsavant controls.

It is a matter of considerable interest, and possibly of considerable importance, that a number of people at the genius or near-genius level in the "normal" population have also exhibited some signs of autism. Many of the eccentricities—the "absent-minded professor" habits—of geniuses such as Newton and Einstein fall into the category of autistic traits. A few years ago, chess champion Bobby Fischer impressed the world not only with his skills at chess but with many bizarre habits and mannerisms—strikingly like those seen in autistic individuals. Fischer was reported to have been immersed in working out chess problems on his miniature board during the ceremonies at which he was crowned World Chess Champion. The brilliant inventor and entrepreneur Howard Hughes was reported to have kept a ruler near at hand during his last two years to make sure that the chocolate cakes he had delivered to him each day measured exactly 12 inches on each side. Any cake that deviated from a 12-inch square would be promptly sent back to the kitchen. Insistence on the preservation of sameness is regarded as one of the cardinal signs of autism. It is at least possible that some autistic individuals are incipient geniuses whose eccentricities are so severe and incapacitating that all but minimal participation in the normal world is precluded:

> He reads and understands books on electronics and uses the theories to build devices. He recently put together a tape recorder, fluorescent light and a small transistor radio with some other components so that music from the tape was changed to light energy in the light and then back to music in the radio. By passing his hand between the recorder and the light, he could stop the music. He understands the concepts of electronics, astronomy, music, navigation and mechanics. He knows an astonishing amount about how things work and is familiar with technical terms. By the age of 12, he could find his way all over the city on his bike with a map and compass. He reads Bowditch on navigation. Joe is supposed to have an IQ of 80. He does assembly work in a Goodwill Store. (Letter dated February 16, 1978 from a parent to B. Rimland)

The Institute for Child Behavior Research Study of Autistic Savants

The Institute for Child Behavior Research (ICBR) in San Diego serves as a world registry of cases and as a clearinghouse for information on autism and related disorders. The ICBR files contain data on many thousands of autistic children throughout the United States and many foreign countries. Detailed questionnaires, completed by the parents of the children, provide information on many topics, including "special abilities" the children may display. Our data from the ICBR study that we conducted on autistic savants (Rimland, 1978b; Rimland & Hill,

TABLE 25-1. Incidence of Idiot–Savant Individuals, by Sex, in Population of "Autistic" persons

	N	Percent
Base population of autistic or autisticlike cases	5,400	100.0
Boys with idiot–savant abilities	414	7.7
Girls with idiot–savant abilities	117	2.2
Total cases with idiot–savant abilities	531	9.8
Ratio of boys to girls in base population	3.16:1	
Ratio of boys to girls in idiot–savant sample	3.54:1	

Note. Adapted from Rimland (1978b) in Serban, G. (Ed.) Cognitive Defects in the Development of Mental Illness (p. 46) N.Y.: Brunner/Mazel, with the permission of the editor.

1984) provide a rich phenomenology of talents seen and permit a first estimate of incidence data.

At the time the ICBR savant study was conducted, the data bank contained case files on approximately 5,400 autistic children. A search of the data bank for children reported to have special abilities produced the records for some 561 cases. Thirty of these cases were rejected from the savant study when examination of the case files indicated that the skills possessed were insufficiently remarkable to warrant "savant" status. The remaining 531 cases (9.8%) are tabulated in Table 25-1.

The approximately 10% incidence of savant skills in the autistic population may be compared with the value of 0.06% reported by Hill (1974) in his survey of several hundred residential facilities for the retarded. Of the 300 facilities queried, only 111 responded. These 111 facilities served approximately 90,000 retardates, of whom 54 were reported to display savant skills. Hill's finding of approximately 1 idiot savant per 2,000 retardates contrasts sharply with our finding of savant skills

TABLE 25-2. Frequency of Kinds of Idiot–Savant Skills in Autistic-type Individuals (Follow-up Sample)

Skill	Boys ($N = 91$)	Girls ($N = 28$)	Total ($N = 119$)	Percent Girls
Music	43	20	63	31.7
Memory	41	7	48	14.5
Art	16	7	23	14.5
Pseudoverbal	16	3	19	15.7
Mathematics	12	5	17	29.4
Mechanical	14	0	14	0
Directions, paths, etc.	13	0	13	0
Coordination	11	5	16	31.2
Calendar calculations	10	3	13	23.0
"Extrasensory perception"	3	1	4	25.0

Note. From Rimland (1978b) in Serban, G. (Ed.). Cognitive Defects in the Development of Mental Illness (p. 47) N. Y.: Brunner/Mazel with the permission of the editor.

in 1 out of 10 autistic individuals. (It must be acknowledged, however, that institutions are not the ideal settings in which to foster or recognize unusual talents.)

In the earlier Rimland (1978b) report on the ICBR study of autistic savants, it was noted that among the subgroups of autistic children who fit the definition of classical early infantile autism (Kanner syndrome), the incidence of savant skills was considerably higher than in the larger population of children who displayed autism, as it is more loosely (and commonly) defined. The identification of children with classical early infantile autism was made through the use of Rimland's Diagnostic Checklist, Form E2. Interested readers are referred to the original report (Rimland, 1978b) for a discussion of this matter.

After identifying the children with savant abilities, he wrote to the parents to obtain further information. The questionnaire covered such areas as varieties of special performance; examples of the child's performance; presence of multiple abilities; age pattern of onset and, where applicable, decline of performance; manner in which the child acquired interest in the activities; and familial occurrence of related superior ability. Usable replies were received from 119 parents in time for analysis. Table 25-2 presents a breakdown, by sex, of the various kinds of skills reported for the savants in the sample.

Music and Memory Skills

Table 25-2 reveals that music and memory skills are by far the most common. The musical skill of these children is primarily a memory ability—auditory memory—but their musical skills are by no means limited to mere auditory memory. Nor are the memory skills limited to auditory materials, as is shown by the following examples:

Music

"Can play anything he hears *once* on a piano or any instrument with keys, has perfect pitch."

"She can sing any note you tell her to and can tell what note (and key) is being played. Ilene woke up singing as an infant and never let up. Ilene knows practically every song written—who wrote it, what show it is from (or film), who first recorded it, in what year it was popular, etc. She also has a large command of the classical repertoire. She composes at the piano and has taught herself to play the guitar as one would play a zither—on her lap—sliding her finger up and down all the strings at once."

"First noted musical and photographic ability at age 2. With 'tape recorder' accuracy, she would explode from her silence with a total song with words—long verses—pages read, etc."

Memory

"Photographic memory when 'switched on.' Can recollect incidents of early childhood, can quote time and place of minute trivial incidents. Seems to *remember in pictures* which he can 'look at' at will."

"One really unusual thing about his memory is how it works. The first time Russ ever became involved in a game with me was with the alphabet. He said A to me. I said B to him. He went on to C and so we continued to the end. Then he started with AB, so I said CD and so on to the end. After that he said ABC, I went to DEG, etc. But what floored me was what he did next. He said Z. For fun I said Y and he went to X. I couldn't go further and asked him what came next. On a hunch I asked him to say the alphabet backwards. He went from Z to A with hardly a hesitation."

"Exceptional memory—almost photographic—I say almost because he has to be interested in a subject to even bother with it. Recently after the final episode of the television program 'Roots', the credits were run fairly quickly. Todd rarely watches television so he wasn't familiar with any of the actors. But he could tell us what actor played each part. Even the actors with unfamiliar African names. It really amazed us."

Art

Table 25-2 shows art to be in third place, far behind music and memory as a skill common in autistic savants. It is of special interest that in the autistic savants' production of works of art, *just as is the case in music and memory performances*, close fidelity to the physical stimulus characterizes the savants' efforts. It is not unusual for a drawing of a house by an autistic savant to be carried out in such detail that even the pull rings at the bottoms of the window shades are depicted. One mother of an autistic savant noted that even at age 3 her son could draw cars and trucks with wheels that were so round that neither she nor her husband could match the little boy's skill.

Pseudoverbal skills

Pseudoverbal skills refer to the child's unusual ability to produce or reproduce words by reading and/or writing, including perfect spelling. Despite this ability, the child has a very limited capacity to *understand* words. Some examples from parents' reports:

"He never forgets a word, its meaning or spelling, so his vocabulary is that of a highly educated person. His IQ is 80."

"She can type pages, error-free. No typographical errors, no spelling errors." [The father sent a page of very long and difficult sentences the girl (at 18) had typed from memory after having seen it only once $1\frac{1}{2}$ years earlier.]

"He writes beautifully in Japanese, can print in Old English as fast as he can print normally. He has a knack for foreign accents, is excellent at languages, but of course has the same base communication problem he has in English. He has a working knowledge of French, Spanish, Japanese and Russian—knows at least the alphabet and pronunciations of Arabic, Hebrew and several others."

Other Skills

The following quotations from the parents' reports illustrate the various other types of skills that have been reported:

Mathematics

"Age 11, worked out all primes to c. 1100, could tell you of any odd number, whether it was a prime; if not, gave prime factors. Many remarkable examples of factorization, which she did obsessively."

"Could multiply numbers in his head at age 5, compute square roots in his head at age 9."

Mechanical Skills

"Richie's mechanical skills have always been outstanding. At age 3, he preferred to play with cast-off appliances donated by friends and relatives—clocks, radios, TV's, vacuum sweepers, etc. He could take them apart and put them back together without error."

Directions

"If we travel in summer to the country, and we have made the trip before, Herbert can lead you to the lodge; i.e. when you leave the highway and must find your way here and there down dirt roads, etc., he can name every turn, every street you will pass, every landmark and do this without error."

Coordination

"He is very, very good at swimming; his teacher says he is a 'natural' but he could never race—he forgets what he is doing."

"Swam like a fish from age three months."

"Jim had a fantastic ability to balance things, even seemingly to defy gravity. At 18 months, he built elaborate structures with blocks that seemed not to be able to stand. He balanced round coasters that we challenged adults to do and they couldn't. He'd make elaborate piles of favorite possessions that should have collapsed."

"Once he even walked around the rail of his crib. I can't believe that now, but I saw it with my own eyes."

Extrasensory Perception

A surprising outcome of our study was the four reports by parents who claimed, often with disbelief, that their children had exhibited, consistently, signs of extrasensory perception. Here are three examples:

"Teachers have also noticed that George probably has ESP. He seems to be very psychic. We would decide to pick up George from school suddenly, if we were in the area (he usually rode the bus). He would tell the teacher we were coming, and would come to open the door when we arrived. So he has many special abilities, but cannot write his name or read a sentence."

"An extraordinary ability to hear conversations out of the range of hearing, and to pick up thoughts not spoken."

"Possesses verified ESP. First observed around age 4. Accurately related an accidental occurrence known only to her father. His watch crystal fell out in the bathroom and was immediately replaced. Michelle accurately related entire incident back to father a short time thereafter. Several dozens of similar "clairvoyant" incidents have occurred since this first incident. Statistical probability of coincidental knowledge nil."

Chess

To our surprise, none of the parents listed special abilities in chess or checkers. This may have been an artifact of the way in which our questionnaire was worded, but it is more likely to be a consequence of the noncompetitiveness of autistic persons. In view of the autistic person's characteristic indifference to others, it should not surprise us that interpersonal competitiveness is not a strong motive. One parent who tried to teach his son chess found that although the rules were quickly understood, the game was played very passively, with no motivation to win. The competitiveness—desire to win—that is seen even in small children and that we take for granted was not there.

On the other hand, in other contexts, parents have reported to one of us (B. R.) autistic individuals who have easily outperformed much brighter than average adults on various tasks. One autistic young woman consistently solved anagram problems presented in the daily newspaper immediately upon being shown them. She was much faster at solving the anagrams than her brother (a law student) and her father (a college-educated businessman). An autistic young man, very retarded by most standards, was consistently able to solve problems (consisting of familiar sayings, phrases, or song titles that were presented to contestants gradually, only a few letters at a time) on a television game show (*Wheel of Fortune*) much faster than any of the contestants and any of the other viewers in his family at home. These situations were not necessarily perceived as being competitive by the autistic individuals, however.

Multiple Skills

One of the differences between autistic savants and idiot savants appears to be the relatively higher frequency of multiple skills in the former. Two examples from parents' reports:

"He has apparently total recall for statistics, such as baseball, football, hockey, basketball scores, individual records, etc. He knows capitals and heads of governments for all countries of the world, their flags, can make a good outline map of any of them (and keep them current). He reads almanacs, encyclopedias and dictionaries. You never have to look anything up if Peter is around. He remembers dates, birthdays, etc. He seems also to be quite artistic—draws quite well, and the last couple of years has shown some originality (not much but a step forward). Is inclined to copy. Peter could do calendar calculating, but won't do it anymore. He could draw an outline of the 48 states and place the capital cities when he was two years old."

"I noticed when George was $2\frac{1}{2}$ years of age that he had a special ability in sense of direction. He would mention the place he wanted to go, and if we decided to go someplace else first, the tantrums of self-destruction would start. He knew the minute the route was changed. His motor development is excellent, such as tumbling, riding bicycles, swimming, kicking balls, etc. He taught himself all of this since no one could teach him. He excels on the trampoline, and it would be hard for a normal child or adult to compete with him in this. He has been able to read from age 4 to present things or places that meant something to him such as Food Giant, Safeway, etc. He started talking around $2\frac{1}{2}$ or 3 years of age, but only says what he wants, does not carry on a conversation."

Inspection of the forms returned to us show that more than half (53%) of the children have multiple special abilities. One child was reported to have five special skills, 7 children had four skills, 13 had three skills, and 38 had two skills. Only 56 of the 119 (47%) exhibited a single skill.

As might be expected, most of the combinations of skills were reported in children with unusually retentive memories, a combination of unusual musical ability and memory being by far the most common pair. In normal populations, musical and mathematical ability are frequently found in association, 6 of the 17 autistic savants with mathematical skills also had unusual musical ability.

Familial Tendencies

When asked about familial tendencies toward the unusual skills seen in the autistic children, a number of parents reported that some close relatives of the child showed similar talents, especially in music, art, and mathematics. Of special interest were the fathers of our five mathematically talented autistic savant girls. Two of the five fathers are physicists, one is a farmer, and the fourth is a factory worker. (One listed no occupation.)

Age-Related Cognitive Changes

Rimland (1968) had reported that many autistic children show a remarkable, but difficult-to-characterize, change in their cognitive ability at approximately $5\frac{1}{2}$ years of age. Partly to investigate this phenomenon, but also because of our interest in the developmental history of the savant skills, we asked the parents to draw a graph depicting the age at which the child's special abilities were first noted, the age at which the abilities reached their peak, and, for those cases in which the abilities had declined, the age-related course of the decline. Figure 25-1 shows the age of onset, for both sexes combined, for savant musical abilities. As the figure shows, there was a very sharp rise in the appearance of musical skills at age 2. By age 4, fully two thirds of the savants with musical skills had made their skills manifest.

Savant Sex Ratios

The data in Table 25-1 on autistic savants show a ratio of 3.51 males to each female. This is approximately the same male-to-female ratio as is found in the autistic population in general.

Hill (1974) reported a 6:1 male-to-female ratio based on his analysis of 63 published reports covering 105 individuals who were described as idiot savants.

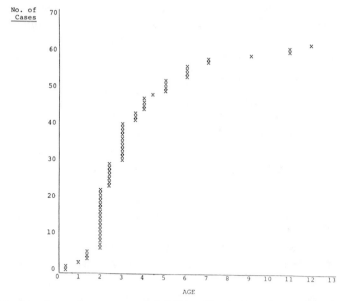

FIGURE 25-1. Age of onset for savant musical abilities. Xs, number of cases. From Rimland (1978). In G. Serban (Ed.), Cognitive defects in the development of mental illness. New York, Brunner/Mazel. Courtesy of the editor and publisher.

Since there are many more severely retarded males than females, it is possible that among idiot savants, as among autistic savants, the male-to-female ratio approximates that in the general autistic and severely retarded populations.

New Varieties of Savant Performance

Subsequent to the completion of the ICBR autistic savant study, two new varieties of savant performance were reported to the ICBR that are of sufficient interest to warrant their being recorded here:

Visual Measurement
     "[Alan could] accurately determine an object's dimensions—a room, a fence, a driveway, etc.—by just glancing at it. These amazing skills did not appear to be attached to an extensive general mathematical ability, but rather seemed isolated. This special skill was limited to a particular range of numbers. His accuracy of estimating dimensions of items larger than 50 feet in size was better than average, but much less precise than his ability to estimate the size of smaller objects. . . . His accuracy in guessing the size of things smaller than 20 feet was usually accurate within $\frac{1}{4}$ inch."

Sense of Time
     "[An institutionalized adult] could report the time of day or night to within a minute or so, even if he had not seen a watch or clock for an extended period."

An autistic child also had this same ability, even in his sleep: "When I went into his room late at night to close the window, because it had started to rain or grow cold, he would awaken slightly and say 'It's 2:14 A.M.,' then go back to sleep."

Suggested Neural Mechanisms

We would like to suggest three types of possible neural mechanisms for the extraordinary savant skills displayed by some autistic children, each of which can be related to theories proposed by other authors in this book. These are not meant to be mutually exclusive but may coexist in any combination.

Attentional Systems

Various abnormalities of attention have long been noted in the autistic clinical picture, and some of the earliest cognitive theories of autism have focused on this domain (Hutt, Hutt, Lee, & Ounsted, 1965; Rimland, 1964). Rimland (1964, 1978), in speculating on how autistic savants perform their feats, suggests that the autistic child's pathological inability to broaden his or her focus of attention results in the gating out of external stimuli distractors, thus resulting in intense mental energy being devoted to an internal preoccupation. Judging from the products of the autistic child's skills, he concludes that the child's attention is focused on "high-fidelity" reproduction of the *physical* characteristics of stimuli rather than on abstract, conceptual ideas. He cites as examples the autistic savant's ability to faithfully reproduce complex visual or auditory stimuli after one exposure. Rimland (1964) argues strongly that these two aspects of attention can be separated theoretically and cites research going back to Galton's experiments on imagery to bolster his case. One can be quite undistractible while attending to either physical or conceptual stimuli (see, e.g., Rimland's 1978b anecdote about Newton's absorption in his theories). We shall return to the question of abstract versus image-bound concrete thought in the next section. For now, we shall focus on the question of distractibility.

There is ample clinical and experimental literature (Ornitz, Guthrie, & Farley, 1978; Rimland, 1964; Wing, 1976) to indicate that a primary early symptom of autism, even though it is not found in formal diagnostic criteria, is deficient orienting behavior. The very term "autism" (reverie state) implies such deficiency. One consequence of a persistent depressed or distorted orienting response may be a persistent state of hypodistractibility.

Deficient orienting, we are suggesting, may lead to overly efficient gating out of external stimuli and consequent overfocus on internal processes. But it may have another relevant consequence as well. Orienting may form the primitive biological basis for later development of curiosity, exploration, and novelty-seeking behavior, which is also obviously lacking or reduced in young autistic children. If one thinks in terms of the balance between opposing behavioral tendencies (Kinsbourne & Bemporad, 1983), then the lack of a drive for novelty may allow the opposing behavioral tendency, namely, the drive for repetition and familiarity, to hold sway.

This would reinforce the practice of the skill at the expense of a more varied and flexible behavioral repertoire.

Ericsson and Faivre (Chapter 24, this volume) propose that large amounts of practice alone can account for the extraordinary performance of many skills, including domain-specific memory. We took an informal poll of about 20 psychologists, posing the question of how much an individual with average intelligence could increase his or her digit span of 7, given practice for many hours a week for a year. Many guessed there would be no increase; most said it might be increased to 10–15; no one guessed higher than 20. In fact, Ericsson and Faivre report that one such subject reached a digit span of over 100 and that another reached a span of over 80. Thus there can be a remarkable and counterintuitive potential effect of practice, even where it is not immediately obvious that there is a skill or algorithm that is being practiced. It seems that where there is an apparent skill or algorithm that might be practiced (such as in calendar calculation or memory of specific facts), the effects of focused practice might be even more potent. In fact, extensive practice in calendar calculation over a long period enabled a college student to duplicate the feats of George, the famous savant twin (Rimland, 1978a).

The neural mechanisms for orienting and other relevant features of behavior, such as selective attention and inner versus outer stimulus focus, are not sufficiently understood to postulate a specific site of dysfunction. It is clear that the mechanisms governing the deployment of attention are extremely complex and must involve brain systems at virtually every level of the central and autonomic nervous systems, from the brain-stem reticular activating system, through thalamic and hypothalamic nuclei, to the highest levels of parietal and frontal cortex (see, e.g., Heilman, Watson, & Valenstein, 1985, for a brief recent discussion). Although no attentional mechanism is well understood, one particular structure has been suggested to have a particularly important role in orienting—the hippocampus (Vinogradova, 1975). Furthermore, the hippocampus is hypothesized to have a tonic inhibitory effect on brain-stem arousal mechanisms. This inhibited brain-stem arousal mechanisms, as suggested by Rimland (1964), and reduced orienting behavior should be reflective of *hyperhippocampal*, rather than *hypohippocampal*, functioning. We shall return to discussion of this idea in the final section of this chapter.

Another important facet of this notion of overfocused, intense, undistractible deployment of attention relates to another clinical population that may share this feature. DeLong and Aldershof (Chapter 21, this volume) present data on special skills in children with manic–depressive illness and speculate on a similar attentional mechanism in these children. Rimland (1964) had suggested both a theoretical and familial link between autism and depressive illness and had provided preliminary data (1968) to support the idea. New data obtained by Dwyer and Delong (1985) are confirming a high incidence of manic–depressive disorder in families with autistic members. Thus there may be a genetic link between the several disorders that share this attentional feature. What remains unexplained, however, is the different nature of the preoccupations. The manic–depressive children in Delong and Aldershof's sample (this volume) tended to be preoccupied with affectively charged topics, whereas the autistic children were preoccupied with neutral subjects like train timetables. Clearly, the very different expressions of the preoccupations in the two disorders are not simply a matter of degree; other motivational factors must be in play in the elaboration of autistic symptomatology.

Cortical Rededication

The second notion regarding neural mechanisms in autistic children is that certain cortical areas are reorganized or rededicated in ways that lend themselves to the high-level performance of a particular skill. Theories along these lines are posed in this volume by Waterhouse (Chapter 26) and by Matthysse and Greenberg (Chapter 23). There are several variants of the idea that may relate to autism in particular.

Waterhouse's basic premise is as follows:

> A wide range of special talents . . . all spring from the same global, preconscious, specific set of skills, namely, the ability to generate accurate and elaborate mental representations of images and/or sounds, and to store, manipulate, and recall these sounds, as well as—and more important—the ability to "see" or "hear" complex patterns in those mental sights and sounds. . . . specializations that generate special talents may be hypothesized to operate at an 'end station' of the auditory or visual processing systems, and may consist of a distinctive and/or more extensive organization of the sensory association cortex, or polymodal association cortex . . . the pattern-recognition organization of the visual cortex or auditory/cortex is displayed in association as an open field ready to be used for complex patterning of mental representations. (p. 495, this volume)

Waterhouse's suggested phenomenon would seem to predispose the invidivual to image-bound, concrete, "high-fidelity" thought as opposed to abstract, cross-modal conceptual thought, as differentiated by Rimland (1964, 1978). Thus this reorganization of polysensory cortex to serve the pattern-recognition system of visual or auditory pathways would form a possible basis for this type of thinking.

It is also possible, however, that Waterhouse's mechanism, namely, the dedication of potentially polysensory cortex to the higher processing of information from a particular sensory modality, is accurate but that it rests on functional rededication with no architectural reorganization. The cortical area she mentions, the parietal-occipital-temporal junction, is juxtaposed to the secondary association cortex of both the auditory and the visual systems. Perhaps it comes to serve as (an) additional level(s) of processing for one or both of these systems, serving higher pattern recognition, with architecturally normal structure.

One rare autistic savant skill that would be admirably explained by this mechanism was shown by the autistic twins described in this volume by Matthysse and Greenberg (Chapter 23) and described in detail by Sacks (1985). Aside from the astounding ability they both showed for producing astronomically large prime numbers (discussed by Matthysse and Greenberg), Sacks reports that both of them were also able to determine instantly the number of objects in a very large array (over 100; for other examples of this ability, see Smith, Chapter 2, this volume). They produced the number much too quickly for it to be the result of counting; it seemed, rather, to be a direct perception, much as a normal person might apperceive directly the number of objects in a very small array of three, four, or five items. Waterhouse (Chapter 26, this volume) reports on the visual pattern-recognition skills of another autistic boy who seems to perceive directly patterns that most of us would need to analyze consciously. Leslie Lemke's ability to reproduce Tchaikovsky without practice may represent an auditory analogue of the same phenomenon.

One other variant of the basic thesis is that areas of cortex other than the tertiary association cortex suggested by Waterhouse are rededicated to serve this higher sensory pattern-recognition function. Perhaps the areas of cortex normally dedicated to the most social of tasks are given over in autistic children to this fundamentally asocial process of pattern recognition. Normal children find intrinsically interesting the faces and voices of other people and pay them much attention in the early months and years of life. Perhaps a primary motivational abnormality, that of social disinterest, leads the autistic child at an early age to disregard the faces and speech of other people. The language-comprehension (left temporal) and face-recognition (bilateral inferotemporal) cortical areas may need a wide and varied base of input in early life in order to develop their highly specialized mechanisms for comprehension and recognition. In the motivationally based absence of such input, such areas may not be strongly dedicated to these functions and may thus be available to serve the higher but nonsocial pattern-recognition functions of the auditory and visual systems that they, respectively, adjoin. The autistic child would thus have to rely on general learning mechanisms in order to extract the meaning from speech and faces; indeed, the laborious and artificial language and social learning of some autistic children seems consistent with this idea.

The pictorial productions of such autistic artists as Richard Wawro (Blank, 1983) and Nadia (Selfe, 1977) appear to have a marvelous sense of color and/or form, but both are remarkable for their inept representations of the human face.

Hippocampal Functioning

The third theory regarding neural mechanisms in autistic children relates back to the structure mentioned in the discussion of the first theory—the hippocampus. Some of these ideas were developed in a paper presented by Fein and Waterhouse (1985).

Functions of the hippocampus in animal and clinical literature are very much a subject of controversy (Berger & Orr, 1983; Gray & McNaughton, 1983; Isaacson, 1982; O'Keefe & Nadel, 1978). However, several of the major theories of hippocampal function relate directly to some of the positive symptoms of autism. For example, it has been suggested that the hippocampus is fundamental in the mapping of space, in place learning, in encoding memories contextually, in gating out irrelevant stimuli, and in suppressing the orienting reflex. Deficits in orienting behavior and in gating out external stimuli (sometimes to the point of obliviousness) were discussed earlier. Many autistic children are obsessed with the association between object and place, with spatial layouts, and with routes, and they often have phenomenal visual memories. In addition, when an autistic child produces a memory, it often seems to be a total memory of an episode, complete with date, weather, clothing, and events, rather than being coded in terms of semantic properties. In this regard, it is opposite to the memory deficit of the amnesic with hippocampal damage, who may recognize that something is familiar but be unable to identify it or place it in context. It seems to us, therefore, that one could conceive of autistic memory functioning as having an overly contextual, episodic form of encoding, perhaps consistent with overdependence on hippocampus.

Oscar-Berman (Chapter 9, this volume) has independently arrived at a very similar notion to explain the hypermnestic performances described by Brown and Deffenbacher (Chapter 8, this volume). She suggests that disinhibition or over-stimulation of the hippocampal mechanisms for preserving the record of the stream of consciousness might lead to supranormal memory of the "experiential" type.

Our suggestion of hyperhippocampal functioning has come from an admittedly selective reading of the literature. There are some hippocampal lesion effects, such as fixation of predominant behavioral dispositions and reduced exploratory behavior, that make autistic symptomatology seem more consistent with hippocampal *dysfunction*. It is possible that only some of the complex functions of the hippocampus are overrepresented in autistic behavior and that others are dysfunctional. This division might follow anatomical lines, or the division might be in terms of neurotransmitters. One provocative finding in the animal literature (Plaznik, Danysz, & Kostowski, 1983) is that noradrenaline and serotonin injected into hippocampus may have some opposing behavioral effects. If this is so, it is the results of serotonin injection, including lessened response to pain and less exploratory activity in an open field, that mimic autistic symptoms. In fact, it has been suggested that some autistic children have hyperserotonemia (Young, Kavanagh, Anderson, Shaytwitz, & Cohen, 1982) and other abnormalities of the serotonin system (Boullin, Coleman, & O'Brien, 1970).

Another possible mechanism for hyperhippocampal function is raised by the theories of Mishkin (Mishkin, Malamut, & Bachevalier, 1984; Murray & Mishkin, 1985). He suggests that the amygdala and hippocampus together form a system for laying down conscious memories. Each structure alone has specialization, the hippocampus for place learning and the amygdala for the making of cross-modal association, but each is able to do basic within-modality association. Perhaps deficiencies in amygdala (which has been shown to be intimately and consistently associated with changes in social behavior—Isaacson, 1982; Mirsky, 1960; Mishkin, personal communication, 1985, June) lead the child to an overreliance on hippocampus for basic formation of memories.

Several important developments have been reported recently which shed new light on the neurophysiological basis of autism, and thus, indirectly, on the basis of the unusual talents which are found inordinately often in autistic patients.

Recently, Bauman and Kemper (1985) reported morphological abnormalities in the amygdala and hippocampus as well as in the cerebellum and brain stem nuclei of an autistic young man. This man, however, from the case description, appears to have been very low functioning, with virtually no language, no special skills, no cognitive sparing at all. Perhaps only the high-functioning autistic child, with some of the special skills (especially in memory) discussed earlier, demonstrates hyperhippocampal function. The cerebellar findings are of particular interest, however.

Cerebellar Impairment

Further evidence of cerebellar impairment in autism has been reported by Courchesne and his coworkers. Courchesne, Hesselink, Jernigan and Yeung-Courchesne (1987) have reported finding, through magnetic resonance imaging, striking hypoplasia of the superior posterior vermis of the cerebellum in a high functioning autistic young man. In a subsequent study Courchesne, Yeung-Courchesne, Press, Jernigan and Hesselink (1987) found evidence of vermal cerebellar hypoplasia in 14 of 18 high functioning autistic young men. Courchesne et al. (submitted) speculate that the cerebellar impairment may produce the symptoms of autism by disrupting numerous brainstem and thalamic systems, including, most importantly, the reticular activating system, as well as the vestibular oculomotor system and various other serotonergic, dopaminergic and noradrenergic systems. For a comprehensive discussion of his neurophysiological theory of autism, see Courchesne (1987b, and in press).

Prescott appears to have been the first researcher to implicate faulty cerebellar function in autism (e.g., Prescott 1971, 1975). Prescott based his ideas on theoretical grounds and animal studies, rather than the post-mortem and MRI methods which Bauman and Kemper and Courchesne have used so effectively in demonstrating cerebellar defects in cases of autism. Although Prescott did not address the topic of primary interest in this volume, exceptional talent, his pioneering efforts to show the relationship between cerebellar defect and autism, and the implications of cerebellar defects for the impaired social behavior seen in autistic persons, deserve acknowledgement.

In closing this chapter, a statement written by the first author a quarter of a century ago still seems perfectly apt: "The brain mechanisms postulated in this paper are admittedly very tentative and speculative. However, whether or not these specific hypotheses are in time confirmed, the writer is firm in his belief that Sarason and Gladwin were correct when they wrote of early infantile autism, "The importance of these cases to the development of a science of psychology would seem to be vastly beyond what their relatively rare occurrence in the general population would suggest" (1958, p. 345, 1964, p. 2). And we would add that understanding the abilities of the autistic savant may be of fundamental importance to the understanding of ability in general.

References

Altshuler, K. Z., & Brebbia, D. R. (1968). Sleep patterns and EEG recordings in twin idiot savants. *Psychophysiology*, *5*, 244–245.

Bauman, M., & Kemper, T. L. (1985). Histoanatomic observations of the brain in early infantile autism. *Neurology*, *35*, 866–874.

Berger, T. W., & Orr, W. B. (1983). Hippocampectomy selectively disrupts discrimination reversal conditioning of the rabbit nictitating membrane response. *Behavioral Brain Research*, *8*, 49–68.

Blank, J. P. (1982, October). The miracle of May Lemke's love. *Reader's Digest*, pp. 81–86.

Blank, J. P. (1983, October). I can see feeling good. *Reader's Digest*, pp. 98–104.

Boullin, D. J., Coleman, M., & O'Brien, R. A. (1970). Abnormalities in platelet 5-hydroxytryptamine efflux in patients with infantile autism. *Nature, 226,* 371–372.

Courchesne, E., Hesselink, J., Jernigan, T., & Yeung-Courchesne, R, (1987). Abnormal neuroanatomy in a nonretarded person with autism. *Archives of neurology, 44,* 335–341.

Courchesne, E. (1987b). A neurophysiological view of autism. In E. Schopler & G. Mesibov (Eds.), *Neurobiological issues in autism,* pp. 285–324. New York: Plenum Publishing Corp.

Courchesne, E. Neuroanatomical systems involved in infantile autism: Implications of cerebellar abnormalities. In G. Dawson (Ed.), *Autism: new perspectives in diagnosis, nature, and treatment.* New York: The Guilford Press, in press.

Courchesne, E., Yeung-Courchesne, R., Press, G., Jernigan, T. & Hesselink, J. (1987). Hypoplasia of cerebellar vermal lobules VI and VII in infantile autism. Submitted for publication.

Duckett, J. (1976). *Idiot savants: Super specialization in mentally retarded persons.* Unpublished doctoral dissertation, University of Texas at Austin.

Dwyer, J., & DeLong, G. R. (1985, November). *Families of the autistic syndromes: Preliminary report of an ongoing study.* Paper presented at the Northeast Regional meeting of National Society for Autistic Children, Portland, Maine.

Fein, D., & Waterhouse, L. (1985, June). *Infantile autism: Delineating the key deficits.* Paper presented at the International Neuropsychological Symposium, North Berwick, Scotland.

Gray, J. A., & MacNaughton, N. (1983). Comparison between the biobehavioral effects of septal and hippocampal lesions: A review. *Neuroscience and Biobehavioral Reviews, 7,* 119–188.

Heilman, K., Watson, R. T., & Valenstein, E. (1985). Neglect and related disorders. In K. M. Heilman, & E. Valenstein (Eds.), *Clinical neuropsychology* (pp. 243–294). New York: Oxford University Press.

Hill, A. L. (1974). Idiot savants: Rate of incidence. *Perceptual and Motor Skills, 44,* 12–13.

Hill, A. L. (1978). Savants: Mentally retarded individuals with special skills. In N. Ellis, (Ed.), *International review of research in mental retardation* (pp. 277–298). New York: Academic Press.

Hill, A. L. (1982, April). *The performance of idiot savants on the WAIS.* A poster presented at the meeting of the Eastern Psychological Association, Baltimore.

Horwitz, W. A., Kestenbaum, C., Person, E., & Jarvik, L. (1965). Identical twin idiot savant calendar calculators. *American Journal of Psychiatry, 121,* 1075–1079.

Hutt, S., Hutt, C., Lee, D., & Ounsted, C. (1965). A behavioral and EEG study of autistic children. *Journal of Psychiatric Research, 3,* 181–198.

Isaacson, R. L. (1982). *The limbic system* (2nd ed.). New York: Plenum Press.

Kinsbourne, M., & Bemporad, B. (1983). Lateralization of emotion: A model and the evidence. In N. Fox, & R. Davidson (Eds.), *The psychobiology of affect* (pp. 254–291). Hillsdale, NJ: Erlbaum.

Mirsky, A. (1960). Studies of the effects of brain lesions on social behavior in *Macaca mulatta*: Methodological and theoretical considerations. *Annals of the New York Academy of Sciences, 85,* 785–794.

Mishkin, M., Malamut, B., & Bachevalier, J. (1984). Memories and habits: Two neural systems. In G. Lynch, J. L. McGaugh, & N. M. Weinberger (Eds.), *Neurobiology of learning and memory* (pp. 65–79). New York: Guilford Press.

Monte, S (1981). *May's boy.* Nashville: Thomas Nelson.

Murray, E. A., & Mishkin, M. (1985). Amygdalectomy impairs crossmodal association in monkeys. *Science, 228,* 604–605.

O'Keefe, J., & Nadel, L. (1978). *The hippocampus as a cognitive map*. Oxford: Oxford University Press.

Plaznik, A., Danysz, W., & Kostowski, W. (1983). Some behavioral effects of microinjections of noradrenaline and serotonin into the hippocampus of the rat. *Physiology & Behavior, 31*, 625–631.

Prescott, J. W. (1971). Early somatosensory deprivation as an ontogenetic process in the abnormal development of the brain and behavior. In I. Goldsmith & J. Moor-Jankowski (Eds.), *Medical primatology*, New York: S. Karger, pp. 1–20.

Prescott, J. W. (1975). Developmental neuropsychophysics. In J. W. Prescott, Read & Coursin (Eds.), *Brain function and malnutrition: Neuropsychological methods of assessment*, New York: John Wiley & Sons, pp. 325–358.

Rimland, B. (1964). *Infantile autism. The syndrome and its implications for a neural theory of behavior*. New York: Appleton-Century-Crofts.

Rimland, B. (1968). On the objective diagnosis of infantile autism. *Acta Paedopsychiatrica, 35*, 146–161.

Rimland, B. (1978a, August). Inside the mind of the autistic savant. *Psychology Today*, pp. 68–80.

Rimland, B. (1978b). Savant capabilities of autistic children and their cognitive implications. In G. Serban (Ed.), *Cognitive defects in the development of mental illness*. New York: Brunner/Mazel.

Rimland, B., & Hill, A. L. (1984). Idiot Savants. In J. Wortis, (Ed.), *Mental retardation and development disabilities*, Volume 13, pp. 155–169. New York: Plenum.

Sacks, O. (1985). The twins. In *The man who mistook his wife for a hat*. New York: Summit Books.

Selfe, L. (1977). *Nadia: A case of extraordinary drawing ability in an autistic child*. New York: Harcourt Brace Jovanovich.

Spitz, H. H., & LaFontaine, L. (1973). The digit span of idiot savants. *American Journal of Mental Deficiency, 77*, 757–759.

Vinogradova, O. S. (1975). The hippocampus and the orienting reflex. In E. N. Sokolov & O. S. Vinogradova, (Eds.), *Neuronal mechanisms of the orienting reflex* (pp. 217–235). Hillsdale, NJ: Erlbaum.

Wing, L. (1976). Diagnosis, clinical description and prognosis. In L. Wing (Ed.), *Early childhood autism* (2nd ed., pp. 15–64). Oxford: Pergamon Press.

Young, J. G., Kavanagh, M. E., Anderson, G. M., Shaytwitz, B. A., & Cohen, D. J. (1982). Clinical neurochemistry of autism and associated disorders. *Journal of Autism and Developmental Disorders, 12*(2), 147–165.

26

Speculations on the Neuroanatomical Substrate of Special Talents

Lynn Waterhouse

Current Models of Intelligence

Current theories of the origin and nature of intelligence include a wide variety of models. The basis for normal human intelligence is seen by some to be essentially innate, where brain functions that govern intelligent behavior develop with environmental influence operating only negatively, to harm or distort development (Gazzaniga, 1985). Others see individual variation in human intelligence as a basis for theorizing that genotype-environment interactions yield phenotypical intelligence (DeFries *et al.* 1979; Scarr & Carter-Saltzman, 1982). Still others view the source of intelligence as largely a product of environment, wherein higher intelligence results from a more positive and more stimulating environment (Diamond, Johnson, Protti, Ott, & Kajisa, 1985; Flynn, 1984; Kamin, 1981).

The nature of the structure of human intelligence can be seen as a separate question from the question concerning the source of human intelligence. What human intelligence consists of is one of the great questions of 20th-century science. It has been a major concern in such various fields as developmental psychology, cognitive psychology, the neurosciences, sociology, and education. In general, it is fair to say that older unitary models, such as Spearman's *g*, have given way to a faculty model of intelligence, which outlines discrete or overlapping sets of functions, collocations of processes, areas of localization, distinct abilities, modules of functioning, and the like.

Sternberg and Powell (1982) have argued that notions of human intelligence are currently at the third stage of model building. They hypothesized that Stage 1 was the posing of the initial question—the debate whether there is a unitary intelligence or multiple distinct intelligences or skills (e.g., Thurstone's primary mental abilities). They proposed as Stage 2 the process involving combinatorial notions, wherein unitary models were joined with multiple-skill and multiple-ability models. They offer as an example of Stage 2 Sternberg's (1980) own model, which claims that an executive function (unitary) exists for human intelligence and that

Lynn Waterhouse. Child Behavior Study, Trenton State College, Trenton, New Jersey.

the job of this executive function is to supervise a set of processes (multiple functions). Sternberg states that we are now at Stage 3 in theorizing about human intelligence, in which theorists have the job of designing models in which "circumplicially related abilities are not hierarchically ordered but rather are arranged circularly, with adjacent abilities essentially shading off into each other. Thus, adjacent abilities may be seen as overlapping each other so that, for example, numerical ability shades off into reasoning ability" (Sternberg & Powell, 1982, p. 989).

Sternberg's stage model might have to treat such theoretical notions of human intelligence as Fodor's (1983) modularity of mind and Gardner's (1983) notion of multiple intelligences as "throwback" theories. Both Fodor's and Gardner's models resolve the issue of the overlap of skills and processes by treating skills and processes as two separate vectors—skills being the vertical vector and processes being the horizontal vector. A modular theory of mind proposed by Gazzaniga (1985) also offers the notion of skills versus processes but resolves the issue more radically, in favor of duplicated and encapsulated modules of function. Gazzaniga states:

> The normal brain is organized into modular-processing systems, hundreds of them or maybe even thousands, and . . . these modules can usually express themselves only through real action, not through verbal communication. Most of these systems . . . can remember events, store affective reactions to those events, and respond to stimuli associated with a particular memory. . . . These activities are the elements that a functioning mental system draws upon for complete mental life. (p. 77)

Theories of the source and structure of intelligence *per se* are part of the playing field for theories of special abilities. Gardner, for example, argues that each of a set of seven discrete abilities can run the range of being virtually absent to being vastly superior. These seven abilities—linguistic, musical, logical–mathematical, spatial, bodily-kinesthetic, knowledge of others, and knowledge of self—all are in the vertical vector of skills and depend on the horizontal vector of memory association, recall, and the like for their functioning.

For Gardner's model, then, special talents represent the end points of a set of distinct abilities. The hereditary basis for special abilities would then be part and parcel of the hereditary basis for intelligence in general. There would exist a separate normal distribution of talent in each of the separately identified intelligences. Offspring would tend to be somewhat like their parents in each of the distinct abilities or faculties identified (with allowance for regression toward the mean across generations), but every so often (rarely) an individual with a particular genotype would arise who would have such special skills in a specific domain that this individual would be identified as a genius in that domain.

Another theory of the source of special abilities is the notion of special training for a particular skill, which would lead to the development of a special ability. Ericsson and Faivre (Chapter 24, this volume) have argued that each one of us can be a genius in terms of digit-span memory if we simply practice and develop strategies for memorizing larger units of numbers. It is their belief that sustained attention and effort lead to extraordinary skills but that most people find such sustained effort aversive and therefore few actually do develop special talents. Ericsson and Faivre further suggest that unique environmental circumstances, such as an intensely structured environment controlled by a parent or teacher, or the evolution of some unique psychological isolation, can foster a state in which intense efforts cease to be aversive to the individual. Thus they see practice effects leading to the development of special strategies (through intense effort) as the central source of special abilities.

Recently, a possible biological basis for special abilities was argued by Diamond and Scheibel (1985). In work covering the past 20 years, Diamond and colleagues (Diamond et al., 1985; Diamond et al., 1966) found evidence to suggest that environmental factors can alter the development of the neocortex of the rat's brain. Analysis of the brains of rats who were raised in an enriched and stimulating environment compared with the brains of rats who were not raised in such an environment revealed increased numbers of glial cells and a greater proliferation of dendritic spines on neurons. Diamond and Scheibel (1985) recently analyzed tissue sections from Brodmann areas 9 and 39 of Einstein's brain and found that the ratio of glial cells to neurons in area 39 approached that of twice the ratio found in sections of control brains. It is their belief that Einstein's genius stemmed at least in part from the enhanced metabolic functioning that an increased number of glial cells may provide.

In the Diamond and Scheibel model, genius feeds itself. Special talent may arise from an enriched environment, but the enriched environment (for their model in Einstein's case, presumably this is constituted by intense thinking) leads to a permanent positive set of brain-cell changes, which in turn support the development of "genius."

This brief review is an attempt to suggest the range of theories currently under consideration concerning intelligence and the relationship of intelligence to special abilities. It is my purpose in this chapter to add another theory concerning the relationship between intelligence and special abilities.

A New Theoretical Model

This chapter outlines a model of the organization and structure of special abilities that is distinct from those just reviewed. The central thesis is that special cognitive talents or abilities are different in source from human intelligence in general. I hypothesize that special cognitive abilities are based on a set of skills that involve the acutely accurate and extremely extensive representation of visual images and sounds, and the rapid recognition and facile manipulation of patterns involving those visual and auditory representations. The principal claims to support this model are as follows:

   1. Special cognitive talents are not the extreme ends of the normal distribution of multiple intelligences but are separately and uniquely determined.

2. A wide range of special talents, including music, art, mathematics, poetry, and prodigious memory, all spring from the same global, preconscious, specific set of skills, namely, the ability to generate accurate and elaborate mental representations of images and/or sounds, and to store, manipulate, and recall these sounds, as well as—and more important—the ability to "see" or "hear" complex patterns in those mental sights and sounds.

3. Special talents will not arise in areas of dedicated tissue such as brain regions specialized for the control of language perception, processing, and production, or brain regions dedicated to the control of visual processing (visual cortex), because the parameters of functioning and the control of behavior have been tightly set through evolution for human adaptive necessity.

4. The potential for special talents is essentially innate, and the brain functions that give rise to special talents may originate from a variety of sources, including (a) pathological development (as in the Geschwind and Galaburda model, 1985, (b) Mendelian trait transmission, (c) as a rare multigene effect, or, possibly, (d) as a result of some accidental mutation or change.

5. In terms of brain morphology, the functional specializations that generate special talents may be hypothesized to operate at an "end station" of the auditory or visual processing systems, and may consist of a distinctive and/or more extensive organization of the sensory association cortex, or polymodal association cortex (e.g., the temporo-parieto-occipital junction). In the present hypothesis the pattern-recognition organization of the visual or auditory cortex is displayed in association cortex as an open field ready to be used for complex patterning of mental representations.

6. Environmental enrichment provides crucially necessary material for the expression of special abilities, and intense efforts often, but not always, accompany the expression of special talents; enriched environment and practice however, do not cause or generate special abilities. Furthermore, it may be that unique patterns of internal rewards are associated with the functioning of those qualitatively different areas that are here hypothesized to determine special abilities.

7. General mechanisms of enhanced brain function, such as globally or locally increased ratios of glial cells to neurons, increased EEG site-to-site amplitudes (Perecman, 1983), or increased dendritic growth, may be causally related to generally better learning, memory or association, but these general mechanisms will not be the basis for the formation of special abilities. Enhanced brain function may give rise to general giftedness, as in high IQ and the like (Spearman's g correlated test scores, etc.), but it is not likely that it will generate a basis for special abilities, because special abilities are isolated in the behavioral repertoire of individuals.

Detailing and Evaluating the Arguments for the Model

Each of the seven claims for the model needs explanation and justification. As each claim is considered here, supporting arguments and evidence will be presented, and some competing notions will be reviewed.

Claim 1

Special talents do not represent the extreme ends of a distribution of different "multiple intelligences."

The essential problem with theorizing that special talents are the end of a continuum of each of a set of discrete intelligences lies in the notion of discrete intelligences. In the early part of the 20th century, Thurstone argued for the existence of seven primary mental abilities, and recently, Gardner has argued that there are seven domains of intelligence.

The first problem to note is validity. Faculty theories of intelligence tell us more about context than about brain function, because they are developed on the basis of what is salient either through testing or through cultural focus. Thurstone's model is test-bound, and Gardner's model is culture-bound. Thurstone's model reflects what can be measured by neuropsychological tests, and Gardner's model reflects what is of value to modern human culture. Gardner's model could, as he points out in fact, be extended. The model could include not seven sorts of intelligence but many sorts, such as olfactory and gustatory intelligences (wine tasters, great chefs, perfumers) or stereognostic intelligence. There is at least one known olfactory savant who can make remarkable odor discriminations (Dr. Wayne Silverman, personal communication, March 1986). Not only can the list be lengthened, but within currently hypothesized types of intelligence there could be subdivisions, again, as Gardner acknowledges. In other words, the linguistic intelligence could be divided into prosodic intelligence, articulation intelligence, vocabulary intelligence, and the like. Visual intelligence similarly, could be divided into subskills to include eidetic savants such as Stromeyer and Psotka's (1970) subject.

In fact, Gall's 19th-century phrenological faculty theory of intelligence did evolve into a hydra of over 100 heads, collapsing from the weight of the proliferating faculties (Clarke & Dewhurst, 1972).

The second problem is the idea that each discrete module of intelligence has an implicit normal distribution. While the skills are divided categorically (i.e., Gardner's seven types of intelligence), the mental processes that constitute these skills are divided both categorically (i.e., memory versus association) and continuously (degree of memory skill). But to argue that all functions give way to a continuous range is fallacious. There are either–or recognition functions that operate in the olfactory, auditory, gustatory, and visual-sensory areas, and there are specific categorical functions in smell and taste.

It is generally understood that the more complex the skill to be measured, the more likely it is that the function will show a normal distribution, and this, in turn, is likely to be a function of the interaction of multiple factors. However, if each separate faculty of intelligence is normally distributed, then the top end of each normal distribution should show a long, slow, smooth declining curve. In fact, some studies of more generally conceived and tested skills, such as SAT math tests and some nonverbal IQ tests, suggest a distribution that shows a small bump at the upper end of the curve (Benbow & Stanley 1980; Stanley, Keating, & Fox, 1974; Stanley 1976, 1982; Stanley & Benbow 1982). This suggests the possibility of a separate distribution of skills at the top end. I would argue that this type of finding does provide support for a categorical difference in degree of talent.

A possible specific genetic mechanism has been hypothesized that would account for these findings. Bock and Kolakowski (1973) outlined a model wherein skill in spatial visualization or representation is determined in part by many autosomal alleles and also by some (as yet unidentified) recessive gene on the X chromosome. The differential presence of the recessive gene in combination with the autosomal alleles could thus generate the phenotypical trait of enhanced ability. Moreover, the finding that the "bump" scores are generated by males is explained in this model by the fact that females would need to have two of the special recessive X's in order to have a chance to generate enhanced ability.

In general, although individuals may express peaks and valleys in cognitive skill profiles, there is no good evidence to support the notion of clear separate heritability of distinct measurable skills (Loehlin & Nichols, 1976). With the notable exception of spatial ability (as discussed earlier), "intelligence" would appear to have a polygenetic base. The various subskills constituting intelligence are correlated with one another and generate a normal distribution suggestive of complex polygene inheritance.

Furthermore, what makes the expression of special abilities so special—and makes special abilities different from functioning at the top end of a distribution—is a combination of salient elements. These elements include speed of function, accuracy of function, novelty of the expression of that function, and the apparent encompassing scope of the expression of that function. Moreover, the early expression of speed, accuracy, novelty, and scope of a special ability is particularly salient. Thus child prodigies stand out as they reveal "mature" expression of a skill at a stage too early to have benefited from a massive practice effect.

Claim 2

Special talents depend on the ability to store, generate, and manipulate accurate, complex, and novel visual images and sound patterns, and, most important, the ability to perform large-scale pattern generation and pattern recognition on these internal representations.

Recent work in cognitive psychology has led to intriguing hypotheses about the nature of internal representation. Kosslyn, Holtzman, Farah, and Gazzaniga (1985) recently concluded the following:

> Imagery is not a simple event and it does not take place entirely within a single part of the brain. Attempts to localize the imagery system, as an undifferentiated whole, to one neurolocus have not been successful . . . more recent attempts to bring order to the effects of brain damage on visual imagery have been more successful by breaking imagery down into component imagery abilities such as image generation . . . the discovery of dissociations suggests that the theoretical analysis is in fact a description of how functions are actually organized in the brain. (p. 313)

Kosslyn et al. (1985) developed a three-part component model of image processing in which the three component parts include the following:

> A PICTURE processing module that activates stored visual information, a PUT processing module that looks up and interprets a description of how parts are to be

arranged . . . and a FIND processing module that locates the foundation part . . . the PUT module uses the location information in conjunction with the description of the relation . . . to set the processing module so that the two images are correctly juxtaposed. (p. 313)

My argument for the nature of special abilities is not specifically designed to include the Kosslyn *et al.* model, but I do propose that the existence of special abilities depends on a qualitatively different level of functioning of such theorized modular programs as "PICTURE, PUT, and FIND" as well as on a vastly elaborated organization for the control of pattern generation and pattern recognition.

In the remainder of this section, I will argue that pattern generation and pattern recognition of accurate and complex visual and auditory representations form the core of special abilities. One line of reasoning stems from an anlaysis of anecdotes regarding eminent individuals with apparent special abilities, which have been reported by themselves and by others. Another line of reasoning stems from an analysis of the products of special talents. The reasoning is also based on an examination of the special abilities shown by idiot savants.

THE CORE OF SPECIAL ABILITIES

A great number of people with notable talents, and some idiot savants (Sacks, 1985), report seeing vast patterned images in their "mind's eye" or hearing polyphonic patterned sounds (music) in memory. In a recent review Fincke (1985) concluded that research on visual-mental imagery supports the notion that visual (mentally imagined) images do resemble actual perception in some fundamental respects. Fincke states that normal individuals both remember previously seen images and generate new ones: I hypothesize that special talents are characterized by (1) a prodigious memory for sights or sounds, (2) a prodigious generating of new mental images and mental sounds, and (3) an associated faculty of pattern recognition operating on those remembered or created mental images and sounds.

Gardner (1983) reports on the life of Stravinsky, who at age 2 could repeat songs exactly as they had been sung, immediately after he had heard them. Gardner also discusses Nikola Tesla, whose generation of mental imagery apparently was so powerful that he could both build and test complex machines in his mind. Sacks (1985) considers idiot–savant twins who could generate prime numbers apparently from a visual-mental array of some sort.

In an article entitled "Mozart's Brilliance Is Not Dimmed by Analysis," Donal Henehan (1985) concludes that we can never really know the source of a special talent like that of Mozart. In this conclusion he is stating the familiar "genius-is-a-mystery" argument. In coming to this conclusion Henahan invokes the notion of perceptual chunking as was first outlined by Miller (1956) for language:

Mozart memorized in the same way we all do when trying to store complex material in our minds. That is, he identified musical patterns based on his already vast experience and remembered unfamiliar groups of sounds by hearing them not as strings of individual notes but as familiar units or chunks of sound. A good sight reader works exactly this way. He does not go from note to note but takes in whole measures and phrases at a gulp. (Henahan, 1985, p. 17)

While Henahan alludes to the possibility that Mozart's special ability to retain music in his mind was based on a kind of photographically accurate eidetic imagery, he also argues that all musicians can visualize a particular page of a familiar score when at work on it. However, Henahan reviews evidence to suggest that chess players and musicians have something in common—their ability to pick out recurring strategic patterns. Just as a chess master may know thousands of patterns of chess-piece movements, a musician will know episodic structures in music. Thus Henahan concludes that Mozart's talent was different in degree, but not in kind, from that of amateur musicians.

However, the plethora of anecdotes about famous musicians suggests that there is more to the story. Not only Stravinsky and Mozart but also Toscanini, Verdi, Bach, and Handel had the abilities to work rapidly, remember whole pieces, and perform them immediately. Beethoven, in particular, was able to continue to compose in complete deafness, apparently by generating musical scores and musical sounds in his head. Mozart is reported to have said that music was always in his head; Beethoven said it (music) "thundered in."

In addition, anecdotes about great talent always include great talent that is very early expressed. Mozart was 4 when he wrote a concerto—a concerto for harpsichord that was too difficult for anyone to play but that was a complete, well-composed piece of music. It is true that Mozart's father was driven to train and exploit his son's talent, with the result that Mozart became one of the most celebrated child prodigies ever known in Europe; however, the manifestation of his talent came early—earlier than would be expected were such talent to be a function of practice and training. In fact, for those who argue that training is the basis of special talent, a counterargument is provided by the persistent presence of prodigies like Mozart, Clara Schumann, and Picasso, whose talent arose before massive training effects could be expected to have an impact.

Furthermore, Galton, Einstein, Mozart, Handel, Matisse, van Gogh, Proust, Joyce, and many others who may be presumed to have special abilities have *all* been reported to have possessed prodigious memory for forms of mental representation, particularly visual images and auditory patterns.

Such great geniuses may be presumed to possess not only the underlying special talent of pattern recognition for visual and auditory representations but also the ability to be creative with such patterns. There are various other individuals who may have an element or a component of these special abilities—that is, prodigious memory for visual or auditory patterns and pattern recognition—but who are limited in the ability to associate or construct creatively on the basis of such patterns. One such example is Luria's famous subject S., presented in his book *The Mind of a Mnemonist* (1968). This subject (as reported by Brown & Deffenbacher, Chapter 8, this volume) was able to convert a series of words into a series of graphic images. Luria reported that S. always needed to have the words read clearly and distinctly, and not too quickly. Luria argued that S. needed a certain amount of time to convert the words into images. These images were complete, strong, and unlimited. As Luria (1968) reports, "Once we were convinced that the capacity of S's memory was virtually unlimited, that he did not have to 'memorize' the data presented but merely had to 'register an impression' which he could read on a much later date . . . we naturally lost interest in trying to 'measure' his memory capacity" (p. 34).

Luria found that S.'s errors were not defects of memory but in fact defects of perception—confusions, that is, in the visual images that he had created in order to store the information. S. eventually became a mnemonist, and as such, it was his job to entertain people by his feats of memory. In the course of developing his skills for this job, he developed strategies for organizing the visual images. He used these strategies to remember many complex series of bits of information.

S. was not a creative genius, and Luria tried to explain what problems S. had in interpretation and creativity. Luria believed that when S. read poetry, such a cascade of images would be stimulated by the sentences in the poem that S. was both distracted and circumstantial. Furthermore, S., according to Luria, had "synesthetic thinking"—which Luria believed to be the basis for S.'s ability to generate complex images. Such thinking was defined by Luria as connections across the memory systems for separate sensory processes. A taste would trigger a color memory, a sight would sound like something. Luria believed that this cross-sensory memory association made S.'s memories more vivid and thus more lasting. In general, however, synesthetic experiences are associated with pathology. Mishkin (personal communication, December 1985) has argued that synesthetic thinking would be an unlikely basis for prodigy.

Biographers have attributed synesthetic thinking to Proust. However, unlike S., Proust used this skill and his prodigious memory for social experiences to create a famous series of novels. The existence both of Luria's S. and of Proust suggests a dissociation of image generation from associative higher skill pattern manipulation and creativity.

Idiot savants, who have been described in a variety of ways and who are discussed in a number of chapters in this volume, also present a similar problem. They may often show prodigious memory, calculating skills, artistic ability, musical talent, and the like; nonetheless, these talents are most often not generative. They are passive skills, in which the idiot savant is able to perform a given task but is not able to generate a creative product that is unusual or novel on the basis of this skill.

Claim 3

Special cognitive talents (as defined here) develop as a function of tissue—such as the secondary sensory areas or the tertiary association areas—that is not highly elaborated in most individuals but in which, on occasion, a unique organization arises. A corollary of this claim is that special talents do *not* devolve on the function of highly specialized tissues such as the language areas or primary visual cortex.

The rationale for arguing that the tissue underlying special talents should be previously undedicated is based on two related arguments, each from a different field. First, evidence from neuropathological studies suggests that nearly all changes in highly elaborated brain systems are pathological and would thus lead to disruptions in functioning rather than to enhancement of functioning. It is likely that there is both pathological and nonpathological individual variation in neurological organization (Ojemann, 1983). However, this variation has not been found to be the imposition of new organization on tissue but so far appears to be a variation in the relative locations and extent of dedicated tissue areas.

Second, brain systems for vision, audition, and language are highly specialized with distinctive and dedicated tissue because they have evolved over a million years in order to serve human needs. In animals, adaptive evolutionary change tends to reduce variation in the phenotypical functioning of an inherited trait. If a trait function or bit of morphology is successful, its form may become limited.

In humans, for example, all those who function normally follow a very tight time course and fairly rigid sequence of developmental shifts in the unfolding of visual skills (Boothe, Thompson & Teller, 1985). We also follow a fairly rigid course for language acquisition (Lenneberg, 1967). These behavioral developmental limits support the notion of phenotypical constraint.

The phenotypical constraints on vision and language use may be determined by the functioning of specifically organized tissue (e.g., the language areas and visual cortex). Thus it is unlikely that there would be a radical reorganization of these areas for supernormal skills. Moreover, improved adaptive functioning of the visual sensory system or language areas would be most likely to yield incremental efficiency in function rather than a categorically different type of functioning, as special skills are here argued to be.

My claim is that special talents represent fortuitous accidental or multigene effects, or other influences, which give rise to some unique organization of brain tissue in particular areas. This hypothesized organization (which is discussed again in the section on Claim 5) would not require "tabula rasa" tissue but merely that the tissue not be completely function-committed.

If we credit the American poets Wallace Stevens and Emily Dickinson, and the English playwright William Shakespeare, with special talents, their talents would be hypothesized in this model to rest in the power of their individual abilities to generate sounds and images in language. It would not be theorized here that syntax and vocabulary *per se* are the elements of Stevens's poems or Shakespeare's sonnets or plays that so amaze and entrance us. It is in fact the arresting and powerfully vivid images as well as the "music" of the language that make us call their poems and plays works of genius. Schweiger (1985) has shown that the artistic functions of music and painting can be dissociated from language skills. It may also be that the "imagination" of literature, not the syntax, is evidence of genius.

Gazzaniga (1985) and Mattingly and Lieberman (1985) have argued separately for the uniqueness of language functions within a modular theory of mind. Although their arguments differ, the general point they make is shared: the linguistics module, or the source of language behavior in the brain, is the executor of the brain and is dominant over other processing modules. Although Gazzaniga talks about action going on in the brain without attention from the linguistic module, nonetheless, both in Gazzaniga's model and in the theoretical notions of Mattingly and Lieberman, it is suggested that linguistic functions are innate and that they play a "tough-guy" role in dominating other modules of information processing. A long history of evolution of linguistic function in the brain, combined with the relative dominance of language functions, suggests that tissue dedication would reveal tightly committed function. And if the language system does function as an "executor," it would seem that there should be even less functional flexibility and variability (because of the importance of this control function). If language skills constitute an executor, they would be even less likely to be able to generate special skills without impairment to basic and control functions.

Of course, there is clearly a normal distribution of language skills, as measured by various vocabulary tests, reading-comprehension tests, and the like. The normal distribution of these skills suggests either that such tasks involve a very tightly evolved shared unitary function (or module) or that the tasks (i.e., reading comprehension) may devolve on a complex, interrelated set of skills such that the multiple nature of the component skills leads to a normal distribution. In terms of the argument presented here, having a superior vocabulary and superior reading comprehension may be forms of giftedness, but they are not particularly involved in special talents, unless these functions involve visual or auditory imagery.

Similarly, the special motor skills seen in star athletes may be a form of giftedness, but they do not represent special, extraordinary skills. Motor cortex in the brain is very tightly organized, and the expression of motor skills is here argued to be on a normal distribution.

Another issue concerning distribution of skills is that those skills showing a normal distribution (where most people are average, a few are below average, and a few are above average), if based on innate traits, are likely to be polygenic. That is, a normal distribution of phenotypical performance may suggest a multigene basis for the behavior. A sharp peak at the upper end of an otherwise normal distribution, however, may suggest the presence of a single gene effect within the overall polygenic pattern.

Claim 4

Special talents are essentially innate and arise from an altered brain organization, which may originate in pathology, accident, single-gene effects, or multigene effects.

Geschwind and Galaburda (1985) have argued for a model of hormonal influence on fetal brain development, which would yield for some boys a better organization or more mature development of right-hemisphere functions, with less optimal development of the physical structure of the left hemisphere. Their theory postulates that differential hemisphere development is in part a result of the release of testosterone in the fetal system subsequent to the determination of the primary sex characteristics and the beginning of circulating fetal hormones. If the ability to generate images is, for most normal right-handers, a right-hemisphere function, then perhaps the currently noted sex ratio of many more male "geniuses" to female "geniuses" may be theorized to be in part the product of such a process. If males have the possibility of optimizing right-hemisphere development at the expense of left-hemisphere development, it may be that within the framework of this general biological event, there is a greater possibility for both pathology and superior functioning in males. Pathology might arise when left-hemisphere development is so compromised by a deficit in the requisite tissue as to cause a deficit in language-

skill development. It is possible that extreme forms of the biological effect of
testosterone in males in utero may generate idiot savants, whose visuo-spatial skills
are generally extremely high but whose language and social communication skills are
often minimal or absent.

Although sex differences in special talents have often been attributed to the
cultural history of women in both Western and Eastern societies, it is still possible
that such differences may have a biological basis. In addition to cultural constraints,
there may be more biological opportunity in male variability, allowing more males
than females to develop special abilities.

It is also true that certain types of talent appear to run in families. This would
suggest a genotype-environment interaction, in which family members who share
certain essential abilities also share the same environment and thus may come to
share the same expression of skills. Mozart and his sister and father were all
extremely talented musicians. The Wyeth family has produced four generations of
painters, all of whom share similar and recognizable technical expertise in the
realization of forms. What is notable, however, is that extremely superior talents are
not repeated across generations. Mozart was immensely more talented than his
father; Bach was much more talented than his sons. This pattern can be seen in many
family constellations. Biographies of eminent men and women of great talent suggest
that while other family members may be somewhat talented, the eminent individuals
alone possess the unique abilities seen.

The finding of families wherein several members are talented but only one is
a "genius" would seem to support the notion that special talents may be the joint
result of great efforts *and* some innate, but not extra special, abilities. In fact,
however, there is little evidence to suggest that individuals with superior talents
actually have worked harder than those family members with less remarkable
talents.

Another possibility is that there may be some difference in degree of phenotypical expression of the hypothesized genotype that determines brain-area reorganization for auditory and visual image memory and pattern recognition. This difference
in expression might arise in the context of different environments and different
individual patterns of associated traits (such as motivation).

Still another possibility is that in those cases of family talent, there may be a
polygenically determined trait with a range of distribution of expression and that
special talent in the uniquely talented individual is the result of a heritable or
accidental factor operating independently of the family talent trait.

Claim 5

In cytoarchitectonic terms, the specialization that could give rise to special abilities
is hypothesized to come from a unique organization of the tissue areas representing
the end points of the visual and auditory processing systems.

Currently there are a number of models of the neural pathways of the human
sensory systems. Models of both visual and auditory primary sensory processing
systems outline a core processor for the individual modality (auditory or visual)
in which cortical representations of discrete elements of sounds and sights are

automatically registered. Such discrete cortical representations of sounds (tono-topic) and sights (retinotopic) fit a tight, essentially prewired grid, which apparently is a product of the evolution of neural organization for auditory and visual perception. The visual cortex areas are Brodmann areas 17, 18, and 19. The auditory cortex area is 41. At present it is not clear whether core storage and processing areas also serve interpretation of the stored representations.

Srebro (1985) recently concluded from a series of studies that visual recognition of faces and shapes is "subserved by activity in the temporal lobes" (p. 257). However, Srebro goes on to state the following:

> Mishkin *et al.* (1983) proposed that the analysis of the "physical properties" of a visual object "such as its size, colour, texture and shape" is performed in the prestriate occipital cortex and in the posterior temporal lobe cortex but that its recognition as an object requires "funnelling" to the anterior pole of the temporal lobe. This hypothesis was based largely on anatomical evidence, i.e. the existence of the inferior longitudinal fasciculus. The results presented here suggest that the analysis of shape and the recognition of a visual object in humans is subserved by temporal cortex relatively near to the occipital lobe boundary. (p. 257)

The specific location of the hypothesized unique organization may be the secondary or tertiary temporal lobe sensory areas (for the visual system—Brodmann areas 18, 19, 20, 21, 37; for the auditory system—areas 22, 42) or even the parietal polymodal association areas (39, 40). However, if the function of the polymodal association areas is, as is currently theorized, to integrate cross-modal sensory input, then the polymodal association areas would be an unlikely candidate as a source of unique higher order pattern recognition for functioning within one sensory modality.

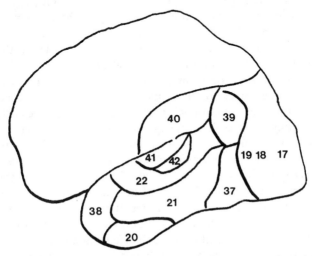

FIGURE 26-1. Brodmann areas 20, 21, 37, and 38 are thought to conduct analyses of visual and auditory input from afferent projections from the primary auditory areas (41, 42), and visual areas (17, 18, 19). Areas 39 and 40 are thought to integrate sense modality information about a stimulus.

Nonetheless, at present the polymodal association areas are thought to be less differentiated in terms of cell layers in the neocortex than are other areas (i.e., the language areas and the primary visual cortex). The polymodal association areas are contiguous to the primary visual cortex; in fact, they lie between the primary visual cortex and the temporal lobe language areas.

I have hypothesized that special abilities may arise when the structure of the tissue at the "end of the line" of visual and auditory processing unfolds developmentally with a pattern-recognition organization similar to that found in primary sensory cortex. In sum, this position claims that tissue that is not directly dedicated to the basic tasks of object or sound processing has an unusual (because it is essentially displaced) cell-assembly structure.

A variety of etiologies may be hypothesized to cause the tissue to take this form. What is important is that these areas be ready to provide (1) areas of within-modality association, (2) a template for prodigious memory, (3) a template for pattern recognition, and (4) a basis for pattern generation. The essential mechanism hypothesized here is that the special organization of primary sensory cortex (which provides retinotopic or tonotopic information) is present in the tissue of the sensory association or polymodal association areas. This organization may provide a template for the recognition and storage of representations, and for the creation and manipulation of patterns based on that storage, where these mental activities are well beyond those of normal ability.

The organizing power of the cell-assembly organization within, for example, the striate cortex is significant. Hubel and Wiesel (1979) found that columnar cell assemblies connect simple cells together with complex cells in a way that allows the system to generate a new, more abstract level of analysis of sensory input. Such organization occurs in both the primary visual and the primary auditory systems.

In the visual system, which has been very well studied, it is known that there are also lower order and higher order hypercomplex cells. The higher order hypercomplex cells can be seen as the "angels at the top of the Christmas tree." These cells look down on, and take in input from, a neural net of various cells in their cell assembly. Furthermore, the interconnection of these "angels" in the sensory systems may subserve the detection of complex patterns.

Another possible hypothesis for the neural substrate of special abilities is that in the subareas of the cortex for those individuals who have special abilities, the hypercomplex cells have an additional set of hyper-hypercomplex cells that are also connected, enabling larger scale pattern recognition than is usual. In this case the special tissue commitments underlying special abilities would be hypothesized to originate not in the secondary sensory association or polymodal association areas but in the primary sensory areas as a special cell differentiation within those areas. However, this possibility is unlikely. Shifting the structure of primary sensory cortex, like the hypothesized shifting of structure in dedicated tissue within the language area or within any other firmly structured area, would more likely lead to impairment rather than to significantly enhanced functioning. Thus still another possibility may be that it is a network of hyper-hypercomplex cells arising *outside* the primary sensory cortex, that subserve special skills. An important caveat remains: feature detection and pattern detection are complex processes whose neural substrate is both multiple and varied. Encoding of selectivity has not been conclusively localized in the primate brain (Van Essen, 1986); therefore the model presented here must be seen as purely speculative.

Yates (1985) recently reconsidered a theorized dichotomy established by Lindsay and Norman (1977). They postulated that visual perception was analyzable either by data driven (bottom-up) pathways or by a concept-driven (top-down) pathway. Yates has argued that perception is essentially data driven, because the adaptive goal of the visual system is to represent the images of things observed. He has, however, argued that conceptual frameworks that are flexible do shape our understanding of our own visual perceptions.

In these terms my model identifies special abilities as being a function of a "bottom-up" system of auditory or visual perception. This model is an argument for a system that simply goes further "up" in analyzing and storing visual or auditory patterns.

Diamond found that there were twice as many glial cells in area 39 in Einstein's brain than were found in area 39 of the normal brains studied. It may be that enhanced metabolism is a factor in generating superior talent; on the other hand, it may in fact be that glial-cell enhancement is a *post hoc* effect of Einstein's greater "use" of an area that was already prepared structurally to do a better sort of mental image pattern analysis than is typical of the average human brain.

Another issue arises if we consider the case of the idiot savant. Individuals who are idiot savants may have good visuo-spatial skills, good memories, or good calculating skills, but they do not have good language skills. Language skills are so impaired in most idiot savants, by definition, that the differential between visual and verbal skills is extreme. It may be in cases such as these that the pattern-recognition organization (with a columnar basis, as in the primary sensory areas) extends across, and thus delimits or impairs in some way, the major language areas of the brain. It may be, too, in such cases that the relative distribution of left- to right-hemisphere tissue can yield a dysfunctional state (as in the Geschwind and Galaburda model).

The main findings that this hypothesized pattern-recognition template would account for would be the evidence in early childhood of great skill at memorizing or learning instantly through a single impression long pieces of music, complex visual patterns, and the like. Young "geniuses", particularly those identified as prodigies before the age of 5, rarely have had—other than the famous John Stuart Mill—exposure to intense training at an early age, and thus what they are evincing so early may be the result of some special brain function. Even Mozart's father didn't begin the training of his son until after he had recognized his son's special talent for musical repetition.

Having the special cell-assembly organization of the primary sensory area extended into the secondary or tertiary sensory association areas may allow for the generation of large-scale visual or auditory patterns easily and instantly, and this may be available to the very young child who has such a talent. Of course, the fullest expression of such a skill would still depend on continuing input from some aspect of the environment.

Claim 6

Environmental enrichment provides crucially necessary material for the expression of special abilities, but practice does not cause special abilities.

There is a great deal of difference among eminence, giftednesss, talent, and special abilities as they are defined here. "Eminence" comes from the social power of giftedness, talent, or special abilities, typically in conjunction with great productivity. "Talent" is defined as above-average skill and/or productivity in any specific area. "Giftedness" is the state of being at the upper end of a normal distribution of general intelligence. "Special abilities," however, are defined here as separate and unique skills that on occasions may be identified as bumps at the end of a distribution of skills but that more often are identified in individuals who are singled out as having notable, amazing, or phenomenal talent involving prodigious memory, recognition, or ability to generate images and sounds.

For special skills to be expressed, there has to be a realm in which the skills may be manifested. Intense devotion to the realm (such as music or mathematics) often suggests that it is the intensity of effort that leads to the development of special abilities. This argument can be turned on its head: special abilities in fact may lead to special efforts of great intensity.

It may be that the exercise of such special abilities is accompanied by internal brain reward, such that the practice of the activity engenders its own particular pleasures. Although Ericsson and Faivre (Chapter 24, this volume) have argued that intense practice is aversive for most people, it may be that special abilities are often associated with a special reward system. It may simply be rewarding for the individual who has the hypothesized special tissue organization to engage in activities in which his or her special abilities come into play.

Mishkin, Malamut & Bachevalier (1984) have outlined two learning mechanisms–rapid and slow—where rapid learning is found to involve single experiences associated with exogenous rewards. These researchers propose that the limbo–thalamic circuit is the basis for the rapid learning, and that while both rapid and slow processes promote learning, the latter lead to "habits" as opposed to "memories."

From their model a simple counter–notion may be proposed: that limbo–thalamic functioning is vastly superior in individuals with special talents. Albeit this notion would suggest a means for rapid consolidation of memory–explaining instant storage as in Luria's S.—it does not help to understand the pattern analysis associated with special abilities as defined here.

More simply, special abilities cannot be noticed unless they are expressed. It is possible that there are people who have the special ability to generate and manipulate powerful mental representations and to work with them creatively but who may not—for whatever reason—generate products that would exhibit the influence of their special talents. Motivation must certainly be a factor, but the source of that motivation—be it environmental, internal, or some complex interaction of the two—is not yet understood.

Claim 7

General mechanisms of enhanced brain function, such as increased numbers of glial cells, increased EEG site-to-site amplitudes, or increased dendritic growth, may be associated with generally enhanced mental functioning but are not associated with "super normal" memory and special abilities.

The argument to support this notion is simply that general mechanisms and general functions (1) provide a basis for learning and (2) are likely to be spread across different modules or areas of the brain. It has yet to be proven that intense activity of a specific area of the brain leads to localized glial-cell enhancement or to area-specific dendritic growth. Furthermore, the possible link between great talent and the ratio of glial cells to neurons in a particular cortical area has as yet been demonstrated in only one human, that is, Einstein. However, it is reasonable to assume that general mechanisms of enhancement may operate throughout a great number of brain areas and, in fact, that such mechanisms may be the underlying basis for such effects as Spearman's g and the intercorrelation of a variety of measures of intelligence within the individual. Cohen (1985) has considered the field theory of memory—selective enhancement processes (LTP, synaptogenesis) for different content of memory—and rejected it (Cohen 1985, p. 425–26). However, he does argue that there is a need to have "functionally defined neuronatomy in which structures are distinguished on functional grounds rather than cytoarchitectonic ones" (Cohen, 1985, p. 426). The present hypothesis posits that displacement of sensory cytoarchitectonic (tissue) organization may in rare instances allow for special functions.

Another argument has been made (Gazzaniga, 1985) against the notion that enhanced brain functioning is a general result of an enriched environment. Gazzaniga claims that the baseline of enrichment studies of animals is actually deprivation and that instead of comparing normal and enriched environments, researchers (such as Diamond and colleagues in their rat studies) are comparing deprivation and a normal state. "Normal" is dependent on being in a state of stimulation; thus a rat in its normal habitat is being enriched. In this sense, if we live in a normal environment, we all have stimulating enrichment and should expect to have elaborate and enhanced systems throughout our brains.

Conclusion

The model proposed here is, of course, extremely speculative. It involves an argument essentially against the notion that special abilities represent the end points of normal distributions of different faculties. It argues against the notion that enrichment and/or intense practice effects lead to the development of special abilities. It also argues that although intense motivation and activity may accompany special abilities, the causal relationship between the two may not be in the direction that is commonly understood: It may be that brain activity involving a special and unique tissue organization is associated with its own special endogenous rewards (just as early language practice appears to be rewarding for normal children).

The arguments presented here in general support modularity models of the mind, and in particular, the notion of the separation of linguistic skills from the rest of our skills. Furthermore, although no specific argument is made about the relationship of left to right hemispheres in special skills, this model is constructed in accord with the notions of Brown (1983), who has argued that hemispheric differences are not absolute in functioning and that processing of complex information may shift across hemispheres in the course of processing. In other words, the model should not be interpreted as an argument for the existence of "right-hemisphere genius."

Finally, this model is not an attempt to be absolutely reductionistic about the nature of special skills, although identifying possible tissue areas and possible mechanisms for tissue allocation and structure are *de facto* reductionistic. The goal of the chapter is simply to argue that special abilities *are* special. They cannot be explained away by an appeal to hypermotivated effort or to the upper end of a normal distribution. Special abilities amaze us all. Shakespeare, Mozart, Einstein, and the idiot savant who knows every name in every phone book in every major city in the United States—these phenomenal minds are exciting and represent a tremendous challenge to those who think about them. The model I have presented is offered in the spirit of enthusiastic interest in the wonderful mystery of the human mind.

References

Benbow, C., & Stanley, J. C. (1980). Sex differences in mathematical ability: Fact or artifact? *Science, 210*, 1262–1264.

Bock, R. D., & Kolakowski, D. (1973). Further evidence of sex-linked major-gene influence on human spatial ability. *American Journal of Human Genetics, 25*, 1–14.

Boothe, R. G., Dobson, V., & Teller, D. Y. (1985). Postnatal development of vision in human and nonhuman primates. *Annual Review of Neuroscience, 8*, 495–545.

Brown, J. W. (1983). Rethinking the right hemisphere. In E. Perecman (Ed.), *Cognitive processing in the right hemisphere* (pp. 41–52). New York: Academic Press.

Clarke, E., & Dewhurst, K. (1972). *An illustrated history of brain function*. Oxford: Sandford.

Cohen, N. J. (1985). Levels of analysis in memory research: the neuropsychological approach. In N. M. Weinberger, J. L. McGaugh & G. Lynch (Eds.), *Memory systems of the brain animal and human cognitive processes* (pp. 419–432). New York: Guilford Press.

DeFries, J. C., Johnson, R. C., Kuse, A. R., McClearn, G. E., Polovina, J., Vandenberg, S. G., & Wilson, J. R. (1979). Familial resemblance for specific cognitive abilities. *Behavior Genetics, 9*, 23–43.

Diamond, M. C., Johnson, R. E., Protti, A. M., Ott, C., & Kajisa, L. (1985). Plasticity in the 904 day old male rat cerebral cortex. *Experimental Neurology, 87*, 309–317.

Diamond, M. C., Law, F., Rhodes, H., Lindner, B., Rosenzweig, M. R., Krech, D., & Bennett, E. L. (1966). Increases in cortical depth and glial numbers in rats subjected to enriched environment. *Journal of Comparative Neurology, 128*, 117–125.

Diamond, M. C., & Scheibel, A. B. (1985, July 28). Research on the structure of Einstein's brain. In W. Reich: The stuff of genius. *The New York Times Magazine*, pp. 24–25.

Fincke, R. A. (1985). Theories relating mental imagery to perception. *Psychological Bulletin, 98*, 236–259.

Flynn, J. R. (1984). The mean IQ of Americans: Massive gains 1932 to 1978. *Psychological Bulletin, 95,* 29–51.

Fodor, V. A. (1983). *The modularity of mind.* Cambridge, MA: The MIT Press.

Gardner, H. (1983). *Frames of mind: The theory of multiple intelligences.* New York: Basic Books.

Gazzaniga, M. (1985). *The social brain.* New York: Basic Books.

Geschwind, N., & Galaburda, A. M. (1985). Cerebral lateralization: Biological mechanisms, associations and pathology: 1. A hypothesis and a program for research. *Archives of Neurology, 42,* 428–459.

Henahan, D. F. (1985, August 25). Mozart's brilliance is not dimmed by analysis. *The New York Times Magazine,* p. 17.

Hubel, D. H., & Wiesel, T. N. (1979). Brain mechanisms of vision. *The Mind's Eye* (pp. 40–52). New York: W. H. Freeman.

Kamin, L. (1981). *The intelligence controversy.* New York: Wiley.

Kosslyn, S. M., Holtzman, J. D., Farah, M. J., & Gazzaniga, M. S. (1985). A computational analysis of mental image generation. *Journal of Experimental Psychology: General, 114,* 311–341.

Lenneberg, E. (1967). *Biological foundations of language.* New York: Wiley.

Lindsay, P. H., & Norman, D. A. (1977). *Human information processing.* New York: Academic Press.

Loehlin, J. C., & Nichols, R. (1976). *Heredity, environment, and personality: A study of 850 sets of twins.* Austin: University of Texas Press.

Luria, A. R. (1968). *The mind of the mnemonist.* New York: Basic Books

Mattingly, I. G., & Leiberman, A. M. (1985). Verticality unparalleled. [Commentary on J. Fodor *Modularity of mind*]. *Behavioral and Brain Sciences, 8,* 24–26.

Miller, G. A. (1956). The magical number seven plus or minus two: Some limits on our capacity for processing information. *Psychological Review, 63,* 81–97.

Mishkin, M., Malamut, B. & Bachevalier, J. (1984). Memories and habits: two neural systems. In G. Lynch, J. L. McGaugh, & N. M. Weinberger (Eds.), *Neurobiology of learning and memory* (pp. 65–77). New York: Guilford Press.

Ojemann, G. A. (1983). Brain organization for language from the perspective of electrical stimulation mapping. *Behavioral and Brain Sciences, 6,* pp. 189–230.

Perecman, E. (Ed.) (1983). *Cognitive processing in the right hemisphere.* New York: Academic Press.

Sacks, O. (1985). Sublime idiot geniuses. In *The man who mistook his wife for a hat.* New York: Summit Books.

Scarr, S., & Carter-Saltzman, L. (1982). Genetics and intelligence. In R. J. Sternberg (Ed.), *Handbook of human intelligence* (pp. 792–900). New York: Cambridge University Press.

Schweiger, A. (1985). Harmony of the spheres and the hemispheres: the arts and hemispheric specialization. In D. F. Benson and E. Zaidel (Eds.), *The dual brain; hemispheric specialization in humans* (pp. 359–374). New York: Guilford Press.

Srebro, R. (1985). Localization of cortical activity associated with visual recognition in humans. *Journal of Physiology, 360,* 247–260.

Stanley, J. C. (1976). Test better finder of great math talent than teachers are. *American Psychologist, 31,* 313–314.

Stanley, J. C. (1982). Identification of intellectual talent. *New Directions for Testing and Measurement, 13,* 97–109.

Stanley, J. C., & Benbow, C. P. (1982). Huge sex ratios at upper end. *American Psychologist, 37,* 972.

Stanley, J. C., Keating, D. P., & Fox, L. H. (Eds.), (1974). *Mathematical talent: Discovery, description and development*. Baltimore: Johns Hopkins University Press.

Sternberg, R. J. (1980). Sketch of a componential subtheory of intelligence. *Behavioral and Brain Sceinces, 3,* 573–584.

Sternberg, R. J., & Powell, J. S. (1982). Theories of intelligence. In R. J. Sternberg (Ed.), *Handbook of human intelligence* (pp. 975–1006). New York: Cambridge University Press.

Stromeyer, C. F., & Psotka, J. (1970). The detailed texture of eidetic images. *Nature, 225,* 346–349.

Van Essen, D. C. *Information processing in primate visual vortex*. Presented at Neural Connections–Mental Computation Conference, Tucson: University of Arizona, February 1986.

Yates, J. (1985). The content of awareness is a model of the world. *Psychological Review, 92,* 249–284.

Index

Tests Employed

Cases of Talent